ISCCM
Textbook of Toxicology

Treating the Critically Ill Poisoned Patient

ISCCM
INDIAN SOCIETY OF CRITICAL CARE MEDICINE

ISCCM
Textbook of Toxicology
Treating the Critically Ill Poisoned Patient

Editors

Ashish Bhalla
MD FRCP (Edinburgh) FRCP (Glasgow) FACMT (Fellow of American College of Medical Toxicology) FICCM FICP FACEE
Professor
Department of Internal Medicine
Postgraduate Institute of Medical Education and Research
Chandigarh, India
Past President, APAMT (Asia Pacific Association of Medical Toxicology)
Commonwealth Fellow (Clinical Toxicology 2015–2016)

Sheila Nainan Myatra
MBBS MD FCCM FICCM
Professor
Department of Anesthesia, Critical Care and Pain
Tata Memorial Hospital
Homi Bhabha National Institute
Mumbai, Maharashtra, India

JV Peter
MBBS MD DNB MAMS FRACP FJFICM FCICM FICCM
Professor
Department of Critical Care Medicine
Christian Medical College
Vellore, Tamil Nadu, India

Pradip Kumar Bhattacharya
MBBS MD ACME FICCM FCCCM FCCM
Professor and Head
Department of Critical Care Medicine
In-charge, Trauma and Emergency
Dean Research and PhD Coordinator
Rajendra Institute of Medical Sciences (RIMS)
Ranchi, Jharkhand, India
President, ISCCM National 2024–25

YP Singh
MBBS MD FICCM FCCM (American College of Critical Care Medicine)
Principal, Director, and Head
Department of Critical Care Medicine
Max Super Specialty Hospital
New Delhi, India

Forewords

Michael Eddleston
Kent R Olson
Paul I Dargan
Winai Wananukul

JAYPEE BROTHERS MEDICAL PUBLISHERS
The Health Sciences Publisher
New Delhi | London

Jaypee Brothers Medical Publishers (P) Ltd.

Headquarters
Jaypee Brothers Medical Publishers (P) Ltd
EMCA House, 23/23-B
Ansari Road, Daryaganj
New Delhi 110 002, India
Landline: +91-11-23272143, +91-11-23272703
+91-11-23282021, +91-11-23245672
Email: jaypee@jaypeebrothers.com

Corporate Office
Jaypee Brothers Medical Publishers (P) Ltd
4838/24, Ansari Road, Daryaganj
New Delhi 110 002, India
Phone: +91-11-43574357
Fax: +91-11-43574314
Email: jaypee@jaypeebrothers.com

Overseas Office
JP Medical Ltd.
83, Victoria Street, London
SW1H 0HW (UK)
Phone: +44 20 3170 8910
Fax: +44 (0)20 3008 6180
Email: info@jpmedpub.com

Website: www.jaypeebrothers.com
Website: www.jaypeedigital.com

Inquiries for bulk sales may be solicited at: jaypee@jaypeebrothers.com

ISCCM Textbook of Toxicology: Treating the Critically Ill Poisoned Patient

First Edition: **2025**

ISBN: 978-93-5696-574-4

Printed at: Samrat Offset Pvt. Ltd.

Contributors

Aarushi Sahni MBBS MD
Senior Resident
Department of Transfusion Medicine
Postgraduate Institute of Medical Education and Research
Chandigarh, India

Abhisheksingh R Rajput MBBS MD
Fellow
Division of Critical Care
Tata Memorial Hospital
Homi Bhabha National Institute
Mumbai, Maharashtra, India

Ahmad Khaldun Ismail
MBBCh BAO BMedSci (Medicine) DrEmMed (Emergency Medicine)
Professor Madya & Consultant Emergency Physician
Department of Emergency Medicine
Universiti Kebangsaan Cheras
Kuala Lumpur, Malaysia

Alisha Chaudhury
MBBS MD (Pulmonary Medicine) IDCCM EDIC FSM (Sleep Medicine)
Consultant
Department of Critical Care and Sleep Medicine
Sum Ultimate Medicare, A Unit of SOA
Bhubaneswar, Odisha, India

Amarnath P MBBS MD
Senior Resident
Department of Medicine
Jawaharlal Institute of Postgraduate Medical Education and Research
Puducherry, India

Ananya Ray MBBS MD(Anesthesia)
Fellowship in Solid Organ Transplant Anesthesia (Anesthesia and Critical Care)
Assistant Professor
Department of Anesthesia
Dr BR Ambedkar State Institute of Medical Sciences
Mohali, Punjab, India

Anas Mohammed Muthanikkatt
MBBS MD (Emergency Medicine) DNB (Emergency Medicine)
Senior Resident
Department of Emergency Medicine and Trauma
Jawaharlal Institute of Postgraduate Medical Education and Research
Puducherry, India

Angel Miraclin T MBBS MD DM
Associate Professor
Department of Neurological Sciences
Christian Medical College
Vellore, Tamil Nadu, India

Anupam Kumar Singh
MBBS MD DM (Gastroenterology)
Assistant Professor
Department of Gastroenterology
Postgraduate Institute of Medical Education and Research
Chandigarh, India

Anusha Cherian MBBS MD DNB EDIC
Professor
Department of Anesthesiology and Critical care
Jawaharlal Institute of Postgraduate Medical Education and Research
Puducherry, India

Ashish Bhalla MD FRCP (Edinburgh) FRCP (Glasgow) FACMT (Fellow of American College of Medical Toxicology) FICCM FICP FACEE
Professor
Department of Internal Medicine
Postgraduate Institute of Medical Education and Research
Chandigarh, India
Past President, APAMT (Asia Pacific Association of Medical Toxicology)
Commonwealth Fellow (Clinical Toxicology 2015–2016)

Ashish Kumar Kakkar MBBS MD DM
Associate Professor
Department of Pharmacology
Postgraduate Institute of Medical Education and Research
Chandigarh, India

Ashish Thomas George MBBS
Senior Resident
Department of Pharmacology
Postgraduate Institute of Medical Education and Research
Chandigarh, India

Atul Prabhakar Kulkarni
MBBS MD FISCCM PGDHHM FICCM
Professor and Head
Division of Critical Care Medicine
Department of Anesthesiology, Critical Care Medicine and Pain
Tata Memorial Hospital
Homi Bhabha National Institute
Mumbai, Maharashtra, India

Ayushi Saxena MBBS MD
Senior Resident
Department of Anesthesiology and Critical Care
Jawaharlal Nehru Medical College
Aligarh Muslim University (AMU)
Aligarh, Uttar Pradesh, India

Badria Ali Alhatali
MBBS MD FACMT FRCP
Emergency Medical and Toxicology Consultant
Head of the Poison Control Section
Ministry of Health—Sultanate of Oman
President of Middle East and North Africa Clinical Toxicology Association (MENATOX)

Balaji Venkatachalam
MBBS DNB (Gen. Medicine) Dip Diab MRCP (UK) IFCCM ED
Critical Care Intensivist
Department of Critical Care Medicine
Vijaya Hospitals
Chennai, Tamil Nadu, India

Banambar Ray MBBS MD FICCM
Head
Department of Critical Care Medicine
SUM Ultimate Medicare, A unit of SOA
Bhubaneswar, Odisha, India

Banani Poddar
MBBS MD (Pediatrics) DNB (Pediatrics)
Professor and Head
Department of Critical Care Medicine
Sanjay Gandhi Postgraduate Institute of Medical Sciences
Lucknow, Uttar Pradesh, India

Bhuvana Krishna MBBS MD IDCCM IFCCM
Professor and Head
Department of Critical Care Medicine
St John's Medical College Hospital
Bengaluru, Karnataka, India

Binila Chacko MBBS MD DNB DM (Critical Care) FICCM FCICM
Professor and Head
Department of Critical Care Medicine
Christian Medical College
Vellore, Tamil Nadu, India

CE Eapen MBBS MD DNB DM MRCP
Professor and Head
Department of Hepatology
Christian Medical College
Vellore, Tamil Nadu, India

Chanaveerappa Bammigatti
MBBS MD (Medicine)
Professor
Department of Medicine
Jawaharlal Institute of Postgraduate Medical Education and Research
Puducherry, India

Charanpreet Singh MBBS MD DM
Senior Research Associate
Department of Clinical Hematology and Medical Oncology
Postgraduate Institute of Medical Education and Research
Chandigarh, India

Cynthia Habib MBBS MD
Senior Emergency Medicine Resident
Department of Emergency Medicine
American University of Beirut
Beirut, Lebanon

Dag Jacobsen MD PhD FACCT FEAPCCT
Consultant
Department of Norwegian Poisons Information Centre
Norwegian Institute of Public Health
Oslo, Norway

Deba Prasad Dhibar MBBS MD
Associate Professor
Department of Internal Medicine
Postgraduate Institute of Medical Education and Research
Chandigarh, India

Dhruva Choudhary
MD (Medicine) DNB (Medicine) DM (Pulmonary and Critical Care Medicine) FAMS FICP FICCM FNCCP
Senior Professor and Head
Department of Pulmonary and Critical care Medicine
Pt BD Sharma Post Graduate Institute of Medical Sciences
Rohtak, Haryana, India

Eepsita Mishra MBBS MD (Psychiatry)
Senior Resident
Department of Psychiatry
Postgraduate Institute of Medical Education and Research
Chandigarh, India

Ezhilkugan Ganessane
MBBS MD (Emergency Medicine & Trauma)
Assistant Professor
Department of Emergency Medicine and Trauma
Sri Manakula Vinayagar Medical College and Hospital (SMVMCH)
Puducherry, India

Firoze Sogiawalla MBBS MD FRCP
Medical Officer (ED)
Royal Melbourne Hospital
Melbourne, Australia

Gaurav Agrawal
MBBS MS DNB PDC FACS FISS
Department of Gastroenterology
Postgraduate Institute of Medical Education and Research
Chandigarh, India

Gaurav Pratap Singh
MBBS DA IDCCM IFCCM
Senior Consultant
Department of Critical Care Medicine
Max Super Specialty Hospital
New Delhi, India

Gunchan Paul
MBBS MD (Anesthesia) IDCCM
Professor
Department of Critical Care Medicine
Dayanand Medical College and Hospital
Ludhiana, Punjab, India

Gurpreet S Wander
MBBS MD (Medicine) DM (Cardiology)
Professor
Department of Cardiology
Dayanand Medical College and Hospital
Ludhiana, Punjab, India

Harsha Vardhini CP
MBBS DNB (Emergency Medicine) DrNB (Critical Care Medicine)
Assistant Professor
Department of Critical Care
ST John's Medical College and Hospital
Bengaluru, Karnataka, India

Indira M MBBS MD (General Medicine) MSc (Medical Toxicology)
Professor
Department of General Medicine
Government Medical College
Ernakulam, Kerala, India

Jasper Rathinam J MBBS MD DM
Assistant Professor
Medical Intensive Care Unit
Christian Medical College
Vellore, Tamil Nadu, India

Jignesh Navinchandra Shah
MBBS MD DNB EDIC IFCCM
Professor
Department of Critical Care Medicine
Bharati Vidyapeeth Deemed University Medical College
Pune, Maharashtra, India

Jonathan Looms
BA (Hons) Oxon BMBCh MRCP (UK) FFICM
Consultant
Department of Anesthesia, West Midlands Poisons Unit
City Hospital, Sandwell and West Birmingham Hospitals NHS Trust
Birmingham, UK

JS Thakur
MBBS MD (CM) DNB (FM) FAMS FIPHA FIAPSM
Professor
Department of Community Medicine and Coordinator, Family Medicine Program, Community Medicine and School of Public Health
Postgraduate Institute of Medical Education and Research
Chandigarh, India

JV Divatia MBBS MD
Professor and Head
Department of Anesthesiology, Critical Care and Pain
Tata Memorial Hospital
Homi Bhabha National Institute
Mumbai, Maharashtra, India

JV Peter MBBS MD DNB MAMS FRACP FJFICM FCICM FICCM
Professor
Department of Critical Care Medicine
Christian Medical College
Vellore, Tamil Nadu, India

Kamal Kajal MBBS MD(Anesthesia)
Associate Professor
Department of Anesthesia
Postgraduate Institute of Medical Education and Research
Chandigarh, India

Karan Kumar MBBS MD
Assistant Professor
Department of Transfusion Medicine and Blood Bank
All India Institute of Medical Sciences
Kalyani, West Bengal, India

Karthik Gunasekaran MBBS MD
Associate Professor
Department of Medicine
Christian Medical College
Vellore, Tamil Nadu, India

Karthikeyan A MBBS
Junior Resident
Department of Emergency Medicine
All India Institute of Medical Sciences
New Delhi, India

Kartik Ganesh MBBS MD DM
Consultant
Department of Nephrology
VPS Lakeshore Hospital
Kochi, Kerala, India

Kashish Garg MBBS MD (Anesthesia)
Assistant Professor
Department of Anesthesia
Postgraduate Institute of Medical Education and Research
Sangrur, Punjab, India

Kathik
MBBS MD (Internal Medicine) DM (Neurology)
Associate Professor
Department of Neurology
Postgraduate Institute of Medical Education and Research
Chandigarh, India

Keyurkumar B Shah MBBS MD
Fellow
Division of Critical Care
Tata Memorial Hospital
Homi Bhabha National Institute
Mumbai, Maharashtra, India

Knut Erik Hovda MD PhD FACMT FEAPCCT
Professor and Senior Consultant
Department of Acute Medicine
Oslo University Hospital
Oslo, Norway
Professor and Senior Consultant
Department of Clinical Medicine
University of Oslo
Oslo, Norway
Professor and Senior Consultant
Department of Norwegian Poisons Information Centre
Norwegian Institute of Public Health
Oslo, Norway

KPP Abhilash MBBS MD
Professor
Department of Emergency medicine
Christian Medical College
Vellore, Tamil Nadu, India

Kushal Rajeev Kalvit
MBBS MD DM EDIC EDEC
Senior Fellow
Department of Critical Care Medicine
Guys and St Thomas' Hospital
London, UK

Lalit Gupta DA DNB
Professor
Department of Anesthesia and Critical Care
Maulana Azad Medical College
New Delhi, India

Lovely Thomas MBBS MD DM
Associate Physician
Division of Critical Care
Christian Medical College
Vellore, Tamil Nadu, India

Maleha Ahmed MBBS MD
Resident
Katihar Medical College
Katihar, Bihar, India

Manish Gupta MBBS MD FNB DM (Critical Care Medicine, SGPGI Lucknow)
Consultant Critical Care
Department of Anesthesia and Critical care
EMC Group of Hospitals
Amritsar, Punjab, India

Manisha Manohar MBBS MD
Associate Professor
Department of Anesthesiology and Critical Care
Pt BD Sharma Post Graduate Institute of Medical Sciences
Rohtak, Haryana, India

Manoj Goyal MBBS MD DM (Neurology)
Professor
Department of Neurology
Postgraduate Institute of Medical Education and Research
Chandigarh, India

Manu Ayyan MBBS MD
Associate Professor
Department of Emergency Medicine and Trauma
Jawaharlal Institute of Postgraduate Medical Education and Research
Puducherry, India

Meera Ekka MBBS MD
Additional Professor
Department of Emergency Medicine
All India Institute of Medical Sciences
New Delhi, India

Michael Eddleston
ScD FRCPEdin FRSE FMedSci
Professor of Clinical Toxicology
The University of Edinburgh
Consultant Clinical Toxicologist
NPIS Edinburgh & Royal Infirmary of Edinburgh, NHS Lothian
Clinical Lead for the UK's National Poisons Information Service
Director, Centre for Pesticide Suicide Prevention
Co-Director, NIHR RIGHT4 Preventing Deaths from Acute Poisoning in LMICs

Mohan Gurjar MBBS MD PDCC
Professor
Department of Critical Care Medicine
Sanjay Gandhi Postgraduate Institute of Medical Sciences
Lucknow, Uttar Pradesh, India

Mohan Kumar Hanumanthappa MBBS MD PGDMLE
Assistant Professor
Department of Internal Medicine
Post Graduate Institute of Medical Education and Research
Chandigarh, India

Mohit Kharbanda
MBBS MD (Medicine) IDCCM FNB (Critical Care) FICCM
Senior Director Critical Care, Senior Consultant Internal Medicine
Department of Critical Care
Desun Hospital
Kolkata, West Bengal, India

Muhammad EMO Elamin MBBS DTM & H PGCert ClinEd MSc MedTox FRCP (UK)
Consultant Physician and Clinical Toxicologist
National Poisons Information Service (Birmingham Unit)
Birmingham, UK

Nagarajan Ramakrishnan AB (IM) AB (CCM) FACP FCCP FCCM FAASM FICCM FISDA
Senior Consultant and Director
Critical Care Medicine
Senior Consultant, Sleep Medicine
Apollo Hospitals
Chennai, Tamil Nadu, India

Naman Agrawal
MBBS MD (Emergency Medicine) FACEE
Assistant Professor
Department of Trauma and Emergency
All India Institute of Medical Sciences
Raipur, Chhattisgarh, India

Narendra Rungta
MBBS MD FCCM FICCM FISCCM
Senior Consultant
Department of Critical Care and Anesthesiology
Rajasthan Hospital
Jaipur, Rajasthan, India

Nayer Jamshed MBBS MD
Additional Professor
Department of Emergency Medicine
All India Institute of Medical Sciences
New Delhi, India

Nita George MBBS MD (Anesthesia) FRCA (UK) EDIC CCT (Oxford) FICCM (Fellow of Indian College of Critical Care Medicine)
Senior Consultant Intensivist and Anesthesiologist
Department of Anesthesiology and Critical Care
VPS Lakeshore Hospital
Kochi, Kerala, India

Pankaj Soni MBBS MD FICCM
Director
Department of Anesthesia and Critical Care
EMC Group of Hospitals
Amritsar, Punjab, India

Parshotam Lal Gautam MBBS MD (Anesthesia) MNAMS FICCM (Critical Care Medicine)
Professor and Head
Department of Critical Care Medicine
Dayanand Medical College and Hospital
Ludhiana, Punjab, India

Pooja Jangid BSc MSc Nursing
Nursing Officer
Department of Internal Medicine
Post Graduate Institute of Medical Education and Research
Chandigarh, India

Prabakaran Parameswaran
MBBS DrNB
Critical Care Intensivist
Department of Critical Care Medicine
Vijaya Hospitals
Chennai, Tamil Nadu, India

Pradip Kumar Bhattacharya
MBBS MD ACME FICCM FCCCM FCCM
Professor and Head
Department of Critical Care Medicine
In-charge, Trauma and Emergency
Dean Research and PhD Coordinator
Rajendra Institute of Medical Sciences (RIMS)
Ranchi, Jharkhand, India
President, ISCCM National 2024–25

Prashant Kumar
MBBS MD MBA FICCM FSNCC
Professor
Department of Anesthesiology and Critical Care
Pt BD Sharma Post Graduate Institute of Medical Sciences
Rohtak, Haryana, India

Prashant Nasa MBBS MD
Professor
Department of Critical Care Medicine
NMC Specialty Hospital
Dubai, UAE

Praveen Agrawal MBBS MD DNB
Professor and Head
Department of Emergency Medicine
ESIC Medical College and Hospital
Faridabad, Haryana, India

Priyadarsini Jayachandran Arcot MBBS MD
Assistant Professor
Department of Transfusion Medicine and Blood Bank
All India Institute of Medical Sciences
Kalyani, West Bengal, India

Puneet Chopra
MBBS MD IDCCM IFCCM EDIC
Associate Director
Department of Critical Care
Satguru Partap Singh (SPS) Hospitals
Ludhiana, Punjab, India

Rajesh Vijayvergiya
MBBS MD DM FSCAI FACC FESC FISES
Professor
Department of Cardiology, Advanced Cardiac Center
Post Graduate Institute of Medical Education and Research
Chandigarh, India

Rakesh Kocchar MBBS MD DM (Gastroenterology) Fellowship in GI Motility (Mayo Clinic, USA)
Professor and Head
Department of Gastroenterology
Postgraduate Institute of Medical Education and Research
Chandigarh, India

Ramya Iyadurai MBBS MD DNB MRCP
Professor and Head
Department of Medicine
Christian Medical College
Vellore, Tamil Nadu, India

Ranajit Chatterjee
MBBS MRCPI FRCPI EDIC DA FIACM
Head Critical Care, CMO SAG
Department of Anesthesia and Critical care
Swami Dayanand Hospital
New Delhi, India
Honorary Consultant, Critical Care
RKM Hospital
Vrindavan, Uttar Pradesh, India

Ravikar Ralph MBBS MD
Professor
Clinical Toxicology Unit and Poisons Information Center
Christian Medical College
Vellore, Tamil Nadu, India

Rawan Eskandarani MBBS MD
Adult Emergency Medicine and Toxicology Consultant
Emergency Medicine Residency Program Director
King Fahad Medical City
Saudi Arabia

Ritushree MBBS MD DM (Neurology)
Department of Neurology
Post Graduate Institute of Medical Education & Research (PGIMER)
Chandigarh, India

Riyaz Sogiawalla MBBS MD
Medical Officer (ED)
Royal Melbourne Hospital
Melbourn, Australia

Rohit Bhowmick MBBS MD (Pediatrics) DM (Pediatric Critical Care) DrNB (Pediatric Critical Care)
Assistant Professor
Department of Pediatrics
All India Institute of Medical Sciences
Kalyani, West Bengal, India

S Raghunathan MBBS MD PG Dip in Higher Education MBA (Hospital Management)
Professor of Medicine
Madras Medical College
Chennai, Tamil Nadu, India

Sandeep Dewan DA DNB IDCCM
Senior Director and Head
Critical Care and ECMO Programme
Fortis Memorial Research Institute
Gurgaon, Haryana, India

Saswati Sinha
MBBS MD (Medicine) IDCCM EDIC
Senior Consultant
Department of Critical Care
Manipal Hospital
Kolkata, West Bengal, India

Saurabh Chaturvedi MPharm (Pharmacology) PhD (Immunopharmacology)
Division of Medical Laboratory Technology
School of Allied Health Sciences
Delhi Pharmaceutical Sciences and Research University
New Delhi, India

Saurabh Jain MBBS DA IDCCM IFCCM
Senior Consultant
Department of Critical Care Medicine
Max Super Specialty Hospital
New Delhi, India

Seema Singhal MBBS MD
Assistant Professor
Department of Microbiology and Infection Control Officer
MM College of Medical Sciences and Research
Ambala, Haryana, India

Sheila Nainan Myatra
MBBS MD FCCM FICCM
Professor
Department of Anesthesia, Critical Care and Pain
Tata Memorial Hospital
Homi Bhabha National Institute
Mumbai, Maharashtra, India.

Shivakumar Sankarnarayanan Iyer
MBBS MD DNB EDIC FICCM MSc Palliative Medicine
Professor and Head
Department of Critical Care Medicine
Bharati Vidyapeeth Deemed University Medical College
Pune, Maharashtra, India

Shruti Sharma MBBS DNB (Anesthesia) IDCCM (Critical Care Medicine)
Associate Professor
Department of Critical Care Medicine
Dayanand Medical College and Hospital
Ludhiana, Punjab, India

Shubh Mohan Singh MBBS MD (Psychiatry)
Professor
Department of Psychiatry
Postgraduate Institute of Medical Education and Research
Chandigarh, India

Shyam Charan Meena MBBS MD
Senior Resident
Department Anesthesia and Intensive Care
Postgraduate Institute of Medical Education and Research
Chandigarh, India

Siju V Abraham MBBS MD
Associate Professor
Department of Emergency Medicine
Jubilee Mission Medical College and Research Institute
Thrissur, Kerala, India

Soorya Suresh MBBS MD
Senior Resident
Department of Emergency Medicine
All India Institute of Medical Sciences
New Delhi, India

SP Kalantri MBBS MD MPH
Director-Professor of Medicine
Mahatma Gandhi Institute of Medical Sciences
Wardha, Maharashtra, India

Stuti Pramod MBBS MD (CM)
Senior Resident
Department of Community Medicine
Coordinator
Family Medicine Program, Community Medicine and School of Public Health
Postgraduate Institute of Medical Education and Research
Chandigarh, India

Suchet Sachdev MBBS MD
Additional Professor
Department of Transfusion Medicine
Postgraduate Institute of Medical Education and Research
Chandigarh, India

Sumedha Vashishth MBBS MD
Associate Professor
Department of Anesthesiology and Critical Care
Pt BD Sharma Post Graduate Institute of Medical Sciences
Rohtak, Haryana, India

Suneeth Kuriakose
MBBS MD (General Medicine)
Assistant Professor
Department of General Medicine
Government Medical College
Ernakulam, Kerala, India

Syed Moied Ahmed
PhD MD FICCM FCCP FICM FIMSA MNAMS
Professor
Department of Anesthesiology and Critical Care
Jawaharlal Nehru Medical College
Aligarh Muslim University
Aligarh, Uttar Pradesh, India

Tarun Sharma MBBS MD
Associate Professor
Department of Internal Medicine
All India Institute of Medical Sciences
Bilaspur, Himachal Pradesh, India

Tharwat El Zahran MBBS MD
Associate Professor
Department of Emergency Medicine
Medical Toxicologist
Co-director of Toxicology Service
Beirut, Lebanon

Thomas Sudarsan MBBS MD
Associate Professor
Department of Critical Care
Christian Medical College
Vellore, Tamil Nadu, India

Tushar Kumar MBBS PDCC (Neuroanesthesia)
Assistant Professor
Department of Anesthesiology
Rajendra Institute of Medical Sciences
Ranchi, Jharkhand, India

Vaishnavi RR Pemmaraju
MBBS MD (Emergency Medicine)
Senior Resident
Department of Emergency Medicine
All India Institute of Medical Sciences
New Delhi, India

Veer Thakkar MBBS MD
Assistant Professor
Department of Anesthesiology, Critical Care and Pain
Tata Memorial Hospital, Homi Bhabha National Institute
Mumbai, Maharashtra, India

Vijay Alexander
MBBS MD (Medicine) DM (Hepatology)
Assistant Physician
Department of Hepatology
Christian Medical College
Vellore, Tamil Nadu, India

Vikas Saini MBBS MD
Associate Professor
Department of Anesthesia and Intensive Care
Postgraduate Institute of Medical Education and Research
Chandigarh, India

Vikas Suri MBBS MD
Professor
Department of Internal Medicine
Postgraduate Institute of Medical Education and Research
Chandigarh, India

Vimal Krishnan S
MBBS MD FACEE FAIMER ACME
Professor and Head
Department of Emergency Medicine
Coordinator-Clinical Skills Lab
Kasturba Medical College and Medical Simulation Centre
Manipal Academy of Higher Education
Manipal, Karnataka, India

Vinay Singhal
MBBS MD (Anesthesiology) IDCCM IFCCM
Director and Head
Department of Critical Care & Emergency Services
SPS Hospitals
Ludhiana, Punjab, India

Vinodha Chandrasekar
MBBS MD (Emergency Medicine)
Assistant Professor
Department of Emergency Medicine
Sri Venkateshwara Medical College and Hospital
Puducherry, India

Vivek Gupta
MBBS DA DNB (Anesthesiology) FIACTA (Cardiac Anesthesia) FICCM
Consultant
Department of Cardiac Anesthesia and Intensive Care
Hero DMC Heart Institute
Ludhiana, Punjab, India

YP Singh MBBS MD FICCM FCCM (American College of Critical Care Medicine)
Principal Director and Head
Department of Critical Care Medicine
Max Super Specialty Hospital
New Delhi, India

Yvonne Elisabeth Lao
PhD MSc (Pharm) MSc (Clinical Pharmacy)
Clinical Pharmacist
Department of Acute Medicine
Oslo University Hospital, Oslo, Norway
Clinical Pharmacist
Department of Clinical Pharmacy and Consulting
Oslo Hospital Pharmacy
Oslo, Norway

Foreword

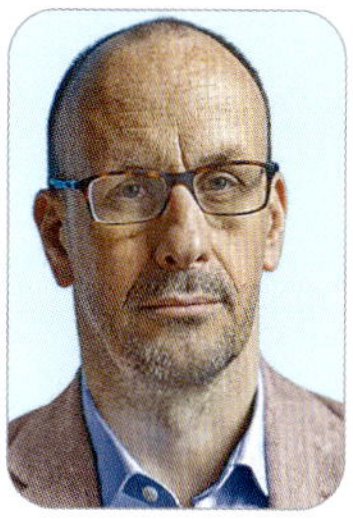

Clinical toxicology in South Asia is easily the most interesting toxicology in the world, with its complex and diverse array of pesticides, venomous snakes and marine creatures, toxic alcohols, drugs, and medicines.

Pesticide poisoning, both unintentional and intentional, is a huge problem in rural India, killing over 50,000 people each year. Medical treatment is difficult, in part because so much has happened before the patient reaches medical care. Pesticide regulation, replacing the most toxic pesticides with less toxic chemicals or non-chemical approaches, is key to reducing deaths. Tens of thousands of people die from snakebite each year; thousands more are severely injured and never fully recover. Early use of effective and safe antivenoms will save lives as promoted by the Indian zero snakebite death initiative. Methanol poisoning is a major but underappreciated problem across India, exacerbated by the difficulty of identifying the poisoning. Novel diagnostic approaches, accompanied by the availability of affordable fomepizole therapies, will save thousands of lives every year.

Early high-quality medical treatment of patients, with stabilization and antidotes before decontamination, is essential to improve patients' outcomes. Critical care plays a major role in this effort to save lives from poisoning and envenoming. While antidotes can be key, especially atropine and antivenom, it is the provision of excellent supportive care and nursing care that will save most lives.

Clinical toxicology problems are often neglected across the globe due to a lack of understanding of the immense burden and of the political will to address the issue. Lack of training and lack of awareness regarding the toxic potential of some chemicals potentiate morbidity and mortality. Unintentional exposure while pesticide spraying and chronic low-dose exposure are important health issues that need to be addressed. Intentional self-harm results in an avoidable loss of individuals in the prime of their lives. Restricting highly lethal means of suicide, in particular highly hazardous pesticides, has been shown by the WHO to be highly effective methods of preventing deaths.

I am therefore happy that Professors Ashish Bhalla and JV Peter, and their team, have addressed in this book many of the common toxicological problems faced by clinicians across South East Asia, especially the Indian subcontinent. I hope that their efforts to educate doctors, particularly intensive care specialists, will address many of the toxicological issues they face. I am glad to note that the authors emphasize a comprehensive psychological evaluation of individuals with self-harm.

I would finally like to emphasize to doctors reading this book the importance of being public health activists, of identifying problems with their individual patients, and then seeing the bigger picture. Of working with communities, healthcare systems, and government to find solutions to the toxicological problems illustrated in this book. This will be an important legacy of the book.

Michael Eddleston ScD FRCPEdin FRSE FMedSci
Professor of Clinical Toxicology
The University of Edinburgh
Consultant Clinical Toxicologist
NPIS Edinburgh & Royal Infirmary of Edinburgh, NHS Lothian
Clinical Lead for the UK's National Poisons Information Service
Director, Centre for Pesticide Suicide Prevention
Co-Director, NIHR RIGHT4 Preventing Deaths from Acute Poisoning in LMICs

Foreword

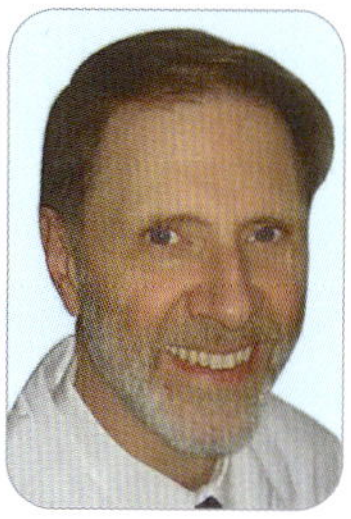

I am pleased to comment on this new textbook on poisoning authored by physicians in the Indian subcontinent. A comprehensive guide with an emphasis on poisons more common in low- and middle-income countries with large rural/agricultural populations, this book will be especially welcomed by practitioners who are more likely to treat a patient with phosphide ingestion than one who has overdosed on paracetamol. The authors recognize that the time and distance to reach tertiary hospital care may impact the choice of initial treatment in a rural clinic. Also, even when caring for patients with poisonings that are more commonly ingested in "western" countries, clinicians in developing countries may have little or no access to expensive treatments (e.g., hemodialysis, ECMO, liver transplantation) or antidotes (e.g., fomepizole, digoxin-specific antibodies). Recognizing this, the creators of this textbook have tried to include alternate treatments that might be employed (e.g., plasma exchange in patients with toxic hepatitis when liver transplantation is not an option, ethanol to block methanol poisoning when fomepizole is not available).

Kent R Olson MD FAPAMT FACMT
California Poison Control System
University of California
San Francisco, California, USA

Foreword

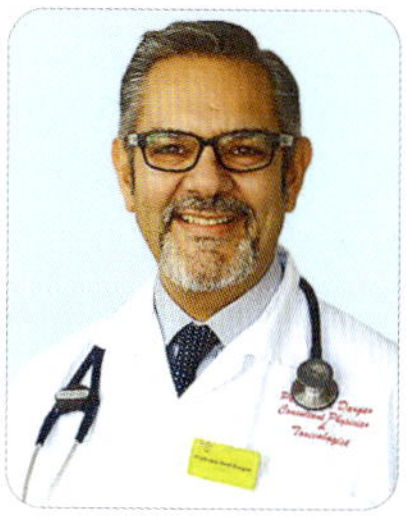

In this textbook, Professors Ashish Bhalla and JV Peter have brought together an impressive group of authors, many of whom are international opinion leaders in the topic of their chapters. Poisoning is an important cause of critical care admission with a wide range of different toxins causing severe clinical features requiring specific management in a critical care environment. This textbook provides a practical and authoritative overview of the toxins responsible for severe toxicity. It will serve toxicologists, emergency physicians, and critical care physicians as a reference source on this important topic.

Best wishes.

Paul I Dargan
FRCPE (Edinburgh) FACMT FRCP (London) FAACT FEAPCCT FBPhS
Professor of Clinical Toxicology and Consultant Physician
Caldicott Guardian/Guy's & St Thomas' NHS Foundation Trust
Professor of Clinical Toxicology
King's College London
London, UK
President, EAPCCT (European Association of Poisons
Control Centers and Clinical Toxicologists)

Foreword

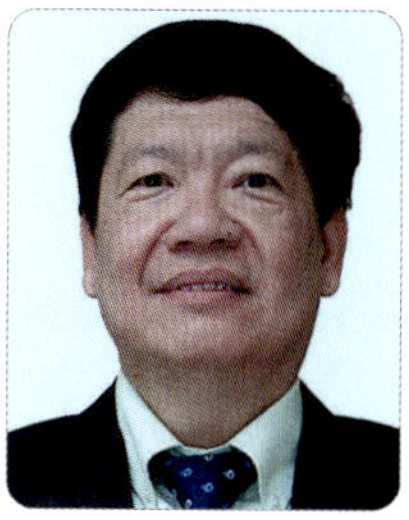

Poisoning remains a significant public health challenge, particularly in regions with limited resources where the severity of illness can be exacerbated. Unlike other medical specialties, clinical toxicology often lacks the extensive knowledge base and human resources.

This textbook addresses a crucial gap by providing comprehensive coverage of the majority of poisoning cases encountered in India and the Asia-Pacific region. The detailed exploration of the pathophysiology of various poisonings is a standout feature, offering readers a deep understanding of the underlying mechanisms, clinical presentations, and the rationale behind management strategies.

This textbook is commendable. It will undoubtedly enhance the knowledge and capabilities of healthcare professionals who utilize it, ultimately benefiting poisoned patients, the public, and the healthcare systems in the countries.

Winai Wananukul MD FACMT
Professor
Department of Medicine
Ramathibodi Poison Center
Faculty of Medicine
Ramathibodi Hospital
Mahidol University
Bangkok, Thailand
Past President, Asia Pacific Association of Medical Toxicology

Preface

It give us immense pleasure to introduce this textbook on the management of critically ill poisoned patient. This book is an important initiative to address the issues related to severe poisonings encountered in South East Asia, especially focused on problems in the Indian subcontinent.

The book has been divided into 4 sections with the first section focusing on approach to a poisoned patient, clinical and laboratory diagnosis, and resuscitation in the emergency room as well as intensive care units. There is an important aspect discussed here that focuses on dealing with the comprehensive psychiatric assessment of the victim.

The second section focuses on the individual toxins and covers the pathophysiology, clinical presentation, and management in a more detailed fashion. The emphasis here is on the specific management issues related to commonly encountered local toxins like pesticides, herbicides, commonly encountered household toxins, envenomation, plant poisons, heavy metal, and Complementary and Alternate Medicine (CAM) toxicities. There is an important aspect discussed here dealing with the comprehensive psychiatric assessment of the victim. The threats of chemical and biological terrorism are also covered here, which is the need of the hour.

The third section deals with supportive care of poisoned patients, with special reference to the intensive care unit. This section addresses the nuances of cardiovascular support, ventilatory support, renal replacement therapy, plasma exchange, and endoscopic management.

The last section deals with individual antidotes. The issues regarding the dose and duration of individual antidotes have been adequately addressed here.

This is indeed a herculean effort by the editors in addressing common issues in toxicology. We wish this book succeeds in its endeavor.

Best of luck.

Ashish Bhalla
JV Peter
Sheila Nainan Myatra
Pradip Kumar Bhattacharya
YP Singh

Contents

SECTION 1: COMPREHENSIVE EVALUATION OF A POISONED PATIENT

Section Editors: *Ashish Bhalla, Dhruva Choudhary, Parshotam Lal Gautam*

SECTION 2: SPECIFIC POISONS

Section Editors: *JV Peter, Ashish Bhalla, Shivakumar Sankarnarayanan Iyer*

SECTION 3: SUPPORTIVE THERAPY IN POISONING

Section Editors: *Vivek Gupta, Sandeep Dewan, Ranajit Chaterjee*

SECTION 4: ANTIDOTES

Section Editors: *Binila Chacko, Narendra Rungta, Syed Moied Ahmed*

Antidotes Acting on the Toxin

Antidotes Acting on the Toxin Binding Site

Antidotes that Decrease Toxic Metabolites

Antidotes that Counteract Toxic Effects

1

SECTION

Comprehensive Evaluation of a Poisoned Patient

Section Editors: *Ashish Bhalla, Dhruva Choudhary, Parshotam Lal Gautam*

1.1 Triage of Poisoned Patients (in the Emergency Department and Intensive Care Unit)

Praveen Agrawal, Vaishnavi RR Pemmaraju

INTRODUCTION

The word "triage" originated from the French word "trier" meaning "to sort" and was used anciently in England and France for assigning some ranked value or priority to what was being sorted. In emergency care setting, triage is practiced to prioritize patients and is an important tool in deciding the further management of the patient. The standard triage categories that are used in many emergency departments (EDs) are red, yellow, and green. The patients triaged *red* are the ones requiring immediate attention as they have a high potential to deteriorate rapidly. The patients triaged *yellow* suffer from illnesses that are not immediately life threatening but require urgent, if not emergent, attention where treatment can be delayed for a limited period. And the patients who are triaged *green* can be managed once other categories have been taken care of.[1]

TRIAGE OF POISONED PATIENTS IN EMERGENCY DEPARTMENT

Acute poisoning is a global health problem, and prevention of mortality is essential in both intentional and accidental poisonings. Prediction of prognosis in patients with acute poisoning has clinical significance, i.e., it helps in timely and appropriate treatment.

When it comes to triaging poisoned patients, the type of drug or toxin, quantity, route of exposure (ingestion/inhalation/cutaneous exposure), intent of poisoning (suicidal/accidental/homicidal), time since exposure, vital signs, clinical appearance of the patient, and associated comorbidities play important roles in determining the severity of intoxication and outcome of the patient. Additionally, the toxic substances and their lethality are often unknown to the emergency physicians. However, toxicology research lacks a well-accepted method for assessing the severity of poisoning. Several scoring systems have been used to triage a patient of poisoning in the ED but studies on their effectiveness have shown variable results. In the practice of medical toxicology, vital signs play an important role in assessing and monitoring the overall status of a patient.

ABCD Approach for Initial Triage in the Emergency Department

An initial ABCD approach may help in triaging the poisoned patients in the ED.

Airway

Patients with a threatened or compromised airway should be given priority and immediately managed by securing a definitive airway. It has been reported that every year, nearly 16% of patients with drug overdose require intubation. The requirement of endotracheal intubation (ETI) is most commonly seen after ingestions of atypical antipsychotics, benzodiazepines, antidepressants, and opioids.[2] In pediatric patients, ETI requirement has most commonly been seen after ethanol, clonidine, and paracetamol ingestions.[3]

Poisoned patients requiring ETI may present with an altered mental status due to loss of airway reflexes, or because the predicted clinical course anticipates the risk of aspiration and further deterioration leading to an inability to protect the airway.[4] Airway protection may also be required in agitated patients or patients with refractory seizures requiring sedation or high dose of antiepileptics to facilitate treatment.[5] There are numerous poisonings leading to clinical conditions which may require emergency ETI, some of which are highlighted in **Table 1**.

Breathing

Toxic exposures may lead to respiratory insufficiency due to direct lung or orotracheal injury or decreased respiratory drive.[6] The next in-line priority patients are those with breathing difficulty which may be due to failure of oxygenation from various causes such as poisoning-induced atelectasis, acute respiratory distress syndrome (ARDS), and pulmonary edema. ARDS may occur due to aspiration of gastric contents, hemodynamic instability, multiorgan dysfunction, and certain poisonings such as opioids, barbiturates, and salicylates. Such patients must be immediately managed by providing adequate oxygenation by nasal prongs or face mask or noninvasive ventilation (NIV) based on the clinical requirement of the patient.

TABLE 1: Clinical conditions and causative toxic agents requiring endotracheal intubation.

Depressed mental status	*Severe agitation*	*Tracheal/oropharyngeal injury*
• Cholinergics • Sympatholytics • Sedative–hypnotics • Hypoglycemic agents • Carbon monoxide • Cyanide • Salicylates • Lithium	• Anticholinergics • Sympathomimetics • Withdrawal from alcohol and sedative–hypnotics	• Trauma related—toxin-induced seizures (cyclic antidepressants, alcohol and sedative–hypnotics withdrawal, isoniazid, *Gyromitra* mushrooms) • Ingestion of corrosives • Inhalation of hydrocarbons

Note: These are only a few examples; the complete list is exhaustive.

Circulation

A thorough clinical evaluation must take place to identify patients with hemodynamic instability. Patients should be placed on a cardiac monitor with recording of pulse and blood pressure and a 12-lead electrocardiogram (ECG) taken. A definitive intravenous (IV) line must be secured and, based on the requirement, patients should be started on either IV fluids or inotropic support. In case of failed IV access, intraosseous or a central line placement must be attempted. Some cases may require antidysrhythmic therapy (e.g., atropine, sodium bicarbonate).

Disability

Disability assessment should be a brief assessment with immediate determination of blood glucose (point-of-care testing), rapid neurological assessment by Glasgow Coma Scale (GCS), and assessment of pupils. Seizures must be managed by benzodiazepines, pyridoxine, barbiturates, or propofol (phenytoin is avoided). Patients with GCS ≤13 should be triaged as "red."

Once ABCD of the patient are not compromised, further assessment is made by taking history and detailed evaluation.

Ingestion of Minimally Toxic Substances

If, after evaluation, the patient is deemed to have exposure to minimally toxic on nontoxic substance, he or she may be triaged under "green" category and may be discharged from the ED. Minimally toxic or nontoxic exposures have certain characteristics listed in **Boxes 1 and 2.**[7-9] However, decisions regarding patient disposition should consider the patient's intent, symptoms, and social environment. In addition, individual patient circumstances (e.g., pregnancy, preexisting medical conditions) need to be considered before discharge.

BOX 1: Characteristics of a minimally toxic substance.

- Physician has confidence in the accuracy of history obtained
- Physician has a reasonable estimation of the maximum amount involved in the exposure
- Risks of adverse reactions or expected effects are acceptable, benign, and self-limiting

BOX 2: Characteristics of a nontoxic substance.

- Absolute identification of the product
- Absolute assurance that only one product was ingested
- No signal word (danger, poison, warning, caution) on the container
- A good approximation of the amount ingested
- Assurance that the victim is free of symptoms
- Ability to call back at intervals to determine that no symptoms have developed

Poisoning Severity Score for Triaging Poisoned Patients in Emergency Department

Poisoning Severity Score (PSS) is a severity grading scale adopted by the International Programme on Chemical Safety (IPCS) for grading the severity of poisoning. PSS recorded at admission can be used to predict outcome of poisoning. It is a score for grading the severity of poisoning which allows qualitative evaluation of morbidity caused by poisoning without considering the type and number of agents involved.[10] The score considers the overall clinical course and is based on the patient's most severe symptoms or signs **(Table 2)** of nine different organs or systems. The gastrointestinal tract, respiratory system, nervous system, cardiovascular system, metabolic balance, liver, kidney, hemopoietic system, muscular system, local effects on the skin, local effects on the eye, and local effects from bites and stings are evaluated for PSS. It is often a retrospective process, requiring follow-up of cases. Although PSS is not intended as a prognostic score, a few studies have suggested the utility of PSS in prognosticating poisoned patients.[11]

TABLE 2: Poisoning Severity Score: severity grades.

None (0)	No symptoms or signs related to poisoning
Mild (1)	Mild, transient, and spontaneously resolving symptoms
Moderate (2)	Pronounced or prolonged symptoms
Severe (3)	Severe or life-threatening symptoms
Death (4)	Death

However, there are several limitations of PSS:

- It has several subjective criteria (e.g., mild cough, mild hemolysis, infrequent seizures, pronounced vomiting) reducing its inter-rater agreement.
- It is time consuming to calculate the score as it includes a large number of data points from 12 different organ systems.
- It is of little use in some types of poisonings [e.g., aluminum phosphide (ALP), paraquat].
- It requires laboratory data to have all 12 dataset values which is not possible while performing triage in ED.
- Occurrence of similar features by two different toxins may indicate vastly different levels of toxicity (e.g., coma produced by benzodiazepines and that by tricyclic antidepressants).

Due to several limitations of PSS, it is not a useful triage scoring system for poisoned patients in ED.[12]

New Poisoning Mortality Scoring System

This scoring system includes several variables available at the time of presentation to the ED. The New Poisoning Mortality Scoring System (new-PSS) comprises age, sex, type of substance, intent of poisoning, route of poisoning, systolic blood pressure (SBP), heart rate, respiratory rate, mental status (based on AVPU scale—A: alert; V: verbal response; P: pain response; U: unresponsive), and body temperature. The total score ranges between 0 and 117. The patients are grouped into 4 categories—0–27 points: very low risk; 28–40 points: low risk; 41–55 points: intermediate risk (1.82% mortality); and ≥56 points: high risk (18.6% mortality).[13] Patients with new-PSS score of 0–27 can easily be discharged from the ED.

Triage for Snakebites

Snakebite envenoming is a serious but neglected problem in India. Poisonous snakebites are broadly classified as hemotoxic and neurotoxic.

Snakebite Severity Score

Snakebite Severity Score (SSS) was developed in 1996 for crotalid snakebite which ranges from 0 to 20 points and assesses the respiratory, cardiovascular, hematological, gastrointestinal, central nervous system (CNS), and other systems and local wound to assign points for each. The hematological parameters include prothrombin time (PT), activated partial thromboplastin time (aPTT), platelets, or fibrinogen. The SSS has been shown to provide an objective instrument for the evaluation of severity and progression of envenomation in patients with crotalid snakebite.[14] SSS has also been used as a prognostic score for both hemotoxic and neurotoxic bites in one study reported from India, but a formal validation is unavailable.[15] If the ED has a point-of-care hemogram analyzer for platelet count, SSS could be used to triage patients with crotalid snakebites into minimal (score ≤3) and more severe (score >3) envenomation.

However, the SSS has several limitations: it combines both neurotoxic and hemotoxic manifestations; includes several laboratory results including PT, aPTT, platelets, or serum fibrinogen which are usually not available at primary care settings; and common elapid neurological signs like ptosis do not figure in the score. Furthermore, nausea, vomiting, diarrhea, dizziness, fainting, and tachycardia may be consequences of fear of snakebite by a nonpoisonous snake. Pain and swelling can be the consequence of a tight tourniquet.[16]

TRIAGE OF PATIENTS FOR INTENSIVE CARE UNIT ADMISSION

Patients are often admitted to the intensive care units (ICUs) because of abnormal vital signs or ingestion of a significant amount of toxins. However, poisoned patients are sometimes admitted to the ICUs because of unwillingness of hospitals to manage these patients in the general wards. Most patients with overdose admitted to the ICU are discharged within 1–2 days without any complications. Unnecessary ICU admission of stable poisoned patients places a constraint on already limited number of beds available in the ICUs. Therefore, it is important to triage patients properly so that only deserving patients are shifted to the ICUs which will increase the available ICU beds for other critically ill patients.

Common Indications of Triaging Poisoned Patients to the Intensive Care Units

Vital signs are important parts of toxidromes and play an important role in assessing the severity of poisoned patients. Triage SBP, heart rate, temperature, and respiratory rate have been shown to correlate with mortality either in the ED or in the ICU. Heart rate <35 or >120/min, SBP <100 or >150 mm Hg, respiratory rate <16 or >20/min, and body temperature <36 or >37°C have been shown to be independently associated with bad prognosis, and, therefore, can be used in the ED to decide disposition of the patient, either to the general ward or to the ICU.[17]

Box 3 mentions some of the common indications for ICU admission of poisoned patients.[18-22]

Triaging Patients with Pesticide Poisoning to Intensive Care Unit

Organophosphate Poisoning

Acute organophosphate compound (OPC) pesticide poisoning is a significant global health problem in developing countries, especially in India. As OP poisoning carries a high mortality, early recognition of severe cases may allow institution of intensive therapy in ICUs.

The Peradeniya organophosphorus poisoning (POP) scale is based on clinical parameters without the need of laboratory investigations.[23] It also does not rely on patient cooperation and hence can be applied to severely ill as well as unconscious patients. In this scale, five common clinical manifestations of OP intoxication, representing muscarinic, nicotinic, and CNS features, at the initial presentation of patients are taken into consideration **(Table 3)**. The maximum possible score is 11 and the severity of poisoning can be graded as mild (score 1–3), moderate (score 4–7), or severe (score 8–11).

The scale has been validated in a few studies by correlating scores with three outcomes, namely, death, need for ventilatory support, and the total dose of atropine required in the first 24 hours after admission. Those with mild poisoning can be admitted in the ward while others can be admitted in the ICU. However, in some other studies, many patients with mild poisoning as per the POP scale required mechanical ventilation.[24,25] Therefore, the POP scale may not be a good scale for ED use to accurately predict triaging patients to ICUs or general wards.

BOX 3: Common indications for ICU admission of poisoned patients.

- Respiratory depression (e.g., $PaCO_2$ >45 mm Hg)
- Endotracheal intubation in ED
- Seizures
- Cardiac arrhythmia (second- or third-degree atrioventricular block)
- Systolic blood pressure <90 mm Hg
- Unresponsiveness to verbal stimuli
- Glasgow Coma Scale score ≤13
- Need for emergency dialysis, hemoperfusion, or extracorporeal membrane oxygenation
- Increasing metabolic acidosis
- Pulmonary edema induced by toxins (including inhalation)
- Hypothermia or hyperthermia, including neuroleptic malignant syndrome
- Tricyclic or phenothiazine overdose that manifests anticholinergic signs, neurological abnormalities, QRS duration of greater than 0.12 seconds, or QTc that is greater than 0.5 seconds
- Body packers and stuffers
- Concretions and bezoars caused by drugs (verapamil, nifedipine, theophylline, clomipramine, enteric-coated aspirin)
- Emergency surgical intervention
- Need for continuous infusion of naloxone
- Hypokalemia secondary to digitalis overdose
- Exposure to any supposedly toxic pharmaceutical or recreational drug that can induce organ failure

(ED: emergency department; ICU: intensive care unit)

TABLE 3: Peradeniya organophosphorus poisoning scale

Parameter	*Score*
• Pupils	
– Pupil size >2 mm	0
– Pupil size ≤2 mm	1
– Pinpoint pupils	2
• Fasciculations	
– None	0
– Present but not continuous or generalized	1
– Generalized and continuous	2
• Respiration	
– Respiratory rate ≤20/min	0
– Respiratory rate >20/min	1
– Respiratory rate >20/min with central cyanosis	2
• Pulse rate	
– Pulse rate >60/min	0
– Pulse rate 41–60/min	1
– Pulse rate ≤40/min	2
• Level of consciousness	
– Conscious and rational	0
– Impaired, responds to verbal commands	1
– Impaired, no response to verbal commands	2
• Seizures	
– Absent	0
– Present	1
Total	11

Pesticide Poisoning

Several studies have compared the efficacy of various scoring systems, including the GCS, Acute Physiology and Chronic Health Evaluation II (APACHE II), Sequential Organ Failure Assessment (SOFA), and PSS, in predicting the outcomes of commonly used pesticides, including OP and ALP. Very few studies have evaluated the use of these scoring systems in predicting the need for ICU admission in pesticide-poisoned patients. In one study, the median APACHE II, Modified Early Warning Score (MEWS), and PSS scores were 11, 5, and 3, respectively, in acute ALP-poisoned patients who required ICU admission. The median APACHE II, MEWS, and PSS scores were 22, 5, and 3, respectively, in OP-poisoned patients who required ICU admission.[26]

However, some studies have failed to show sufficient predictive value of any of the severity scores (SOFA, APACHE, Simplified Acute Physiology Score) in the ED to allow the need for ICU admission.[27]

Aluminum Phosphide Poisoning

The prognosis in ALP toxicity depends on the amount ingested, form in which it is consumed (pellet vs. powder), and whether the formulation was exposed to atmospheric moisture. However, history is often unreliable in all these aspects. Furthermore, there is no specific antidote for ALP poisoning. The only treatment available is intensive supportive care. Therefore, early triage of patients with ALP poisoning to ICU is required. Most of the scoring tools mentioned above and used in poisoned patients have been devised for the assessment of multiorgan dysfunction in critical medical or surgical conditions. ED physicians do not routinely use them during management of poisoned patients, mostly because of the perceived difficulty and time needed to perform calculations and the requirement of the many laboratory tests. Hence, a simple score is critical in ALP poisoning.

In patients with ALP poisoning, three simple parameters, namely, blood pH <7.25, GCS score <13, and SBP <87 mm Hg, have a strong association with in-hospital mortality. With similar importance and 1 point awarded to each variable, a simple prognostic scoring system has been devised [PGI score—low pH (P), low GCS (G), impaired SBP (I)], ranging from 3 (worst) to 0 (best).[28] There is a good correlation between the PGI score, SOFA score, and APACHE-II score. Mortality is only 10.7% if score at admission is "0."[29] Therefore, PGI, a simple and easily available scoring system, can be used in almost every ED to assess whether a patient with ALP poisoning requires admission in ICU.

TABLE 4: VENOM score.

Parameter	*Points*
Female gender	1
Capillary leak syndrome	2
Time from bite to ASV > 6.5 hours	1
Overt bleeding	3
Systolic blood pressure <100 mm Hg	2
Hemoglobin <10 g/dL	1
Urine output <20 mL/h in 24 hours	2

(ASV: anti-snakebite venom; VENOM: Viper ENvenOming Mortality)

Triaging of Snakebite Patients

Viper ENvenOming Mortality Score

The Viper ENvenOming Mortality (VENOM) score includes parameters as assessed at 24 hours of admission and may help in determining whether the patient requires transfer to an ICU. The seven parameters (six at admission and one after 24 hours) include overt bleeding (presence of bleeding from the oral cavity, persistent bleeding from bite site hematuria, epistaxis, bleeding from IV puncture sites, hematemesis or melena, fresh bleeding per rectum, abnormal uterine bleeding or intracranial hemorrhage), hemoglobin at admission <10 g/dL, bite to antivenom time >6.5 hours, SBP at admission <100 mm Hg, presence of signs of capillary leak syndrome (conjunctival chemosis, parotid swelling, or periorbital puffiness with clinical evidence of pleural effusion or ascites), urine output <20 mL/h in the first 24 hours, and female gender.[30] Points allotted in VENOM score are given in **Table 4**. Patients with a score >6 should be admitted/transferred to ICU for appropriate care and reducing mortality.

CONCLUSION

Acute poisoning is a common emergency all over the world. When poisoned patients present to the ED, the first priority is stabilization of ABCD, and initial triage decisions are based on unstable ABCDs. The emergency physician should be aware of various pointers in poisoned patients which place them in the "red" or "immediate" category. All patients who are in the "red" category are transferred o ICU for further management. There are several scoring systems available which can guide emergency physicians to triage other patients to various categories as well as admission to ICU or general ward.

REFERENCES

1. Christian MD. Triage. Crit Care Clin. 2019;35:575-89.
2. Beauchamp GA, Hendrickson RG, Hatten BW; Toxicology Investigators Consortium (ToxIC). Endotracheal intubation for toxicologic exposures: a retrospective review of Toxicology Investigators Consortium (ToxIC) Cases. J Emerg Med. 2016;51:382-8.
3. Even KM, Armsby CC, Bateman ST. Poisonings requiring admission to the pediatric intensive care unit: a 5-year review. Clin Toxicol. 2014;52:519-24.
4. Duncan R, Thakore S. Decreased Glasgow Coma Scale score does not mandate endotracheal intubation in the emergency department. J Emerg Med. 2009;37:451-5.
5. Thundiyil JG, Rowley F, Papa L, Olson KR, Kearney TE. Risk factors for complications of drug-induced seizures. J Med Toxicol. 2011;7:16-23.
6. Rollin M, Jaulim A, Vaz F, Sandhu G, Wood S, Birchall M, et al. Caustic ingestion injury of the upper aerodigestive tract in adults. Ann R Coll Surg Engl. 2015;97:304-7.
7. McGuigan MA; Guideline Consensus Panel. Guideline for the out-of-hospital management of human exposures to minimally toxic substances. J Toxicol Clin Toxicol. 2003;41:907-17.
8. Kwon WY, Rhee JE, Gang HS, Shin SD, Cho JH, Song HG, et al. Triage method for out-of-hospital poisoned patients. J Korean Med Sci. 2007;22:336-41.
9. Mofenson HC, Greensher J, Caraccio TR. Ingestions considered nontoxic. Clin Lab Med. 1984;4:587-602.
10. Persson H, Sjöberg G, Haines J, Pronczuk de Garbino J. Poisoning Severity Score: grading of acute poisoning. J Toxicol Clin Toxicol. 1998;36:205-13.
11. Casey PB, Dexter EM, Michell J, Vale JA. The prospective value of the IPCS/EC/EAPCCT poisoning severity score in cases of poisoning. J Toxicol Clin Toxicol. 1998;36:215-7.
12. Schwarz ES, Kopec KT, Wiegand TJ, Wax PM, Brent J. Should we be using the poisoning severity score? J Med Toxicol. 2017;13:135-45.
13. Han KS, Kim SJ, Lee EJ, Shin JH, Lee JS, Lee SW. Development and validation of new poisoning mortality score system for patients with acute poisoning at the emergency department. Crit Care. 2021;25(1):29.
14. Dart RC, Hurlbut KM, Garcia R, Boren J. Validation of a severity score for the assessment of crotalid snakebite. Ann Emerg Med. 1996;27:321-6.
15. Padhiyar R, Chavan S, Dhampalwar S, Trivedi T, Moulick N. Snake bite envenomation in a tertiary care centre. J Assoc Physicians India. 2018;66:55-9.
16. Nishioka SA. Limitations of the snakebite severity score. Ann Emerg Med. 1996;28:371-2.
17. Yu JH, Weng YM, Chen KF, Chen SY, Lin CC. Triage vital signs predict in-hospital mortality among emergency department patients with acute poisoning: a case control study. BMC Health Serv Res. 2012;12:262-9.
18. Mégarbane B, Oberlin M, Alvarez JC, Balen F, Beaune S, Bédry R, et al. Management of pharmaceutical and recreational drug poisoning. Ann Intensive Care. 2020;10(1):157.
19. Brandenburg R, Brinkman S, de Keizer NF, Kesecioglu J, Meulenbelt J, de Lange DW. The need for ICU admission in poisoning patients: a prediction model. Clin Toxicol. 2017;55:4-11.
20. Beaune S, Juvin P, Beauchet A, Casalino E, Megarbane B. Deliberate drug poisonings admitted to an emergency department in Paris area—a descriptive study and assessment of risk factors for intensive care admission. Eur Rev Med Pharmacol Sci. 2016;20:1174-9.
21. Novack V, Jotkowitz A, Delgado J, Novack L, Elbaz G, Shleyfer E, et al. General characteristics of hospitalized patients after deliberate self-poisoning and risk factors for intensive care admission. Eur J Intern Med. 2006;17:485-9.
22. Maignan M, Pommier P, Clot S, Saviuc P, Debaty G, Briot R, et al. Deliberate drug poisoning with slight symptoms on admission: are there predictive factors for intensive care unit referral? A three-year retrospective study. Basic Clin Pharmacol Toxicol. 2014;114:281-7.
23. Senanayake N, de Silva HJ, Karalliedde L. A scale to assess severity in organophosphorus intoxication: POP scale. Hum Exp Toxicol. 1993;12:297-9.
24. Malaviya NB, Parikh R, Pancholi K, Belim OB. Assessment of the Peradeniya organophosphorus poisoning scale as a severity and prognostic marker in patients with acute organophosphorus poisoning presenting to an emergency medicine department. Cureus. 2023; 15(6):e40277.
25. Shabari G, Kalyan K, Reddy YJ. To assess the severity of organophosphorus compound poisoning clinically by using Peradeniya score. Indian J App Res. 2016;6:617-9.
26. El-Sarnagawy GN, Abdelnoor AA, Abuelfadl AA, El-Mehallawi IH. Comparison between various scoring systems in predicting the need for intensive care unit admission of acute pesticide-poisoned patients. Environ Sci Pollut Res Int. 2022;29:33999-4009.
27. Ebrahimi K, VaisiRaigani AA, Jalali R, Rezaei M. Determining and comparing predictive and intensity value of severity scores - "Sequential Organ Failure Assessment Score," "Acute Physiology and Chronic Health Evaluation 4," and "Poisoning Severity Score" - in short-term clinical outcome of patients with poisoning in an ICU. Indian J Crit Care Med. 2018;22:415-21.
28. Pannu AK, Bhalla A, Sharma A, Sharma N. "PGI score": a simplified three-point prognostic score for acute aluminium phosphide poisoning. Indian J Crit Care Med. 2020;24:790-3.
29. Pannu AK, Jhuria L, Bhalla A, Sharma N. PGI score: prospective validation and correlation with SOFA, SAPS-II, and APACHE-II scores for predicting outcomes in acute aluminum phosphide poisoning. Toxicol Res (Camb). 2022;11:361-6.
30. Gopalakrishnan M, Saurabh S, Sagar P, Bammigatti C, Dutta TK. A simple mortality risk prediction score for viper envenoming in India (VENOMS): a model development and validation study. PLoS Negl Trop Dis. 2022;16(2):e0010183.

1.2 Airway Management in a Poisoned Patient

Ananya Ray, Kashish Garg, Kamal Kajal

INTRODUCTION

Airway management is a fundamental aspect of critical care medicine, and its significance becomes even more pronounced when dealing with a poisoned patient. Poisoning, whether accidental or intentional, can lead to a wide range of clinical features and complications that may hamper a patient's ability to maintain a patent airway and adequate ventilation. Effective airway management in poisoned patients is paramount to ensure their survival and minimize the risk of complications. This section explores the complexities of airway management in poisoned patients and highlights the strategies and considerations that clinicians must be aware of.

TOXICOLOGY CONSIDERATION

In managing the airway of poisoned patients, understanding the toxicological effects of the ingested or exposed substance is important **(Table 1)**. Most of the poisoning occurs through the oral route. However, it can also occur through inhalational exposure to volatile compounds or suspended particles. High-dose exposure can affect multiple components of the airway from the point of air entry to the level of gas exchange.

REQUIREMENT OF ARTIFICIAL AIRWAY IN A POISONED PATIENT

Endotracheal intubation may be required for the following reasons:

- Altered mental status causing an inability to maintain airway reflexes
- Imminent threat to airway patency, especially due to mucosal edema from exposure to irritant gases
- Respiratory insufficiency due to central hypoventilation or inadequate muscle power or paralysis

TABLE 1: Common poisons and their mechanisms of action.

Category	*Examples*	*Mechanism*
Asphyxiant	Carbon dioxide, nitrogen, methane	Oxygen displacement from hemoglobin leading to CNS symptoms and hypoxia
Water-soluble irritant	Ammonia, chlorine, sulfur dioxide, chloramines	Predominant upper respiratory symptoms
Water-insoluble irritant	Oxides of nitrogen, phosgene	Predominantly delayed-onset lower respiratory symptoms
Dyshemoglobinemia	Carbon monoxide, MetHb inducers	Impaired oxygen delivery to tissues, secondary pulmonary toxicity
Cellular asphyxiant	Mitochondrial toxicity from cyanide, salicylate, phosphine	Impaired oxygen tissue utilization, secondary pulmonary toxicity
Transfer of systemic toxins	• Multiple • Metal fume fever	• Systemic delivery of toxins through pulmonary route • Metal oxides induce cytokine-mediated pulmonary inflammation (flu-like illness)
Unique mechanism	Hydrocarbons, paraquat, asbestos, silica, beryllium	• Each agent causes characteristic clinical or radiographic feature • *Paraquat:* Progressive pulmonary fibrosis • *Asbestos:* Restrictive lung disease and malignancy
Respiratory depression	Sedative–hypnotic drugs like opioids, benzodiazepines	
Thermal/physical	Heat, caustics	Direct thermal or caustic injury causing upper airway burns
Acid–base imbalance	Salicylates such as aspirin	Metabolic acidosis and hyperventilation

(CNS: central nervous system; MetHb: methemoglobinemia)

- Laryngospasm and bronchospasm due to irritant substances
- Acute lung injury (ALI), aspiration of gastric contents, acute respiratory distress syndrome (ARDS), pulmonary edema due to offending agent
- Arterial blood gas parameters showing hypercapnia, hypoxia, or acidosis

ASSESSING THE POISONED PATIENT

Airway management in poisoned patients begins with a thorough assessment. It is essential to establish the cause and extent of poisoning. The assessment should include:

- *History and clinical presentation:* Obtain a detailed history, including the type and amount of the toxin ingested or exposed to, the time of exposure, and any coexisting medical conditions. The patient's clinical presentation may vary from asymptomatic to severe, so recognizing the signs and symptoms is critical. Airway edema from irritant gases develops within a few hours; hence, time of exposure is paramount.
- *Airway assessment:* Evaluate the patient's airway patency, including the presence of foreign objects, secretions, or any physical obstruction. It is very essential to predict a threatened airway, compromised airway, or difficult airway during airway assessment so that appropriate measures can be taken.
- *Breathing:* Monitor the patient's respiratory rate, depth, and effort.
- *Circulation:* Assess blood pressure, heart rate, and oxygen saturation to determine the patient's hemodynamic stability. Some toxins can cause profound cardiovascular depression which may lead to circulatory failure and lactic acidosis.
- *Level of consciousness:* Assess the patient's level of consciousness using the Glasgow Coma Scale (GCS) to determine whether airway management interventions are needed urgently. A GCS score of ≤8 is usually an indication for endotracheal intubation.

RECOGNIZING THREATENED AIRWAY AND COMPROMISED AIRWAY IN THE EMERGENCY AREA

Compromised Airway

A compromised airway is a condition in which there is an existing partial or complete obstruction of the airway leading to difficulty in breathing, hypoxia, and ultimately hypoxic cardiac arrest if left untreated.

Threatened Airway

A threatened airway is a condition that puts the patient *at risk* for developing acute upper airway obstruction, although the patient can breathe normally. It is important to recognize the signs of a threatened airway and take appropriate action to prevent imminent complications.

Common causes of threatened and compromised airways in cases of poisoning include airway edema, foreign body obstruction, blood and secretions, and neurological conditions like neuromuscular insufficiency, altered mental status, or seizures.

Clinical Features

- Dyspnea
- Inspiratory stridor
- Hoarseness
- Snoring
- Cyanosis (one of the last signs to appear after airway compromise)
- Ineffective cough or gag reflex

Management

- Assess the patient's airway, breathing, and circulation.
- Call for help.
- Supplement oxygen via face mask. A non-rebreathing mask with oxygen flow at 15 L/min can provide a fraction of inspired oxygen up to 1.0.
- Position the patient in a head-up position to maximize airflow. Maintaining adequate oxygenation is the primary goal.

Specific Maneuvers

- If sensorium allows, encourage coughing to clear any potential obstruction.
- Perform the Heimlich maneuver in case of suspected foreign body aspiration.
- In an obtunded patient, a simple head-tilt and chin-lift maneuver can restore patency **(Fig. 1)**. The head-tilt maneuver can be performed by tilting the head back by applying pressure with the palm of one hand on the forehead. The chin-lift maneuver can be performed by lifting the chin up with the forefinger of the opposite hand. A jaw-thrust maneuver can also increase airway patency by pulling the soft tissues of the oropharynx upwards **(Fig. 2)**.
- In a patient with secretions/vomitus/blood in the airway, suction to clear the airway. Availability of

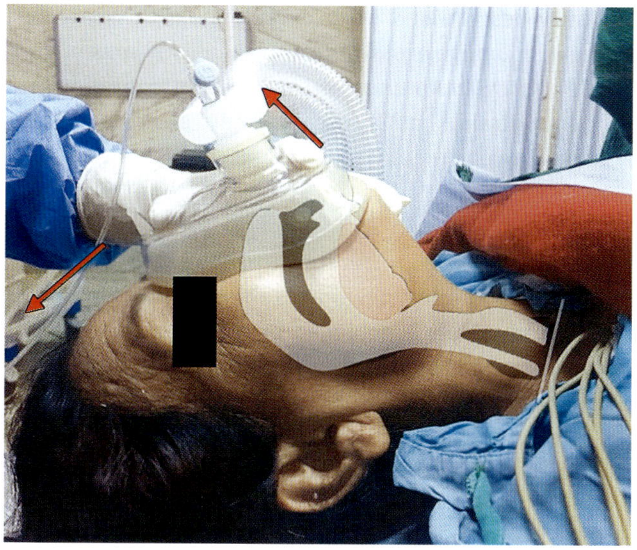

Fig. 1: Technique of performing 'head-tilt' and 'chin lift'.

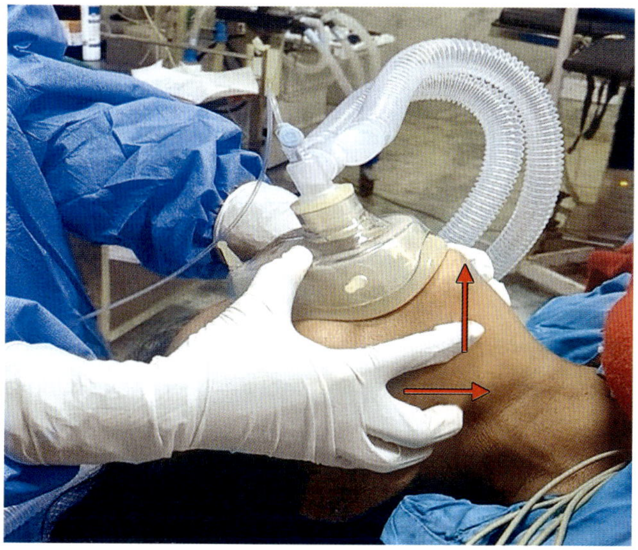

Fig. 2: The jaw-thrust maneuver.

a suction is essential in this subset of patients as they often have increased secretions and may be full-stomach.

- Assist ventilation with a bag and mask ventilation with an Ambu bag or breathing circuit (e.g., Bains circuit).
- Airway adjuncts
  - Nasopharyngeal and oropharyngeal airways may be used to maintain patency of the airway in upper airway obstruction since they prevent the tongue and soft tissues from falling backward. Nasopharyngeal airways must not be used in the presence of base of skull fractures, nasal masses, or epistaxis. The size of the nasopharyngeal airway is estimated by measuring the length from the nares to the tragus, and the size of the oropharyngeal airway can be estimated by measuring the distance between the incisor and the angle of the jaw.
  - Laryngeal mask airway (LMA) may be used to ventilate a patient in case of an emergency or in a difficult airway situation since it is easy to insert and serves as an alternative means of ventilation. It is a device originally designed based on cadaver studies to bypass the upper airway and rest above the laryngeal inlet. It may be cuffed or uncuffed and may have a separate port for gastric suction.
  - If a difficult intubation is encountered, a gum elastic bougie is often helpful in guiding a railroaded endotracheal tube (ETT) into the trachea. The bougie has a curved tip which is atraumatic and bent anteriorly to pass easily into an anterior larynx.
- In recent times, videolaryngoscopes are being used for intubation. They are shaped like conventional Magill or Macintosh direct laryngoscopes, with a few modifications, and have a camera at the tip that projects the view or the larynx onto a screen. They have been proven to enable intubation in cases of difficult intubation and are useful in most scenarios except in cases of limited mouth opening and presence of copious amounts of blood and secretions in the upper airway.[1]
- Prepare for advanced airway management such as intubation or surgical airway when indicated.
  - The ideal location is the operating room.
  - There should be a formal time-out in which the intended course of steps and actions is announced to ensure the team completely understands the plan.
  - Brief introduction of the team
  - In case of a difficult airway, the patient's neck should be prepared for possible surgical access.
  - The patient's cricothyroid membrane (CTM) should be identified.
  - At least one surgeon should be present in case of a difficult airway. Communication between the anesthetist/intensivist and the surgical team is essential.
  - Tracheostomy instrument set should be made available in addition to the airway equipment cart.

INTUBATION

Pharmacological Preparation

Under ideal circumstances, a combination of sedatives and amnestic agents, antisialagogues, and muscle relaxants is used to facilitate optimal conditions for securing the airway. However, the choice of agents varies with the clinical condition, the drug ingested, and the indication for intubation. In a poisoned patient, the use of pharmacological agent will vary with the indication of intubation.

- Altered mental status will preclude the requirement for sedation if GCS is <8. In the presence of delirium, the sedatives of choice will be intravenous propofol (up to 1 mg/kg), ketamine (0.2–0.75 mg/kg), etomidate (0.1 mg/kg), and thiopentone (1.5–3.5 mg/kg). Midazolam is known to cause further delirium in the critical care setting,[2] hence must be used with caution. In the presence of seizures, barbiturates may be the drug of choice. Rapid-onset and short-acting muscle relaxants like succinylcholine may be used in the absence of hyperkalemia as in digoxin toxicity and rhabdomyolysis.
- *Imminent threat to airway patency, especially due to mucosal edema:* Due to the imminent risk of airway collapse, spontaneous ventilation is best preserved such that loss of tone of upper airway muscles does not further compromise the patency of the airway. In this case, sedation must be carefully titrated so as not to abolish spontaneous respiration and muscle tone. Ketamine is an agent that preserves spontaneous ventilation as well as airway reflexes but has the unwanted effects of sialorrhea, tachycardia, and hypotension. (This makes it unfavorable for use in organophosphate poisoning and in patients with preexisting cardiac disease.) Intermediate- and long-acting muscle relaxants are best not used and short-acting muscle relaxants like succinylcholine (1–1.5 mg/kg) should also be used with caution only.
- *Respiratory insufficiency from central hypoventilation, inadequate muscle power, or paralysis:* Depending on the clinical scenario, muscle relaxation or mild sedation may be administered judiciously.
- *Laryngospasm and bronchospasm:* Premedication in such conditions must be with agents which are not irritant to the airway, like propofol and ketamine. Thiopentone is notorious for causing bronchospasm and is best avoided. Muscle relaxation in this case must be adequate to avoid worsening of airway spasm.
- *ALI/ARDS/pulmonary edema:* These conditions do not contraindicate any agent in the absence of other organ involvement.

Position

The "sniffing position" is optimal as it aligns the oral, pharyngeal, and laryngeal axes to provide a clear view of the larynx. This is achieved by elevating the patient's head, extending the head at the neck, and aligning the ears horizontally. In morbidly obese patients, the "ramp" position is used, for which rolls may be utilized to align the external auditory meatus with the sternal notch.

Rapid Sequence Intubation

Rapid sequence induction is essential since the patient in the emergency department is unlikely to be in nil per oral status.

Preoxygenation

When intubation is elective, preoxygenation with a high fraction of inspired oxygen replaces the alveolar air of the lungs with 100% oxygen which can maintain blood oxygen levels during the period of apnea, providing valuable time for intubation.

Technique

After making the sniffing position, the heel of one hand is placed on the forehead and the forefinger is used to open the mouth. The laryngoscope is held with the other hand. The blade of the laryngoscope is then inserted into the oral cavity and the tongue is swept to the opposite side and the tip of the blade is made to rest at the base of the epiglottis. The epiglottis is then lifted with an anterior, upward, and leftward force, taking care not to hinge the blade on the teeth of the patient. This reveals the larynx, and an ETT is inserted into the laryngeal inlet.

Confirmation

The correct placement of the ETT is confirmed by:

- Bilateral chest rise
- Misting of the ETT
- Bilateral air entry into the chest on auscultation
- No sound on auscultation of the stomach
- A sustained graph on end-tidal CO_2 monitor
- Tracheal ultrasound

DIFFICULT AIRWAY

The difficult airway has been defined as the clinical situation in which a conventionally trained anesthesiologist experiences difficulty with facemask ventilation of the upper airway, difficulty in tracheal intubation, or both, or supraglottic airway device insertion.

Before intubation, one should be able to answer the following:

- Will I be able to mask ventilate?
- Will I be able to perform laryngoscopy?
- Will I be able to intubate?
- Is there a high risk of aspiration?
- If difficulty is predicted, should I opt for awake intubation?
- Should I plan for cricothyroid access, if needed?
- What equipment shall I keep ready?

Various parameters may be indicative of potential difficulty in achieving mask ventilation:

- *Predicting difficult mask ventilation (DMV):* Body mass index >26 kg/m^2, age >55 years, macroglossia, presence of beard, lack of teeth, history of snoring, increased Mallampati grade (MPG), and lower thyromental distance are potential DMV risk factors.[3]
    - Thyromental distance is the distance from the mentum to the thyroid notch while the patient's neck is fully extended. A value of <6 cm predicts difficult laryngoscopy or intubation.
    - MPG: This test is performed with the patient sitting, with the head in a neutral position, the mouth open, and the tongue protruding out.
        - Class I: Visualization of the soft palate, fauces, uvula, and anterior and posterior pillars
        - Class II: Visualization of the soft palate, fauces, and uvula
        - Class III: Visualization of the soft palate and base of the uvula
    - In Samsoon and Young's modification (1987) of the Mallampati classification, class IV was added.
        - Class IV: Only the hard palate is visible. The soft palate is not visible at all. Mallampati classes III and IV suggest difficult laryngoscopy. Class III or IV suggests a significant chance that the patient will be difficult to intubate.
- *Predicting difficult laryngoscopy:* Limited mouth opening is a barrier to insertion of all airway devices. Assessment of the interincisor gap must be estimated while selecting the device to be used. An interincisor gap of approximately 3 cm is normally required for Macintosh blade. The rescue devices then are slimmer supraglottic devices and fiberoptic bronchoscopes. A narrow or high arching palate also indicates decreased space in the oropharynx. Large, barrel chests and large breasts can hinder laryngoscope insertion by decreasing maneuverability of the handle, necessitating a "ramping" position. Limited neck extension and retrognathia also predict difficult laryngoscopy.
- Predicting difficult intubation: Laryngeal tumors, vocal cord palsies, and subglottic stenosis hinder ETT insertion. Stridor should alert the intensivist to these potential pathologies as well.

Managing the Anticipated Difficult Airway

- Have a preformulated plan. Weigh the risks and benefits of awake intubation, intubation with sedation with spontaneous respiration preserved, and intubation with the use of muscle relaxants.
- Keep airway adjuncts and backup equipment ready.
- Be aware of the patient's vitals, number of attempts, and time taken[4] **(Fig. 3)**.

Managing Unanticipated Difficult Airway

See **Figure 4**.

ROLE OF POINT-OF-CARE ULTRASOUND

The portability and high diagnostic accuracy of point-of-care ultrasound (POCUS) in a wide variety of scenario has secured the role of POCUS in resuscitation.

Upper airway ultrasound can aid in identification of the upper airway structures such as the trachea, esophagus, tracheal rings, cricoid cartilage, CTM, thyroid cartilage, vocal cords, hyoid bone, epiglottis, and tongue.

Five views are used to assess the upper airway **(Table 2)**:

1. Suprahyoid
2. Thyrohyoid
3. Thyroid
4. Cricothyroid
5. Suprasternal

Endotracheal Tube Placement Confirmation

Endotracheal tube placement can be detected reliably by POCUS.[7] The transducer is placed in transverse position in

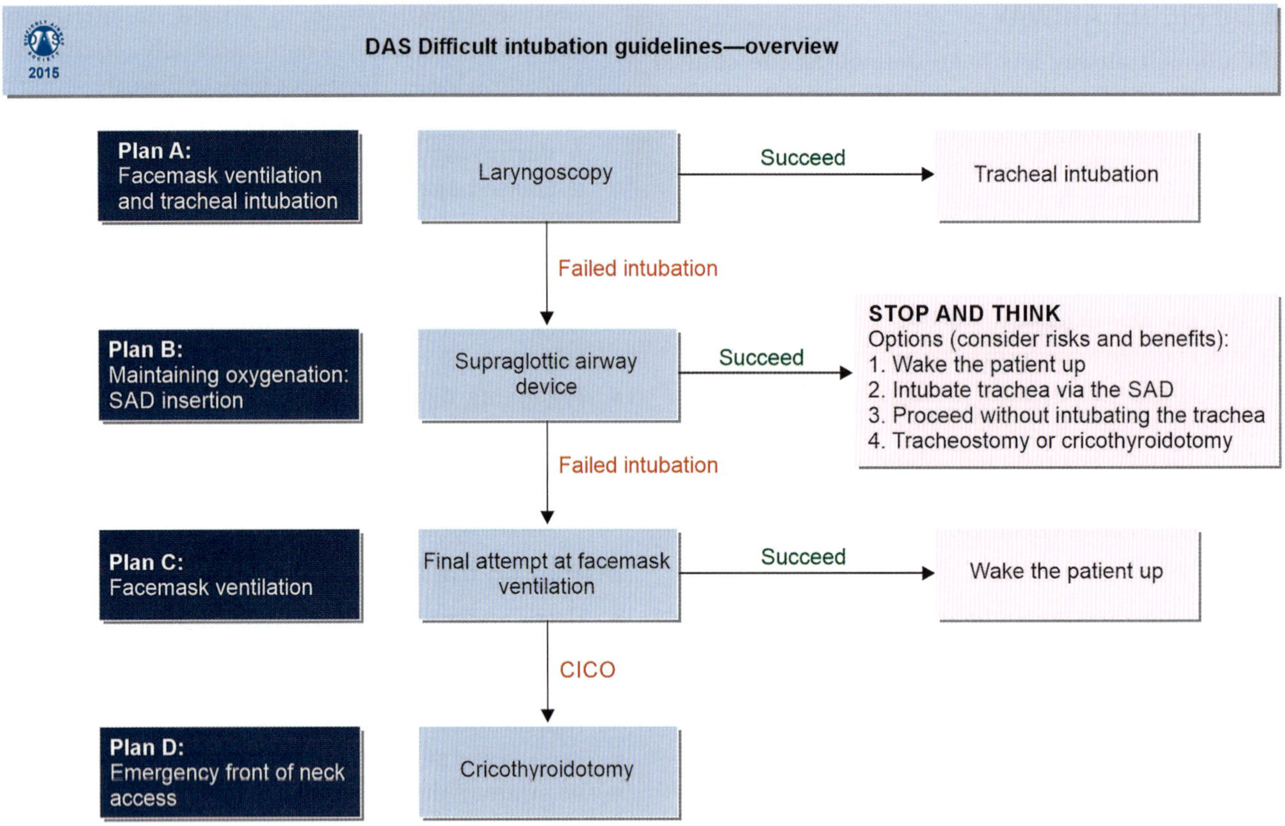

This flowchart forms part of the DAS Guidelines for unanticipated difficult intubation in adults 2015 and should be used in conjunction with the text

Fig. 3: Difficult Airway Society guidelines, 2015. (DAS: Difficult Airway Society; SAD: supraglottic airway device)
Source: Reproduced from Frerk C, Mitchell VS, McNarry AF, Mendonca C, Bhagrath R, Patel A, et al. Difficult Airway Society 2015 guidelines for management of unanticipated difficult intubation in adults. Br J Anaesth. 2015;115(6):827-48.

the suprasternal notch. Movement in the trachea appearing like a snowstorm as the ETT passes across the probe, called the "snowstorm sign," confirms correct ETT placement. If the ETT enters the esophagus, the "double tract sign" is seen.[8]

CONCLUSION

- The poisoned patient may present with various situations that mandate securing the airway including altered mentation, hypoxemia, airway edema, etc.
- Maintaining airway patency is of paramount importance and can be facilitated by various rescue maneuvers and adjuncts.
- Optimal intubating conditions must always be ensured which may include use of various amnestic/anesthetic agents and neuromuscular blockers, however, the choice of drug and dose must be carefully adjudged.
- An airway assessment must always be performed when conditions permit to be able to anticipated a difficult airway.
- Airway ultrasound is a non-invasive adjunct to clinical assessment of the airway and can assist in placement of an endotracheal tube, as well as performing cricothyroidotomy.

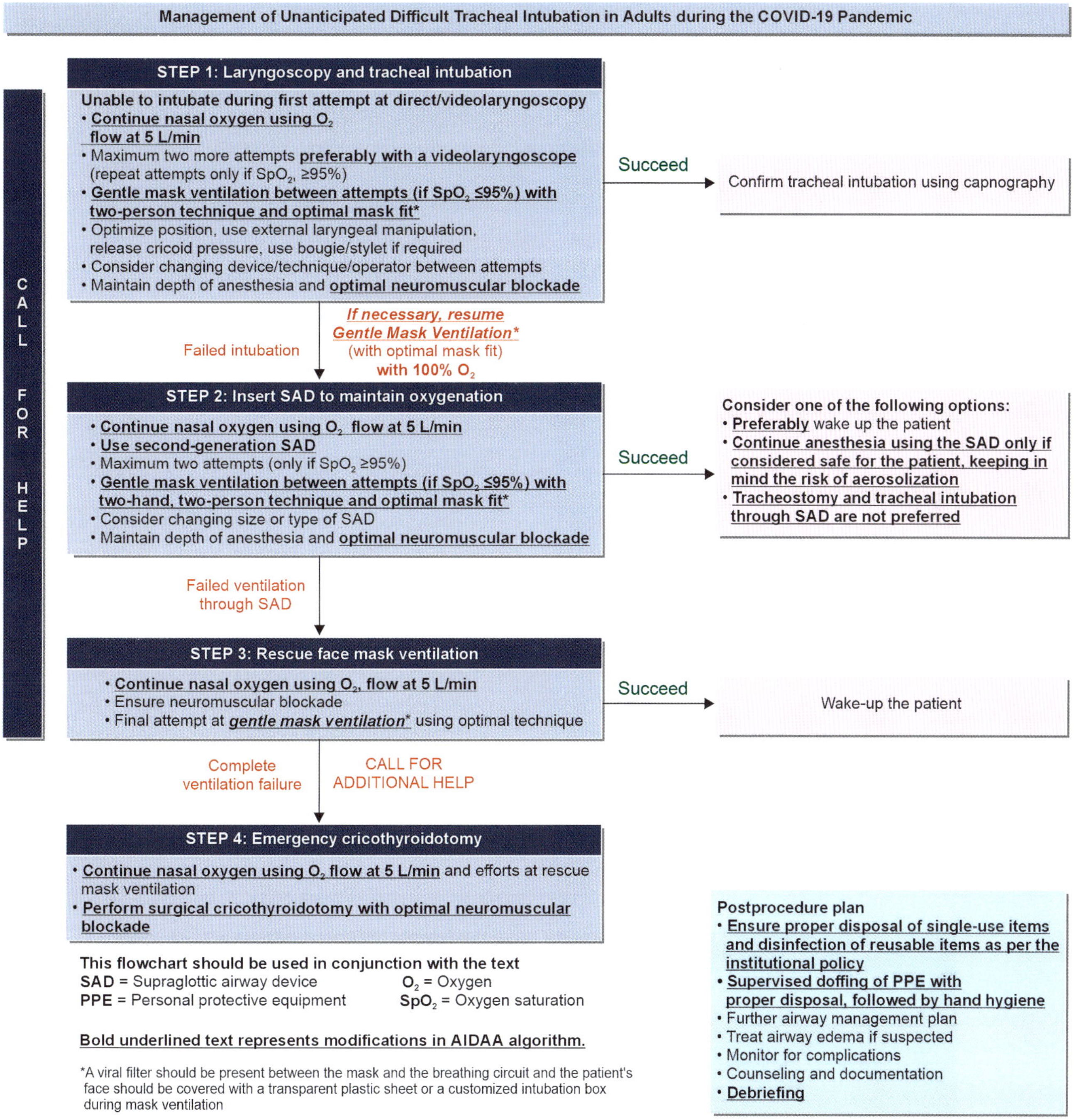

Gement of unanticipated difficult tracheal intubation in adults during the COVID-19 pandemic-Algorithm

Fig. 4: All India Difficult Airway Society algorithm for management of unanticipated difficult airway.[5]
(AIDAA: All India Difficult Airway Society)

TABLE 2: Ultrasound probe placement and image acquired for various views during airway ultrasonography.[6]

Anatomical structure	*Probe position and image acquisition*	*Sonographic appearance*
Tongue	Midsagittal, below the mentum	Fan shaped with intrinsic muscles giving striated appearance; hyperechoic line of dorsal surface from A-M interface
Hyoid bone	Transverse over the neck; slide caudad from the mentum	Superficial, hyperechoic, inverted U-shaped, linear structure
	Sagittal or parasagittal	Narrow curved structure, casting acoustic shadow
Epiglottis	Transverse above the thyroid cartilage through the thyrohyoid membrane window	Hypoechoic transverse curvilinear structure, with hyperechoic pre-epiglottic space and bright A-M interface delineating the posterior border
	Sagittal in most subjects	Hypoechoic longitudinal curvilinear structure
Thyrohyoid membrane	Transverse between the hyoid bone and the thyroid cartilage	Hyperechoic line between the hyoid bone and the thyroid cartilage
	Parasagittal	Hyperechoic line between the hyoid bone and the thyroid cartilage
Thyroid cartilage	Transverse on thyroid prominence	Inverted V-shaped hypoechoic, with varying age-related hyperechogenicity and intraglottic structures
	Parasagittal over the thyroid cartilage	Linear hypoechoic structure with varying calcification
Cricothyroid membrane	Transverse using TACA technique **(Figs. 5A to D)**	Hyperechoic transverse line between the thyroid and cricoid cartilages
	Midsagittal probe above the suprasternal notch and slide cephalad	Longitudinal hyperechoic line between the thyroid and cricoid cartilages
Cricoid cartilage	Transverse over the cricoid cartilage	Superficial, thick hypoechoic arch-shaped structure
	Sagittal, probe above the suprasternal notch	Hypoechoic oval structure larger than the tracheal rings
Trachea	Transverse over the suprasternal notch	Inverted U-shaped hypoechoic rings on transverse view
	Midsagittal over the suprasternal notch	Hypoechoic oval structures (string of pearls/beads appearance)
Esophagus	Transverse over the suprasternal notch sliding laterally (usually to left)	Collapsed muscular structure lateral to trachea; swallowing facilitates its identification

(A-M: air–mucosa; TACA: thyroid–airline–cricoid–airline)

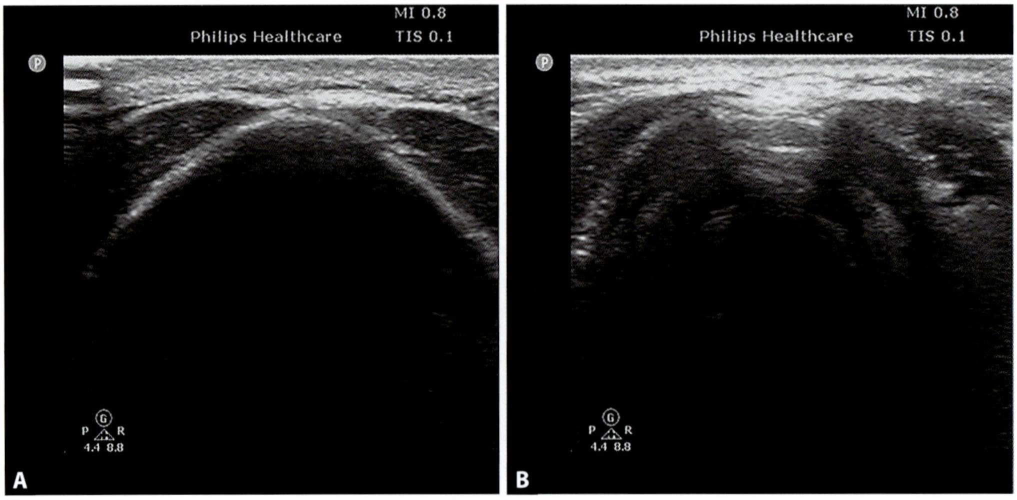

Figs. 5A and B

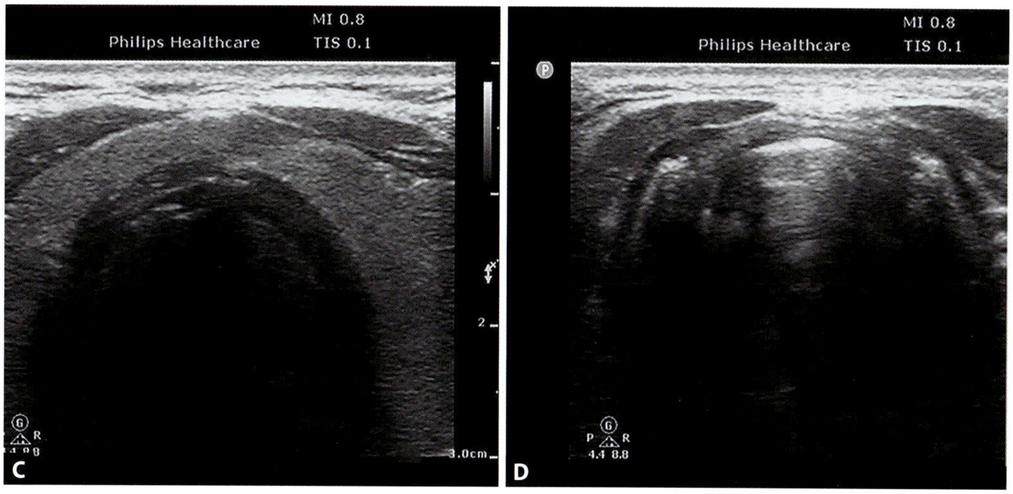

Figs. 5C and D

Figs. 5A to D: (A) Transverse view of the Thyroid cartilage; (B) Transverse view showing the air interface at the cricothyroid membrane; (C) Transverse view of the Cricoid cartilage; (D) Cricothyroid membrane and the air interface seen once again.

REFERENCES

1. Asai T, Jagannathan N. Videolaryngoscopy is extremely valuable, but should it be the standard for tracheal intubation? Anesth Analg. 2023;136(4):679-82.
2. Shi HJ, Yuan RX, Zhang JZ, Chen JH, Hu AM. Effect of midazolam on delirium in critically ill patients: a propensity score analysis. J Int Med Res. 2022;50(4):3000605221088695.
3. Langeron O, Masso E, Huraux C, Guggiari M, Bianchi A, Coriat P, et al. Prediction of difficult mask ventilation. Anesthesiology. 2000;92:1229-36.
4. Apfelbaum JL, Hagberg CA, Connis RT, Abdelmalak BB, Agarkar M, Dutton RP, et al. 2022 American Society of Anesthesiologists practice guidelines for management of the difficult airway. Anesthesiology. 2022;136:31-81.
5. Myatra SN, Shah A, Kundra P, Patwa A, Ramkumar V, Divatia JV, et al. All India Difficult Airway Association 2016 guidelines for the management of unanticipated difficult tracheal intubation in adults. Indian J Anaesth. 2016;60(12):885.
6. Kolli S, Singh M. POCUS spotlight: airway. ASRA News. 2021;46, Table 1.
7. Chou H-C, Chong K-M, Sim S-S, Ma MH-M, Liu S-H, Chen N-C, et al. Real-time tracheal ultrasonography for confirmation of endotracheal tube placement during cardiopulmonary resuscitation. Resuscitation. 2013;84(12):1708-12.
8. Chou H-C, Tseng W-P, Wang C-H, Ma MH-M, Wang H-P, Huang P-C, et al. Tracheal rapid ultrasound exam (T.R.U.E.) for confirming endotracheal tube placement during emergency intubation. Resuscitation. 2011;82(10):1279-84.

1.3 Breathing Component of Airway, Breathing, Circulation, and Disability in a Poisoned Patient

Pradip Kumar Bhattacharya, Tushar Kumar

INTRODUCTION

Deaths and morbidity due to poisoning are increasing every day globally. In India, about 1.6 people out of 100,000 population die because of poisoning.[1] Poisoning, whether intentional or unintentional, is a serious health issue and is among the most common reasons for admission to the emergency department.[2] Resuscitation of critical patients with basic life support is a talisman and the same is followed for poisoned patients. The airway, breathing, and circulation maintenance is the primary goal along with the safety of health care personnel and preserving the operational integrity of the health center. Physicians in emergency departments are expected to have a systematic approach toward the evaluation and management of poisoned patients. Initial management should encompass airway, breathing, and circulation on acute stabilization and supportive care till the causative agent is identified. Management should include supportive care, halting further poison absorption, using antidote if applicable, and expediting elimination of causative agent.

The breathing component of stabilization primarily depends on the correction of altered physiology due to poisoning. Acute respiratory failure is the most common cause of mortality, affecting either central or peripheral pathway.[3] According to the World Health Organization (WHO), pesticides are the most common cause of unintentional deaths across the world while antidepressants, tranquilizers, and analgesics are intentional causes of poisoning.[4,5] In this chapter, we will discuss about the approach toward and management of poisoned patients in respiratory failure.

ACUTE CLINICAL PRESENTATION

Poisoned patients often present with headache, dyspnea, nausea, vomiting, eye pain, altered sensorium, and shock in severe cases.[6] Severe respiratory depression leading to hypoxia and ventilatory failure, bronchospasm, and bronchorrhea are hallmarks of malfunction in breathing components.[7]

Organophosphorus (OP) poisoning and opioid poisoning present with a different spectrum of symptoms, converging into respiratory failure and death.

PATHOPHYSIOLOGY

In OP poisoning, M3 receptor stimulation along with nicotinic and M2 receptor stimulation causes contractions of bronchial smooth muscles, which results in bronchospasm.[8]

It is not uncommon that opioid overdose causes massive release of histamine, thereby causing bronchospasm and pulmonary edema.[9]

Bronchorrhea from OP poisoning results from neuronal and non-neuronal cholinergic stimulation of the mucus glands, cilia, and cells producing periciliary fluid.[10] The excess fluid in the interstitium hampers in oxygen therapy in spite of treatment.

Acute respiratory distress syndrome (ARDS) has been reported in several cases of OP insecticide poisoning as well as opioid poisoning.[9,11] It may result directly from pulmonary complications of poisoning, such as aspiration or inhalation, or indirectly via hematogenous exposure to OP compounds. ARDS frequently remains undiagnosed in nonpoisoning cases; it further remains unnoticed in poisoning cases.[12]

The increased pulmonary capillary permeability due to hypoxemia, immense histamine release, and respiratory acidosis caused by depression of medullary respiratory centers may cause pulmonary edema and ARDS.[13]

Organophosphorus nerve agents act within minutes and may cause death within 5 minutes, thus raising suspicion of the involvement of central pathways directly, leading to respiratory failure. However, the mechanism of OP-induced central respiratory depression is unknown. The proposed respiratory center pacemaker—the pre-Bötzinger complex—in the ventrolateral medulla has glutamatergic and muscarinic control. Excess acetylcholine may alter the function of the pre-Bötzinger complex or other linked hindbrain areas to depress respiratory activity.[14]

On the other hand, opioid-induced respiratory depression (ORID) occurs via activation of μ-opioid receptors at specific sites in the central nervous system (CNS) including the pre-Bötzinger complex, affecting respiration rhythm-generating capacity.[3]

In OP poisoning, an excess of acetylcholine at neuromuscular junctions (NMJs) can lead to fasciculations and flaccid paralysis due to a depolarizing block leading to respiratory muscle weakness. This further worsens ventilatory drive and hypoxia.[15]

MANAGEMENT

Patients with OP poisoning present with acute, delayed, and late manifestations. Acute manifestations occur within minutes and last up to 24 hours. In this phase, patients present with weakness, fasciculations, cramps, paralysis, salivation, lacrimation, urination, defecation, gastric cramps, emesis, bradycardia, hypotension, miosis, bronchospasm, anxiety, restlessness, convulsions, and respiratory depression. In the delayed presentation, which spans from 24 hours to 2 weeks, patients present with intermediate syndrome, cholinergic symptoms like bradycardia, miosis, salivation, coma, and extrapyramidal manifestations. After 2 weeks, in the late phase, peripheral neuropathy starts.[16]

The management of the breathing component is challenging during the acute phase of presentation.

Patients may present with mild to severe respiratory failure. Bronchospasm, bronchorrhea, and respiratory failure ultimately lead to hypoxia and death in severe cases. Another important aspect of poisoning is that self-poisoning is often more dangerous to life than accidental poisoning.[17]

During the primary survey, a quick assessment of airway, breathing, circulation, and disability (ABCD) should be done along with placement of Guedel's airway to ensure airway patency and left lateral decubitus position in a slight head-low position to reduce the risk of aspiration.[17] Neck extension will help in keeping the airway open. A baseline Glasgow Coma Scale (GCS) should be recorded to guide the extent of neurological deficit.

A routine assessment revealing miosis, excessive sweating, poor air entry into the lungs due to bronchorrhea and bronchospasm, bradycardia, and hypotension indicates the use of atropine. If the clinical presentation is not clear, administer atropine 0.6–1 mg. A marked increase in heart rate (>20–25 beats/min) and flushing of the skin suggest that the patient does not have significant cholinergic poisoning and further atropine is not required. In case of obvious clinical features, then administer 1.8–3 mg of atropine.

Although injection atropine takes time to reverse the effects, ensure that the two intraventricular (IV) drips have been set up (one for fluid and drugs, the other for atropine). Give 500–1,000 mL (10–20 mL/kg) of isotonic saline over 10–20 minutes.

After 3–5 minutes of giving atropine, check for reversal of symptoms. Reversal of all five parameters is important and not just of one. Some centers have a preference of glycopyrrolate over atropine as it has lesser CNS penetration and produces less central anticholinergic toxicity in overdose.[18] However, the central effects of poisoning are also spared in such cases.

Pralidoxime, an oxime acetylcholinesterase (AChE) reactivator, is another widely recommended and most commonly used drug across the world.[19]

The lungs of poisoned patients are filled with bronchial secretions in OP poisoning. Bronchorrhea and bronchospasm will make the transport of gases difficult. Atropine will reverse the effects, dry the secretions, and relieve bronchial muscles.

Role of Bronchodilators

Salbutamol may help in relieving bronchospasm through beta-2 agonism. During atropine resuscitation, atropine only stops the secretions but removal of fluid takes time. Salbutamol might also work to increase fluid elimination from the lungs. Bronchorrhea during acute cholinergic crisis can be treated with atropine but it does not speed its removal from the lung. Beta-agonists like salbutamol help in increasing removal, augmenting atropine's cessation of fluid production, thereby enhancing effective oxygenation.

Salbutamol can be used in either intravenous or nebulized form. In a recent BALTI-2 (Beta-Agonist Lung injury TrIal-2) study, the role of beta-2 agonists was studied in patients with lung injury for 7 days via intravenous routes. The study concluded that there is no clinical benefit seen but it might help in poisoned patients when used through nebulized routes during resuscitation in the acute phase.[20] However, there is a problem that salbutamol has to cross lung secretions to reach the alveolar epithelium in order to act.

In severely poisoned patients, endotracheal intubation is warranted. The decision of endotracheal intubation depends on clinical findings and history. Endotracheal intubation helps in clearing up bronchial secretions, oxygen therapy, and nebulization with bronchodilators.

In OP poisoning or opioid poisoning, pharmacotherapy is the cornerstone for treatment; however, to maintain oxygenation, ventilatory support may be required. In case of bronchospasm not responding to pharmacotherapy, patients should be managed on mechanical ventilation. There is no role of noninvasive ventilation (NIV) in poisoned patients. In pressure support ventilation (PSV), the initial pressure support should not be high and the target tidal volume can be around 6–8 mL/kg.[21] In severe bronchospasm, intensivists should see any signs for auto-positive end-expiratory pressure (auto-PEEP) and dynamic hyperinflation.[21] Sedation with benzodiazepines also helps in preventing patient–machine asynchrony and seizure prophylaxis, especially in opioid poisoning.[18]

The management of ARDS is often vital as it is often missed in poisoned patients. Aspiration of gastric content after any illicit drug overdose or poisoning is common.[22] As patients are comatose, there are high chances of silent aspiration and developing pneumonia and further worsening to ARDS. The cornerstone of treatment is symptomatic and reducing further harm to the patient. Antibiotics should be given to inhibit microbial colonization.[23] Hypoalbuminemia, creatinine, lactate, or C-reactive protein serum levels have a poor prognosis associated with ARDS in OP poisoning.[24]

In opioid overdose, naloxone is the antidote used. Naloxone can be used safely via injectable or intranasal spray form. There is no standard dose for naloxone; however, the recommended dose is 1-2 mg/kg IV.[25]

Management of carbon monoxide (CO) poisoning is another challenge for intensivists. It is a colorless and odorless gas which is sometimes considered in differential diagnosis. Depending on the concentration and the duration of exposure, patients present with headache and dizziness, loss of orientation, symptoms of cardiac angina, loss of consciousness, and death. The diagnosis is based on the patient history, clinical features, acidosis, low or normal plasma oxygen in arterial blood gas analysis, and raised cardiac biomarkers.[26] In the preclinical phase, ensure 100% oxygenation and prevent acidosis. There is 50% mortality associated with pH <7.2. There is a mixed opinion on the use of hyperbaric oxygen therapy and normobaric oxygen therapy in CO poisoning. There is a paucity of randomized controlled data to conclude the superiority of any treatment.

CONCLUSION

Poisoning can be intentional or accidental. Intentional exposure is often associated with poor prognosis as the amount and duration is higher than in accidental exposure. OP poisoning is often accompanied by bronchorrhea, bronchospasm, and respiratory failure leading to hypoxia and death. Opioid overdoses present with bronchospasm, aspirations, and ARDS leading to death. CO poisoning should be considered in differential diagnosis and should be treated promptly with 100% oxygen. There should also be awareness about inhalational organophosphates like sarin, in view of bioterrorism. The cornerstone of maintaining breathing is early pharmacological treatments along with ensuring proper oxygenation. Mechanical ventilation has a vital role in maintaining oxygenation in poisoned patients.

REFERENCES

1. Sharma R, Neelanjana, Rawat N, Panwar N. Mortality and morbidity associated with acute poisoning cases in north-east India: a retrospective study. J Family Med Prim Care. 2019;8(6):2068-72.
2. Dash SK, Raju AS, Mohanty MK, Patnaik KK, Mohanty S. Sociodemographic profile of poisoning cases. J Indian Acad Forensic Med. 2005;27:133-8.
3. Hulse EJ, Davies JO, Simpson AJ, Sciuto AM, Eddleston M. Respiratory complications of organophosphorus nerve agent and insecticide poisoning. Implications for respiratory and critical care. Am J Respir Crit Care Med. 2014;190(12):1342-54 [Erratum in Am J Respir Crit Care Med. 2019;200(7):946-8].
4. Konradsen F, Dawson AH, Eddleston M, Gunnell D. Pesticide self-poisoning: thinking outside the box. Lancet. 2007;369:169-70.
5. McClure GM. Suicide in children and adolescents in England and Wales 1970-1998. Br J Psychiatry. 2001;178:469-74.
6. Okumura T, Takasu N, Ishimatsu S, Miyanoki S, Mitsuhashi A, Kumada K, et al. Report on 640 victims of the Tokyo subway sarin attack. Ann Emerg Med. 1996;28:129-35.
7. Lotti M. Clinical toxicology of anticholinesterase agents in humans. Handb Pesticide Toxicol. 2001;2:1043-85.
8. Wess J, Eglen RM, Gautam D. Muscarinic acetylcholine receptors: mutant mice provide new insights for drug development. Nat Rev Drug Discov. 2007;6:721-33.
9. Lusk JA, Maloley PA. Morphine-induced pulmonary edema. Am J Med. 1988;84(2):367-8.
10. Takemura Y, Helms MN, Eaton AF, Self J, Ramosevac S, Jain L, et al. Cholinergic regulation of epithelial sodium channels in rat alveolar type 2 epithelial cells. Am J Physiol Lung Cell Mol Physiol. 2013;304:L428-37.
11. Akgur S, Veral A, Ege B. Adult respiratory distress syndrome in human organophosphate poisoning cases. Toxicol Environ Chem. 2008;90:493-9.
12. Ferguson ND, Frutos-Vivar F, Esteban A, Fernández-Segoviano P, Aramburu JA, Nájera L, et al. Acute respiratory distress syndrome: underrecognition by clinicians and diagnostic accuracy of three clinical definitions. Crit Care Med. 2005;33:2228-34.
13. Edston E, van Hage-Hamsten M. Anaphylactoid shock—a common cause of death in heroin addicts? Allergy. 1997;52(9):950-4.
14. Gaspari RJ, Paydarfar D. Dichlorvos-induced central apnea: effects of selective brainstem exposure in the rat. Neurotoxicology. 2011;32:206-14.
15. Boom M, Niesters M, Sarton E, Aarts L, Smith TW, Dahan A. Non-analgesic effects of opioids: opioid-induced respiratory depression. Curr Pharm Des. 2012;18(37):5994-6004.
16. Peter JV, Sudarsan TI, Moran JL. Clinical features of organophosphate poisoning: a review of different classification systems and approaches. Indian J Crit Care Med. 2014;18(11):735-45.
17. Eddleston M, Dawson A, Karalliedde L, Dissanayake W, Hittarage A, Azher S, et al. Early management after self-poisoning with an organophosphorus or carbamate pesticide—a treatment protocol for junior doctors. Crit Care. 2004;8:R391.
18. Eddleston M, Chowdhury FR. Pharmacological treatment of organophosphorus insecticide poisoning: the old and the (possible) new. Br J Clin Pharmacol. 2016;81(3):462-70.
19. Eyer P, Eddleston M, Thiermann H, Worek F, Buckley NA. Are we using the right dose? A tale of mole and gram. Br J Clin Pharmacol. 2008;66:451-2.

20. Gao Smith F, Perkins GD, Gates S, Young D, McAuley DF, Tunnicliffe W, et al. Effect of intravenous beta-2 agonist treatment on clinical outcomes in acute respiratory distress syndrome (Balti-2): a multicentre, randomised controlled trial. Lancet. 2012;379:229-35.
21. Thille AW, Cabello B, Galia F, Lyazidi A, Brochard L. Reduction of patient-ventilator asynchrony by reducing tidal volume during pressure-support ventilation. Intensive Care Med. 2008;34:1477-86.
22. Son YG, Shin J, Ryu HG. Pneumonitis and pneumonia after aspiration. J Dent Anesth Pain Med. 2017; 17(1):1-12.
23. Raghavendran K, Nemzek J, Napolitano LM, Knight PR. Aspiration-induced lung injury. Crit Care Med. 2011;39:818.
24. Ramadori GP. Organophosphorus poisoning: acute respiratory distress syndrome (ARDS) and cardiac failure as cause of death in hospitalized patients. Int J Mol Sci. 2023;24(7):6658.
25. Rzasa Lynn R, Galinkin JL. Naloxone dosage for opioid reversal: current evidence and clinical implications. Ther Adv Drug Saf. 2018;9(1):63-88.
26. Eichhorn L, Thudium M, Jüttner B. The diagnosis and treatment of carbon monoxide poisoning. Dtsch Arztebl Int. 2018;115(51-52):863-70.

1.4 Circulation in Poisoning

Naman Agrawal, Karthikeyan A, Nayer Jamshed

INTRODUCTION

The circulatory system, comprising the cardiovascular and lymphatic systems, constitutes a sophisticated anatomical and physiological framework responsible for the orchestrated transport of oxygen, nutrients, and metabolic by-products. Poisons and toxins can cause disruption in the circulatory homeostasis and early recognition of a poison's circulatory impact is crucial, given that these disturbances may rapidly result in hemodynamic instability, shock, and multiorgan dysfunction.[1] A structured approach is essential to tailor interventions to the specific toxicological insult and the individual patient's hemodynamic profile.

India, with its diverse population, poses unique challenges in the management of critically sick poisoned patients. Factors such as availability of poisons over the counter, varied toxic exposures, resource limitations, and sociocultural influences necessitate a tailored approach. Acknowledging these challenges is vital for developing effective strategies to optimize circulatory support in poisoned patients in the Indian healthcare setting.

NORMAL CIRCULATION

Cardiac Cycle

The cardiac cycle, a rhythmic sequence, commences with atrial contraction, initiating ventricular filling, succeeded by ventricular contraction propelling blood into circulations. Diastole, the relaxation phase, allows ventricular filling, creating a cyclic repetition of events.[2]

The cardiac impulse, originating in the sinoatrial (SA) node, coordinates the cycle. Sodium ions (Na^+) move through funny channels, establishing a pacemaker potential. Calcium ion (Ca^{2+}) influx prompts depolarization, modulated by autonomic stimulation. Repolarization involves potassium efflux. The atrioventricular (AV) node introduces a controlled delay, and the bundle of His and Purkinje fibers transmit the impulse, ensuring ventricular contraction.[3]

The cardiac myocyte action potential consists of phases involving sodium and calcium movements, ensuring the heart's coordinated contraction and relaxation.[4] Excitation–contraction coupling involves L-type calcium channels, calcium-induced calcium release (CICR), and active calcium reuptake, ensuring effective cardiac muscle contractions.[5] Regulation of cardiac function involves inotropy, chronotropy, and factors affecting stroke volume (SV). Autonomic control, hormonal influence, and ion concentrations modulate inotropy and chronotropy. SV depends on preload, afterload, contractility, heart rate (HR), venous return, and ejection fraction, orchestrating optimal circulation and hemodynamic stability.[6]

Oxygen Delivery to Tissues

Tissue oxygen delivery is a dynamic process influenced by cardiac output, hemoglobin concentration (Hb), arterial oxygen saturation (SaO_2), and the efficiency of oxygen extraction. The equation for cardiac output is as follows: Cardiac output = heart rate (HR) × stroke volume (SV), highlighting the importance of HR and SV in determining the volume of oxygenated blood reaching tissues. Hb significantly impacts oxygen-carrying capacity, and the oxygen content (CaO_2) is calculated using the following equation: $CaO_2 = (Hb \times 1.34 \times SaO_2) + (0.003 \times PaO_2)$, where 1.34 is the oxygen-carrying capacity of hemoglobin, SaO_2 is arterial oxygen saturation, and PaO_2 is arterial oxygen partial pressure.[7]

Arterial oxygen saturation influences the oxygen-hemoglobin dissociation curve, impacting oxygen binding and release. Oxygen extraction ratio (O_2ER) is a critical factor, calculated as follows: $[(CaO_2 - CvO_2)/CaO_2] \times 100$, representing the proportion of oxygen delivered and utilized by tissues.[8]

Mechanisms of Circulatory Alterations in Poisoned Patients

See **Table 1**.

TABLE 1: Mechanisms of circulatory alterations in poisoned patients.

Mechanisms of circulatory alterations in poisoned patients	***Specific toxins and effects***
Myocardial toxicity	
Direct cardiotoxic agents	*Digitalis (e.g., foxglove):* Increased intracellular calcium, arrhythmias, impaired contractility
Ischemic injury	*Cocaine:* Coronary vasospasm, elevated risk of myocardial infarction
Arrhythmogenic effects	• *Certain antiarrhythmics:* Disruption of normal cardiac conduction system, potentially fatal arrhythmia • *Sympathomimetics (e.g., cocaine, amphetamines):* Precipitation of tachycardia due to sympathetic stimulation
Delayed effects	*Heavy metals and certain toxins:* Delayed cardiac effects, requiring prolonged monitoring and follow-up
Vascular effects	
Vasospasm	• *Ergot alkaloids:* Vasoconstriction, impaired tissue perfusion • *Sympathomimetics (e.g., cocaine):* Vasoconstriction, contributing to tissue ischemia and organ dysfunction
Vasodilation	• *Calcium channel blockers, beta-blockers:* Widespread vasodilation, drop in systemic vascular resistance • *Peripheral pooling of blood:* Exacerbates hypotension, necessitating aggressive interventions
Capillary leak syndrome	*Toxins and venoms:* Induce capillary leak syndrome, leading to fluid and protein extravasation, resulting in edema, hypovolemia, and compromised tissue perfusion
Coagulation abnormalities	*Warfarin, certain rodenticides:* Inhibit vitamin K–dependent clotting factors, increasing the risk of bleeding or thrombosis

CLINICAL EVALUATION OF CIRCULATION IN ACUTE CARE

Clinical assessment involves understanding the nature and dose of the poison, time since exposure, and any coingestions. Like any other critically sick patient in the emergency, poisoned patients must be evaluated in a structured template of primary survey (ABCDE approach). The assessment of circulatory status in critically ill poisoned patients is a cornerstone of emergency and critical care medicine.[9]

This includes vital signs, physical examination, and a focused bedside assessment by ultrasound and point-of-care testing (POCT) labs.

Heart Rate

Alterations in HR may be an early pointer to potential hemodynamic instability in poisoned patients. Tachycardia reflects sympathetic activation. However, bradycardia may also occur **(Table 2)**. Unstable tachyarrhythmias/bradyarrhythmias will require immediate stabilization. Serial monitoring of HR provides valuable insights into the evolving clinical course.

Blood Pressure

Hypotension is a red flag for circulatory compromise and may indicate severe poisoning. Elevated blood pressure (BP) may be observed **(Table 2)**. BP trends guide fluid resuscitation, vasopressor therapy, and antidote response, when administered.

Respiratory Rate

Respiratory compromise may occur due to direct respiratory depressant effects or secondary to cardiovascular collapse. Tachypnea may result from acid-base

TABLE 2: Change in ABG parameters and their significance.

ABG parameter	Significance
Anion gap calculation	Elevated anion gap points toward specific toxins (MUDPILES)
Lactate levels	Monitoring aids in assessing shock severity and guiding resuscitation; elevated levels suggest certain toxins (e.g., cyanide, CO poisoning)
Pattern recognition	Identifying acid–base patterns inform about underlying toxins (e.g., respiratory alkalosis and metabolic acidosis in salicylate toxicity)
Other pearls and pitfalls	• Tricyclic antidepressants have increased toxicity in acidic milieu and hence acidosis must be aggressively treated • Patients with severe metabolic acidosis may land into peri-intubation cardiac arrest if minute ventilation is not maintained after paralysis

(ABG: arterial blood gas; CO: carbon monoxide)

disturbances or hypoxia, underscoring the need for respiratory support.

Temperature

Hyperthermia or hypothermia may accompany certain poisonings, influencing metabolic demands and exacerbating cardiovascular instability **(Table 2)**.

Oxygen Saturation

Continuous monitoring of oxygen saturation (SpO_2) is essential, particularly in cases where respiratory compromise is anticipated. It guides the need for supplemental oxygen and provides insights into the adequacy of tissue oxygenation.

Capillary Refill Time

Prolonged capillary refill time (CRT) is indicative of impaired peripheral perfusion. This simple yet informative bedside test aids in assessing the adequacy of cardiac output and vascular tone.

Skin and Mucous Membranes

Evaluation of skin color, temperature, and moisture provides insights into perfusion status and type of poison. Sympathomimetic and cholinergic toxidromes manifest as sweaty skin, whereas anticholinergic agents lead to dry and flushed skin. Cyanosis, mottling, or cool extremities may indicate compromised tissue perfusion.

Point-of-Care Ultrasound

Point-of-care ultrasound (POCUS) is a pivotal tool in rapidly assessing the cause of shock at the patient's bedside.[10-13]

Point-of-care ultrasound facilitates the identification of hypovolemia by assessing the inferior vena cava, detects pericardial effusion, and evaluates cardiac chambers and valves. Additionally, it assesses pulmonary causes, identifies deep venous thrombosis, and performs focused abdominal assessments.[14]

Various well-established ultrasound protocols like RUSH (Rapid Ultrasound in Shock and Hypotension) and FALLS (Fluid Administration Limited by Lung Sonography) may be leveraged for assessment and emergency management of poisoned patients who are in shock.[15-17]

Point-of-care ultrasound also aids in monitoring fluid responsiveness, guiding procedural interventions, and providing real-time insights for intervention assessment. However, its effective use requires clinician expertise and integration with clinical context for accurate shock diagnosis and management.[18]

ACID–BASE ALTERATIONS

Poisoned patients presenting with shock often exhibit complex acid–base disturbances, providing valuable insights into the underlying poison and guiding resuscitation strategies.[19-23]

ELECTROCARDIOGRAM CHANGES

Electrocardiogram (ECG) changes in poisoned patients can provide critical insights into the toxic effects on the cardiovascular system. These alterations may range from mild abnormalities to life-threatening arrhythmias. Understanding the mechanisms behind these ECG changes is crucial for prompt recognition and appropriate management. **Table 3** mentions the various ECG changes in poisoned patients.[24-26]

PRINCIPLES OF RESUSCITATION IN ACUTELY POISONED PATIENTS

The overall schematic for the circulatory resuscitation in poisoned patients is shown in **Flowchart 1**.

Fluids

Fluids have conventionally been the first treatment of choice for the management of shock. There is no high-quality evidence to guide the fluid therapy in toxin-related shock. Evidence from Surviving Sepsis Campaign guidelines of 2021 for patients with septic shock suggests the use of 30-mL/kg intravenous bolus.[27]

TABLE 3: Important ECG changes in poisoning.

ECG change	*Mechanism*	*Examples of toxins*
QT prolongation	• Inhibition of cardiac repolarization (K^+ blockade) • Risk of TdP	• Antiarrhythmics (quinidine) • Antibiotics (macrolides) • Tricyclic antidepressants
Bradyarrhythmias	Blockade of the cardiac conduction system	• Beta-blockers • Calcium channel blockers • Digoxin
Tachyarrhythmias	Increased sympathetic stimulation	• Cocaine • Amphetamines • Theophylline
• QRS widening • Right-axis deviation • Tachyarrhythmias	Sodium channel blockade	• Tricyclic antidepressants • Carbamazepine • Antiarrhythmics • Cocaine • Insecticides
ST-segment changes	Induction of ischemic or nonischemic conditions affecting myocardium	• Cocaine • Digitalis toxicity
Osborn (J) waves	Hypothermia, hypercalcemia	Sedatives, alcohols

(ECG: electrocardiogram; TdP: torsades de pointes)

This recommendation of 30-mL/kg fluids is based on PROCESS, PROMISE, and ARISE trials, which used the 30-mL/kg fluids for resuscitation.[28-30]

Our primary goals are to increase the preload to the heart, increase the ventricular filling, and improve the tissue perfusion. Aggressive fluid resuscitation may result in an increased risk of pulmonary edema and poor outcomes.[31,32] Using pulse index continuous cardiac output (PiCCO)-based fluid resuscitation does not improve outcomes as compared with central venous pressure–based management of sepsis and patients with septic shock with fluid resuscitation.[33] Thus, we recommend giving fluid boluses and continuous assessment of multiple end points of tissue perfusion and POCUS guidance. The choice of intravenous fluids has been a matter of debate for decades. In general, crystalloids are favored over colloids based on the literature from other patient populations. There is some evidence to favor balanced salt solution over normal saline;[34,35] however, some evidence suggests no such benefit.[36]

Antidotes

Most poisoned patients will require supportive management with fluids, vasopressors, etc. However, some poisons respond promptly to the administration of their antidotes. These agents (remembered as ABCDEN) must be readily available to the treating physician if the clinical condition demands **(Table 4)**.

Vasopressors

Vasopressors are useful for patients who have persistent shock after fluid resuscitation, or those patients who are not hypovolemic. The usual initial vasopressor of choice

Flowchart 1: Management approach to circulatory shock in poisoned patients.

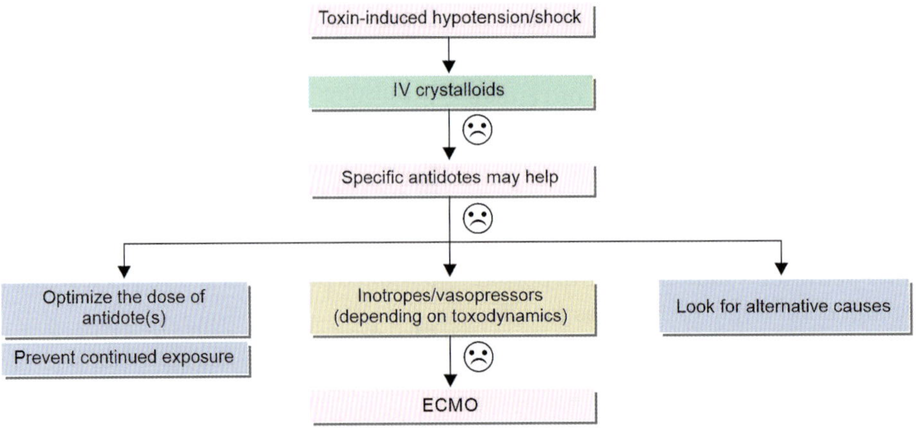

(ECMO: extracorporeal membrane oxygenation; IV: intraventricular)

TABLE 4: Specific antidotes in poisoning.

Resuscitation antidotes	*Useful in poisoning of*
Atropine	• Organophosphates • Beta-blocker, calcium channel blocker overdose
Antivenom (polyvalent)	Hemotoxic/vasculotoxic snake bite
Bicarbonate	Sodium channel blocking agents (tricyclic antidepressants, carbamazepine, etc.)
Calcium gluconate	• Life-threatening hyperkalemia • Hydrofluoric acid
Cyanide kit	Cyanide poisoning
DigiFab	• Digoxin overdose • Oleander poisoning
Dextrose	Hypoglycemic agents (insulin, sulfonylureas, valproate, salicylates, etc.)
Emulsion (intralipids)	Local anesthetic systemic toxicity (LAST)
Naloxone	Opioid overdose

is norepinephrine (0.1–2 μg/kg/min), epinephrine (2–10 μg/min) being the second-line vasopressor. Dopamine is out of favor as a preliminary choice of vasopressor as it has no role in renal protection and has an increased risk of tachyarrhythmias.[27] Dobutamine can be used where there is myocardial dysfunction, or low cardiac output despite fluid therapy. The evidence for the use of vasopressors is extrapolated from patients with septic shock as the data on poisoned patients are lacking. Phenylephrine is usually not used due to a greater risk of reduced cardiac output and reduced tissue perfusion.[37]

The role of inodilators like milrinone in patients with cardiac failure due to toxicological causes is weak and has no robust evidence.[38] Levosimendan is a calcium channel sensitizer with additional phosphodiesterase 3 (PDE3) inhibitory properties; its use in calcium channel blocker toxicity with circulatory failure is supported by case reports but robust evidence is lacking.[39] Similarly, the role of methylene blue in calcium channel blocker toxicity is supported by a few case reports of improving the mean arterial pressure when given along with conventional therapies and vasopressors.

There are data available that favor the use of high-dose insulin dextrose therapy (1–10 U/kg/h) doses in beta-blockers, and calcium channel blocker toxicities.[40-42] Insulin is an ionotropic agent and is a potent vasodilator, thereby reducing systemic vascular resistance and increasing the cardiac output in poisoned patients.

Extracorporeal Interventions

There is building evidence that poisoned patients with refractory shock managed on venoarterial (VA) extracorporeal membrane oxygenator have a lower mortality compared with patients managed on antidotal therapy and supportive medication because the multiorgan dysfunction is prevented in the extracorporeal membrane oxygenation (ECMO) subset and the kidneys and liver recover over time to flush the toxins out of the system.[43] So VA-ECMO may be used in patients with refractory shock and refractory dysrhythmias leading to cardiovascular collapse in poisoned patients.

MONITORING THE ACUTELY ILL POISONED PATIENT

The resuscitation must continue till the microcirculatory end points are reached. **Table 5** includes common clinical monitoring parameters to be considered. However, the monitoring must be individualized to the patient's clinical condition. End points of resuscitation are mentioned in **Table 6**.

COMMON CAUSES OF HEMODYNAMIC COLLAPSE IN TOXICOLOGY

Calcium Channel Blockers

Calcium channel blockers are a leading cause of mortality in poisoning patients.[44] There are two major types of calcium channel blockers—the dihydropyridines (DHPs) and non-DHPs. These act on the slow voltage-gated L-type calcium channels; however, at supratherapeutic doses, the difference of action between the non-DHP and DHP varieties is not maintained. Sinus bradycardia is the common presentation of calcium channel blocker toxicity, although all types of heart blocks can occur with no particular pattern or predilection. Calcium channel blockade can also lead to sodium channel blockade leading to a delay in phase 0 depolarization, resulting in rhythms like ventricular premature contractions and sometimes asystole.[24] Class 1 recommendation is to start vasopressors in conjunction with high-dose insulin therapy. Administering calcium is a class 2a recommendation and VA-ECMO is a class 2a recommendation. The role of intravenous lipid emulsion is placed at class 3 recommendation with no role in the management of calcium channel blocker toxicity.[45]

TABLE 5: Clinical monitoring parameters in poisoned patients.

Parameters	*Monitoring strategy*	*Clinical significance*
Vital signs	Continuous monitoring of BP, HR, and RR	Early indicators of shock, guide fluid resuscitation
Continuous cardiac monitoring	Continuous ECG monitoring	Detects arrhythmias, guides targeted interventions
Hemodynamic monitoring	CVP monitoring, arterial catheterization	Provides insights into intravascular volume status, guides vasopressor use
Oxygenation and ventilation	Pulse oximetry, end-tidal CO_2 monitoring	Assess oxygenation status, detect changes in respiratory status
Temperature monitoring	Continuous temperature monitoring	Identifies hyperthermia or hypothermia
Neurological monitoring	GCS	Evaluates neurological status, detects changes in mental status
Blood gases	Serial blood gas analysis, lactate levels	Provides insights into acid–base status, assesses tissue perfusion
Fluid balance and urine output	Hourly urine output monitoring, fluid input and output monitoring	Assesses renal perfusion, prevents fluid overload
Clinical assessment	Serial clinical examination	Detects subtle changes indicative of ongoing shock

(BP: blood pressure; CVP: central venous pressure; ECG: electrocardiogram; GCS: Glasgow Coma Scale; HR: heart rate; RR: respiratory rate)

TABLE 6: End points of resuscitation in poisoned patients.

Category	*Parameter*	*End points*
Peripheral perfusion	• Capillary refill time • Skin mottling • Peripheral temperature	• <3 seconds • Absent • Warm
Venous oxygen saturation	• Central • Mixed	• ≥65–70% • ≥60–65%
Lactate	• Absolute value • Lactate clearance	• <2 mmol/L • >2 mmol/h
Urine output		>0.5 mL/kg/h

Cocaine Toxicity

It produces a sympathomimetic syndrome because of the effect cocaine has on multiple channels across the spectrum. Tachycardia is because by postsynaptic beta-receptor agonism with hypertension due to postsynaptic alpha-adrenergic agonism, it blocks the reuptake of norepinephrine and serotonin in the central nervous system (CNS) leading to neuropsychiatric manifestation.[46,47] Cocaine blocks sodium channel receptors leading to the prolongation of phase 0 of the cardiac cycle increasing the risk of wide complex tachycardias; the potassium efflux blockade leads to QT prolongation. Class 1 recommendation is to start external cooling if there is hyperthermia; class 2a recommendations are to give sodium bicarbonate if there are wide complex tachycardias and also lidocaine. Given the vasospasm and hypertensive emergency it produces, calcium channel blockers and nitrates are class 2a recommendations. Beta-blockers are not recommended.[45]

Sympathomimetic Toxicity

Sympathomimetics result in tachycardia, hypertension, agitation, seizures, hyperpyrexia, rhabdomyolysis, and acidosis.[48,49] Cardiac rhythm anomalies like ventricular tachycardia, fibrillation, pulseless electrical activity,[49,50] or myocardial infarction with normal coronaries can occur; takotsubo cardiomyopathy is a dreaded complication, although it resolves spontaneously within weeks and requires supportive circulatory care.[51]

Class 1 recommendation is controlling agitation and external cooling in cases of hyperthermia.[45]

Organophosphate and Carbamate Toxicity

In organophosphate and carbamate (OPC) poisoning, class 1[45] recommendation will be early administration of atropine at doses of 1–2 mg intravenous dose with doubling the dose every 5 minutes and, once atropinization is reached, then starting 10–20% of the atropinization dose as infusion till 48 hours of symptom resolution.[52] Early use of atropine is indicated in suspected OPC poisoning leading to bronchorrhea, bradycardia, cardiac arrest, and bronchospasm. Atropinization is defined by a clear chest on auscultation, a HR greater than 80, and systolic BP greater than 80 mm Hg.

Sodium Channel Blocker Toxicity

These agents cause prolongation of phase 0 of the cardiac cycle leading to QRS prolongation, ventricular arrhythmias, and, in extreme poisoning, sine wave and asystole. The patient is also prone to developing ventricular arrhythmias due to intraventricular conduction delays and conduction blocks. Bradyarrhythmias are not common but are possible due to their effects on the pacemaker cells. Intraventricular conduction delays with a right-terminal R deviation in aVR lead are characteristic ECG changes in tricyclic antidepressant (TCA) toxicity **Figure 1**.[53] The class 1 indication would be using sodium bicarbonate at a dose of 100–150 mEq bolus followed by infusions at 1–3 mL/kg/h of 150 mEq/L sodium bicarbonate solutions. Management is continued till hypotension improves and the dysrhythmia ceases. pH should be maintained between 7.50 and 7.55, and serum sodium between 150 and 155 mEq/L. Lidocaine as a class 2 recommendation for ventricular dysrhythmia is recommended. VA-ECMO can be tried if there is refractory cardiogenic shock despite the best medical management.[45] The role of lipid emulsions is questionable and is suggested if all treatment modalities fail.

Cardiac Glycosides

Cardiac glycosides include a variety of compounds like digoxin, digitoxin, yellow oleander, and toad toxins. They are versatile in causing any type of dysrhythmia. Digitalis effect is a flattened T wave with a scooped ST-segment depression. The toxic effects of digitalis are because of increased automaticity with prolonged AV conduction. Premature ventricular contractions are very commonly found in digitalis toxicity.[24] Apart from that, AV blocks, tachyarrhythmias like paroxysmal atrial tachycardia with associated AV blocks, accelerated junction tachycardia, or atrial fibrillation with a slow ventricular rate are characteristic ECG findings of cardiac glycoside toxicity. Class 1 recommendation is using digoxin fab to reverse the effects of the offending agent **(Fig. 2)**. Class 2 recommendations advise using digoxin fab to treat yellow oleander toxicity **(Fig. 3)**. Extracorporeal hemoperfusion hemodialysis or plasmapheresis is designated as having no role in the management of the above-mentioned poisoning.[45]

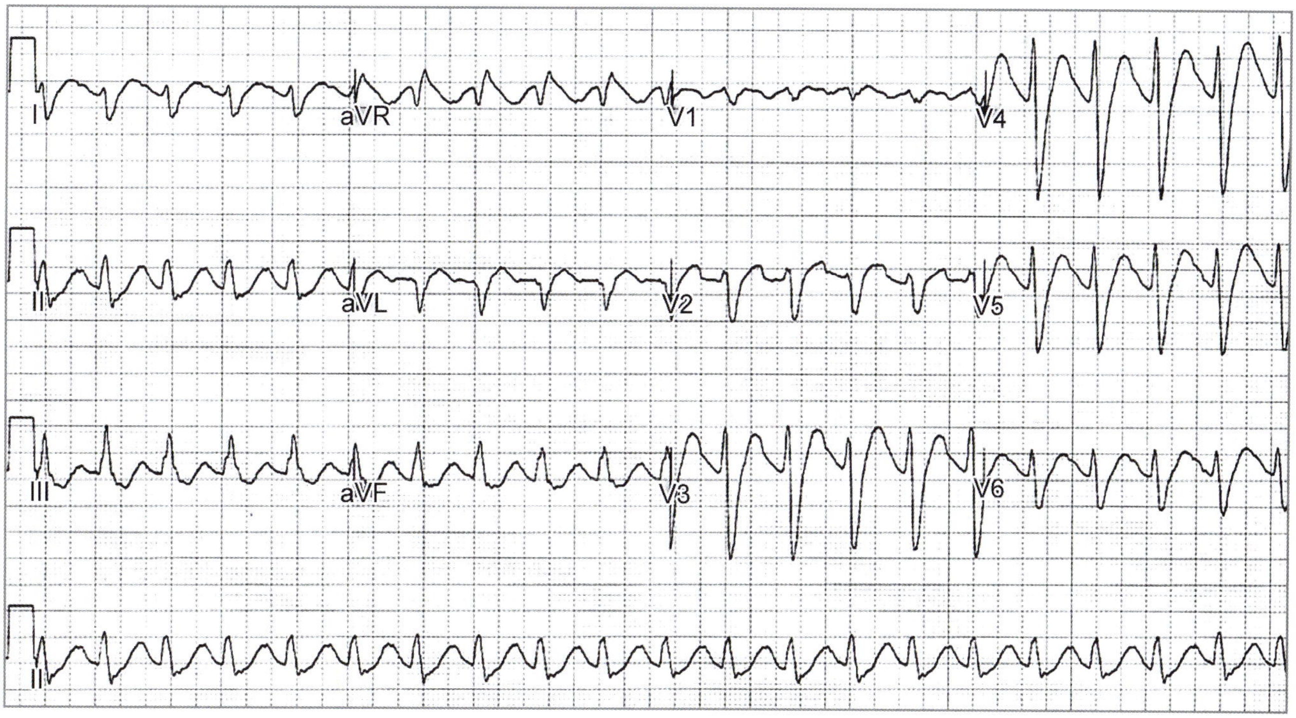

Fig. 1: TCA overdose. (TCA: tricyclic antidepressant)

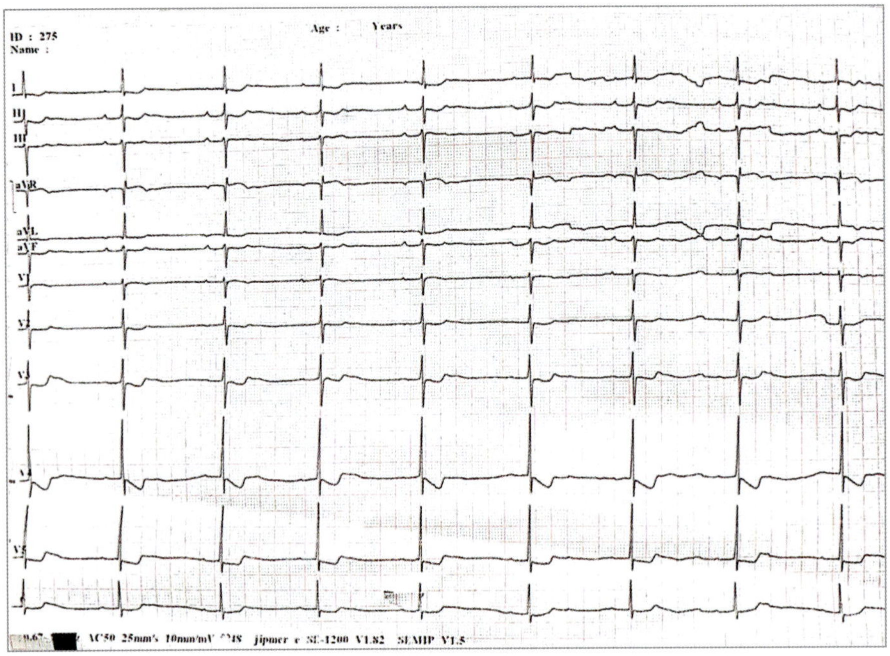

Fig. 2: Reverse tick digoxin effect.

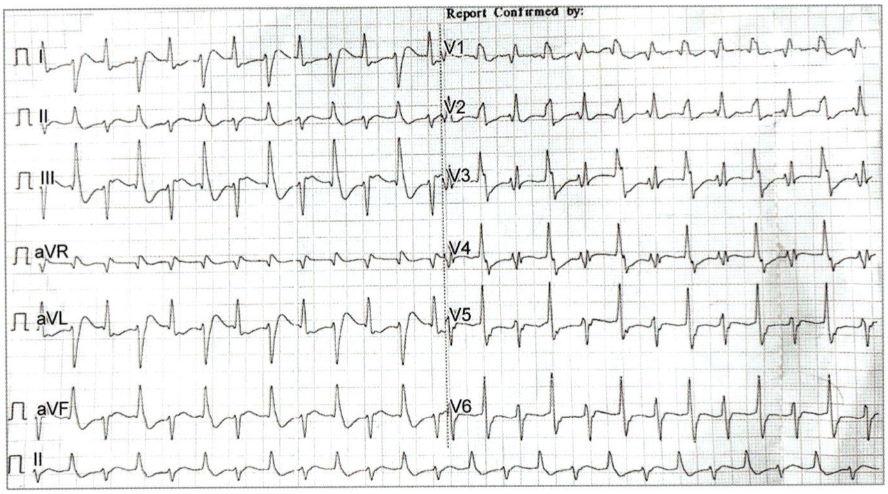

Fig. 3: Bidirectional VT of digoxin toxicity. (VT: ventricular tachycardia)

Local Anesthetic Systemic Toxicity

In local anesthetic systemic toxicity, we get CNS effects in 77–89% cases while (32–55%) will have cardiovascular symptoms. Bupivacaine is the most cardiotoxic local anesthetic because of its predilection to affect the cardiac calcium channels leading to conduction delays and reentry arrhythmias like ventricular fibrillation.[54] Acidemia and hypoxia lead to a worsening of the toxicity of local anesthetics.[55] Bradycardia is the first sign that the local anesthetic toxicity will lead to cardiovascular compromise. Class 1 recommendation is to use in vascular lipid emulsions of 20% at the dose of 1.5 mL/kg and then an infusion of 0.25 mL/kg/min for 30 minutes. Class 2 recommendations include using sodium bicarbonate for broad complex tachycardias and atropine for bradycardias. Avoidance of acidemia and hypoxia also precedes this step, with the American Heart Association (AHA) advising to use benzodiazepines to control seizures as a class 1 indication.[45]

Cyanide Toxicity

Cyanide is another mitochondrial toxin we need to keep in mind when dealing with cases that present with unexplained acidosis, cardiovascular collapse, and lactatemia. It is an obscure diagnosis.[56,57] Class 1 indication is the administration of hydroxocobalamin 5 g intravenous stat. Sodium nitrate is also a class 1 indication but the complications of methemoglobinemia have to be kept in mind during sodium nitrate administration.[45]

Beta-blocker Toxicity

Beta-blocker toxicity is a common cause of mortality in toxicology.[24] Patients can present with hypotension, bradycardia, and cardiovascular collapse. The AHA recommends the use of high-dose insulin therapy as a class 1 indication of hypotension along with vasopressor support. Glucagon is recommended as a class 2 recommendation for bradycardia management in this subset with no role for intravenous lipid emulsion.[45]

CONCLUSION

- Any discrepancies in paired occurrences, orthostatic hypotension, sudden onset of hypotension or hypertension, and suspicion of a toxin affecting the circulation should be thought of.
- ECGs are primordial in evaluating any case of poisoning.
- Preload augmentation and initiation of vasopressors are advised but early initiation of specific antidotal agents or high-dose insulin therapy is recommended at the earliest for better outcomes and to reduce the need for vasopressor support.
- Increasing evidence and recommendation for the use of extracorporeal systems in cases of refractory cardiogenic shock after maximal medical management.
- Tissue perfusion-based end points for resuscitation seem to be better and easier in continuous monitoring and also give a physiological basis for monitoring of the resuscitative efforts in circulatory failure.

REFERENCES

1. Singh O, Deepak D. Poisoning induced circulatory failure. Principles and Practice of Critical Care Toxicology. New Delhi: Jaypee Brothers Medical Publishers; 2019. p. 167.
2. Luisada AA, MacCanon DM. The phases of the cardiac cycle. Am Heart J. 1972;83(5):705-11.
3. Iaizzo PA, Laske TG. Anatomy and physiology of the cardiac conduction system. Cardiac Electrophysiology Methods and Models. New York: Springer-Verlag; 2010. pp. 73-89.
4. Walker CA, Spinale FG. The structure and function of the cardiac myocyte: a review of fundamental concepts. J Thorac Cardiovasc Surg. 1999;118(2):375-82.
5. Stern MD. Theory of excitation-contraction coupling in cardiac muscle. Biophys J. 1992;63(2):497-517.
6. Stergiopulos NI, Meister JJ, Westerhof NI. Determinants of stroke volume and systolic and diastolic aortic pressure. Am J Physiol Heart Circ Physiol. 1996;270(6): H2050-9.
7. Morisaki H, Sibbald WJ. Tissue oxygen delivery and the microcirculation. Crit Care Clin. 2004;20(2):213-23.
8. Vincent JL. Determination of oxygen delivery and consumption versus cardiac index and oxygen extraction ratio. Crit Care Clin. 1996;12(4):995-1006.
9. McGrath A, Cox CL. Cardiac and circulatory assessment in intensive care units. Intensive Crit Care Nurs. 1998;14(6):283-7.
10. Jones AE, Tayal VS, Sullivan DM, Kline JA. Randomized, controlled trial of immediate versus delayed goal-directed ultrasound to identify the cause of nontraumatic hypotension in emergency department patients. Crit Care Med. 2004;32(8):1703-8.
11. Volpicelli G, Lamorte A, Tullio M, Cardinale L, Giraudo M, Stefanone V, et al. Point-of-care multiorgan ultrasonography for the evaluation of undifferentiated hypotension in the emergency department. Intensive Care Med. 2013;39:1290-8.
12. Boyd JH, Sirounis D, Maizel J, Slama M. Echocardiography as a guide for fluid management. Crit Care. 2016;20:1-7.
13. Shokoohi H, Boniface KS, Pourmand A, Liu YT, Davison DL, Hawkins KD, et al. Bedside ultrasound reduces diagnostic uncertainty and guides resuscitation in patients with undifferentiated hypotension. Crit Care Med. 2015;43(12):2562-9.
14. Sasmaz MI, Gungor F, Guven R, Akyol K, Kozaci N, Kesapli M. Effect of focused bedside ultrasonography in hypotensive patients on the clinical decision of emergency physicians. Emerg Med Int. 2017;2017:6248687.
15. Keikha M, Salehi-Marzijarani M, Nejat RS, Vahedi HS, Mirrezaie SM. Diagnostic accuracy of rapid ultrasound in shock (RUSH) exam; a systematic review and meta-analysis. Bull Emerg Trauma. 2018;6(4):271.
16. Lichtenstein D. FALLS-protocol: lung ultrasound in hemodynamic assessment of shock. Heart Lung Vessels. 2013;5(3):142.
17. Lichtenstein D. Fluid administration limited by lung sonography: the place of lung ultrasound in assessment of acute circulatory failure (the FALLS-protocol). Expert Rev Respir Med. 2012;6(2):155-62.
18. Lewis D, Rang L, Kim D, Robichaud L, Kwan C, Pham C, et al. Recommendations for the use of point-of-care ultrasound (POCUS) by emergency physicians in Canada. Can J Emerg Med. 2019;21(6):721-6.
19. Hamdi H, Hassanian-Moghaddam H, Hamdi A, Zahed NS. Acid-base disturbances in acute poisoning and their association with survival. J Crit Care. 2016;35:84-9.
20. Jones A. Metabolic effects of poisoning. Medicine. 2012;40(2):55-8.

21. Liu JH, Chou CY, Liu YL, Liao PY, Lin PW, Lin HH, et al. Acid-base interpretation can be the predictor of outcome among patients with acute organophosphate poisoning before hospitalization. Am J Emerg Med. 2008;26(1):24-30.
22. Bernal W, Donaldson N, Wyncoll D, Wendon J. Blood lactate as an early predictor of outcome in paracetamol-induced acute liver failure: a cohort study. Lancet. 2002;359(9306):558-63.
23. Gabow PA, Anderson RJ, Potts DE, Schrier RW. Acid-base disturbances in the salicylate-intoxicated adult. Arch Intern Med. 1978;138(10):1481-4.
24. Delk C, Holstege CP, Brady WJ. Electrocardiographic abnormalities associated with poisoning. Am J Emerg Med. 2007;25(6):672-87.
25. Holstege CP, Eldridge DL, Rowden AK. ECG manifestations: the poisoned patient. Emerg Med Clin. 2006;24(1):159-77.
26. Skolnik A, Monas J. The crashing toxicology patient. Emerg Med Clin. 2020;38(4):841-56.
27. Dellinger RP, Levy MM, Rhodes A, Annane D, Gerlach H, Opal SM, et al. Surviving Sepsis Campaign: international guidelines for management of severe sepsis and septic shock: 2012. Crit Care Med. 2013;41(2):580-637.
28. ProCESS Investigators, Yealy DM, Kellum JA, Huang DT, Barnato AE, Weissfeld LA, et al. A randomized trial of protocol-based care for early septic shock. N Engl J Med. 2014;370(18):1683-93.
29. ARISE Investigators, ANZICS Clinical Trials Group, Peake SL, Delaney A, Bailey M, Bellomo R, et al. Goal-directed resuscitation for patients with early septic shock. N Engl J Med. 2014;371(16):1496-506.
30. Mouncey PR, Osborn TM, Power GS, Harrison DA, Sadique MZ, Grieve RD, et al. Trial of early, goal-directed resuscitation for septic shock. N Engl J Med. 2015;372(14):1301-11.
31. Jozwiak M, Silva S, Persichini R, Anguel N, Osman D, Richard C, et al. Extravascular lung water is an independent prognostic factor in patients with acute respiratory distress syndrome. Crit Care Med. 2013;41(2):472-80.
32. Zhang Z, Lu B, Ni H. Prognostic value of extravascular lung water index in critically ill patients: a systematic review of the literature. J Crit Care. 2012;27(4):420.e1-8.
33. Zhang Z, Ni H, Qian Z. Effectiveness of treatment based on PiCCO parameters in critically ill patients with septic shock and/or acute respiratory distress syndrome: a randomized controlled trial. Intensive Care Med. 2015;41(3):444-51.
34. Semler MW, Self WH, Wanderer JP, Ehrenfeld JM, Wang L, Byrne DW, et al. Balanced crystalloids versus saline in critically ill adults. N Engl J Med. 2018;378(9):829-39.
35. Self WH, Semler MW, Wanderer JP, Wang L, Byrne DW, Collins SP, et al. Balanced crystalloids versus saline in noncritically ill adults. N Engl J Med. 2018;378(9):819-28.
36. Young P, Bailey M, Beasley R, Henderson S, Mackle D, McArthur C, et al. Effect of a buffered crystalloid solution vs saline on acute kidney injury among patients in the intensive care unit: the SPLIT Randomized Clinical Trial. JAMA. 2015;314(16):1701-10.
37. Vincent JL, De Backer D. Circulatory shock. N Engl J Med. 2013;369(18):1726-34.
38. Unverzagt S, Wachsmuth L, Hirsch K, Thiele H, Buerke M, Haerting J, et al. Inotropic agents and vasodilator strategies for acute myocardial infarction complicated by cardiogenic shock or low cardiac output syndrome. Cochrane Database Syst Rev. 2014;(1):CD009669.
39. Varpula T, Rapola J, Sallisalmi M, Kurola J. Treatment of serious calcium channel blocker overdose with levosimendan, a calcium sensitizer. Anesth Analg. 2009;108(3):790-2.
40. Holger JS, Engebretsen KM, Marini JJ. High dose insulin in toxic cardiogenic shock. Clin Toxicol (Phila). 2009;47(4):303-7.
41. Shepherd G, Klein-Schwartz W. High-dose insulin therapy for calcium-channel blocker overdose. Ann Pharmacother. 2005;39(5):923-30.
42. Greene SL, Gawarammana I, Wood DM, Jones AL, Dargan PI. Relative safety of hyperinsulinaemia/euglycaemia therapy in the management of calcium channel blocker overdose: a prospective observational study. Intensive Care Med. 2007;33(11):2019-24.
43. Masson R, Colas V, Parienti JJ, Lehoux P, Massetti M, Charbonneau P, et al. A comparison of survival with and without extracorporeal life support treatment for severe poisoning due to drug intoxication. Resuscitation. 2012;83(11):1413-7.
44. Gummin DD, Mowry JB, Beuhler MC, Spyker DA, Bronstein AC, Rivers LJ, et al. 2020 annual report of the American Association of Poison Control Centers' National Poison Data System (NPDS): 38th annual report. Clin Toxicol (Phila). 2021;59(12):1282-501.
45. Lavonas EJ, Akpunonu PD, Arens AM, Babu KM, Cao D, Hoffman RS, et al. 2023 American Heart Association focused update on the management of patients with cardiac arrest or life-threatening toxicity due to poisoning: an update to the American Heart Association guidelines for cardiopulmonary resuscitation and emergency cardiovascular care. Circulation. 2023;148(16):e149-84.
46. Pergolizzi JV, Magnusson P, LeQuang JAK, Breve F, Varrassi G. Cocaine and cardiotoxicity: a literature review. Cureus. 2021;13(4):e14594.
47. O'Leary ME, Hancox JC. Role of voltage-gated sodium, potassium and calcium channels in the development of cocaine-associated cardiac arrhythmias. Br J Clin Pharmacol. 2010;69(5):427-42.
48. Potocka-Banaś B, Janus T, Majdanik S, Banaś T, Dembińska T, Borowiak K. Fatal intoxication with α-PVP, a synthetic cathinone derivative. J Forensic Sci. 2017;62(2):553-6.
49. Bosak A, LoVecchio F, Levine M. Recurrent seizures and serotonin syndrome following "2C-I" ingestion. J Med Toxicol. 2013;9(2):196-8.

50. Packe GE, Garton MJ, Jennings K. Acute myocardial infarction caused by intravenous amphetamine abuse. Br Heart J. 1990;64(1):23-4.
51. Chen JP. Methamphetamine-associated acute myocardial infarction and cardiogenic shock with normal coronary arteries: refractory global coronary microvascular spasm. J Invasive Cardiol. 2007;19(4):E89-92.
52. Abedin MJ, Sayeed AA, Basher A, Maude RJ, Hoque G, Faiz MA. Open-label randomized clinical trial of atropine bolus injection versus incremental boluses plus infusion for organophosphate poisoning in Bangladesh. J Med Toxicol. 2012;8(2):108-17.
53. Bruccoleri RE, Burns MM. A literature review of the use of sodium bicarbonate for the treatment of QRS widening. J Med Toxicol. 2016;12(1):121-9.
54. Gitman M, Barrington MJ. Local anesthetic systemic toxicity: a review of recent case reports and registries. Reg Anesth Pain Med. 2018;43(2):124-30.
55. Gosselin S, Hoegberg LCG, Hoffman RS, Graudins A, Stork CM, Thomas SHL, et al. Evidence-based recommendations on the use of intravenous lipid emulsion therapy in poisoning. Clin Toxicol (Phila). 2016;54(10): 899-923.
56. Baud FJ, Barriot P, Toffis V, Riou B, Vicaut E, Lecarpentier Y, et al. Elevated blood cyanide concentrations in victims of smoke inhalation. N Engl J Med. 1991;325(25):1761-6.
57. Petrikovics I, Budai M, Kovacs K, Thompson DE. Past, present and future of cyanide antagonism research: from the early remedies to the current therapies. World J Methodol. 2015;5(2):88-100.

1.5 Disability Assessment in a Critically Ill Poisoned Patient

Manoj Goyal, Ritushree, Kathik, Ashish Bhalla

INTRODUCTION

Management of a patient with impaired consciousness (i.e., brain failure) represents one of the most challenging clinical scenarios and demands an urgent remedial action, more so as alteration of sensorium often indicates impending irreversible brain damage. Intoxication with drugs accounts for approximately one third of all patients presenting with coma to the emergency department.[1]

INITIAL RESUSCITATION

The first step in management of any critically ill poisoned patient (as is true for any patient presenting with altered sensorium irrespective of etiology) is quick assessment along with maintenance of airway, breathing, and circulation.[2] In any patient with stupor or coma, intubation is necessary to protect airway and prevent aspiration. Many drugs/poisons reduce ventilatory drive per se, resulting in CO_2 narcosis, further depressing the central nervous system (CNS). Often, patients in the emergency department are placed on high-flow oxygen therapy, resulting in adequate oxygen saturation values despite poor ventilatory drive. Thus, wherever possible, arterial blood gas measurement should be included as standard of care for management of patients with altered sensorium.

For maintenance of circulation, all patients with drug-induced coma and hypotension shall have two intravenous lines: One large-bore peripheral intravenous catheter and second intravenous line placed in either the peripheral or the central circulation.[3] For a poisoned patient, attention shall be given to specific poison while choosing the vasopressor agent if needed. Norepinephrine may be a better drug for hypotension secondary to poisoning.[3,4]

Many of the poisoned patients present with deep coma (opiates, sedative-hypnotics) and poor respiratory efforts. These patients need securing of the airway and ventilation as initial resuscitation. Seizures are common in organophosphate (OP) poisoning and opiate, sedative, and alcohol withdrawal and may be aborted. Benzodiazepines are the drug of choice for aborting and controlling toxic seizures.

ASSESSMENT AND DIFFERENTIAL DIAGNOSIS (TABLES 1 AND 2)

History

The first step in the evaluation of any patient with altered sensorium is to obtain good history. As most patients with altered sensorium cannot give history, it shall be obtained from relatives or friends. Whenever possible, try to obtain

TABLE 1: Common toxidrome in clinical practice.[5]

Class of drugs	*Examples*	*CNS features*
Anticholinergic drugs	Atropine, antispasmodics, antihistaminics, antiparkinsonian anticholinergic agents, phenothiazines, scopolamine, tricyclic antidepressants	Agitation, hallucinations, dilated pupils, abnormal movements—plucking at bedclothes
Cholinergic drugs	Cholinesterase inhibitors, insecticides—organophosphates and carbamate	Constricted pupils, urinary/fecal incontinence, weakness, muscle fasciculations, LMN paralysis, delayed neuropathy
Opioid drugs	Codeine, fentanyl, heroin, hydrocodone, hydromorphone, morphine, oxycodone, propoxyphene	CNS depression, coma, constricted pupils, hyporeflexia, seizures
Sedative–hypnotic drugs	Barbiturates, benzodiazepines, chloral hydrate, ethanol, ethchlorvynol, meprobamate, nonbenzodiazepine GABA agonists	CNS depression, hyporeflexia
Sympatho-mimetic drugs	Amphetamines, cocaine, ephedrine, phenylephrine, pseudoephedrine, psychostimulants	Agitation, paranoia, hallucinations, dilated pupils, piloerection
Neuroleptic drugs	Chlorpromazine, fluphenazine, haloperidol, olanzapine, perphenazine, prochlorperazine, promethazine, quetiapine	Oculogyric crisis, trismus, dystonia, ataxia, parkinsonism, neuroleptic malignant syndrome
Serotonergic drugs	Buspirone, dextromethorphan, fentanyl, monoamine oxidase inhibitors, selective serotonin reuptake inhibitors, tramadol, tricyclic antidepressants	Akathisia, tremor, agitation, central hyperthermia, hypertonia, hyperreflexia, clonus

(CNS: central nervous system; GABA: gamma-aminobutyric acid; LMN: lower motor neuron)

history from a person who lives with or is directly involved in caring for the sick patient. Enquire about the mode of onset (e.g., stroke—sudden onset; metabolic/toxic/infections—gradual onset) and associated symptoms (e.g., sudden thunderclap headache—subarachnoid hemorrhage; fever—neuroinfections; diplopia—brainstem lesion; hemiparesis—supratentorial lesion; seizures—encephalitis/supratentorial brain lesion). Obtain past history about diabetes, renal failure, and liver failure, and personal history about alcoholism, illicit drug use, etc. In the authors' experience, two questions which yield maximum information but are often enquired casually include:

1. When was the patient last well?
2. Does the patient have access to psychotropic drugs or insecticides/pesticides at home? Always enquire whether any of the patient's relative or his/her roommate is on any psychotropic drugs.

General Physical Examination

The next step is to carry out a quick and focused general physical examination.

Look for any signs of head trauma (black eyes, blood behind the tympanic membrane, nasal bleed, or subcutaneous blood over the mastoid region) and signs of meningeal irritation. Note that signs of meningeal irritation disappear once coma deepens **(Box 1)**.

Carefully examine the skin for signs of chronic disease, needle marks (illicit drug use), pressure sores (long-standing illness, bullae—phenobarbitone intoxication), petechiae (meningococcal meningitis/intravascular coagulation), etc.

Level of Consciousness

The next step is to determine the level of sensorium.

Correct assessment of the level of sensorium is important both for tailoring the initial management and prognostication and for monitoring the response to treatment.

Agitation, hallucinations, and tremors are commonly seen with anticholinergic overdose, serotonergic drug overdose, and sympathomimetic drug overdose. Withdrawal from opiates and alcohol may also cause agitation and tremors.

Traditionally, Glasgow Coma Scale (GCS) is used to assess the level of sensorium **(Box 2)**.[6] Its utility has been proven in numerous studies. It is easy to perform and record and is reproducible. However, authors recommend

TABLE 2: CNS signs in common toxidrome.[5]

Class of drugs	***Pupils***	***Agitation***	***Muscle weakness***	***Depression/ coma***	***Reflexes***	***Other CNS features***
Anticholinergic drugs	Dilated	++	–	–	Normal or hyporeflexia	Abnormal movements—plucking at bedclothes
Cholinergic drugs	Constricted	–	++ (LMN) fasciculation	–	Hyporeflexia/ absent	Urinary/fecal incontinence, delayed neuropathy
Opioid drugs	Constricted	–	–	+++	Hyporeflexia	Seizures
Sedative–hypnotic drugs	Normal	–	–	++	Hyporeflexia	Sleepiness
Sympathomimetic drugs	Dilated	++	–	–	Normal	Paranoia, piloerection
Neuroleptic drugs	Oculogyric crisis	+	–	–	Normal	Trismus, dystonia, ataxia, parkinsonism, neuroleptic malignant syndrome
Serotonergic drugs	Normal	++	+	–	Hyperreflexia, clonus	Hypertonia, akathisia, tremor, agitation, central hyperthermia

(CNS: central nervous system; LMN: lower motor neuron)

BOX 1: Clinical evaluation of patients with coma.[2]

- *History (from relatives, friends, or attendants):*
  - Onset of coma (abrupt, gradual)
  - Recent complaints (e.g., headache, depression, focal weakness, vertigo)
  - Recent injury
  - Previous medical illnesses (e.g., diabetes, renal failure, heart disease)
  - Previous psychiatric history
  - Access to drugs (sedatives, psychotropic drugs)
- *General physical examination:*
  - *Vital signs:* Respiration, blood pressure, heart rate
  - Evidence of trauma
  - Evidence of acute or chronic systemic illness
  - Evidence of drug ingestion (needle marks, alcohol on breath)
  - Nuchal rigidity (assuming that cervical trauma has been excluded)
- *Neurological examination:*
  - Verbal response
  - Eye opening
  - Fundus examination
  - Pupillary examination
  - Spontaneous eye movements
  - Oculocephalic and oculovestibular responses
  - Corneal responses
  - Respiratory pattern
  - Motor responses
  - Deep tendon reflexes
  - Skeletal muscle tone
  - Plantar responses
  - Abnormal movements (seizures, chorea, myoclonus, etc.)

BOX 2: Glasgow Coma Scale.[6]

- *Eye response:*
  - 4: Eyes open spontaneously
  - 3: Eye opening to verbal command
  - 2: Eye opening to pain
  - 1: No eye opening
- *Motor response:*
  - 6: Obeys commands
  - 5: Localizing pain
  - 4: Withdrawal from pain
  - 3: Flexion to pain
  - 2: Extension to pain
  - 1: No motor response
- *Verbal response:*
  - 5: Oriented
  - 4: Confused
  - 3: Inappropriate words
  - 2: Incomprehensible sounds
  - 1: No verbal response

recording the sensorium in a more detailed manner, clearly noting down the degree of stimulus and level of response rather than just noting down GCS. For instance, a person who fails to opens his/her eyes after his/her name is called repeatedly and loudly is considered highly impaired compared with a person who opens his/her eyes after his/her name is called only once, although both will come under category E3. *So, response shall be recorded clearly, "After I vigorously shook his arm, he opened his eyes slightly and immediately closed them again."*

Pupillary Responses

An extremely important and easy-to-perform bedside examination which can help immensely in differentiation between metabolic and structural coma is examination of pupils including pupillary light reflex. This is related to two facts:

1. The anatomy of pupillary reflexes is closely intertwined with ascending arousal pathways.
2. Pupillary pathways are among the most resistant to metabolic insult.

While examining the pupils, first observe pupils in ambient light and look for their size and shape. Remember that 8–18% of normal individuals have anisocoria >0.4 mm. *Also remember that pupils of stuporous or comatose patients are usually smaller than normal pupils in awake subjects.*

After noting their shape and size, note down pupillary light reflex with a bright light. A common finding in patients with altered sensorium is the *presence of small reactive pupils. Although this pattern can result from diencephalic injuries, it is also seen in almost all forms of metabolic encephalopathies and is thus of limited localizing value*. On the other hand, the presence of a unilateral, small, reactive pupil accompanied by ipsilateral ptosis (Horner's syndrome) or a new-onset unilateral, fixed, and dilated pupil (in the absence of instillation of Atropine/homatropine/scopolamine eye drops), almost always suggests structural brain injury.

Preserved pupillary light responses in a comatose patient suggest a metabolic/toxic cause for the coma except for 15–20 minutes following a seizure when pupils can dilate and react poorly to light in the absence of structural damage to the brain. Although most drugs which affect sensorium cause small, reactive pupils, poisoning with cholinergic drugs may lead to large, poorly reactive pupils.[2] Opiate intoxication, on the other hand, results in pinpoint pupils that resemble those seen in pontine hemorrhage. Small pinpoint pupils may also be noted in OP poisoning and 2,4-D poisoning (herbicide).

Dilated pupils are seen with anticholinergic poisoning and sympathomimetic poisoning. It is important to note whether someone has already dilated the pupils with drugs for fundus evaluation. It is also needed to serially evaluate vision and optic nerve as toxic alcohol poisoning may have visual disturbances and optic neuritis as the clinical findings. Patients with dilated pupils may complain of hazy vision and photophobia.

Oculomotor Responses

Just like pupillary reflexes, neurological pathways which control eye movements lie closely intertwined with the ascending arousal system. Accordingly, eye movements are invariably affected in patients with structural coma. With rare exception (e.g., a comatose patient with a congenital strabismus), *asymmetric oculomotor function is suggestive of a structural rather than a metabolic cause of coma.*

In a patient with stupor or coma, oculomotor examination usually includes examining position of eyes and eyelids at rest, spontaneous movements of eyes or eyelids, and reflex ocular movements (oculocephalic and oculovestibular movements). In coma, eyelids are closed due to tonic contraction of the orbicularis oculi muscles.

Next, gently raise and then release the eyelids, noting their tone. The eyelids of a comatose patient close smoothly and gradually, a movement that cannot be duplicated by an awake individual simulating unconsciousness. Absence of tone or failure to close either eyelid indicates facial motor weakness or very deep coma.

Presence of blepharospasm, on the other hand, suggests feigned coma, although occasionally lethargic patients with either metabolic or structural lesions may resist eye opening, as do some patients with a nondominant parietal lobe infarct. Tonically retracted eyelids (Collier's sign) suggest dorsal midbrain damage.

The corneal reflex can be tested in stupor or coma by gently dropping two to three drops of sterile saline from a height of 4–6 inches. A normal blink response suggests that pathways from the trigeminal nerve and spinal trigeminal nucleus through the lateral brainstem tegmentum to the oculomotor and facial nuclei are intact. Any asymmetry in blink reflex may be more suggestive of a structural lesion as bilateral suppression of blink may occur in advanced stages of coma.

Next, observe the primary position of eyes. *It is worthwhile to note that most patients with altered sensorium show slight exophoria irrespective of the cause of altered sensorium.* Look for spontaneous eye movements and perform oculocephalic (both horizontal and vertical) and oculovestibular maneuvers. *It is unusual for patients with structural coma to have normal oculocephalic reflexes or doll's eye responses and so preserved doll's eye movements in a patient with stupor or coma shall raise the possibility of metabolic coma.* But doll's eye responses have been found to be absent in patients with deep metabolic coma and in these patients more intense vestibular stimulation may be obtained by testing caloric vestibulo-ocular responses. In contrast, patients with hepatic encephalopathy often demonstrate exaggerated oculocephalic responses. In patients with severe neuroparalysis, all oculocephalic movements may be lost and pupils may be dilated and unresponsive, confusing the physicians. In some patients, even caloric vestibulo-ocular responses may be lost, giving a false impression of brain death.

Absent oculovestibular responses during caloric stimulation do not always imply brainstem dysfunction. Bilateral transient vestibular failure occurs with phenytoin/phenobarbitone or tricyclic antidepressant toxicity. Also, phenytoin and phenobarbitone as well as several other antiepileptic drugs do result in ophthalmoplegia. *In authors' experience, absent oculocephalic or oculovestibular reflexes with normally reacting pupils are almost always indicative of drug intoxication.*

Interpretation of Abnormal Ocular Movements

As mentioned earlier, most individuals with depression of sensorium will have mild exophoria. Also, depression of sensorium may unmask a previously latent strabismus or worsen preexisting strabismus. Hence, always obtain information about the presence of baseline strabismus. However, gross exophoria or esophoria with failure of one eye to follow its mate during spontaneous or evoked eye movements does suggest structural lesion as the cause of coma.

Conjugate horizontal or vertical deviation of eyes or skew deviation (one eye displaced downward and the other upward) usually suggests a structural lesion as the cause of coma.

Some spontaneous eye movements such as ocular bobbing, ocular dipping, inverse ocular bobbing, ping-pong gaze, or roving eyeball movements are nonspecific and may be seen in coma due to both metabolic and structural causes.

Motor Responses

The motor examination in a stuporous or comatose patient is limited to assessment of motor tone, motor responsiveness, reflexes, and identifying abnormal motor patterns, such as hemiplegia or abnormal posturing. The main focus is on observation of any asymmetry of motor responses obtained from the right or left side of the body and any specific patterns which point to a specific metabolic or structural cause of coma. More stress is however placed on any asymmetries rather than on specific patterns as even decorticate and decerebrate posturing (though classically described with brainstem lesions at different levels) are seen in patients with metabolic encephalopathies. *The presence of bilateral asterixis, tremor, or multifocal myoclonus often suggests metabolic/toxic cause as an etiology of coma.*

It is very important to record tone, muscle twitching, reflexes, and, in conscious patients, sensations. It is important to note that in OP poisoning, fasciculation may be noted and it may be lost initially due to severe muscle involvement; however, later in the course, neuropathy may set in. Opiates and sedative-hypnotic overdose may result in hyporeflexia and hypotonia, whereas serotonergic drug overdose will result in hyperreflexia and clonus. In patients suspected of having club drug/recreational drug overdose, ankle clonus should always be looked for.

Severe ethanol intoxication, toxic alcohol overdose, and neuroleptic drug overdose will invariably result in ataxia. This needs to be distinguished from severe myopathy or neuropathy leading to disturbed gait.

One must always be on the lookout for autonomic disturbances in patients with toxic overdoses. Anticholinergic drug overdose and cocaine withdrawal may result in abnormal movements like plucking at the shin. Bruxism is common with serotonergic drug and neuroleptic drug overdose.

Sensory Examination

Sensory examination may be difficult in an acutely toxic patient; however, symptoms like weakness, ataxia, recurrent trauma to the lower limbs, burning pain, or numbness may point toward a possible neurological involvement, especially sensory neuropathy. Most of the toxic neuropathies are sensory axonopathy; however, some toxins may cause pure motor or mixed polyradiculopathy.[7] One must be aware of the associated CNS symptoms, which may provide a clue to the diagnosis. These include encephalopathy, tremors, myopathy, and associated optic nerve involvement.

Heavy metals and pharmaceutical agents are important culprits. Among the commonly used drugs, antitubercular and anticancer agents are notorious to result in peripheral neuropathies **(Table 3)**.[7]

In most of the cases, a good clinical examination is sufficient to make the diagnosis of neuropathy; however,

TABLE 3: Toxic neuropathies.[7]

Phenotype	*Common causes*	*Other causes*
Sensory dominant	• Ethanol • Pyridoxine deficiency (B_6) • Glue sniffing • Cadmium	• INH, ethambutol • Ethylene oxide • Phenytoin, thalidomide, bortezomib • Calcineurin inhibitors • Linezolid, metronidazole • Leflunomide • Metronidazole • Triazole antifungals
Distal motor weakness	• Organophosphates • Lead • Arsenic • Thallium • Glue sniffing	• Vinca alkaloids • Nitrofurantoin • Amiodarone • Dapsone
Dominant pain (neuropathic)	• Ethanol • Mercury • Thallium	• Thalidomide, bortezomib • Linezolid • Metronidazole • Nitrofurantoin • Co-trimoxazole
GBS-like picture	• Thallium • Arsenic • Diethylene glycol • Glue sniffing	• Seafood toxin • Nitrofurantoin • Calcineurin inhibitors • Immune checkpoint inhibitors • TNF inhibitors
Associated encephalopathy	• Ethanol, methanol • Lead, arsenic, mercury • Glue sniffing	• Phenytoin • Metronidazole
Associated tremors	• Mercury • Calcineurin inhibitors	Alcohol withdrawal
Optic neuropathy	• Toxic alcohol • Lead, mercury, thallium	• Ethambutol, INH • Linezolid • Chloroquine, dapsone

(INH: isoniazid; TNF: tumor necrosis factor)

it is a good practice to get an objective documentation by performing nerve conduction studies along with testing for myopathy. Serial nerve conduction studies may help in assessing response to therapy. In some situations like OP poisoning, repetitive nerve stimulation and recording of the muscle response may be an important indicator for diagnosis of intermediate syndrome. In patients with OP poisoning, careful record of nerve conduction at discharge and on follow-up may be an important indicator for delayed-onset OP neuropathy.

Neuroimaging/Lumbar Puncture/ Electroencephalography

Three most important neurological investigations which aid in the diagnosis of coma of undetermined etiology include neuroimaging, cerebrospinal fluid examination, and electroencephalography. Neuroimaging is ubiquitous and shall always be carried out in any patient with depressed sensorium of undetermined etiology. Even in patients with known intoxication, neuroimaging may be ordered in the presence of focal deficits, papilledema, meningeal signs, or lack of expected response to treatment. Neuroimaging may also reveal brain lesions consistent with exposure to particular toxins such as bilateral putaminal hemorrhage in methanol intoxication, carbon monoxide poisoning, or cocaine overdose. Features suggestive of posterior reversible encephalopathy syndrome may be seen in cyclosporine/tacrolimus overdose or cocaine intoxication. In patients with nonresponsive coma to dextrose and naloxone, a noncontrast computed tomography (NCCT) head must always be ordered. MRI may show typical changes in the basal ganglia in patients with CO or gas geyser poisoning. It should be ordered in patients with unexplainable coma or neurological signs.

Cerebrospinal fluid examination likewise may be carried out if the etiology of coma remains obscure even after performing neuroimaging and if a neuroinfection is strongly suspected. It shall be noted that people with intravenous drug abuse are more prone to neuroinfections and if immunocompromised they may not develop fever or meningeal signs even in the presence of neuroinfections. The main role of electroencephalography in evaluation of coma of undetermined etiology is in ruling out nonconvulsive status epilepticus. However, it may help in clinching the diagnosis by showing specific patterns such as periodic lateralized epileptiform discharges in herpes encephalitis, periodic sharp- and slow-wave complexes in subacute sclerosing panencephalitis, and periodic 1-Hz generalized sharp-wave discharges in drug-induced encephalopathies such as due to lithium, isoniazid, hydralazine, and cyclosporine.

CONCLUSION

Assessment of neurological disability in a critically ill poisoned patient is an art which can be achieved by following a stepwise algorithm. Careful history followed by general physical, systemic, and neurological examination along with relevant investigations will help not only in reaching at a diagnosis and give clues about the nature of poisoning, but also in formulating a proper treatment plan and follow-up.

REFERENCES

1. Posner JB, Saper CB, Schiff ND, Claassen J. Plum and Posner's Diagnosis and Treatment of Coma, 5th edition. Oxford, New York: Oxford University Press; 2019. pp. 1-502.
2. Holstege CP, Dobmeier SG, Bechtel LK. Critical care toxicology. Emerg Med Clin NA. 2008;26(3):715-39.
3. Boyle JS, Bechtel LK, Holstege CP. Management of the critically poisoned patient. Scand J Trauma Resusc Emerg Med. 2009;17:29.
4. Tran TP, Panacek EA, Rhee KJ, Foulke GE. Response to dopamine vs norepinephrine in tricyclic antidepressant-induced hypotension. Acad Emerg Med. 1997;4(9):864-8.
5. Mégarbane B. Toxidrome-based approach to common poisonings. Asia Pac J Med Toxicol. 2014;3:2-12.
6. Jain S, Iverson LM. Glasgow Coma Scale. 2023. In: StatPearls. Treasure Island, FL: StatPearls Publishing; 2024.
7. Smyth D, Kramarz C, Carr AS, Rossor AM, Lunn MP. Toxic neuropathies: a practical approach. Pract Neurol. 2023;23:120-30.

1.6 Clinical Diagnosis of Poisoning (Toxidrome—Pearls and Pitfalls; Eyes and Skin)

Parshotam Lal Gautam, Gunchan Paul, Shruti Sharma

INTRODUCTION

Self-harm and accidental poisoning from both licit and illicit substances is among the leading causes of mortality, morbidity, and societal issues worldwide, particularly in the young victims.[1-3] Overdose, both intentional and unintentional, has also become the leading global healthcare challenge. The incidence and pattern of poisoning is increasing and changing due to ease in availability of drugs and toxic agents, increasing substance abuse, cultural change, and stress of life. This mortality rate is exceeding the number of deaths due to firearms, falls, or motorized vehicle accidents or other diseases.[4] We need an organized and multidimensional approach to address this global threat through healthcare facility and government policies. Another concern is manipulation of circumstantial evidence by the patient and family to avoid legal problems, social stigma, etc. However, circumstantial evidence provides important clues to having suspicion and reaching the diagnosis.

Severely poisoned patients may present in life-threatening conditions and mimicking the other medical conditions. Suspecting and recognition of poisoning, rescue resuscitation, and identifying the toxin and antidote are not less than a Herculean task. The clinical profile depends on several factors, such as the ingested dose, characteristics of the poison, time of initial medical support, quality of rescue resuscitation, route of intake, accidental or intentional, and the preexisting comorbid conditions. The management of the poisoned victim is challenging. This is further challenged by alterations in clinical presentation secondary to coexistent medical conditions, antipsychotic medications in psychiatric patients, polypharmacy in geriatric patients, adulteration in illicit drugs, and altered facts in alleged history by the patient or family. The complexity of these critically ill patients demands integrated multidisciplinary management for a good outcome. The integration of all possible medical tools is required to reach the diagnosis in the absence of clinical history, and the implementation of early management strategies is necessary to restore physiological functions. In this chapter, we shall focus on the clinical diagnosis and care of these patients, mainly focusing on toxidromes and the role of epidemiological factors and circumstantial evidence.

CLINICAL DIAGNOSIS

The clinical behavior of poisonings in the critically ill patient is atypical. About 10–15% of severe poisoning cases present to the intensive care unit (ICU) with multiple organ failure and high risk of death due to the severity of poisoning or comorbidities that worsen the clinical course of the patients.[5] The physicians must have an in-depth knowledge of the behavior and pathophysiology of the toxins when making the diagnosis of poisoning in the critically ill patient.

The toxicological diagnosis in settings outside the ICU is largely based on the findings of the physical examination, by associating the set of clinical signs with the possible agents. This process is also called a toxidromic approach.[6] If we miss the diagnosis, we miss the opportunity for specific lifesaving interventions. Emergency and general physicians handling poisoned patients in the early phase play an important role.

ROLE OF TOXIDROMIC APPROACH IN IDENTIFICATION OF AGENT

In most patients with unclear symptoms and an incomplete medical history, the diagnosis of poisoning is made through suspicion, by matching the symptoms or findings that are compatible with toxidromes. A toxidrome is a set of clinical signs and symptoms typical of certain specific xenobiotics with similar mechanisms of action.[7] Toxidromes are a navigation chart for the clinician to carry out the differential diagnosis within the multiple potentially causative toxic agents through physical examination. They also provide a guideline for initiating laboratory tests and treatment.

Based on the predominant effects on central and autonomic nervous systems, they can be classified as stimulants [cocaine, amphetamine, mephedrone and derivatives, 3,4-methylenedioxymethamphetamine (MDMA) and derivatives—ecstasy], depressants [alcohol, benzodiazepines, barbiturates, opioids], or drugs with variable effects [cannabinoids and synthetic cannabinoids, lysergic acid diethylamide (LSD), ketamine].[8] The best way to find out the class of drugs is a syndrome approach, but currently physicians are challenged with overlapping features secondary to polymedication, locally produced products, and adulteration or preexisting medications. Common toxidromes are enlisted in **Table 1** and an algorithmic approach to poisoning with focus on eyes and skin is depicted in **Flowchart 1**.

TABLE 1: Common toxidromes.

Toxidromes	*Vitals: Temperature, heart rate and blood pressure, respiration*	*Mental status*	*Pupils*	*Skin*	*Other findings*
Anticholinergics: Antihistamines, atropine, hyoscine, antispasmodics, atypical antipsychotics (e.g., chlorpromazine, risperidone, quetiapine), tricyclic antidepressants	Hyperthermia, tachycardia, hypertension, tachypnea/ no change	Confusion, delirium, hallucinations, agitation, seizures	Mydriasis	Dry and flushed skin, *hot as a hare, mad as hatter, blind as a bat, dry as a bone, red as a beet*	Urinary retention
Cholinergic: Organophosphates, nerve agents, carbamates, certain mushrooms, physostigmine	Hypothermia, bradycardia, hypotension/ normal tachycardia, hypertension/normal tachypnea, bronchorrhea, bronchospasm	Confusion, weakness, muscle fasciculations, seizures	Miosis	Diaphoresis	Salivation, lacrimation, urinary incontinence, defecation, GI upset, emesis
Opioid: Opiates including fentanyl, morphine, heroin, oxycodone, propoxyphene, tramadol, dextromethorphan	Hypothermia, bradycardia, hypotension/normal bradypnea	Altered mental status, hyporeflexia, coma	Miosis	Dry skin	Decreased bowel motility, respiratory or circulatory arrest, pulmonary edema
Sympathomimetic: Cocaine, amphetamines, methamphetamine, phenylpropanolamine, ephedrine	Hyperthermia, tachycardia, hypertension, tachypnea	Delusions, paranoia, hyperreflexia, seizures, anxiety	Mydriasis	Sweating	Piloerection, increased bowel motility

Contd...

Contd...

Toxidromes	***Vitals: temperature, heart rate and blood pressure, respiration***	***Mental status***	***Pupils***	***Skin***	***Other findings***
Sedative/hypnotic: Barbiturates, benzodiazepines, antipsychotics, alcohols, Soma/carisoprodol	Hypothermia, bradycardia, hypotension, bradypnea/apnea	Coma, stupor, confusion, hyporeflexia, sedation, CNS depression	No change	Dry/variable	Decreased bowel motility, respiratory depression with hypotension, especially in multiple substance abuse
Hallucinogens: Substituted amphetamines, MDMA/ecstasy, LSD, cannabis, phencyclidine, psilocybin	Hyperthermia, tachycardia, hypertension, tachypnea	Disorientation, hallucinations, panic, and seizures	Mydriasis, nystagmus	Sweating, diaphoresis	Hyperactive bowel movements, nausea and vomiting, loss of appetite
Serotonin syndrome: MAO inhibitors, SSRIs, meperidine, dextromethorphan	Hyperthermia, tachycardia, hypertension, tachypnea/normal	Confused, agitated, coma, hyperactive reflexes	Mydriasis	Sweating, diaphoresis	Tremors, myoclonus, trismus, rigidity

(CNS: central nervous system; GI: gastrointestinal; LSD: lysergic acid diethylamide; MAO: monoamine oxidase; MDMA: 3,4-methylenedioxy-methamphetamine; SSRI: selective serotonin reuptake inhibitor)

Flowchart 1: Algorithm depicting toxidrome approach to poisoning with focus on eyes and skin changes.

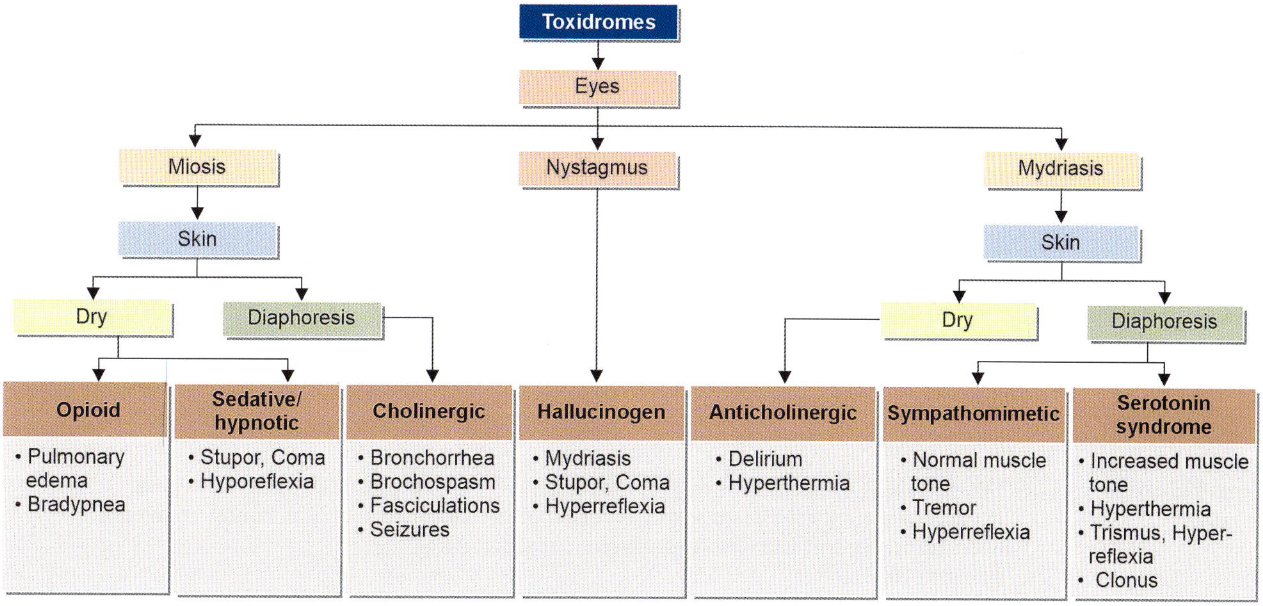

Assessing and monitoring vital signs must be interpreted with consideration of each patient's physiological, psychiatric, and premorbid conditions. Tachycardia may indicate drug toxicity, but it is not uncommon in patients with anxiety or schizophrenia. Serial monitoring of changes in vital signs is more informative than interpretation of vital signs at a particular time point, especially in the early phase of poison exposure.[9] **Table 2** represents the changes

TABLE 2: Alterations in vital physiological parameters caused by poisons along with clinical differentials to be excluded.

Symptoms	*Toxicology*	*Clinical mimics*
Bradycardia 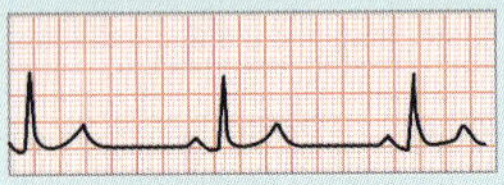	OPC poisoning and anticholinesterase drugs, beta-blockers, clonidine, calcium channel blockers, antiarrhythmics, alcohol, opioid	Sick sinus syndrome, hypothyroidism, raised ICP, complete AV block, inferior wall MI, etc.
Tachycardia 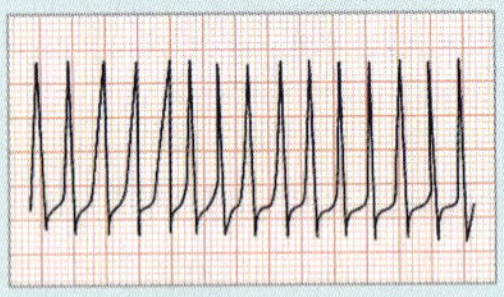	Sympathomimetics (cocaine, caffeine, amphetamine), antihistaminic, antipsychotic, theophylline, thyroid hormone, TCA	Thyrotoxicosis crisis, anxiety, hypovolemia, cardiac arrhythmia, etc.
Hypothermia 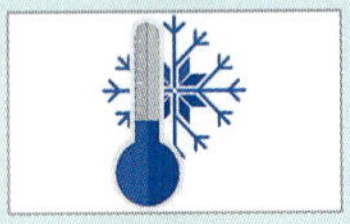	Alcohol, sedatives and hypnotics, hypoglycemic agents, opioids, carbon monoxide	Hypothyroidism, environment exposure in elderly
Hyperthermia 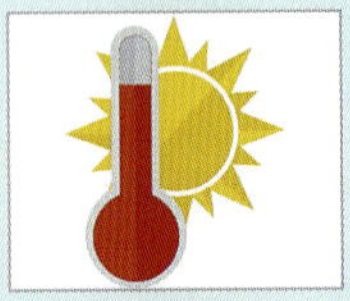	Anticholinergics, antidepressants, antipsychotic, antihistaminic, salicylate, alcohol withdrawal, antihypertensives, rodenticides, sedatives, opiates, heroin	Sepsis, neuroleptic malignant syndrome, intracerebral bleed, thyrotoxicosis crisis
Hypertension 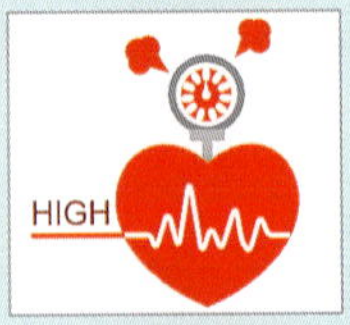	Thyroid hormone, cocaine, sympathomimetic, caffeine, anticholinergic, nicotine	Hypertensive emergencies, thyrotoxicosis, phaeochromocytoma, Cushing's disease, intracranial SOL
Tachypnea 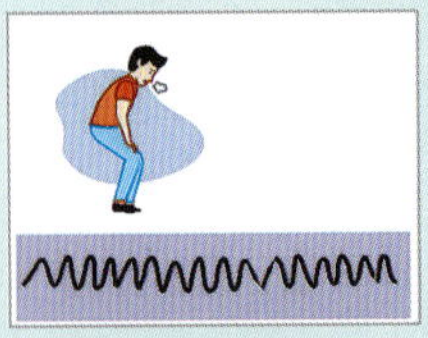	OPC poisoning, chemical pneumonitis, salicylate toxin leading to metabolic acidosis, nerve agents, paraquat	Sepsis, anxiety, thyrotoxicosis, etc.
Slow respiration 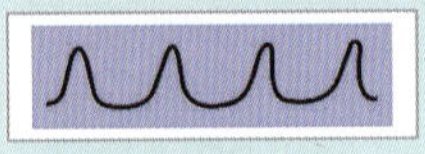	Sedatives, alcohol, opioids, marijuana	Hypothyroidism, altered sensorium
Coma and altered sensorium 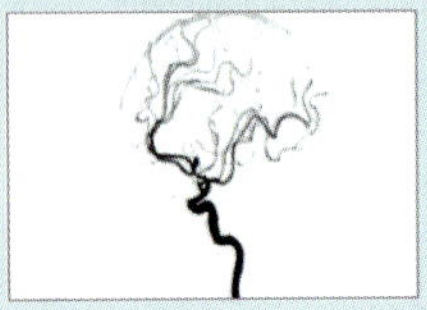	OPC poisoning, alcohol, ethylene glycol, tricyclic antidepressant, anticonvulsant agents, antipsychotics, antidepressants, antihistaminic, hypoglycemic agents, isoniazid, heavy metals	Cerebrovascular accidents, hepatic encephalopathy, metabolic conditions

Contd...

Contd...

Symptoms	***Toxicology***	***Clinical mimics***
Seizure 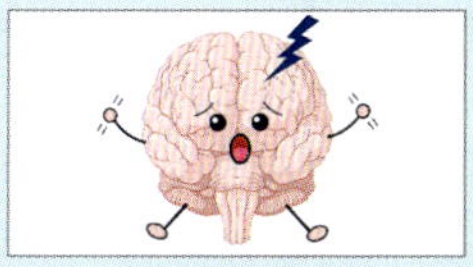	OPC poisoning, hypoglycemic agents, isoniazid, salicylate, tricyclic antidepressant, ethanol withdrawal	SOL in brain, electrolyte disturbances, fever, infective pathologies of brain and meninges
Miosis 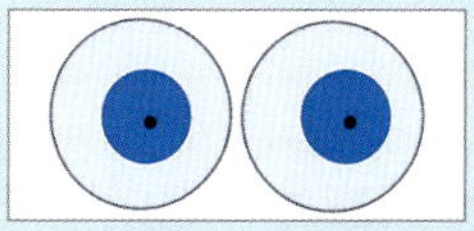	OPC and other cholinergic agents, carbamates, opiates, clonidine, phenothiazine, sedatives	Pontine hemorrhage, head injury
Mydriasis 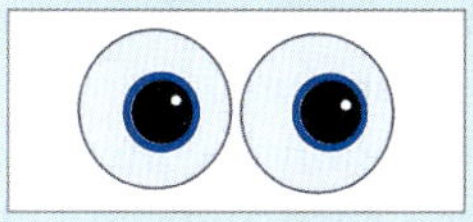	Anticholinergic (datura, atropine), sympathomimetics	Head injury, stroke, tumor
Diaphoresis 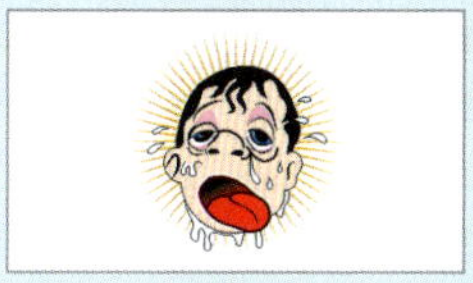	OPC poisoning, salicylates, sympathomimetics	Vasovagal syndrome, acute coronary syndrome
Dry skin 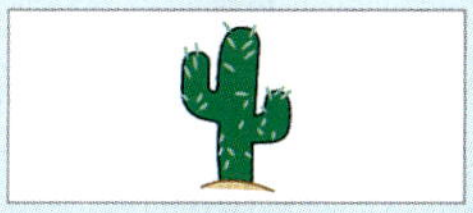	Antihistamines, anticholinergic	Diabetic patients, seborrheic dermatitis, psoriasis
Cyanosis 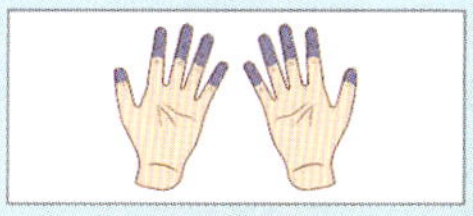	Dapsone, aniline dyes, nitrate, ergotamine, MetHb	Cyanotic heart disease, asthma, chronic obstructive pulmonary disease, polycythemia, peripheral vascular disease
Odor 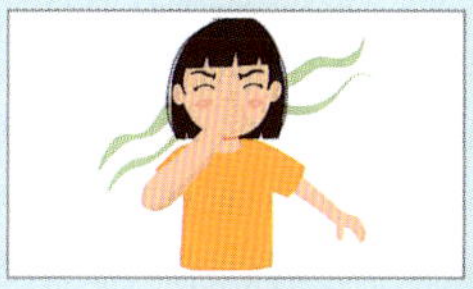	Garlic—OPC, gasoline—petroleum products, alcohol	Diabetic ketoacidosis (fruity odor)
Oropharyngeal ulceration	Paraquat, herbicides, corrosives, acids, alkalis	Autoimmune diseases, viral stomatitis, traumatic ulceration

(AV: atrioventricular; ICP: intracranial pressure; MetHb: methemoglobinemia; OPC: organophosphorus compound; SOL: space-occupying lesion; TCA: tricyclic antidepressant)

in vital signs associated with common poisonings which may be helpful in shortlisting the offending agent.

Anticholinergic

Drugs with anticholinergic action act by inhibiting muscarinic receptors that are associated with the parasympathetic nervous system, located in different organs such as the skin, eyes, heart, respiratory system, gastrointestinal tract, and bladder.[10] These agents act as competitive antagonists to acetylcholine at muscarinic receptors, producing a decrease in the activity of acetylcholine and, finally, decreasing its release.

Clinical Pearls

- Arterial hypertension and arrhythmias such as atrial fibrillation, atrioventricular (AV) blocks, supraventricular tachycardia, and even QT prolongation may occur in critically ill patients.[11]
- Dryness is observed in the areas where the greatest number of sweat glands is concentrated, leading to hyperthermia due to the inability to sweat.

Cholinergic

By binding to the active site of acetylcholinesterase (AChE) enzyme, the acetylcholine gets rapidly hydrolyzed to choline and acetyl and then these products dissociate from AChE so that the enzyme is free. But substances like organophosphates and carbamates prevent the inactivation of acetylcholine, generating overstimulation with acetylcholine, presenting as cholinergic crisis.[12] As acetylcholine, a neurotransmitter, is found throughout the central nervous system (CNS), including sympathetic and parasympathetic autonomic ganglia, the postganglionic system of the parasympathetic nervous system and the motor endplate of skeletal muscle, both muscarinic and nicotinic actions, lead to a wide range of clinical effects.

Clinical Pearls

- Acute toxicity from organophosphorus compounds (OPCs) commonly presents as cholinergic excess. Most fatal symptoms can be remembered with three Bs—bronchorrhea, bronchospasm, and bradycardia.[13]
- Seizures are frequently seen in severe cholinergic poisonings due to effects of the excess of acetylcholine in the CNS.
- The onset and duration of AChE inhibition vary depending on the route of absorption, enzymatic conversion to active metabolites, lipophilicity, and rate of AChE inhibition by the organophosphorus agent.
- Cholinergic toxidrome memorized as mnemonics (DUMBELLS/SLUDGES) helps in making the diagnosis easy; however, 10% of patients may present with odd presentations such as hypertension, mydriasis, and tachycardia.[14] This is due to norepinephrine release from the adrenal gland through cholinergic receptors.
- OPCs may produce a clinical entity named the intermediate syndrome, the mechanism of which is not well clarified. It is characterized by proximal paralysis of the cranial nerves, flexors of the neck, and respiratory muscles after 24–96 hours of intoxication.[15,16]

Adrenergic or Sympathomimetic

Cocaine, amphetamines, mephedrone, MDMA, and methylphenidate share the ability to produce CNS excitation by stimulation and activation of the sympathetic nervous system through various mechanisms.[17] Neurotransmitter norepinephrine then acts at β_1-, β_2-, α_1-, and α_2-adrenergic receptors, found in the skin, eyes, heart, lungs, gastrointestinal tract, exocrine glands, and some neuronal segments in the CNS.[18]

Clinical Pearls

- MDMA, commonly known as "ecstasy", "Molly," and "club drug," is popular among teens and young adults at bars and "raves" (all-night dance parties) to heighten sensory perceptions and reduce inhibitions.
- These drugs are usually taken orally as powder, capsules, or tablets, but may be crushed and snorted, occasionally smoked, but rarely injected.
- People who abuse these drugs also use other drugs at the same time, like alcohol, marijuana, and LSD.
- Taking "Molly" can be fatal; deaths have been reported after first-time use also.[19]

Opioids

Opioids produce their effects via μ (mu), κ (kappa), and δ (delta) opioid receptors.[20] Analgesia, euphoria, sedation, respiratory depression, gastrointestinal dysmotility, and physical dependency are all mediated by μ receptors. μ receptors reduce the medullary response to hypercarbia and the respiratory response to hypoxia, which reduces the impulse to breathe and leads to the development of apnea.[21] Analgesia, diuresis, miosis, and dysphoria are all mediated by κ receptors. Cough suppression, dopamine release inhibition, and analgesia are mediated by δ receptors. Often, opioids have their effect through μ receptors; however, presentation may vary as agents have different affinity profiles for receptors and there may also be product interactions.

Clinical Pearls

- Overdosage in reformed addicts is also common. Some of these patients may switch over to alternative compounds leading to unpredictable effects.
- Typical features of opioid overdose are pinpoint pupil, slow respiratory rates, hypercarbia in blood gas.
- In patients with pinpoint pupil, always screen for three differentials—OPC poisoning, opioid overdose, and pontine hemorrhage.

Sedatives and Hypnotics

They are potent CNS depressants and include benzodiazepines, barbiturates, and ethanol. With chronic use, the patient can develop tolerance; however, abrupt cessation or reduction in the amount of the drugs may precipitate a life-threatening withdrawal syndrome.[22] Clinical features also depend on whether it is drug overdose or withdrawal which produces reciprocal features to the effects of the drug.

Benzodiazepines (BDZ) potentiate gamma-aminobutyric acid (GABA)-A transmission causing CNS depression. Barbiturates attach to the GABA-A receptor complex and prolong the chloride channel opening, in contradistinction to benzodiazepines, which increase the frequency of opening.[23] Benzodiazepines have a very wide toxic therapeutic window while for barbiturates it is very narrow.[24]

Clinical Pearls

- Coma with normal vital signs is the hallmark of benzodiazepine overdose. As there is low density of GABA-A receptors in the brainstem, respiratory depression or cardiovascular instability rarely occurs with oral overdose.
- Nonresponse to noxious stimuli, hypotension, and respiratory depression indicates coingestion of other substances.
- The duration of stupor depends on the half-life of the agent. Oral ingestion of phenobarbitone or primidone takes 1–2 hours to reach clinical toxicity, but the coma may persist for days or weeks.[25]
- Antidepressants, antipsychotics, other sedative-hypnotic medications, and narcotics should also be considered in the differential diagnosis.
- Urine and blood qualitative screening may offer confirmation of exposure but may not detect newer benzodiazepines (clonazepam, nitrazepam) or those in low concentrations.[26]
- Window time for toxic detection varies according to the substance; hence, it is rarely useful in altering the management.[27]

Serotonergics

Serotonin is responsible for regulating mood, social behavior, sleep, memory, and even digestion. Multiple drugs may precipitate serotonin toxicity by a variety of mechanisms.[28] Selective serotonin reuptake inhibitors (SSRIs) (citalopram, escitalopram) and some other drugs like meperidine, tramadol, valproate, carbamazepine, and dextromethorphan inhibit the reuptake of serotonin from the synaptic cleft into the presynaptic neuron. Tricyclic antidepressants also inhibit serotonin reuptake, whereas monoamine oxidase inhibitors (MAOIs) inhibit serotonin metabolism and produce severe and prolonged toxicity.[29] Amphetamines, cocaine, and MDMA increase serotonin release. Some newer opiates, such as fentanyl, and some antiparkinsonian agents may also produce serotonin syndrome.

Clinical Pearls

- Apart from intentional overdose, serotonin syndrome may occur as a consequence of therapeutic medication use and interactions between medications and recreational drugs (addition of one or more of the above medications in patients who are previously stable on a serotonergic agent).
- Since many drugs may cause this syndrome, careful medication history is very important before addition of a new drug.

Hallucinogens

Hallucinogens are substances that cause a variety of physical and psychological manifestations. They were used to induce an altered state of consciousness for religious and spiritual purposes but nowadays they are popular for recreational purposes.[30]

ROLE OF CIRCUMSTANTIAL EVIDENCE

Suspecting and identifying the poison is the first important step to successful management. It is obvious that circumstantial evidence along with clinical profile is very important to suspect and confirm the poisoning along with laboratory workup.

All attempts should be made to obtain history in a conscious patient before they decompensate. Direct, leading questions asked in a confidential and secretive manner by moving the relative away from bedside can be helpful. On many occasions, the critically ill patient is not able to provide history that contributes to making the diagnosis of poisoning very challenging. Even if available, the history should be interpreted with caution and cross-checked with information from other sources, especially in patients with known psychiatric illness, suicidal attempt, or malicious poisoning.[31] History from the patient's employer, friends, primary care clinician, as well as medical records (use of "sleeping pills") and pharmacists (treatment for opioid use disorder) may give some clue to intentional overdose. Other factors that raise alarms of possible poisoning include concerns regarding discordant relationship at home or with friends, acute behavioral changes, alteration in sleep-wake cycles, or earlier episodes of overdose.

The importance of taking the detailed history cannot be overemphasized that may be supported by circumstantial evidence (pills, empty strips or bottles, transdermal patches, etc.), linear track marks indicating injection drug use, signs of trauma (self-inflicted or accidental), etc.

Clinical Pearls

- High index of suspicion is sometimes needed to clinch the diagnosis.
- Inadvertent poisoning may occur when opioid users misjudge dose-tolerance dynamics, e.g., when tolerance is lost following recent detoxification/ incarceration and the patient takes the previous drug dose.
- Tampering of preparations to achieve a high like crushing an extended-release preparation, swallowing fentanyl patch, or injecting oral preparations may result in poisoning.

ROLE OF EPIDEMIOLOGY

The pattern of poisoning and agents used shows a diverse outline in different countries and also different regions within the country. The regional variations and sociodemographic factors therein play a vital role in determining the pattern of poisoning. Pesticides are used commonly in the Asian region for self-poisoning, particularly in rural areas.[32,33] Medicinal poisonings are common in the urban population and are influenced by availability of various toxic substances, over-the-counter drugs, stress, financial problems, influence of mass media, and also peer pressure.[34] Paracetamol poisoning is uncommon in India, but frequent in Europe; on the other hand, OPCs and paraquat are very common in India.[8] Opioid overdosage is common in northern states of India. Occult snake bite in the rainy months of July is very common in Punjab which may get confused with sedative overdosage.

A recent nationwide survey had reported prevalence of the current use of various substances—alcohol, 14.6%; cannabis, 2.8%; opioids, 2.1%; sedatives, 1.1%; solvents, 0.9%; amphetamine-type stimulants (ATSs), 0.2%; cocaine, 0.1%; and hallucinogens, 0.1%.[35] A report from Kerala, Indian, which is much different from other states with respect to literacy, health care, agricultural characteristics, and social and developmental metrics, until recently, happened to have the highest suicide rate in the country. Even the latest statistics show a suicide rate of above twice the national average. The most common poisons used were pharmaceutical drugs; polymedication was found to be the major pattern of poisoning and most were suicide attempts due to familial conflicts.[36] In contrast to above study, from PGI, Chandigarh, reported that corrosives were the most commonly consumed poison during lockdown among patients from Punjab (45%), Himachal Pradesh (22%), Haryana (14%), and Chandigarh UT (16%).[37]

Clinical Pearls

Similar to the knowledge of an antibiogram in the emergency room (ER), the epidemiology of poisoning in the region is a vital key to reach the diagnosis.

PITFALLS OF TOXIDROMIC APPROACH

- The toxidromic approach is challenged by overlapping features secondary to coadministration of another compound or preexisting medication or patient characteristics/comorbidities.
- The effect of poisoning agents may be altered by locally produced products and adulteration.
- The clinical conditions which overlap for the toxic signs should be considered in differential diagnosis. In such cases, investigations help to confirm or rule out the diagnosis.
- Many poisonings are unique and do not fit into typical toxidromes (e.g., paraquat, household chemicals, corrosive ingestion); hence, diagnosis of every patient should be based on history, investigation, and point-of-care testing rather than solely relying on toxidromes.

CLINICAL BEHAVIOR OF A CRITICALLY ILL POISONED PATIENT

The critically ill patients with intoxication in the ICU may not have a well-established predictable clinical course; thus, monitoring of clinical patterns is the most crucial action.[38] The clinical manifestations may vary related to the patient's general health and comorbidities. The natural course of poisoning can evolve into a critical condition that includes neurological compromise, circulatory instability, and multiorgan failure leading to death.[39] These are common in the critically ill ICU patients regardless of the agent causing the condition and, hence, deserve admission to the ICU. According to the potential complications resulting as a consequence of the toxidromes, the critically ill can be grouped as those with:[5]

- *Respiratory failure:* In case of cholinergic toxidrome, a patient with characteristically increased salvation and bronchorrhea, along with depressed mental state, and muscle weakness may present as hypoxemic, hypercapnic, or mixed respiratory failure. In an opioid toxidrome, respiratory depression causing type II failure is the most life-threatening pathophysiology, but significant deterioration of the sensorium necessitates intervention for airway protection.
- *Circulatory shock:* In case of cholinergic manifestations, intestinal and extraintestinal losses characteristically lead to hypovolemic shock but it may be of dual origin, cardiogenic component caused by bradycardia and hypovoluemia. However, in opioid and hypnotic-sedative toxidrome, shock is mainly distributive due to the loss of sympathetic tone. Additionally, multiple agents in the setting of preexisting medication intake or comorbidity can impair heart rhythm, making electrocardiography an essential investigation in case of the patient being critically ill after poisoning.[40]
- *Hypertensive emergency:* Drugs that act over the CNS as anticholinergic, sympathomimetic, and serotonergic toxidromes may increase in the pressor response outside the self-regulation range of blood pressure. This may be aggravated by a state of psychomotor agitation.
- *Acid-base and electrolyte disturbances*: Multiple agents can affect the acid-base and electrolyte state resulting in neurological manifestations and compensatory responses that demand ICU admission and ventilatory support.[41] Hence, an arterial blood gas not only helps to assess the severity of the poisoning but also evaluates perfusion disorders and makes specific diagnosis for some substances. An elevated anion gap (>12 mEq/L) is caused by acetylsalicylic acid, ethanol, methanol, ethylene glycol, and paraldehyde. If anion gap is normal (8-12 mEq/L), poisoning by carbonic anhydrase inhibitors or ion exchange resins is suspected.[42] Hyperlactatemia occurs in carbon monoxide, cyanide, or methanol poisoning. Hyponatremia is seen in SSRIs and lithium overdose. Topiramate can cause hyperchloremic acidosis while methylxanthines cause hypokalemia. Alcohol poisonings typically cause an increased osmolar gap.[43]

An adequate control of neurological status, circulation, and acid-base balance is necessary for the critically ill poisoned patient to be managed in the ICU. Also, evaluation and re-evaluation are required.

CONCLUSION

It is a challenging task to identify poison in a suspected poisoning patient. Any medicines or an agent can be potentially toxic when taken in overdose or by the wrong route. High index of suspicion, circumstantial evidence and clinical toxidromes are the key factors to reach diagnosis. Aggressive resuscitation, general supportive and specific management with antidote if available are the other pillars of active management of poisoning. Toxicological screening is more or less supportive. Enhanced elimination and antidote therapy is helpful in selected specific poisoning.

REFERENCES

1. Gummin DD, Mowry JB, Beuhler MC, Spyker DA, Brooks DE, Dibert KW, et al. Annual report of the American Association of Poison Control Centers' National Poison Data System (NPDS): 37th annual report. Clin Toxicol (Phila). 2020;58(12):1360-541.
2. United Nations. (2023). Online World Drug Report 2023—latest data and trend analysis. [online] Available from https://www.unodc.org/unodc/en/data-and-analysis/wdr-2023-online-segment.html [Last accessed August, 2024].
3. Kumar R, Sheikh NA, Bashar MA, Vasudeva A, Kumar A, Yadav A, et al. Epidemio-toxicological profile of fatal poisoning cases autopsied at a tertiary care centre of North India. J Family Med Prim Care. 2023;12(4):701-7.
4. Lawrence WR, Freedman ND, McGee-Avila JK, Berrington de González A, Chen Y, Emerson MA, et al. Trends in mortality from poisonings, firearms, and all other injuries by intent in the US, 1999-2020. JAMA Intern Med. 2023;183(8):849-56.
5. Brent J, Burkhart K, Dargan P, Hatten B, Megarbane B, Palmer R, et al. Critical Care Toxicology. Diagnosis and Management of the Critically Poisoned Patient. New York: Springer; 2017.
6. Thompson TM, Theobald J, Lu J, Erickson TB. The general approach to the poisoned patient. Dis Mon. 2014; 60(11):509-24.
7. Mellema MS. Initial management of the poisoned patient. Small Animal Toxicology. Amsterdam: Elsevier; 2012. pp. 63-71.
8. Shukla L, Ghadigaonkar DS, Murthy P. Poisoning with drugs of abuse: identification and management. Indian J Crit Care Med. 2019;23(Suppl 4):S296-304.

9. Erickson TB, Thompson TM, Lu JJ. The approach to the patient with an unknown overdose. Emerg Med Clin North Am. 2007;25(2):249-81.
10. Holstege C, Borek H. Toxidromes. Crit Care Clin. 2012;28(4):479-98.
11. Tisdale JE, Chung MK, Campbell KB, Hammadah M, Joglar JA, Leclerc J, et al. Drug-induced arrhythmias: a scientific statement from the American Heart Association. Circulation. 2020;142:e214-33.
12. Gupta RC, Sachana M, Mukherjee IM, Doss RB, Malik JK, Milatovic D. Organophosphates and carbamates. Veterinary Toxicology: Basic and Clinical Principles. Amsterdam: Elsevier Inc; 2018. pp. 495-508.
13. Eddleston M, Buckley NA, Eyer P, Dawson AH. Management of acute organophosphorus pesticide poisoning. Lancet. 2008;371:597-607.
14. Lotti M. Clinical toxicology of anticholinesterase agents in humans. In: Krieger R (Ed). Handbook of Pesticide Toxicology, 2nd edition, vol. 2. San Diego: Academic Press; 2001. pp. 1043-85.
15. De Bleecker J. Intermediate syndrome in organophosphate poisoning. Toxicology of Organophosphate and Carbamate Compounds, 1st edition. Amsterdam: Elsevier; 2006. pp. 371-80.
16. Indira M, Andrews MA, Rakesh TP. Incidence, predictors, and outcome of intermediate syndrome in cholinergic insecticide poisoning: a prospective observational cohort study. Clin Toxicol. 2013;51(9):838-45.
17. Green AR, O'shea E, Isabel Colado M. A review of the mechanisms involved in the acute MDMA (ecstasy)-induced hyperthermic response. Eur J Pharmacol. 2004;500(1-3):3-13.
18. King A, Dimovska M, Bisoski L. Sympathomimetic toxidromes and other pharmacological causes of acute hypertension. Curr Hypertens Rep. 2018;20:8.
19. Kariisa M, Scholl L, Wilson N, Seth P, Hoots B. Drug overdose deaths involving cocaine and psychostimulants with abuse potential—United States, 2003–2017. MMWR Morb Mortal Wkly Rep. 2019;68(17):388.
20. Hoorn EJ, for the Paediatric Death Review Committee, Office of the Chief Coroner of Ontario. A fatal case of ecstasy poisoning. Paediatr Child Health. 2001;6(7):491.
21. Doran KM, Raja AS, Samuels EA. Opioid overdose protocols in the emergency department: are we asking the right questions? Ann Emerg Med. 2018;72(1):12-5.
22. Schiller EY, Goyal A, Mechanic OJ. Opioid overdose. In: StatPearls. Treasure Island, FL: StatPearls Publishing; 2022.
23. Schmitz A. Benzodiazepine use, misuse, and abuse: a review. Ment Health Clin. 2016;6(3):120-6.
24. Lu CY, Chang CI, Huang HH, Yen DH. Clinical predictors for intensive care unit admission in patients with benzodiazepines poisoning in the emergency department. J Acute Med. 2018;8(4):168178.
25. Santos C, Olmedo RE. Sedative-hypnotic drug withdrawal syndrome: recognition and treatment. Emerg Med Pract. 2017;19(3):1-20.
26. Kent R, Smollin CG, Anderson IB, Benowitz NL, Blanc PD, Kim-Katz SY, et al. Poisoning and Drug Overdose: Comprehensive Evaluation and Treatment. New York: McGraw-Hill; 2018.
27. Bertholf RL, Sharma R, Reisfield GM. Predictive value of positive drug screening results in an urban outpatient population. J Anal Toxicol. 2016;40(9):726-31.
28. Raouf M, Bettinger JJ, Fudin J. A practical guide to urine drug monitoring. Fed Pract. 2018;35(4):38-44.
29. Wang RZ, Vashistha V, Kaur S, Houchens NW. Serotonin syndrome: preventing, recognizing, and treating it. Cleve Clin J Med. 2016;83(11):810-7.
30. Buckley NA, Dawson AH, Isbister GK. Serotonin syndrome. BMJ. 2014;348:g1626.
31. Hardaway R, Schweitzer J, Suzuki J. Hallucinogen use disorders. Child Adolesc Psychiatr Clin N Am. 2016;25:489-96.
32. Soslow AR. Acute drug overdose: one hospital's experience. Ann Emerg Med. 1981;10:18.
33. Wright N. An assessment of the unreliability of the history given by self-poisoned patients. Clin Toxicol. 1980;16:381.
34. Chan YC, Fung HT, Lee CK, Tsui SH, Ngan HK, Sy MY, et al. A prospective epidemiological study of acute poisoning in Hong Kong. Hong Kong J Emerg Med. 2005;12:156-61.
35. National Crime Records Bureau. Accidental Deaths and Suicides India. New Delhi: Open Government Data Platform India; 2015.
36. Ambekar A, Agrawal A, Rao R, Mishra AK, Khandelwal SK, Chadda RK. On behalf of the group of investigators for the National Survey on Extent and Pattern of Substance Use in India. Magnitude of Substance Use in India. New Delhi: Ministry of Social Justice and Empowerment, Government of India; 2019.
37. Bonvoisin T, Utyasheva L, Knipe D, Gunnell D, Eddleston M. Suicide by pesticide poisoning in India: a review of pesticide regulations and their impact on suicide trends. BMC Publ Health. 2020;20:1-16.
38. Behera A, Singla N, Sharma N, Sharma N. Paradigm shift in pattern and prevalence of poisoning during COVID-19 pandemic. J Fam Med Prim Care. 2022;11(1):208-14.
39. Nelson LS, Hoffman RS, Howland MA, Lewin NA, Goldfrank LR. Goldfrank's Toxicologic Emergencies. New York: McGraw-Hill Professional; 2018.
40. Rasimas J, Sinclair C. Assessment and management of toxidromes in the critical care unit. Crit Care Clin. 2017;38:521-41.
41. Pinsky MR, Teboul JL, Vincent JL. Hemodynamic Monitoring. New York: Springer International Publishing; 2019.
42. Faulkner N, Mtsa R. Factors associated with admission to the intensive care unit following referral: prospective examination of referrals to a critical care unit in a tertiary centre. Intensive Care Society State of the Art. Intensive Care Soc. 2018;19.
43. Sood P, Paul G, Puri S. Interpretation of arterial blood gas. Indian J Crit Care Med. 2010;14(2):57-64.

1.7 Laboratory Diagnosis of Poisoning (Point of Care, Toxic Screens, Gaps in Diagnosis)

Vinay Singhal, Puneet Chopra, Seema Singhal

INTRODUCTION

Outcomes in medical toxicology are highly dependent on early and appropriate diagnosis to confirm a particular poison exposure or withdrawal. In the absence of gold standard tests for the diagnosis of poisoning, a detailed history and clinical examination comprise the backbone of effective management of the patient. Tests on blood and body fluids can be performed at the bedside or in the laboratory. Once we get all the information, it can be amalgamated to make a final clinical diagnosis. The main aim of this exercise is to differentiate the medical toxicological diagnosis from other conditions with which it has an overlap like metabolic syndromes and cardiac, neurological, or pulmonary disorders.

The time taken to reach this diagnosis is as important as the diagnosis itself. Early intervention can save lives. Point-of-care testing (POCT) or bedside testing is clinical laboratory testing that is conducted close to the place of care of the patient.[1] It usually provides test results immediately that helps clinicians in reaching a particular differential/provisional diagnosis, ensuring appropriate treatment, or managing a reversible biochemical alteration. Toxicology screening can identify many substances from a sample; it has a role and impact in patient management in acutely ill patients who have exposure to toxins. It can detect many drugs and urine is a preferred sample.[2]

There are considerable limitations in the available tests despite technological advancements. It is nearly impossible for any clinical laboratory to provide a full spectrum of tests for toxicological analysis. Although nonspecific toxicological screening has a limited recommendation for the majority of cases by Alberta Medical Association Laboratory guidelines,[3] for peripheral centers, there are still some recommendations for these screening tests.[4]

In this chapter, we will be discussing the use of POCT devices in the field of toxicology, toxic screen, and their limitations in the diagnosis and management of the patients.

POINT-OF-CARE TESTING

Point-of-care testing was initiated in England in the 1950s as on-site testing of near-patient testing.[5] The term "point-of-care testing" was introduced in the 1980s for the use of biosensors in the monitoring of ionized calcium in whole blood.[6] Over the years, with the advancement in technology, we have seen better, more accurate, and smaller POCT devices.

The unique features of POCT devices[7] are that they should be simple to use and affordable with a high sensitivity and specificity, have a longer shelf life, results should be in concurrence with standard laboratory norms, and should be safe for the user during use. Various POCT devices in current use are blood gas analysis machines, infectious disease markers, cardiac markers, blood sugar monitoring devices, etc.

Point-of-Care Testing in Toxicology

In cases of exposure to unknown poisoning or drug overdose, it is difficult to get a definitive diagnosis on the basis of any single clinical sign, symptom, or laboratory abnormality. Rather, it is the pattern recognition and presence or absence of signs and symptoms along with laboratory data (toxidrome) that leads to an accurate diagnosis. Diagnostic testing in these situations may add value in not only in diagnosis but also in determining the severity of illness. These diagnostic tests can be nonspecific POCT [electrocardiogram (ECG), echocardiography, blood gas analysis], bedside toxin screen (presumptive test), or definitive laboratory testing.

Electrocardiogram

Electrocardiogram monitoring is important for early diagnosis for cardiotoxin exposure, as cardiac dysrhythmias are an important cause of morbidity and mortality in such patients. ECG may show tachycardia, bradycardia, ventricular dysrhythmia, and QRS/QTc prolongation. Tricyclic antidepressant (TCA) overdose manifests as prolongation of PR and QRS/QTc intervals.

Serial ECG during treatment in TCA poisoning may help in monitoring the improvement or worsening of the patient.

Echocardiography

Availability of facilities of cardiac function monitoring noninvasively is an important tool in the hands of new-age clinicians. Placement of vascular catheters, hemodynamic assessment, fluid resuscitation, and monitoring of cardiac chamber size and contractility are made easier with the bedside availability of a sonography machine.

Blood Gas Analysis

Blood gas analysis is a nonspecific test in case of toxic exposure/overdose. It adds valuable information in the evaluation and watching the progress of management. Arterial blood gas (ABG) analysis provides an assessment of the patient's acid–base status, oxygenation, and ventilation (pCO_2). It also provides quick assessment of electrolytes and lactate levels. Venous blood samples can be quickly obtained and repeated. It avoids repeated arterial puncture. Acid–base imbalance monitoring can be useful for the diagnosis of certain poisoning and also help in guiding therapeutic intervention. Normal and high anion gap metabolic acidosis are associated with certain poisonings **(Table 1)**. Presence of increased osmolar gap (normal osmolar gap 5 ± 7 standard deviation mOsm/L) is associated with the ingestion of alcohols or glycols such as ethanol, methanol, isopropanol, ethylene glycol, or propylene glycol. Presence of increased oxygen saturation gap (>5%) is an indicator of the presence of abnormal hemoglobin (associated with carbon monoxide, cyanide, sulfhemoglobinemia, hydrogen sulfide, methemoglobin).

TABLE 1: Drug- and toxin-induced metabolic acidosis (normal anion gap 6–12 mEq/L).

Increased anion gap		***Normal/decreased anion gap***
Methanol, ethanol	Metformin	Hypermagnesemia
Ethylene glycol	Paraldehyde	Hypercalcemia
Salicylates	Phenol	Bromide
Isoniazid	Colchicine	Nitrates
Iron	Toluene	Lithium
Glycol ethers	Propylene glycol	Iodide
NSAIDs	Benzyl alcohol	Spironolactone
Sympathomimetics: • Cocaine • Theophylline • Caffeine • Albuterol	*Cellular asphyxiants:* • Carbon monoxide • Cyanide • Hydrogen sulfide • Methemo-globinemia	Acetazolamide Ammonium chloride

(NSAID: nonsteroidal anti-inflammatory drug)

Osmolal Gap and Anion Gap

Serum osmolality is measured in laboratory by freezing point depression method. Calculated osmolality is obtained by an equation incorporating the concentration of principal osmotically active substances (sodium, glucose, blood urea nitrogen). Osmolal gap is the difference between measured and calculated osmolality, which is usually elevated in the presence of exogenous osmotically active substances, such as toxic alcohols, e.g., ethylene glycol and methanol. Serious sequalae of toxic alcohol exposure can be prevented by early diagnosis and initiation of antidotal therapy. However, few hospitals have the facility to perform gas chromatography, the gold standard diagnostic test for toxic alcohol poisoning. An osmolal gap of >10 has a high sensitivity and negative predictive value for identification of patients who require antidotal therapy for toxic alcohol poisoning. However, a high osmolal gap lacks specificity as it is also elevated in other conditions including circulatory shock, diabetic ketoacidosis, and alcoholic acidosis. It is important to consider the relevant information pertaining to ingestion history, clinical features, and other laboratory parameters to reach an accurate diagnosis.[8] Methanol poisoning is seen with illegal spirits consisting of ethanol contaminated with methanol and presents with metabolic acidosis, visual disturbances, and respiratory and cardiovascular failure. Formic acid formed by methanol metabolism leads to metabolic acidosis with a high anion gap. During early stages of methanol poisoning, osmolal gap is high, and as the methanol metabolism progresses, osmolal gap decreases, while anion gap increases due to accumulation of formic acid. Toxic alcohol poisoning is one of the few conditions presenting with both high osmolal and anion gap, which can be useful in making an early diagnosis and management of suspected cases.[9]

Toxin-specific Tests

Blood and urine are the most common samples taken for analysis of various toxins and drugs directly. Other samples that are commonly sent to laboratory are hairs, nail clippings, etc. Comprehensive stool analysis may also be beneficial to assess the body's ability to eliminate the toxin. There are certain tests which are performed not only to diagnose but also either to gauze the progression or for prognostication for certain poisonings. In case of paraquat intoxication, urine sodium dithionite assay is time consuming. It is observed in experimental and clinical studies that portable surface-enhanced Raman scattering (SERS), paper-based devices, and machine learning for paraquat poisoning are promising.[10] Likewise, a bedside 20-minute whole-blood clotting test (20WBCT) helps to diagnose venom-induced consumption coagulopathy. Alternatively, bedside monitoring of international normalized ratio (INR) and D-dimer can be done using point-of-care devices.[11] Blood lead level (BLL) screening can be done using LeadCare II, a US Food and Drug Administration (FDA)-approved POC device using capillary or venous blood. Once it shows a high level of lead, the results must be confirmed by the laboratory method.

Urine sodium dithionate test for paraquat poisoning: Paraquat is a commonly used herbicide, and its acute toxicity carries a high fatality rate. The proposed mechanism of paraquat poisoning includes generation of intracellular oxidative stress as it undergoes redox cycling, leading to multiorgan failure, particularly involving the lungs and kidneys. The systemic manifestations of paraquat toxicity depend on the quantity ingested, and the treatment is supportive in the absence of a specific antidote. Plasma and urine paraquat concentrations within 24 hours can be used to predict outcomes following paraquat toxicity. However, plasma paraquat concentration is not readily available in hospitals due to expense and associated technical issues.[12] About 90% of absorbed paraquat is excreted unchanged in the urine within 12–24 hours of ingestion. Systemic paraquat toxicity can be confirmed at bedside by qualitative test using sodium dithionate. Under alkaline conditions, sodium dithionate reduces paraquat to blue radical. If urine paraquat concentration is >1 mg/L, the urine will turn blue on adding sodium dithionate and this finding indicates a poor prognosis.[13]

TOXIC SCREENS

Exposure to toxin is one of the most important reasons to visit a healthcare facility, and on most of the occasions, history by the patient or relatives gives us a lead toward the diagnosis. Alcohol intoxication is by far the common exposure apart from rising rates of opioids, cocaine, marijuana, and other synthetic drugs. Serum and urine are the most common samples for the toxin screening and must be collected at the earliest.

Toxic screens conventionally use methods such as gas chromatography and radioimmunoassay (RIA); they have given way to enzyme-linked immunosorbent assay (ELISA) and cloned enzyme donor immunoassay (CEDIA).[14] This migration is largely due to quicker results and ease of use. However, they have a limitation of having a lesser sensitivity and specificity. Urine is the preferred sample over blood as it is easier to obtain and many drugs show up in either of them.[2] Toxic screen assays can detect multiple drugs of abuse from a single patient sample, saving time and efforts with effective screening. An ideal toxic screen should be able to check for one specific drug or a number of different drugs at once.[4] Most of the available test kits detect common toxins such as morphine, cocaine, amphetamine, methamphetamine, cannabinoids, phencyclidine (PCP), tricyclidine, benzodiazepine, barbiturate, methadone, and nicotine.

Serum-based tests are usually for the over-the-counter drugs, which can be ingested, and the patient presents with an overdose. These tests are commonly used for acetaminophen, aspirin, salicylates, and ethanol. These tests are commonly quantitative unlike urine tests. Among alcohols, ethanol is detectable, but other toxic alcohols like methanol, ethylene glycol, and isopropyl alcohol are not detectable.[15]

GAPS IN THE DIAGNOSIS

Like any monitoring or investigations, the POCT and toxic screens are being tested for their sensitivity and specificity. Potential pitfalls of these tests are primarily related to their poor sensitivity and specificity of results as compared with traditional laboratory tests **(Table 2)**. These can be directly related to the inherent technology, techniques, training issues, and poor control over variables[16] **(Table 3)**.

Although these new-generation devices are simple to use and have a rapid turnaround time, they still have limitations of having a low sensitivity and specificity. This leads to false-negative and false-positive results. There is also a limitation that in screens detecting multiple toxins, some commonly used or misused drugs (like gabapentin) or other psychoactive substances may be missing. Alcohol and commonly used pesticides and herbicides are also not a component of most of these screen tests.

TABLE 2: Advantages and disadvantages of conventional laboratory testing.

Advantages	*Disadvantages*
Low cost	Slow turnaround time
No issues of quality control and quality assurance	Specimen transport issues
Large number of drugs can be tested	Chain of custody to ensure proper results
Ability to detect adulteration	Delays in decisions
Easy reporting and documentation, and the results are authentic	

TABLE 3: Advantages and disadvantages of POCT (toxicology screening kits).

Advantages	*Disadvantages*
Reasonable cost	Specimen collection issues
Rapid turnaround time	Limited number of drugs can be tested
Large number of drugs can be tested	Operator dependent
Performance nearly similar to that of automated immunoassays	Subjective result interpretation
Easy reporting and documentation	Quality control issues
Does not require extensive personnel training	Inability to detect specimen adulteration
Chain of custody is not an issue	Cross-reactivity

(POCT: point-of-care testing)

LIMITATIONS OF URINE TOXIC SCREEN (TABLE 4)[17]

Urine toxic screens are qualitative and they can detect the presence of multiple agents. The illicit drugs may remain detectable in the urine for varying amounts of time. This fact needs to be kept in mind while interpreting and clinically correlating the results.

- *Cocaine:* The test detects the metabolite benzoylecgonine quite accurately, but the metabolite may be present up to 3 days after use. This may render the test useless in an acute setting if the patient is a chronic user.
- *Amphetamines:* Antihistamines, decongestants, antidepressants, or acid blockers may give a false-positive result as amphetamine on urine toxic screen. The test may remain positive for up to 1–3 days after use.

TABLE 4: Limitations of POCT (toxicology screening kits).

Drug tests	*False positive*	*False negative*
Benzodiazepines	Positive till 30 days (metabolites)	Lorazepam, alprazolam, midazolam, clonazepam
THC	Positive for up to 30 days	Synthetic cannabinoids (K2, Spice)
Cocaine	Positive up to 3 days (inactive metabolite)	
Amphetamines	• Nasal decongestants • Bupropion • Trazadone	• MDMA • Methamphetamine
Phencyclidine	• Tramadol • Diphenhydramine • Dextromethorphan	Quality control issues
Opioids	Poppy seeds	• Tramadol • Fentanyl • Methadone • Buprenorphine

(MDMA: 3,4-methylenedioxymethamphetamine; POCT: point-of-care testing; THC: tetrahydrocannabinol)

- *Marijuana:* Tetrahydrocannabinol is usually detected in the urine of marijuana abusers. Commonly used analgesics like ibuprofen and naproxen can cross-react with this assay, creating false positives.
- *PCP:* False-positive results are expected with ibuprofen, dextromethorphan, and tramadol. The metabolites can be detected for up to 1–2 weeks after use.
- *Opioids:* Many opioids can be missed on routine screening, generating significant false negatives, and there are reports of false-positive results in the presence of poppy seeds and quinolone antimicrobials. Opioids are detectable for 1–4 days after use.
- *Benzodiazepines:* These results are likely among the least clinically useful screens. Diazepam is metabolized to oxazepam and would be identified for up to 4 weeks after use. On the other hand, midazolam, lorazepam, and alprazolam remain undetected.

CONCLUSION

Patients present with exposure or overdose of toxins, and on many occasions, there is a diagnostic dilemma. It can be due to partial or incomplete history. The patient may have an accidental or unintentional exposure, and early accurate diagnosis can help to guide acute management or chronic treatment. Point-of-care tests and toxic screens have variability in the sensitivity and specificity that limits their clinical utility. Positive screen tests may still reflect prior use and mislead a clinician for a definitive diagnosis, and a negative screen test is often not able to exclude the use or exposure of the toxic substance.

REFERENCES

1. Price CP. Point of care testing. BMJ. 2001;322(7297):1285-8.
2. Wu AH, McKay C, Broussard LA, Hoffman RS, Kwong TC, Moyer TP, et al. National Academy of Clinical Biochemistry laboratory medicine practice guidelines: recommendations for the use of laboratory tests to support poisoned patients who present to the emergency department. Clin Chem. 2003;49(3):357-79.
3. Wu AH, McKay C, Broussard LA, Hoffman RS, Kwong TC, Moyer TP, et al. National academy of clinical biochemistry laboratory medicine practice guidelines: recommendations for the use of laboratory tests to support poisoned patients who present to the emergency department. Clin Chem. 2003;49(3):357-79.
4. Bhalla A. Bedside point of care toxicology screens in the ED: utility and pitfalls. Int J Crit Illn Inj Sci. 2014;4(3):257-60.
5. Near Patient Testing Working Party, General Haematology Task Force of BCSH, Thrombosis and Haemostasis Task Force of BCSH. Guidelines for near patient testing: haematology. Clin Lab Haematol. 1995;17(4):301-10.
6. Kost GJ, Jammal MA, Ward RE, Safwat AM. Monitoring of ionized calcium during human hepatic transplantation. Critical values and their relevance to cardiac and hemodynamic management. Am J Clin Pathol. 1986;86(1):61-70.
7. St John A, Price CP. Existing and emerging technologies for point-of-care testing. Clin Biochem Rev. 2014;35(3):155-67.
8. Lynd LD, Richardson KJ, Purssell RA, Abu-Laban RB, Brubacher JR, Lepik KJ, et al. An evaluation of the osmole gap as a screening test for toxic alcohol poisoning. BMC Emerg Med. 2008;8:5.
9. Hovda KE, Hunderi OH, Rudberg N, Froyshov S, Jacobsen D. Anion and osmolal gaps in the diagnosis of methanol poisoning: clinical study in 28 patients. Intensive Care Med. 2004;30(9):1842-6.
10. Wei T-Y, Yen T-H, Cheng C-M. Point-of-care testing in the early diagnosis of acute pesticide intoxication: the example of paraquat. Biomicrofluidics. 2018;12(1):011501.
11. Cubitt M, Armstrong J, McCoubrie D, White J, Williams V, Isbister GK. Point-of-care testing in snakebite: an envenomed case with false negative coagulation studies. Emerg Med Australas. 2013;25(4):372-3.
12. Liu XW, Ma T, Li LL, Qu B, Liu Z. Predictive values of urine paraquat concentration, dose of poison, arterial blood lactate and APACHE II score in the prognosis of patients with acute paraquat poisoning. Exp Ther Med. 2017;14(1): 79-86.
13. Gawarammana IB, Buckley NA. Medical management of paraquat ingestion. Br J Clin Pharmacol. 2011;72(5): 745-57.
14. Mukherji P, Azhar Y, Sharma S. Toxicology screening. In: StatPearls. Treasure Island, FL: StatPearls Publishing; 2024.
15. Posin SL, Kong EL, Sharma S. Mercury toxicity. In: StatPearls. Treasure Island, FL: StatPearls Publishing; 2023.
16. Mirghani RA. Current status of point of are testing in clinical toxicology. Point Care. 2008;7(4):266-70.
17. Larkins MC, Thombare A. Point-of-care testing. In: StatPearls. Treasure Island, FL: StatPearls Publishing; 2023.

1.8 Decontamination Following Exposure to the Toxic Agents

Ashish Bhalla, Deba Prasad Dhibar

INTRODUCTION

Decontamination constitutes an important component of the management guideline for intoxication or poisoning. Unfortunately, due to lack of awareness, the decontamination procedure is often neglected or ignored. It does not require great expensive skills or technology but intelligence and awareness among the healthcare workers (HCWs) and first contact persons. Decontamination not only safeguards the victim from additional exposure to the toxic substance but also prevents absorption of the toxic substance into the systemic circulation. It limits the toxic substance to reach its maximum lethal effects before the poison-specific targeted therapeutic approach is undertaken. Thus, decontamination bridges the golden hour of toxicological emergency between exposure to the toxic substance and poison-specific definitive therapy. Besides the routine risk of domestic or industrial exposure and the toxic substance, the risk of criminal or accidental exposure to the chemical, biological, radiological, or nuclear toxic agents (CBRN) cannot be underestimated.[1] So it is the need of the hour to increase awareness regarding postexposure decontamination of the toxic substances among the general population besides the HCWs. Effective external and internal decontamination can be achieved through exposure prevention, skin decontamination, gastrointestinal (GI) decontamination, and agent-specific or targeted determination.

EXPOSURE PREVENTION

Postexposure, the first step to take is to stop further exposure or ingestion to limit additional exposure to the toxic substance. In case of a chemical or gas, stay away from the source of toxic substance, maintain a safe distance, cover with protective cloths or barrier, or hide in a closed/protective space. External decontamination should start as soon as the further exposure is prevented or source of exposure is under control and subsequently reach or ask for healthcare specialist.

SKIN DECONTAMINATION

The skin (stratum corneum of the epidermis) is the first line of defense against any mechanical, chemical, or biological toxic agents. Decontamination of the skin can be initiated earliest at the point of exposure but unfortunately this is neglected due to lack of awareness as well as due to the fear and anxiety following exposure to the toxic agents. Decontamination of the skin prevents further absorption of the toxic substance through the skin into the systemic circulation and also limits the toxic interaction/penetration at the local site, thereby reducing the toxic effects of the substance following the exposure.[2,3]

The most commonly used and readily available decontamination method is washing with plain water or soap and water. Prompt washing and rinsing generously with water may potentially wipe off the toxic chemical from the skin. Decontamination with water works through mechanical wiping off the chemical substance, dilution of the chemical agents, decreasing the rate of absorption or chemical interaction or metabolism, and restoring of the dermal pH in chemical burn.[2-4]

However, the traditional method of decontamination with water does not always work and may be disadvantageous sometimes. With the application of water or soapy water, the toxic substance may be more solubilized, enhancing skin absorption rather than wiping it off, called the wash-in effect. The lipophilic agents may have limited dissolution rates in water rendering them very difficult to be removed, requiring a large amount of water and detergents. To prevent the "wash-in" effect, application of a dry decontamination agent prior to flushing with water or soapy water is recommended.[2-4] Readily available adsorbent materials such as talcum powder, flour, or clays may be used as dry decontaminants during the emergency situations. Fuller's earth (FE) is a commonly used dry decontaminant during military and chemical warfare.

GASTROINTESTINAL DECONTAMINATION

Gastrointestinal decontamination is the practice of removing a poisonous substance from the GI tract. This is done with an intention to reduce the absorption and hasten its clearance to prevent continued absorption.

Forced emesis or aspiration/lavage of the ingested poison, administration of binding agents to prevent the absorption, and speeding up the toxin's transmission through the GI tract to reduce transit time are the standard approaches. With an increased understanding of the gut physiology and characteristics of poisonous substances, there has been a better understanding of the efficacy, and the understanding/recognitions of the risky practices have been abandoned over time.

There have been few clinical studies addressing the risks and benefits of the "routine" practices of GI decontamination. Over time, it has been observed that morbidity and mortality of using these routine interventions in poisoned patients is limited. Still, there are many specific situations/poisons in which GI decontamination may help reduce their absorption.[5-8]

Physiology of Gastrointestinal Emptying

The gastric emptying is a complex physiological pressure, which aims at delivering ingested gastric contents (liquids, digestible solids, indigestible food residues) into the duodenum. The rate of gastric emptying varies with the physical characteristics and caloric density of the food.[9] Water and liquids leave the stomach at a faster rate, with only 50% remaining in the stomach at 10 minutes. The stomach gets rid of nearly 99% liquids by 120 minutes.[9] Digestible and indigestible solids begin to leave the stomach after a lag period, and remain in the stomach for a longer time varying between 3 and 6 hours **(Figs. 1A and B)**.[9] This understanding of gastric emptying

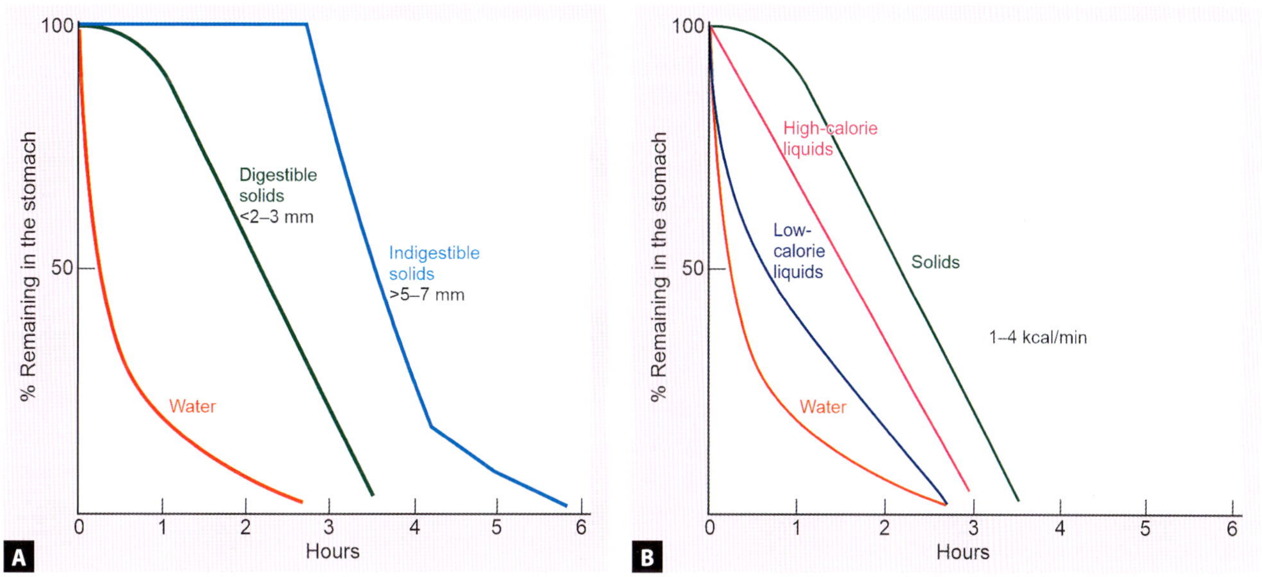

Figs. 1A and B: Gastric emptying rates vary with physical characteristics and caloric density of the food. (A) Effects of the physical characteristics of the food. Water and 5% dextrose leave the stomach at a faster rate. Digestible food particles leave after a lag period, slowly. Indigestible solids leave the stomach after the digestive period. They stay for a long period and then leave rapidly; (B) Water leaves very fast with only 50% remaining at the end of 10 minutes. High-calorie liquids leave the stomach slowly, with >50% remaining in the stomach at the end of 2 hours. Low-calorie liquids leave the stomach at an intermediate rate, 50% emptying by 1 hour.
Source: Adapted from Goyal et al. (2019).[9]

physiology is important to consider gastric lavage in a poisoned patient. It is logical to consider that poisons ingested in liquid form (pesticides) would not be available in the stomach after 2 hours, whereas indigestible solids (plants, seeds, pharmaceutical drugs) would stay in the stomach for a longer period, up to 6 hours, making them conducible to be removed with gastric lavage.

The decision to perform GI decontamination should always be based on the following:

- The type of poison ingested (specific poison)
- Physical form of the poison ingested (solid/liquid)
- Interval between ingestion and presentation at a healthcare facility
- Presenting symptoms
- Perceived or predicted severity of poisoning

Gastrointestinal (GI) decontamination is most likely to benefit when:

- Patients present soon after ingestion (within 1-2 hours).
- Nature of the poisonous substance ingested (solid/liquid) is known.
- Amount ingested is potentially toxic.
- Clinical condition is conducive to perform decontamination.

Gastrointestinal decontamination should *not* be performed:

- If the substance is likely to be nontoxic.
- If the amount ingested is nontoxic.
- If the agent is rapidly absorbed.
- If there is delayed presentation.
- If the substance ingested is not amenable to decontamination.

The decision to decontaminate the GI tract should be taken by an experienced practitioner. The risk of performing decontamination of the GI tract should be weighed against the potential benefits of removing the toxin and the complications likely to result from the intervention.

SYRUP OF IPECAC

Forced emesis is a common first response of the family members and is usually performed by them in turn to clear/empty the stomach. Forced emesis using syrup of ipecac is no longer recommended by the American Academy of Clinical Toxicology (AACT), the European Association of Poisons Centers and Clinical Toxicologists (EAPCCT), or the American Association of Pediatrics (AAP)[10,11] as an intervention in hospitalized patients. Injury and aspiration are the most feared risks associated.

GASTRIC LAVAGE

It is an intervention aimed at emptying the stomach by means of a large-bore orogastric tube. This is followed by repetitive instillation of a neutral liquid (water/saline) and attempted aspiration, using small aliquots of fluid. The aim is to attempt aspiration of toxins from within the stomach. This modality is largely being abandoned due to unclear benefit of the intervention coupled with the risk of serious respiratory complications.

Indications

International societies and experts have recommended that gastric lavage should not be employed routinely in the management of poisoned patients.[12] The decision to consider gastric lavage needs to be individualized if the lethal dose has been consumed orally and the patient reports early (within 12 hours) of the alleged consumption.[13] The clinicians should be aware of the doubtful benefits and associated risks. Since many pharmaceutical agents have a tendency to form bezoars in the stomach, gastric lavage should be avoided. If possible and available, endoscopic removal of the toxin may be considered. Endoscopic gastric evacuation may also be considered if seeds, button batteries, large tablets/capsules, or sharp-edged solids have been ingested.

Some of the poisonings in which early (within 2 hours) gastric lavage may be considered are the following:

- Pesticide ingestion
- Herbicide ingestion
- Energy drinks
- Recreational drugs/club drugs

Contraindications

Gastric lavage should never be performed in patients with the following:

- Unprotected airway
- Caustic ingestion (ingestion of corrosive)
- Hydrocarbon ingestion (due to high aspiration risk)
- Patients at risk of GI hemorrhage or perforation:
  - Recent surgery
  - Known anatomic abnormality or pathology
  - Significant coagulopathy

Complications

Gastric lavage may lead to complications such as the following[12-14]:

- Aspiration pneumonia
- Esophageal or gastric perforation
- Laryngospasm
- Hypoxia
- Dysrhythmia
- Fluid or electrolyte imbalance

Gastric lavage may also push toxic substances beyond the pylorus, thereby facilitating systemic toxicity and decreasing effectiveness of activated charcoal (AC).[15]

ENDOSCOPY

Endoscopic removal of poisons can be considered if a life-threatening poisonous substance has been ingested and it is not possible to remove it by gastric lavage. This includes lethal amounts of heavy metals or sustained-release agents forming bezoars.

Surgical removal is indicated in body packers (ingestion of large drug packets). Risk of rupture and subsequent potential for toxicity makes endoscopy risky in body packers.[16]

CATHARTICS

Cathartics (magnesium sulfate, sorbitol, mannitol) are not routinely recommended as single-agent therapy.[17] Adverse effects of cathartic preclude their administration. They can result in abdominal pain, vomiting, diarrhea, and dehydration. Electrolyte abnormalities may be life threatening in critically ill patients and may potentiate toxicity of ingested poisons.

DILUTION/NEUTRALIZATION

Dilution/neutralization for acidic or alkaline ingestion may result in tissue damage and is hence not recommended.

WHOLE BOWEL IRRIGATION

This is reserved for patients who have ingested toxic foreign bodies (e.g., drug packets), sustained-release or enteric-coated pharmaceutical agents, or toxic materials not bound by AC (e.g., heavy metals).[18]

This intervention is aimed at preventing the absorption of toxins by reducing its contact with the intestinal mucosa. This is achieved by increasing GI motility and hastening the passage of the GI contents through the small/large bowel.[18] Whole bowel irrigation (WBI)/*whole gut lavage* is basically an evolved catharsis concept. A high-molecular-weight substance, generally polyethylene glycol (PEG) solution, is administered orally/via a nasogastric (NG) tube. It is generally combined with intravenous (IV) administration of iso-osmolar electrolyte balanced solution to prevent metabolic side effects of catharsis. This combination tends to prevent systemic electrolyte disturbances that complicate the use of cathartics alone. Large volumes of PEG plus water are administered orally or by a NG tube in a patient who has consumed toxic substances which are indigestible/slow dissolving or may get digested in the small intestine. The administration is continued till rectal effluent is clear.[18]

Important adverse effects associated are nausea, vomiting, and metabolic/electrolyte disturbances. It is also difficult to administer WBI in uncooperative patients and it requires good nursing/supportive care to keep the patient clean.

Whole bowel irrigation is contraindicated in patients with bowel obstruction or perforation. It is also contraindicated in corrosive ingestion.

Whole bowel irrigation may be considered in cases where there has been a long time lag (>2 hours) between ingestion and treatment. Other conditions in which WBI may be indicated are body packers, heavy metal ingestion, or ingestion of a toxic plant (leaves, stem, or seeds).

Whole bowel irrigation should always be performed in a hospitalized setting where vitals and electrolytes can be carefully/continuously monitored. While performing WBI in body packers, clinicians must be vigilant regarding the possible rupture of the drug packets which may result in severe intoxication.

INTERVENTIONS TO DECREASE ABSORPTION OF TOXIN

Activated Charcoal

Activated charcoal is a potential adsorbent powder with a large surface area to soak up the toxins. It is made from superheated, organic material by pyrolysis. The basic principle for administration is the presumption that AC would adsorb the toxins released by poisonous substances ingested for self-harm. It is pertinent to note that not all poisonous substances can be adsorbed; the classic examples are hydrocarbons and heavy metals. In contrast, the degree to which AC is able to bind to toxins in the GI tract is variable. Adsorption would depend on the inherent characteristics of the toxin and the dose of toxin/charcoal administered. In patients with alleged ingestion of pharmaceutical agents and plant poisons, even delayed administration of AC may be beneficial.[5-8]

Contraindications

Contraindications include the following:

- Altered mental status/Glasgow Coma Scale (GCS) <9, with no airway protection (risk of aspiration outweighs the benefit)
- Late presentation (except plant poison/pharmaceuticals)
- Hydrocarbon/pesticides/corrosive/heavy metals/alcohol ingestion
- When endoscopy is needed (likely to impair visibility)
- Presence of intestinal obstruction (absolute contraindication)

Dose

If the amount of poison ingested is known, dose of activated charcoal is in the ratio of 10:1. If an unknown quantity is ingested, follow the below-mentioned regimen:[5]

- Children (up to 1 year): 0.5–1.0 g/kg
- Children (1–12 years): 0.5–1.0 g/kg (maximum dose 50 g)
- Adolescents and adults: 25–100 g

Administration

Activated charcoal is available as both a powder and premixed suspension. Powder should be mixed with water to form slurry.[19,20] AC is also available as suspension premixed with sorbitol, which acts as an adsorbent as well as a cathartic.[21,22]

Complications

Activated charcoal is usually very well tolerated.[5] Common GI side effects are fullness, abdominal pain, nausea, vomiting, and constipation.[5] Chances of aspiration increase if AC and gastric lavage are combined.[23,24]

Multidose Activated Charcoal

In some conditions, a repeat dose of AC may be beneficial. These benefits are reported if:

- Proven or suspected enterohepatic recirculation of toxin
- Ingestion of extended- or delayed-release formulations
- Suspected transluminal diffusion of toxin. Here, AC acts as "gut dialysate."

Multidose AC (MDAC) *may* be helpful if the following are ingested:[6]

- Carbamazepine
- Dapsone
- Phenobarbital

- Quinine
- Theophylline
- Caffeine (energy drinks)
- Acetylsalicylic acid (aspirin)
- Phenytoin

Clinical data are still insufficient to suggest routine use of MDAC in suspected/proven overdose of amitriptyline, digoxin, disopyramide, nadolol, and piroxicam overdose.[6]

Contraindications include the presence of intestinal obstruction (absolute) or concern for decreased peristalsis (relative).

Dose

After the initial loading dose, repeat dose can be administered as 12.5 g/h, or the equivalent. An acceptable regimen is to administer 50 g every 4 hours.[25]

Unusual Circumstances

However, routinely used decontamination method may not work during exposure to the chemical warfare agents (CWAs) and radioactive agents for accidental or criminal events. Very limited available specific decontamination agents should be used during this situation for effective decontamination.

Chemical warfare agents enter the body and systemic circulation very fast due to the ease of skin permeation, producing lethal effects in the exposed person. Decontamination method should be prompt and efficient to minimize the extent of damage. Besides the routinely used water or soapy water, additionally, dry decontamination with an adsorbent material has to be initiated promptly. Commonly used dry decontamination agents during the mass exposure to the CWAs are FE and Canadian reactive skin decontamination lotion (RSDL).

Fuller's earth with a large specific surface area (180 m^2/g) possesses high affinity for the lipophilic molecules with no or minimal skin penetration into. It is very efficacious to remove CWAs after their exposure to the VX (nerve agent) and ^{14}C-methyl salicylate.[26] It can significantly reduce the penetration of the VX, HD (mustard gas), and GD (soman, nerve agent) through damaged and undamaged skin.[27] Potential adverse effects of FE are skin irritation following prolonged contact and may be inhaled, a respiratory health hazard.

Application of RSDL directly on the skin is a standard practice for the adsorption and neutralization of CWAs following exposure to the V-series and G-series nerve agents and sulfur mustard (SM) chemical agents. RSDL contains polyethylene glycol monomethyl ether (mPEG), which adsorbs the chemical agents and a reactive oxime [diacetyl monoxime (DAM)] to neutralize chemical agents. It is highly efficacious against a high concentration of vesicants or nerve agents and it is immediately effective compared with the other decontamination agents.[28,29] But the effectiveness of the RSDL reduces significantly in delayed application of 90–120 minutes after the exposure to the CWA. To extract the best neutralizing effect, it is advisable to apply decontamination agents at the earliest following exposure to the CWA.

Exposure to the radionuclides such as uranium (U), plutonium (Pu), americium (Am), and radioisotopes like technetium-99m (^{99m}Tc), iodine-131 (^{131}I), and thallium-201 (^{201}Tl) can occur as occupational hazards, accidental exposure, or nuclear/criminal warfare.[30] Unfortunately, there is no definitive proven method for cutaneous decontamination following exposure to the radioactive materials. Thus, prevention of further exposure, minimizing the exposure by being at a safer distance or in bunkers, and wearing radiation protective suits or shields at occupational places are the best measures that can be undertaken.[30] Self-decontamination by simple removal of clothes is what is recommended. Double bagging of all radioactive contaminated clothes is needed for safe disposal.[30] Washing of hands, face, and parts of the exposed body with plenty of water and soapy water is encouraged for the external decontamination of a radioactive material following exposure. A gentle shower under the water and application of shampoo to hair can be also considered. Rigorous rubbing or scratching of the skin should be avoided to protect the skin from mechanical tears.[30] Use of chelating agents, such as ethane-1-hydroxy-1,1-biphosphonate (EHBP), diethylenetriaminepentaacetic acid (DTPA), and ethylenediaminetetraacetic acid (EDTA), is still at an experimental level, and the safety and efficacy are yet to be proven in human studies.

CONCLUSION

Decontamination is an important intervention in critically ill poisoned patients. Indiscriminate and improper use of decontamination procedures may lead to serious complications. Simple removal of clothes and washing the skin can take care of nearly 90% of the contamination. Decision to perform gastric decontamination and the modality to be used must be based on the time interval between ingestion and intervention, the nature of the poison, and the presumed benefit of the intervention. The clinicians must carefully weigh the risks and benefits of a particular modality before intervention is initiated. Throughout the procedure, the patient should be carefully monitored for possible complications. Securing the airway just to perform gastric decontamination in a critically ill poisoned patient should not be encouraged, as intubation in an unstable patient may be associated with significant cardiovascular morbidity.

REFERENCES

1. Singh VK, Garcia M, Wise SY, Seed TM. Medical countermeasures for unwanted CBRN exposures: Part I chemical and biological threats with review of recent countermeasure patents., Expert Opin Ther Pat. 2016;26(12):1431-47.
2. Magnano GC, Rui F, Filon FL. Skin decontamination procedures against potential hazards substances exposure. Chem Biol Interact. 2021;344:109481.
3. Chan HP, Zhai H, Hui X, Maibach HI. Skin decontamination: principles and perspectives. Toxicol Ind Health. 2013;29(10):955-68.
4. Hall A, Maibach HI. Water decontamination of chemical skin/eye splashes: a critical review. Cutan Ocul Toxicol. 2006;25:67-83.
5. Chyka PA, Seger D, Krenzelok EP, Vale JA; American Academy of Clinical Toxicology; European Association of Poisons Centres and Clinical Toxicologists. Position paper: single-dose activated charcoal. Clin Toxicol (Phila). 2005;43:61.
6. Position statement and practice guidelines on the use of multi-dose activated charcoal in the treatment of acute poisoning. American Academy of Clinical Toxicology; European Association of Poisons Centres and Clinical Toxicologists. J Toxicol Clin Toxicol. 1999;37:731.
7. Thanacoody R, Caravati EM, Troutman B, Höjer J, Benson B, Hoppu K, et al. Position paper update: whole bowel irrigation for gastrointestinal decontamination of overdose patients. Clin Toxicol (Phila). 2015;53:5.
8. Hoegberg LCG, Shepherd G, Wood DM, Johnson J, Hoffman RS, Caravati EM, et al. Systematic review on the use of activated charcoal for gastrointestinal decontamination following acute oral overdose. Clin Toxicol (Phila). 2021;59:1196.
9. Goyal RK, Guo Y, Mashimo H. Advances in physiology of gastric emptying. Neurogastroenterol Motil. 2019; 31:e13546.
10. Höjer J, Troutman WG, Hoppu K, Erdman A, Benson BE, Mégarbane B, et al. Position paper update: ipecac syrup for gastrointestinal decontamination. Clin Toxicol (Phila). 2013;51:134.
11. American Academy of Pediatrics Committee on Injury, Violence, and Poison Prevention. Poison treatment in the home. American Academy of Pediatrics Committee on Injury, Violence, and Poison Prevention. Pediatrics. 2003;112:1182.
12. Benson BE, Hoppu K, Troutman WG, Bedry R, Erdman A, Höjer J, et al. Position paper update: gastric lavage for gastrointestinal decontamination. Clin Toxicol (Phila). 2013;51:140.
13. Kulig K, Bar-Or D, Cantrill SV, Rosen P, Rumack BH. Management of acutely poisoned patients without gastric emptying. Ann Emerg Med. 1985;14:562.
14. Merigian KS, Woodard M, Hedges JR, Roberts JR, Stuebing R, Rashkin MC. Prospective evaluation of gastric emptying in the self-poisoned patient. Am J Emerg Med. 1990;8:479.
15. Saetta JP, March S, Gaunt ME, Quinton DN. Gastric emptying procedures in the self-poisoned patient: are we forcing gastric content beyond the pylorus? J R Soc Med. 1991;84:274.
16. Trent MS, Kim U. Cocaine packet ingestion. Surgical or medical management? Arch Surg. 1987;122:1179.
17. Position paper: cathartics. J Toxicol Clin Toxicol. 2004; 42:243.
18. Hendrikson RG, Kusin S. Gastrointestinal decontamination in a poisoned patient. [online] Available from https://www.uptodate.com/contents/gastrointestinal-decontamination-of-the-poisoned-patient [Last accessed September, 2024].
19. West L. Innovative approaches to the administration of activated charcoal in pediatric toxic ingestions. Pediatr Nurs. 1997;23:616.
20. Canitrot E, Turgeon AF, Moore L, Diendéré E, St-Onge M. Effect of taste additives on the palatability of activated charcoal: a systematic review. J Med Toxicol. 2023;19:268.
21. Gwilt PR, Perrier D. Influence of "thickening" agents on the antidotal efficacy of activated charcoal. Clin Toxicol. 1976;9:89.
22. Minocha A, Herold DA, Bruns DE, Spyker DA. Effect of activated charcoal in 70% sorbitol in healthy individuals. J Toxicol Clin Toxicol. 1984;22:529.
23. Cooper GM, Le Couteur DG, Richardson D, Buckley NA. A randomized clinical trial of activated charcoal for the routine management of oral drug overdose. QJM. 2005;98:655.
24. Merigian KS, Blaho KE. Single-dose oral activated charcoal in the treatment of the self-poisoned patient: a prospective, randomized, controlled trial. Am J Ther. 2002;9:301.
25. Ilkhanipour K, Yealy DM, Krenzelok EP. The comparative efficacy of various multiple-dose activated charcoal regimens. Am J Emerg Med. 1992;10:298.
26. Thors L, Koch M, Wigenstam E, Koch B, Hägglund L, Bucht A. Comparison of skin decontamination efficacy of commercial decontamination products following exposure to VX on human skin. Chem Biol Interact. 2017;273:82-9.

27. Lydon HL, Hall CA, Dalton CH, Kevin Chipman J, Graham JS, Chilcott RP. Development of haemostatic decontaminants for treatment of wounds contaminated with chemical warfare agents. 3: evaluation of in vitro topical decontamination efficacy using damaged skin. J Appl Toxicol. 2017;37(8):976-84.
28. Schwartz MD, Hurst CG, Kirk MA, Reedy SJD, Braue EH. Reactive skin decontamination lotion (RSDL) for the decontamination of chemical warfare agent (CWA) dermal exposure. Curr Pharm Biotechnol. 2012;13(10):1971-9.
29. Taysse L, Daulon S, Delamanche S, Bellier B, Breton P. Skin decontamination of mustards and organophosphates: comparative efficiency of RSDL and Fuller's earth in domestic swine. Hum Exp Toxicol. 2007;26(2):135-41.
30. Cibulsky SM, Sokolowsky D, Lafontaine M, Gagnon C, Blain PG, Russell D, et al. Mass casualty decontamination in a chemical or radiological/nuclear incident with external contamination: guiding principles and research needs. PLoS Curr. 2015:7.

1.9 Drugs (Drugs Commonly Used to Manage a Sick Patient; Not Antidotes)

Manu Ayyan, Vinodha Chandrasekar, Ezhilkugen Ganessane

INTRODUCTION

Intoxicated patients present with various signs and symptoms. Antidotes directly bind and neutralize specific toxins and are certainly a crucial component of treating poisoning. However, it is important to recognize that many other medications play critical supportive roles in the management of poisoned patients **(Table 1)**. Although they do not directly act as antidotes, these adjunctive therapies can help minimize the morbidity and mortality associated with toxic ingestions or exposures. Also, it may not be always possible to find the toxic agent and hence the antidote. Thus, it is important to know drugs other than antidotes to be used in poisoning.

PHARMACOKINETIC CONSIDERATIONS IN CLINICAL TOXICOLOGY

In overdose situations, the processes of absorption, distribution, metabolism, and excretion (ADME) can be significantly altered compared to therapeutic doses. For example, absorption may be prolonged due to decreased gut motility or saturable transporters. Distribution can be affected by changes in protein binding and pH which impact the free, active concentration of a poison. Metabolism may be saturated at high doses, resulting in nonlinear kinetics. Excretion can also demonstrate capacity-limited processes. A thorough understanding of these toxicokinetic concepts allows for better interpretation of plasma concentrations for risk assessment, determining the required duration of monitoring, optimizing antidote dosing, and evaluating enhanced elimination techniques. They highlight the complex interrelationship between the poison dose, patient factors, and pathophysiological changes in ADME processes. A strong grasp of toxicokinetic and toxicodynamic principles should be an essential skill for all clinicians and researchers taking part in the management of acute poisoning. The altered ADME processes in overdose situations have important implications for risk stratification based on plasma concentrations, poison monitoring times, antidote administration, and enhanced elimination interventions.[1]

DRUGS USED IN RESUSCITATION OF POISONING PATIENTS

Resuscitation in any poisoning is of paramount importance whatever may be the antidote. Resuscitation includes stabilizing the airway, breathing, and circulation. Rapid sequence intubation (RSI) involves the use of medications to facilitate endotracheal intubation in an acute care setting. This may be necessary in poisoning situations when a patient has severely compromised airway reflexes or respiratory drive.

Induction Agents

Etomidate

Etomidate is an imidazole derivative, nonbarbiturate hypnotic agent. It is an ultrashort-acting induction agent and has a rapid onset of action. It acts by potentiating gamma-aminobutyric acid (GABA)-A receptors which

TABLE 1: Supportive drugs other than antidote used to manage poisoned patients.

Drug	***Indication***	***Adult dose***	***Pediatric dose***	***Adverse effects***
Pyridoxine	Isoniazid-induced seizure	5 g	70 mg/kg	Sensory neuropathy—only in chronic use
lidocaine	Ventricular arrhythmias in TCA, cocaine, MAOI	1–1.5 mg/kg	1–1.5 mg/kg	
Amiodarone	Ventricular arrhythmias in MAOI and aconite	150 mg IV	2.5 mg/kg	Hypotension, QT prolongation
Sodium bicarbonate	TCA-induced ventricular arrhythmias	1–2 mEq/kg IV	1–2 mEq/kg IV	Hypokalemia
Magnesium sulfate	• TdP, TCA, digoxin, cocaine, and antipsychotic induce arrhythmias • Methanol and ethylene glycol poisoning	2 g IV	25–50 mg/kg	Respiratory depression
Midazolam	Induction agent, seizure control	0.15–0.4 mg/kg IV (intranasal: 0.2–0.3 mg/kg)	Same as adult	Nausea, vomiting, hypotension
Etomidate	Induction agent for rapid sequence intubation	0.2–0.4 mg/kg IV	Same as adult	Myoclonus, adrenal suppression
Ketamine	Rapid sequence intubation, especially in organophosphorus poisoning	1–2 mg/kg IV	Same as adult	Increased cardiac output and blood pressure, bronchodilation
Propofol	Anesthesia, sedation, seizure control	1–2.5 mg/kg IV	Same as adult	Hypotension, respiratory depression
Succinylcholine	Depolarizing neuromuscular blocker for intubation	1–1.5 mg/kg IV	2 mg/kg in patients weighing <10 kg	Prolonged muscle paralysis, especially in certain poisonings
Rocuronium	Nondepolarizing neuromuscular blocker for intubation	1–1.2 mg/kg IV	Same as adult	Limited physical manifestations of seizures
Vecuronium	Nondepolarizing neuromuscular blocker	Dose varies based on condition 0.08–0.1 mg/kg IV	0.1 mg/kg IV	Increased heart rate and blood pressure
Phenylephrine	Vasopressor in peripheral vasodilatory shock	10–200 µg/min IV	Dose varies based on condition	Reflex tachycardia, headache, hypertension
Norepinephrine	Vasopressor in hypotensive shock	0.5–50 µg/min IV	Dose varies based on condition	Vasoconstriction, hypertension, arrhythmias
Epinephrine	Severe hypotension and shock	0.5–8 µg/kg/min IV	Dose varies based on condition	Tachycardia, arrhythmias, hypertension
Dopamine	Inotrope in hypotension and shock	2.5–20 µg/kg/min IV	Same as adult	Tachyarrhythmias, vasoconstriction
Dobutamine	Inotropic support in heart failure	5–20 µg/kg/min IV	Same as adult	Tachyarrhythmias, hypotension
Vasopressin	Vasoconstrictor in shock	0.01–0.04 U/min IV	0.0002–0.002 U/kg/min	Ischemia, water intoxication

Contd...

Contd...

Drug	Indication	Adult dose	Pediatric dose	Adverse effects
Milrinone	Phosphodiesterase inhibitor in beta-blocker toxicity	Bolus: 50 µg/kg IV, and then 0.375–0.75 µg/kg/min infusion	50 mics/kg IV f/b 0.25–0.75 µg/kg/min	Arrhythmias, hypotension
Lorazepam	First-line anticonvulsant	2–4 mg IV	0.05–0.1 mg/kg IV over 2–5 minutes; not to exceed 4 mg/dose; may repeat q10–15 minutes PRN	Sedation, respiratory depression
Diazepam	First-line anticonvulsant	5–10 mg IV	*Status epilepticus:* • Children >30 days to 5 years: 0.2–0.5 mg slowly q2-5 minutes up to 5 mg maximum (IV preferred) • Children ≥5 years: 1 mg q2-5 minutes up to a maximum of 10 mg	Sedation, respiratory depression
Phenobarbital	Second-line anticonvulsant	15–20 mg/kg IV	Same as adult	Sedation, respiratory depression
Esmolol	Short-acting beta blocker in hypertension	500 µg/kg IV loading, and then 50 µg/kg/min	Same as adult	Hypotension, bradycardia
Nitroprusside	Vasodilator in hypertensive emergencies	0.5–4 µg/kg/min IV	Same as adult	Hypotension, cyanide toxicity
Phentolamine	α-Adrenergic antagonist in hypertensive emergencies	2.5–5 mg IV boluses, and then 0.2–0.5 mg/min	0.1–0.2 mg/kg IV	Reflex tachycardia, hypotension
Ascorbic acid (vitamin C)	Methemoglobinemia	Up to 10 g IV	Dose varies	Transient renal side effects
Cyproheptadine	Serotonin syndrome	12 mg initially, and then 2 mg every 2 hours	Dose varies	Sedation, dry mouth
Chlorpromazine	Serotonin syndrome	• 0.5 mg/kg (maximum 25 mg) in sodium chloride 0.9%, 10 mL/kg (maximum 500 mL) IV, over 30–60 minutes • Repeat the dose every 6–8 hours until symptoms resolve, provided the patient is not hypotensive	–	Hypotension, extrapyramidal symptoms
Dantrolene	Serotonin syndrome, neuroleptic malignant syndrome	1–2.5 mg/kg IV	Same as adult	Muscle weakness, liver toxicity
Bromocriptine	Neuroleptic malignant syndrome	2.5 mg PO 3–4 times a day	Same as adult	Hypotension, nausea, hallucinations
Amantadine	Neuroleptic malignant syndrome	100 mg PO TDS	–	Dizziness, dry mouth

Contd...

Contd...

Drug	Indication	Adult dose	Pediatric dose	Adverse effects
Metadoxine	Ethanol toxicity	900 mg IV	–	Rare, generally well tolerated
Folic acid	Methanol, ethylene glycol poisoning	1 mg/kg IV (up to 50 mg)	Same as adult	Allergic reactions, gastrointestinal discomfort
Thiamine	Ethylene glycol poisoning	100 mg IV	Same as adult	Rare, hypersensitivity reactions
Aspirin	Cocaine-induced acute coronary syndrome	162–325 mg	Same as adult	Gastrointestinal bleeding, allergic reactions
NTG	Cocaine-induced acute coronary syndrome	• S/L NTG: 0.3–0.4 mg • IV: 5–20 mics/min; maximum 400 mics/min	–	Headache, hypotension
Diltiazem	Cocaine-induced acute coronary syndrome	5–20 mg IV	Hypertension: 1.5–2 mg/kg PO	Bradycardia, hypotension
L-Carnitine	Valproic acid poisoning	100 mg/kg IV initially, and then 50 mg/kg every 8 hours	Same as adult	Gastrointestinal discomfort, seizures (rare)
Ipratropium bromide	Organophosphorus poisoning	250 mics	Same as adult	Dry mouth, headache

(f/b: followed by; IV: intravenously; MAOI: monoamine oxidase inhibitor; NTG: nitroglycerine; PO: per os; PRN: pro re nata; S/L: sublingual; TCA: tricyclic antidepressant; TdP: Torsades de Pointes; TDS: thrice a day)

leads to hyperpolarization of chloride channels and neuronal inhibition. Etomidate also potentiates central alpha-2 receptors, hence does not cause cardiovascular instability. The dose of etomidate is 0.2–0.4 mg/kg. Etomidate is also known to cause brief myoclonus. It also can cause adrenal suppression by inhibiting 11-β-hydroxylase enzyme which is transient in nature. It can be widely used in all poisonings.[2,3]

Ketamine

As a phencyclidine derivative, ketamine offers a safe option for RSI in cases of poisoning. The usual dose is 1–2 mg/kg. Ketamine is known to have sympathomimetic effects, thus preserving the cardiac output and blood pressure. Studies also have shown that ketamine due to its bronchodilator effect and antiepileptic property can preferably be used in organophosphorus poisoning.[3-5]

Midazolam

Widely utilized for induction, midazolam is a benzodiazepine that targets GABA receptors. It acts on GABA receptors and increases the frequency of chloride channel opening. This mechanism of action of midazolam is responsible for the properties like anxiolysis, sedation, and antiepileptic and anterograde amnesia. The usual induction dose is 0.15–0.40 mg/kg intravenously (IV). Midazolam can also be given intramuscularly (IM) and intranasally. Intranasal dose is 0.2–0.3 mg/kg commonly used in children. Some adverse effects of midazolam are nausea, vomiting, and hypotension.

Propofol

Used in anesthesia and sedation, propofol acts swiftly and is dosed at 1–2.5 mg/kg. The major adverse effect of propofol is hypotension as it causes vasodilation by antagonizing sympathetic vasoconstriction. Hence, consider avoiding its use in overdoses causing hypotension like organophosphorus, beta-blocker, and calcium channel blocker poisonings.

Neuromuscular Blocking Agents

Succinylcholine is a depolarizing neuromuscular blocker (NMB) used commonly during RSI. It is rapid and short acting. It gives an ideal condition for intubation. The usual dose is 1–1.5 mg/kg. There are few poisonings where succinylcholine is not preferred. It is better to avoid succinylcholine in organophosphorus poisoning, which can lead to prolonged muscle paralysis. This is due to blockage of pseudocholinesterase by organophosphorus compound, which is required for metabolism of succinylcholine. It is also contraindicated in neuromalignant syndrome. The best alternative is rocuronium, a nondepolarizing NMB. The usual dose is 1–1.2 mg/kg. It provides a similar condition as succinylcholine while intubation whose action lasts for 50 minutes. NMB can halt the physical signs of seizure, like muscle contractions, and also can prevent metabolic acidosis, hyperthermia, rhabdomyolysis, and renal failure. However, these NMB cannot stop the abnormal electrical activity in the brain that causes seizures. So after using NMB, antiepileptics should be continued with continuous electroencephalogram (EEG) monitoring. In neuroleptic malignant syndrome and monoamine oxidase inhibitor (MAOI) toxicity, it is advisable to opt for nondepolarizing drugs, such as rocuronium, over depolarizing agents such as succinylcholine. Vecuronium is preferred over pancuronium as pancuronium has the propensity to increase heart rate and blood pressure.

Vasopressors/Inotropes

Phenylephrine

By activating alpha-1 adrenergic receptors on smooth muscle cells in blood vessels, phenylephrine primarily induces vasoconstriction, leading to increased blood pressure. Unlike some other sympathomimetic agents, phenylephrine has little effect on beta-adrenergic receptors, which are found predominantly in heart muscle cells. Therefore, phenylephrine increases blood pressure without directly stimulating cardiac contractility or heart rate like some other adrenergic agonists. The dose of phenylephrine is 10–200 mics/min. The vasoconstriction caused by phenylephrine also increases the volume of blood returning to the heart (venous return). This enhances cardiac preload, further supporting an increase in blood pressure. Administering high-dose phenylephrine is considered an effective and reasonable choice in patients with peripheral vasodilatory shock seen in poisoning by β-adrenergic antagonists such as labetalol, carvedilol, betaxolol, bucindolol, carteolol, celiprolol, and nebivolol. Vasopressin may also be helpful in poisoning by cardiotoxic drugs such as verapamil by increasing systemic vascular resistance and blood pressure.[6]

Norepinephrine

Targeting mainly alpha receptors, with some beta-receptor action, norepinephrine effectively raises blood pressure through vasoconstriction and has additional positive inotropic and chronotropic effects. The dose is 0.5–50 mics/min. It is used in calcium channel blocker and beta-blocker toxicity where hypotension is associated with bradycardia. Norepinephrine is also the preferred inotrope of choice in MAOI-induced hypotension as in MAOI toxicity, the norepinephrine is displaced from the nerve terminals by false neurotransmitters like octopamine leading to hypotension.[6]

Epinephrine

Epinephrine has both alpha- and beta-adrenergic actions. At a dose of 0.5–8 mics/kg/min, its action predominantly is enhancing cardiac contractility. When the dose is >8 mics/kg/min, it causes vasoconstriction. Epinephrine is used in calcium channel blocker and beta-blocker toxicity. Severe MAOI toxicity can cause bradycardia and hypotension and has a poor prognosis. Epinephrine can be used in this situation.[6] Epinephrine is found to be superior to norepinephrine in tricyclic antidepressant (TCA)-induced hypotension especially when combined with sodium bicarbonate as it improves the myocardial perfusion better than norepinephrine.

Dopamine

Dopamine has alpha, beta, and dopaminergic actions. At a dose of 2.5–5 mics/kg/min, dopamine increases cardiac contractility. While increasing the dose to 5–20 mics/kg/min, it has vasoconstrictive action. At a dose <2 mics/kg/min, it has a vasodilatory action. The most common side effect of dopamine is tachyarrhythmias. Dopamine is again preferably used in calcium channel blocker and beta-blocker toxicity. It is relatively contraindicated in MAOI-induced hypotension as its indirect action can have synergistic action with MAOI and can lead to increased adrenergic effect and shoot up the blood pressure. Also, it is avoided as it may not be effective in increasing the blood pressure while there is an alpha blockage which may lead to dopamine-induced vasodilation and thus further reduce the blood pressure.[6]

Dobutamine

Acting as an inodilator, dobutamine primarily targets the beta-1 receptor, enhancing cardiac contractility and stroke volume, while its beta-2-adrenergic effects promote vasodilation and reduce the afterload which again helps in increased cardiac output. The dose ranges from 5 to

20 mics/kg/min. The adverse effect of dobutamine is tachyarrhythmias and rarely can also cause hypotension.[6] Dobutamine can be used in beta-blocker and calcium channel blocker toxicity.

Vasopressin

Vasopressin increases blood pressure primarily by vasoconstriction. It acts on the V1 receptor of the smooth muscles. The usual dose is 0.01–0.04 U/min. Infusion is usually started with the maximum dose and it is not titrated.[6]

Phosphodiesterase Inhibitors

Phosphodiesterase inhibitors such as milrinone have been used to treat beta-blocker toxicity. These agents inhibit the breakdown of cyclic adenosine monophosphate (cAMP), thereby sustaining intracellular calcium levels. In animal models, phosphodiesterase inhibitors produce positive inotropic effects without increasing myocardial oxygen demand but have no appreciable effect on heart rate. Combined with glucagon, phosphodiesterase inhibitors do not provide any additional benefit and therefore have no advantage over glucagon. However, if glucagon is not available or pharmacy stores have been exhausted, a phosphodiesterase inhibitor can be a reasonable alternative. In the setting of a beta-blocker overdose, milrinone can be administered as a continuous IV infusion, starting with a 50-µg/kg IV bolus, followed by an IV infusion of 0.375–0.75 µg/kg/min for milrinone.[7]

ANTIEPILEPTICS

Seizures can manifest in several drug intoxication states as well as during withdrawal. Research indicates that around 6% of new-onset seizures and 9% of status epilepticus cases are caused by drug toxicity. Seizures commonly present in intoxications involving certain pharmacological agents such as TCAs, cocaine, methamphetamine, isoniazid, and tramadol. Furthermore, seizures may arise during the withdrawal stages of medications like opioids and alcohol. The majority of seizures precipitated by pharmacological agents tend to be self-limiting in nature and do not impart long-term neurological consequences. While most drug-induced seizures do not impart long-term consequences, prolonged or repetitive epileptic activity may cause irreversible brain damage. Additionally, other life-threatening systemic complications may arise from uncontrolled seizure states, including hypoxia, hypotension, aspiration pneumonia, hyperthermia, rhabdomyolysis, and metabolic acidosis.

Lorazepam, midazolam, and diazepam are first-line anticonvulsants for treating seizures due to drug toxicity. Typical IV doses are 2–4 mg for lorazepam, 0.05–0.2 mg/kg (or 0.1–0.2 mg/kg IM if IV access is unavailable) for midazolam, and 5–10 mg for diazepam. It is important to rule out other seizure causes like hypoglycemia or electrolyte abnormalities. If seizures continue despite first-line drugs, consider second-line anticonvulsants like phenobarbital (5–15 mg/kg IV) or propofol (1–2 mg/kg IV). If seizures persist even after second-line drugs, start a continuous infusion of midazolam, propofol, or a barbiturate.

Benzodiazepines

When treating drug-induced seizures, benzodiazepines are frequently advised as the first-line anticonvulsant medication. By increasing the frequency of chloride channel opening, benzodiazepines increase GABA-A activity and cause neuronal hyperpolarization. IV midazolam is also commonly used; however, IV lorazepam is the recommended first-line benzodiazepine if it is available. IV lorazepam was found to be more effective for stopping status epilepticus than IV diazepam or IV phenytoin alone, according to a Cochrane review and a sizable randomized controlled study for status epilepticus of any origin. Midazolam has an advantage that it can be administered IM if IV access is not easily accessible.[8-10] Other uses of benzodiazepine in poisoning are sedation and hyperthermia management.

Benzodiazepines for Sedation

Drugs causing agitation: Drugs causing agitation include sympathomimetic drugs, anticholinergic drugs, drug withdrawal like alcohol, benzodiazepine, and other substance withdrawal; and metabolic disturbances caused by poisonings such as salicylate, lithium, and organophosphate poisonings.

Benzodiazepines like lorazepam and diazepam can be the foundation for sedation therapy when there is too much autonomic and brain stimulation. Lorazepam given IV at a dose of 2 mg, or diazepam given IV at 5 mg, can be used as initial doses. Additional doses can then be given and adjusted as needed to decrease the uncontrolled autonomic and neurological hyperactivity. The benzodiazepines work to depress the brain and nervous system functions that have become overactive due to certain toxins or conditions. By slowing down the brain and nerves, the out-of-control symptoms like rapid heart rate, high blood pressure, agitation, and seizures can be controlled. Starting with IV lorazepam at 2 mg or IV diazepam at 5 mg, and repeating as necessary, allows precise titration to gently sedate and calm the central nervous system and sympathetic hyperactivity. This helps restore balance from a state of toxicity-induced neural and autonomic overdrive. Benzodiazepines are often the preferred sedatives in poisoning cases causing agitation. They have few drug interactions and side effects. Flumazenil can reverse them if oversedated. If there is no IV access, give 2–5 mg midazolam IM. With IV access, start with 1–2 mg IV midazolam/lorazepam or 2–5 mg IV diazepam. Double doses can be given if severely agitated with close monitoring.

Antipsychotics such as haloperidol may help by blocking dopamine. But they can worsen seizures, arrhythmias, and temperature regulation. Use antipsychotics cautiously along with benzodiazepines in poisoned patients.

Benzodiazepines for Hyperthermia

Antipyretics are not effective in lowering drug-induced fever. Benzodiazepines such as lorazepam or diazepam are the first-line agents to reduce muscle hyperactivity and thus decrease secondary heat production, e.g., in MAOI toxicity/serotonin syndrome.[11]

Barbiturates

Barbiturates are second-line antiepileptics when seizure does not respond to benzodiazepines. They bind to GABA-A-mediated chloride channel and increase the duration of opening of the channel and hence cause hyperpolarization of neurons; also, certain barbiturates activate the chloride channel directly at high concentrations. Generally, phenobarbital is the preferred medication among the available barbiturates. Although phenobarbital takes a longer infusion period, it is equally efficacious as lorazepam for patients with status epilepticus. Seizures caused by cicutoxin and fluvoxamine that did not respond to benzodiazepines or phenytoin have reportedly been successfully treated with barbiturates. According to experimental studies, phenobarbital is more efficacious in preventing theophylline-induced seizures than phenytoin. The efficacy of barbiturates as a second-line anticonvulsant for drug-induced seizures has not, however, been assessed in any prospective controlled trials.

Propofol

Propofol increases the GABA binding to the chloride channel and also opens the chloride channel with higher concentrations. Barbiturate has synergistic activity with benzodiazepine. In cases when seizures may result from elevated *N*-methyl-D-aspartate (NMDA) activity, propofol's antagonistic action on the NMDA receptor may be advantageous. For individuals with refractory status epilepticus, propofol is typically saved as a last resort. Propofol injection effectively reduced the refractory convulsive activity brought on by amoxapine and star fruit (*Averrhoa carambola*); however, EEG evidence was not mentioned. There are some disadvantages with propofol. First, it is costlier than other antiepileptics; second, prolonged infusion of propofol can cause propofol-related infusion syndrome (PRIS syndrome), which is characterized by bradycardia, hypotension, rhabdomyolysis, and metabolic acidosis.

Pyridoxine

Pyridoxine is the drug of choice for isoniazid-induced seizure and hydrazine-containing *Gyromitra* mushrooms. It inhibits the conversion of glutamate to GABA, hence inducing seizures. Pyridoxine helps in the synthesis of GABA, hence reverses the effect of isoniazid and the effect is immediately seen. The dose of pyridoxine is 5 g IV in adults and 70 mg/kg IV in children. If the dose of isoniazid poisoning is known, pyridoxine should be given equal to isoniazid (grams per grams).[12,13]

Flumazenil-induced Seizure

Flumazenil-precipitated seizures in patients who can be chronically taking benzodiazepines should be treated aggressively with another GABA-A receptor agonist because the benzodiazepine site on the receptor can be antagonized. Anticonvulsants such as phenobarbital or propofol can be recommended for flumazenil-induced seizures.

ANTIHYPERTENSIVES

Hypertension due to Serotonin Syndrome

Serotonin syndrome is a triad of cognitive, autonomic, and neuromuscular effects. It is characterized by agitation, muscle rigidity, myoclonus, tremors, sweating, hyperthermia, etc. Severe forms of serotonin syndrome may present with fluctuating blood pressures and tachycardia.

Thus, short-acting antihypertensives such as esmolol or nitroprusside are recommended in hypertension caused by serotonin agonists.[14-16]

- *Esmolol:* It is a cardioselective beta blocker and a class II antiarrhythmic. It acts on beta-1 receptor, hence has negative chronotropic and inotropic actions. This property of esmolol helps in treating the autonomic instability caused by serotonin syndrome. Esmolol is a rapid- and ultrashort-acting drug. The dose is 500 mics/kg IV loading followed by 50-mic/kg/min infusion.
- *Nitroprusside:* It is a potent vasodilator. It acts by releasing nitric oxide (NO), which activates cyclic guanosine monophosphate (cGMP) intracellularly and inhibits actin–myosin interaction leading to smooth muscle relaxation, thus causing vasodilation. The dose is 0.5–4 mics/kg/min. It is a fast- and short-acting drug, hence is used to treat hypertension due to serotonin syndrome. Some adverse effects are that it can cause profound hypotension, raised intracranial pressure due to cerebral vasodilation, and methemoglobinemia.

Hypertension due to Monoamine Oxidase Inhibitor Overdose

Monoamine oxidase metabolizes neurotransmitters such as norepinephrine, serotonin, dopamine, and tyramine. Hence, the increased catecholamines in the circulation on MAOI toxicity lead to autonomic storm. It is necessary that only short-acting antihypertensives are used to control blood pressure in this situation so as to avoid abrupt hypotension. Thus, phentolamine and nitroprusside are the preferred antihypertensives.[17,18]

- *Phentolamine:* It is a competitive α-adrenergic antagonist. The usual dose administered is 2.5- to 5.0-mg IV boluses every 10–15 minutes until the blood pressure is controlled. It is followed by an infusion of 0.2–0.5 mg/min as a maintenance therapy. The typical adverse effect seen with phentolamine is reflex tachycardia.
- *Nitroprusside:* It is as effective as phentolamine. Prolonged administration of high doses of nitroprusside can predispose to cyanide toxicity.

Beta blockers pose a theoretical risk of increasing blood pressure (through unopposed vasoconstriction) and are relatively contraindicated.

Cocaine-induced Hypertension

Hypertension in cocaine which is not responding to benzodiazepines is treated with phentolamine, nitroprusside, nicardipine, or nitroglycerine. Refractory hypertension is treated with drugs used in any other hypertensive emergencies except for beta blockers, which are contraindicated in cocaine poisoning.[19]

ANTIARRHYTHMICS

Lidocaine

As a class Ib antiarrhythmic, lidocaine is effective in treating wide complex tachyarrhythmias associated with TCA, cocaine, and MAOI toxicity. As lidocaine has some sodium channel blocking property, there is a controversy whether lidocaine can be used in TCA poisoning, but literature says that it has a proven benefit.

Amiodarone

Amiodarone is a class III antiarrhythmic. It is used in wide complex tachyarrhythmias in poisonings like MAOI toxicity as well as aconite poisoning. Amiodarone is preferable to lidocaine in aconite poisoning as aconite poisoning is a sodium channel blocker. Amiodarone should be avoided in TCA poisoning as it can cause QT prolongation. Other drugs like classes IA (quinidine, procainamide, disopyramide) and IC (flecainide, propafenone) are absolutely contraindicated in TCA poisoning as they have actions similar to those of TCA.

Magnesium Sulfate

Magnesium sulfate is the first-line treatment for torsades de pointes. Simultaneously, identify and correct any electrolyte abnormalities that may be contributing to torsades de pointes, such as hypokalemia, hypomagnesemia, or hypocalcemia. Monitoring and repleting potassium levels is particularly important, as hypokalemia is a key risk factor for torsades. After magnesium, antiarrhythmic drugs may be considered for recurrent torsades, but caution is required given their potential to worsen QT prolongation. Eliminating any offending medications that may be causing QT prolongation is also a key step in preventing further episodes of torsades de pointes. Magnesium sulfate can be used in wide complex tachyarrhythmias caused by TCA and digoxin toxicity.[20] In antipsychotic and cocaine poisoning, patients with a QTc interval of >500 milliseconds are at an increased risk for torsades de pointes. Patients taking antipsychotics with QTc interval >500 milliseconds should be given magnesium sulfate 2 g IV over 10 minutes irrespective of the serum magnesium levels.

Benzodiazepines

Benzodiazepines can also be used in treating sinus tachycardia in poisonings such as TCA, cocaine, and MAOI.[21,22]

Sodium Bicarbonate

Sodium bicarbonate is used for alkalinization and thus as an antiarrhythmic agent in TCA poisoning. A systematic review including all animal and human studies has shown that sodium bicarbonate is the most superior agent in treating consequential dysrhythmias and shock. The dose is 1–2 mEq/kg repeated till the pH becomes 7.50–7.55.

Beta Blockers

Beta blockers are used in treating autonomic storm like tachycardia and hypotension induced by serotonin syndrome. Cardioselective beta blockers like esmolol and metoprolol are used in treating atrial fibrillation and supraventricular tachycardia caused by theophylline toxicity. Beta blockers are contraindicated in the treatment of cocaine-induced tachyarrhythmias as they can lead to unopposed alpha-adrenergic action, which can worsen the coronary vasoconstriction and thus precipitate angina. They are also avoided in tachyarrhythmias by TCA poisoning due to their negative inotropic effect.

Calcium Channel Blockers

Calcium channel blocker is used in cocaine-induced atrial fibrillation and narrow complex reentrant tachyarrhythmias. It should be avoided in patients with hypotension.

DRUGS USED IN SPECIFIC POISONING

Methemoglobinemia

- *Ascorbic acid (vitamin C):* It can serve as a reducing agent to lower elevated methemoglobin levels. This makes it a potential treatment option for methemoglobinemia when first-line methylene blue is contraindicated.[23-25] It is indicated in situations where methylene blue should be avoided including glucose-6-phosphate dehydrogenase (G6PD) deficiency, which puts patients at risk for hemolytic anemia, and concurrent use of serotonergic drugs like selective serotonin reuptake inhibitors (SSRIs), where methylene blue can cause serotonin toxicity. In patients with methemoglobinemia with severe symptoms or methemoglobin levels exceeding 30%, IV ascorbic acid up to 10 g total should be administered, given as either a single or multiple divided doses. Compared to methylene blue, ascorbic acid acts more slowly, taking 1–3 days to produce improvement in methemoglobin levels and symptoms.

Serotonin Syndrome

- *Cyproheptadine:* It is an antihistamine and serotonin antagonist with anticholinergic properties. Although not Food and Drug Administration (FDA)-approved for this indication, it has been used off-label to treat serotonin syndrome. However, there is limited clinical evidence supporting its efficacy. Cyproheptadine is available only as oral tablets. The initial dose for serotonin syndrome is 12 mg, followed by 2 mg repeated every 2 hours until the patient improves. While cyproheptadine theoretically counteracts serotonin excess through its serotonin-blocking effects, robust data from human studies are lacking. The benefits and appropriate role of cyproheptadine in treating serotonin toxicity are still unclear.[26,27]
- *Chlorpromazine:* It can be a 5-HT2A serotonin receptor antagonist. Some case reports have described successful use of chlorpromazine to treat serotonin syndrome. A major advantage can be that chlorpromazine comes in an injectable formulation. However, chlorpromazine also has some disadvantages. It can cause hypotension, which can be dangerous in serotonin toxicity. Chlorpromazine blocks dopamine receptors as well, which may worsen neuromuscular symptoms like rigidity. It could also increase seizure risk and precipitate neuroleptic malignant syndrome.[28]
- *Dantrolene:* It is a nonspecific muscle relaxant. It antagonizes the ryanodine receptor and hence reduces the excitation–contraction coupling between actin and myosin. It can be used occasionally in the management of serotonin syndrome, but clinical benefit is unproven. It can also be used in more severe cases of neuroleptic malignant syndrome in which the rigidity is pronounced. It is given in a dose of 1–2.5 mg/kg IV followed by 1 mg/kg every 6 hours. It increase the risk of cardiovascular collapse when administered with calcium simultaneously.[29-31]

Neuroleptic Malignant Syndrome

- *Bromocriptine:* It can be a centrally acting dopamine agonist that can reduce fever and muscle rigidity in neuroleptic malignant syndrome and possibly shorten the duration. This drug is available in an oral preparation and may require administration by a nasogastric tube. Adverse effects such as hypotension, vomiting, and worsening of psychosis can be limiting factors to the routine use of bromocriptine.[32]

- *Amantadine:* It can be similar to bromocriptine in activity and available only in enteral form but can be less likely to cause hypotension.[33]

Ethanol Toxicity

Metadoxine: It increases the ethanol metabolism and hastens recovery. When compared with the patient's own metabolism, metadoxine 900 mg IV is said to double the pace at which ethanol blood levels drop over a period.[34]

Methanol and Ethylene Glycol Poisoning

Vitamin therapy: Despite the lack of conclusive data supporting the necessity or even efficacy of this treatment, supplemental care with B vitamins, especially folate, can be suggested to assist remove the toxic metabolites of methanol and ethylene glycol more quickly. Folic acid in a high dose metabolizes formic acid into carbon dioxide and water. It also hastens the detoxification of formic acid and hence prevents end-organ damage. Recommended dosing is 1 mg/kg (up to 50 mg) IV every 4–6 hours. Adjunctive therapy of ethylene glycol poisoning includes pyridoxine, thiamine, and magnesium which helps in the metabolism of glyoxylate to nontoxic glycine and α-hydroxy-β-ketoadipic acid.[35-38] Magnesium can be given as a single dose of 2 g IV. The dose of thiamine is 100 mg IV and pyridoxine is 50–100 mg IV, both every 6 hours for 2 days.

Cocaine-induced Acute Coronary Syndrome

Aspirin and nitroglycerine can be used in acute coronary syndrome due to cocaine. IV calcium channel blockers (diltiazem, 5–20 mg IV) can be recommended as adjunctive therapy for patients with ST-segment elevation or depression. The use of beta blockers in this setting is controversial. According to the 2014 guidelines by the American Heart Association and the American College of Cardiology, individuals exhibiting symptoms of acute cocaine intoxication should not be given beta blockers.[39]

Digoxin Poisoning

Atropine and/or transvenous cardiac pacing can be used as a temporary treatment for bradyarrhythmias while definitive digoxin-specific antibody fragments are available.

Valproic Acid Poisoning

L-Carnitine is used in valproate overdose patients in order to hasten its metabolism and thus rapid resolution from coma, to prevent hepatic failure, and to reverse mitochondrial metabolic anomalies in individuals experiencing acute intoxication. L-Carnitine 100 mg/kg IV initially followed by infusions of 50 mg/kg every 8 hours can be recommended in cases of valproic acid toxicity with lethargy, coma, hyperammonemia, and hepatic dysfunction.[40,41]

Caustic Ingestions

Systemic steroids: Steroids' capacity to suppress the inflammatory response gave rise to the theory that they may prevent stricture development following caustic consumption; evidence from animal models supports this theory. According to international treatment recommendations, corticosteroids can be used in caustic ingestion, and a prospective human trial revealed statistically significant protection against the development of stricture formation in grade 2B lesions. A further pooled meta-analysis did not find any advantage for injury, and the use of steroids may raise the risk of bleeding, infection, and perforation. Hence, there are conflicting recommendations of its use. One criticism of pooled meta-analysis data is that some individual studies did not clearly distinguish between grade 1 and 2A lesions, which do not typically lead to strictures, and grade 2B and 3 injuries, which might theoretically benefit from steroids.[42-46]

Organophosphorus Poisoning

Ipratropium bromide: It is an anticholinergic medication that blocks acetylcholine receptors. It can be inhaled to help treat organophosphate poisoning. By blocking acetylcholine receptors in the lungs, ipratropium helps dry up respiratory secretions and open up the airways. This improves breathing in organophosphate poisoning, where excess acetylcholine causes profuse airway secretions, bronchoconstriction, and breathing difficulty.[47]

Paraquat Poisoning

A systematic review and meta-analysis suggests that glucocorticoids with cyclophosphamide in addition to standard care may slightly reduce mortality in hospitalized people with oral paraquat poisoning. It is recommended to deliver 8 mg of dexamethasone IV every 8 hours for the first 72 hours, since there may be benefits.[48,49]

Dapsone-induced Methemoglobinemia

Cimetidine, in standard doses, can be used in dapsone poisoning. The hydroxylamine metabolite of dapsone is responsible for the production of methemoglobin by cytochrome P450. Cimetidine inhibits cytochrome P450, thus prevents its formation and methemoglobinemia.[50]

CONCLUSION

Using multiple pharmacological approaches simultaneously gives the best chance of recovery from poisoning. Antidotes neutralize toxins, but additional medications treat and prevent complications while the antidote takes effect. A poisoned patient requires diligent monitoring and tailored drug therapy to maintain vital functions. With proper intensive care and the right combination of drugs, even severe poisoning cases can have positive outcomes. In the fight against poisoning, antidotes are powerful but are strongest when complemented by other pharmacological therapies.

REFERENCES

1. Roberts DM, Buckley NA. Pharmacokinetic considerations in clinical toxicology: clinical applications. Clin Pharmacokinet. 2007;46:897-939.
2. Mohr NM, Pape SG, Runde D, Kaji AH, Walls RM, Brown CA. Etomidate use is associated with a lower incidence of hypotension than ketamine for emergency department sepsis intubation of patients with sepsis: a National Emergency Airway Registry cohort study. Acad Emerg Med. 2020;27:1140-9.
3. April MD, Arana A, Schauer SG, Davis WT, Oliver JJ, Fantegrossi A, et al. Ketamine versus etomidate and peri-intubation hypotension: a National Emergency Airway Registry study. Acad Emerg Med. 2020;27:1106-15.
4. Cornelius BG, Webb E, Cornelius A, Smith KWG, Ristic S, Jain J, et al. Effect of sedative agent selection on morbidity, mortality and length of stay in patients with increase in intracranial pressure. World J Emerg Med. 2018;9:256-61.
5. Gu WJ, Wang F, Tang L, Liu JC. Single-dose etomidate does not increase mortality in patients with sepsis: a systematic review and meta-analysis of randomized controlled trials and observational studies. Chest. 2015;147:335-46.
6. Bangash MN, Kong ML, Pearse RM. Use of inotropes and vasopressor agents in critically ill patients. Br J Pharmacol. 2012;165:2015-33.
7. Sandroni C, Cavallaro F, Caricato A, Scapigliati A, Fenici P, Antonelli M. Enoximone in cardiac arrest caused by propranolol: two case reports. Acta Anaesthesiol Scand. 2006;50:759-61.
8. Fletcher ML, Sarangarm P, Nash J, Smolinske SC, Alunday RL, Seifert SA, et al. A systematic review of second line therapies in toxic seizures. Clin Toxicol (Phila). 2021;59:451-6.
9. Chen H, Albertson TE, Olson KR. Treatment of drug-induced seizures. Br J Clin Pharmacol. 2016;81:412-9.
10. Prasad M, Krishnan PR, Sequeira R, Al-Roomi K. Anticonvulsant therapy for status epilepticus. Cochrane Database Syst Rev. 2014;2014:CD003723.
11. Dean-Paccagnella R, Creed M, Kakollu M, Gopala Pillai SK. Hyperthermia and rigidity following overdose of an unknown drug; a case report and literature review. Bull Emerg Trauma. 2018;6:249-52.
12. Glatstein M, Carbell G, Scolnik D, Rimon A, Banerji S, Hoyte C. Pyridoxine for the treatment of isoniazid-induced seizures in intentional ingestions: the experience of a national poison center. Am J Emerg Med. 2018;36:1775-8.
13. Tajender V, Saluja J. INH induced status epilepticus: response to pyridoxine. Indian J Chest Dis Allied Sci. 2006;48:205-6.
14. Nguyen H, Pan A, Smollin C, Cantrell LF, Kearney T. An 11-year retrospective review of cyproheptadine use in serotonin syndrome cases reported to the California Poison Control System. J Clin Pharm Ther. 2019;44:327-34.
15. Tormoehlen LM, Rusyniak DE. Neuroleptic malignant syndrome and serotonin syndrome. Handb Clin Neurol. 2018;157:663-75.
16. Uddin MF, Alweis R, Shah SR, Lateef N, Shahnawaz W, Ochani RK, et al. Controversies in serotonin syndrome diagnosis and management: a review. J Clin Diagn Res. 2017;11:OE05-7.
17. Zisook S. A clinical overview of monoamine oxidase inhibitors. Psychosomatics. 1985;26:240-6, 251.
18. Linden CH, Rumack BH, Strehlke C. Monoamine oxidase inhibitor overdose. Ann Emerg Med. 1984;13:1137-44.
19. Beckley I, Ansari NAA, Khwaja HA, Mohsen Y. Clinical management of cocaine body packers: the Hillingdon experience. Can J Surg. 2009;52:417-21.
20. Emamhadi M, Mostafazadeh B, Hassanijirdehi M. Tricyclic antidepressant poisoning treated by magnesium sulfate: a randomized, clinical trial. Drug Chem Toxicol. 2012;35:300-3.
21. Part 10.2: toxicology in ECC. Circulation. 2005;112:IV-126.
22. Woolf AD, Erdman AR, Nelson LS, Caravati EM, Cobaugh DJ, Booze LL, et al. Tricyclic antidepressant poisoning: an evidence-based consensus guideline for out-of-hospital management. Clin Toxicol. 2007;45:203-33.
23. Rino PB, Scolnik D, Fustiñana A, Mitelpunkt A, Glatstein M. Ascorbic acid for the treatment of methemoglobinemia: the

experience of a large tertiary care pediatric hospital. Am J Ther. 2014;21:240.
24. Atyabi N, Yasini SP, Jalali SM, Shaygan H. Antioxidant effect of different vitamins on methemoglobin production: an in vitro study. Vet Res Forum. 2012;3:97-101.
25. Topal H, Topal Y. Toxic methemoglobinemia treated with ascorbic acid: case report. Iran Red Crescent Med J. 2013;15:e12718.
26. Lappin RI, Auchincloss EL. Treatment of the serotonin syndrome with cyproheptadine. N Engl J Med. 1994;331:1021-2.
27. Graudins A, Stearman A, Chan B. Treatment of the serotonin syndrome with cyproheptadine. J Emerg Med. 1998;16:615-9.
28. Gillman PK. Successful treatment of serotonin syndrome with chlorpromazine. Med J Aust. 1996;165:345-6.
29. Kaufman KR, Levitt MJ, Schiltz JF, Sunderram J. Neuroleptic malignant syndrome and serotonin syndrome in the critical care setting: case analysis. Ann Clin Psychiatry. 2006;18:201-4.
30. Ngo V, Guerrero A, Lanum D, Burgett-Moreno M, Fenati G, Barr S, et al. Emergent treatment of neuroleptic malignant syndrome induced by antipsychotic monotherapy using dantrolene. Clin Pract Cases Emerg Med. 2019;3:16-23.
31. Frank C. Recognition and treatment of serotonin syndrome. Can Fam Physician. 2008;54:988-92.
32. Dhib-Jalbut S, Hesselbrock R, Mouradian MM, Means ED. Bromocriptine treatment of neuroleptic malignant syndrome. J Clin Psychiatry. 1987;48:69-73.
33. Amantadine and the glutamate hypothesis of schizophrenia experiences in the treatment of neuroleptic malignant syndrome. [online] Available from https://link.springer.com/article/10.1007/BF01245162 [Last accessed September, 2024].
34. Shpilenya LS, Muzychenko AP, Gasbarrini G, Addolorato G. Metadoxine in acute alcohol intoxication: a double-blind, randomized, placebo-controlled study. Alcohol Clin Exp Res. 2002;26:340-6.
35. Barceloux DG, Bond GR, Krenzelok EP, Cooper H, Vale JA, American Academy of Clinical Toxicology Ad Hoc Committee on the Treatment Guidelines for Methanol Poisoning. American Academy of Clinical Toxicology practice guidelines on the treatment of methanol poisoning. J Toxicol Clin Toxicol. 2002;40:415-46.
36. Ghosh A, Boyd R. Leucovorin (calcium folinate) in 'antifreeze' poisoning. Emerg Med J. 2003;20:466.
37. Davis DP, Bramwell KJ, Hamilton RS, Williams SR. Ethylene glycol poisoning: case report of a record-high level and a review. J Emerg Med. 1997;15:653-67.
38. Paasma R, Hovda KE, Jacobsen D. Methanol poisoning and long term sequelae—a six years follow-up after a large methanol outbreak. BMC Clin Pharmacol. 2009;9:5.
39. McCord J, Jneid H, Hollander JE, de Lemos JA, Cercek B, Hsue P, et al. Management of cocaine-associated chest pain and myocardial infarction. Circulation. 2008;117: 1897-907.
40. Lheureux PER, Hantson P. Carnitine in the treatment of valproic acid-induced toxicity. Clin Toxicol (Phila). 2009;47:101-11.
41. Lheureux PE, Penaloza A, Zahir S, Gris M. Science review: carnitine in the treatment of valproic acid-induced toxicity—what is the evidence? Crit Care. 2005;9:431-40.
42. Fulton JA, Hoffman RS. Steroids in second degree caustic burns of the esophagus: a systematic pooled analysis of fifty years of human data: 1956–2006. Clin Toxicol. 2007;45:402-8.
43. Katibe R, Abdelgadir I, McGrogan P, Akobeng AK. Corticosteroids for preventing caustic esophageal strictures: systematic review and meta-analysis. J Pediatr Gastroenterol Nutr. 2018;66:898-902.
44. Mirhashemi SH, Hadizadeh-Neisanghalb M, Salehi M, Rostami P. Research paper: effectiveness of corticosteroid therapy for caustic esophageal injury. Int J Med Toxicol Forensic Med. 2018;8:131-6.
45. Olcay I, Şen N, Soyupak S, Zorludemir U, Okur H, Keskïn E, et al. Does steroid treatment prevent caustic esophageal stricture? A prospective study. Ann Med Sci. 2000;9:56-8.
46. Pelclová D, Navrátil T. Do corticosteroids prevent oesophageal stricture after corrosive ingestion? Toxicol Rev. 2005;24:125-9.
47. Shemesh I, Bourvin A, Gold D, Kutscherowsky M. Chlorpyrifos poisoning treated with ipratropium and dantrolene: a case report. J Toxicol Clin Toxicol. 1988;26:495-8.
48. Li LR, Chaudhary B, You C, Dennis JA, Wakeford H. Glucocorticoid with cyclophosphamide for oral paraquat poisoning. Cochrane Database Syst Rev. 2021;2021:CD008084.
49. Krishnamurthy H, Bharathi S, Bhangari VS. (2023). The corticosteroids in paraquat poisoning—are they the sole life-saving drugs?: a prospective cohort study. J Clin Diagn Res. [online] Available from https://www.jcdr.net//article_fulltext.asp?issn=0973-709x&year=2023&month=July&volume=17&issue=7&page=OC01-OC04&id=18149 [Last accessed September, 2024].
50. Barclay JA, Ziemba SE, Ibrahim RB. Dapsone-induced methemoglobinemia: a primer for clinicians. Ann Pharmacother. 2011;45:1103-15.

1.10 Disposition of Patients with Poisoning from Emergency Room and Intensive Care Unit

Vikas Saini, Shyam Charan Meena, Prashant Nasa

INTRODUCTION

Acute poisoning describes bodily harm resulting from exposure to single or multiple hazardous substances. It represents a substantial problem in both developed and developing countries.[1] Annually, the World Health Organization (WHO) records >3 million acute poisoning cases with 220,000 deaths.[2,3] A recent systematic review on unintentional acute pesticide poisoning concluded that 44% of the farmers' population worldwide is poisoned every year with pesticides. The burden is much higher in developing countries, where pesticide use is unregulated, pesticides constitute a significant cause of poisoning, and many cases stay unreported. The impact of poisoning on morbidity and mortality is also high in this part of the world, with delays in seeking medical attention and a lack of appropriate resources.[4]

History may be unreliable in acute poisoning, especially in patients with suicidal intentions. Myriad offending agents with varied clinical manifestations require multiple laboratory tests to confirm diagnosis. Hence, the disposition of patients with acute poisoning is challenging, especially when there is uncertainty in cause, dose, or duration elapsed since the poisoning. These patients often need continuous, intensive monitoring, warranting admission to an intensive care unit (ICU) or high-dependency unit.[5] A vast majority of patients need only continuous monitoring of vital functions and timely intervention in case of any deteriorating clinical condition, which may be offered in a short-term observation unit in the emergency room (ER). Those needing no definitive therapy can be discharged from the observation area in ER.[6]

Intensive care unit beds are precarious in any healthcare setting, and a rational use ensures equity and contains healthcare costs.[7] Efforts are needed to identify the most likely patients to benefit from ICU admission. These include patients who either need organ support (such as mechanical ventilation, vasopressors, and renal replacement therapy) or are at risk of dying. The timing of transfer to the ICU is a considerable determinant of patient outcomes.[8] Early risk stratification of patients with acute poisoning is essential to identify patients at a higher risk of ICU admission. This will help clinicians make timely decisions about the appropriate level of care.[9]

There are no universally accepted criteria or scoring systems for ICU admissions of patients with acute poisoning. However, for individual agents such as theophylline, certain clinical features (i.e., hallucinations, agitation, and hypotension) could predict an increased risk of clinical deterioration and ICU admission.[10] Similarly, few clinical models have been evaluated in a mixed cohort for prediction of risk of deterioration and ICU admission.[6,11]

The disposition of patients with poisoning from the ER and ICU involves determining the most suitable level of care for a particular patient. It may be admission to a lower level of care area, observation in ER, or in certain situations discharge.[12] This chapter aims to provide an overview of the factors influencing the disposition of poisoned patients, highlighting the importance of a comprehensive approach and evidence-based decision making.

RISK STRATIFICATION AND INTENSIVE CARE UNIT DISPOSITIONS

After initial stabilization, risk stratification plays a crucial role in determining the appropriate disposition. Several factors should be considered, including the ingested substance, dose, time since ingestion, coingestions, patient's age, comorbidities, and clinical presentation. Various methods have been proposed for risk stratification of poisoned patients and the need for admission to ICU.

Clinical Prediction Models

Intensive Care Requirement Score

The Intensive Care Requirement Score (IRS) is a clinical prediction model, including variables such as age, comorbid illness (cirrhosis, respiratory insufficiency, arrhythmia), intoxication type, Glasgow Coma Scale (GCS), heart rate, and systolic blood pressure (SBP). The score was initially developed in a large cohort of >9,500 patients.[6] Among the variables, age >55 years, respiratory failure, and GCS < 6 were found to be strong predictors of ICU admission. This scoring system had a very high negative predictive value of 98.7%, thereby meaning that younger patients with absence or respiratory failure and GCS > 6 should not be admitted in the ICU.[6]

Subsequently, the model was also externally validated in other studies.[13,14] El Gharbi et al. found that IRS < 6 had a high negative predictive value (95%) of excluding the need of ICU admission defined by the need of organ support and/or death during hospital stay.[14] However, the specificity was only 38%, with a positive predictive value of only 21%. Hence, a negative IRS (IRS < 6) accurately excludes the need for ICU admission, but a positive IRS (IRS ≥ 6) cannot be used for risk stratification of poisoned patients.[13,14]

Risk Stratification Nomogram

The Tanta University risk model is a risk stratification nomogram based on the admission clinical and laboratory variables to predict the need for ICU in acutely poisoned patients. The model includes GCS, oxygen saturation, diastolic blood pressure, respiratory rate, and bicarbonate concentration, and was found to have good discrimination with area under the curve (AUC) = 0.92 to determine ICU admission.[11] The external validation of nomograms found a high negative predictive value (98%) to exclude the need for ICU admission.[12]

Recently, new risk stratification nomograms for acute poisoning have been published. El-Gharbawy et al. developed a nomogram to predict the need for ICU admission for acute antipsychotic poisoning. The variables included were seizures, mean blood pressure, oxygen saturation, GCS, and corrected QT interval.[15] Another nomogram for predicting ICU admission was evaluated for acute clozapine poisoning, with an overall accuracy of 96.2%.[16]

External validation of these models is required before they can be recommended in routine clinical practice.[17]

The major drawback of these prediction models is the fact that they have been proposed and validated in developed countries where the patient profile and the toxins/poisons are entirely different from the ones seen in low- and middle-income countries like many South East Asian and African countries.

Scoring Systems

Various conventional scoring systems, such as Acute Physiology and Chronic Health Evaluation II (APACHE II) score, Rapid Emergency Medicine Score (REMS), Modified Early Warning Score (MEWS), Simplified Acute Physiology Score (SAPS II), and Simple Clinical Score (SCS), have been evaluated to predict the need for ICU admission in specific acute poisoning cases. Conventional scoring systems are used to predict outcomes and the need for organ support and ICU admissions in various conditions.

Conventional Scoring Systems

Very few studies have critically evaluated the conventional scoring systems to predict ICU admission with some success. Sagah et al. recommended that SCS can accurately predict ICU admissions and the need for mechanical ventilation in patients with acute theophylline poisoning, with a sensitivity and specificity of 92.9% and 90.9%, respectively.[18] Another study comparing different scores in acute clozapine poisoning found comparable discriminative ability of APACHE II or MEWS for predicting the need for mechanical ventilation and mortality. The authors recommended MEWS as an alternative outcome predictor for clozapine poisoning because of its ease of application, feasibility, and economic implications.[19] MEWS was recommended for predicting ICU admissions for acute pesticide poisoning,[20] while SAPS II performed better for predicting outcomes.[21]

Physicians, especially those working in the emergency department and ICU, are familiar with conventional scoring systems. The familiarity is the main strength of these scoring systems; however, the lack of customization of these scores for acute poisoning is a major limitation. Another major limitation is the fact that these conventional scores only include physiological abnormalities and lack poisoning-specific variables such as the type of poison, route of its exposure, and intent of poisoning, thereby losing specificity for critically ill poisoned patients.

Specific Scoring Systems

Certain scores, such as the Poisoning Severity Score (PSS) or the new-Poisoning Mortality Score (new-PMS) system, have been specifically designed for acute poisoning. These scores can aid in risk stratification and guide disposition decisions.

Poisoning Severity Score: PSS is a widely recognized scoring system used to assess the severity of poisoning cases. The tool was developed through a joint collaboration between the European Association of Poisons Centres and Clinical Toxicologists (EAPCCT), the International Programme on Chemical Safety, and the European Commission in the 1990s.[22] The score was found helpful for accurately predicting severity and identifying patients who could deteriorate further, need a referral to a clinical toxicologist, and warrant follow-up.[22] It takes into account various factors such as the type and amount of toxic substance ingested, clinical manifestations, laboratory findings, and treatment requirements. By assigning numerical values to these parameters, the PSS provides a standardized approach to evaluate the severity of poisoning cases objectively. However, PSS lost its clinical utility due to infrequent use, misinterpretation, and various modifications over time.[23] The PSS was again developed for the different settings and is not practical in different geographic areas with different patient population.

New-Poisoning Mortality Scoring system: The new-PMS including vital signs (SBP, heart rate, respiration rate, body temperature, and mental status), demographics (age and sex), and poisoning-specific variables was developed and validated through the Korea Centers for Disease Control and Prevention (KCDC) database. The new-PMS with a cutoff of 49 was found to have a good accuracy (87.2%) for predicting in-hospital mortality and could be used for clinical decision making for identifying patients requiring ICU admission.[24] Recently, the new-PMS score was externally validated in another large cohort and performed better than MEWS in acute poisoning.[25]

Snakebite Severity Score

The Snakebite Severity Score (SSS) was developed as an objective tool for evaluation of severity and progression of envenomation in patients with crotalid snakebite. It correlated well with the clinical condition of patients bitten by crotalid snakes, and helped the physician decide about antivenom administration.[26] It was later modified to include presenting pain local effect index, as an independent factor predicting additional antivenom requirement.[27] This scoring system was neither developed nor utilized for admitting envenomed patients; however, any patient with clinically significant envenomation, where a decision to administer antivenin has been made, should be admitted in the ICU. If the ICU beds are not available, this patient may be admitted to a ward/unit with facility for observation and monitoring. This scoring system has been developed and validated in management of crotalid snakebite. Its utility for any other type of snake envenomation is questionable.

Peradeniya Organophosphorus Poisoning Scale

This scoring system was envisaged by the authors as a simple and effective system to determine the need for ventilatory support early in the course of admission. It helps in grading the severity of organophosphate (OP) poisoning and can be used to take decisions regarding ICU admission of moderate to severely ill patients. Since OP compound poisoning is a common problem in India, this scale may be helpful in taking such decisions. A study was conducted to validate this in Indian patients.[28] It was observed that when used at presentation in patients with acute OP poisoning, the Peradeniya Organophosphorus Poisoning (POP) scale assists in predicting the need for ventilatory support. Early identification of danger signs may help in taking decisions regarding shifting to ICUs to reduce mortality and morbidity.[29]

PGI Score for Aluminum Phosphide Poisoning

Aluminum phosphide is a grain fumigant, used for storage of grains. It an important cause of mortality and morbidity related to self-harm in India, especially the northern part of India.[30] Three simple parameters—pH < 7.25, score on GCS < 13, and SBP < 87 mm Hg—have been found to be robust predictors of mortality. This score, primarily developed as a prediction model, can help in deciding admission to ICU and management strategies in poisoned patients. Patients with score ≤1 may be kept under observation on a monitored bed, whereas those with score 2 or more, should be admitted to ICU.[31]

Indian Guidelines

Recently the Ministry of Health, Government of India (GOI), has released guidelines for admission to ICUs.[32] These are general guidelines; however, they can be used to identify patients to be shifted to ICUs.

The important considerations for admission to ICU in these guidelines are the following:

- Altered level of consciousness of recent onset
- Hemodynamic instability (e.g., clinical features of shock and arrhythmia)
- Need for respiratory support (e.g., escalating oxygen requirement, de novo respiratory failure requiring noninvasive ventilation, and invasive mechanical ventilation)
- Any medical condition or disease with anticipation of deterioration.

Many poisoned patients at presentation have the need for supportive therapy due to airway compromise, respiratory difficulty, or hemodynamics/cardiovascular instability. Any severely poisoned patient can potentially deteriorate at any given time; therefore, potential deterioration or observed/documented deterioration would be important indications for admission to ICUs.

GUIDING DISPOSITION DECISIONS

Scoring systems assist healthcare professionals in making informed disposition decisions for patients with acute poisoning. Based on the severity assessment provided by scoring systems like PSS or new-PMS, healthcare providers can determine whether a patient can be safely managed in an outpatient setting, requires admission to a general medical ward, or necessitates transfer to an ICU. These disposition decisions are crucial in optimizing patient outcomes and resource utilization.

By objectively assessing the severity of poisoning cases, these scoring systems enable healthcare professionals to allocate appropriate resources and provide optimal care. Incorporating scoring systems into clinical practice enhances patient management and improves outcomes in the field of toxicology.

In the GOI guidelines, the expert group also provided guidance for discharge from ICU. The important determinants are the following[32]:

- Return of physiological aberrations to near-normal or baseline status
- Reasonable resolution and stability of the acute illness that necessitated ICU admission
- The patient/family agrees for ICU discharge for a treatment-limiting decision or palliative care
- Based on lack of benefit from aggressive care.

Among these, return to baseline or near-normal physiology is an important criterion for discharge or shifting to a step-down care unit. Resolution of the life-threatening hemodynamics compromise may guide the physicians to shift to step-down unit for rational use of intensive care facilities. Since most of the poisoned patients in India are young individuals, with relatively normal baseline physiology,[32] every effort should be made to provide intensive care to these individuals. The classic example is severe envenomation by neuroparalytic snakebite, mimicking brain death, which may be completely reversed with timely institution of antivenom and supportive ventilation.[33,34]

CONCLUSION

Disposition of patients with poisoning from the ER and ICU requires a comprehensive approach, considering the severity of poisoning, clinical presentation, and individual patient factors. Collaboration with toxicology specialists, and poison control centers, along with utilization of risk stratification tools or scoring tools can aid in making evidence-based decisions regarding admission, observation, or discharge. Timely and appropriate disposition ensures optimal patient outcomes and reduces healthcare resource utilization.

REFERENCES

1. Mehrpour O, Akbari A, Jahani F, Amirabadizadeh A, Allahyari E, Mansouri B, et al. Epidemiological and clinical profiles of acute poisoning in patients admitted to the intensive care unit in eastern Iran (2010 to 2017). BMC Emerg Med. 2018;18(1):30.
2. Balaraju R, Vallepalli C, Sattari SR, Yenna KR, Vijayagiri KS, Sunkavalli NC, et al. Demographic trends and outcome of acute poisoning in a rural tertiary care hospital of Nalgonda District, Telangana. Indian J Public Health Res Dev. 2020;11(7):652-6.
3. World Health Organization. Guidelines for Poison Control. Geneva: World Health Organization; 1997.
4. Boedeker W, Watts M, Clausing P, Marquez E. The global distribution of acute unintentional pesticide poisoning: estimations based on a systematic review. BMC Public Health. 2020;20(1):1875-89.
5. Chandran J, Krishna B. Initial management of poisoned patient. Indian J Crit Care Med. 2019;23(Suppl 4):S234-40.
6. Brandenburg R, Brinkman S, de Keizer NF, Kesecioglu J, Meulenbelt J, de Lange DW. The need for ICU admission in intoxicated patients: a prediction model. Clin Toxicol (Phila). 2017;55(1):4-11.
7. Van Beusekom I, Bakhshi-Raiez F, de Keizer NF, de Lange DW. The healthcare costs of intoxicated patients who survive ICU admission are higher than non-intoxicated ICU patients: a retrospective study combining healthcare insurance data and data from a Dutch national quality registry. BMC Emerg Med. 2019;19(1):6.
8. Glass G, Hartka TR, Keim-Malpass J, Enfield KB, Clark MT. Dynamic data in the ED predict requirement for ICU transfer following acute care admission. J Clin Monit Comput. 2020;35(3):1-9.
9. Liu V, Kipnis P, Rizk NW, Escobar GJ. Adverse outcomes associated with delayed intensive care unit transfers in an integrated healthcare system. J Hosp Med. 2012;7(3):224-30.
10. Khalifa H, Lashin H. Predictors for intensive care unit admission in acute theophylline intoxicated patients. Ain Shams J Forensic Med Clin Toxicol. 2018;31(2):77-86.

11. Elgazzar FM, Afifi AM, Shama MAE, Askary AE, El-Sarnagawy GN. Development of a risk prediction nomogram for disposition of acute toxic exposure patients to intensive care unit. Basic Clin Pharmacol Toxicol. 2021;129(3):256-67.
12. Schmoll S, Heier EC, Böll R, Zellner T, Romanek K, Eyer F, et al. Independent validation of the Tanta University risk model for intensive care requirement in acutely poisoned adults. Clin Toxicol (Phila). 2023;61(4):266-9.
13. Böll R, Romanek K, Schmoll S, Stich R, Ott A, Stenzel J, et al. Independent validation of the ICU requirement score in a cohort of acutely poisoned adults. Clin Toxicol (Phila). 2018;56(7):664-6.
14. El Gharbi F, El Bèze N, Jaffal K, Sutterlin L, Mora P, Malissin I, et al. Does the ICU Requirement Score allow the poisoned patient to be safely managed without admission to the intensive care unit?—a validation cohort study. Clin Toxicol (Phila). 2022;60(3):298-303.
15. El-Gharbawy DM, Kabbash IA, Ghonem MM. A nomogram proposal for early prediction of intensive care unit admission in patients with acute antipsychotic poisoning. Toxicol Res (Camb). 2023;12(5):873-83.
16. Sharif AF, Aouissi HA, Kasemy ZA, Byeon H, Lashin HI. Development and validation of a risk prediction nomogram for disposition of acute clozapine intoxicated patients to intensive care unit. Hum Exp Toxicol. 2023;42:9603271231186154.
17. Shi Q, Zhang J. Clinical prediction models for intensive care unit admission in patients with acute poisoning: is it time for a comprehensive evaluation of their utility? Toxicol Res (Camb). 2024;13(2):tfae031.
18. Sagah GA, Elmansy AM. Comparison of different scores as predictors of mechanical ventilation and intensive care unit admission in acute theophylline poisoning. Toxicol Res (Camb). 2023;12(5):990-7.
19. Lashin HI, Sharif AF. Evaluation of various scoring systems as predictors of the need for intensive care unit admission and other adverse outcomes among patients with acute clozapine poisoning. Toxicol Res (Camb). 2023;12(3):468-79.
20. El-Sarnagawy GN, Abdelnoor AA, Abuelfadl AA, El-Mehallawi IH. Comparison between various scoring systems in predicting the need for intensive care unit admission of acute pesticide-poisoned patients. Environ Sci Pollut Res Int. 2022;29(23):33999-4009.
21. Dorooshi G, Samsamshariat S, Gheshlaghi F, Zoofaghari S, Hasanzadeh A, Abbasi S, et al. Comparing Sequential Organ Failure Assessment Score, Acute Physiology and Chronic Health Evaluation II, Modified Acute Physiology and Chronic Health Evaluation II, Simplified Acute Physiology Score II and Poisoning Severity Score for outcome prediction of pesticide poisoned patients admitted to the intensive care unit. J Res Pharm Pract. 2024;12(2):49-57.
22. Persson HE, Sjöberg GK, Haines JA, Pronczuk de Garbino J. Poisoning Severity Score. Grading of acute poisoning. J Toxicol Clin Toxicol. 1998;36(3):205-13.
23. Schwarz ES, Kopec KT, Wiegand TJ, Wax PM, Brent J. Should we be using the Poisoning Severity Score? J Med Toxicol. 2017;13(2):135-45.
24. Han KS, Kim SJ, Lee EJ, Shin JH, Lee JS, Lee SW. Development and validation of new Poisoning Mortality Score system for patients with acute poisoning at the emergency department. Crit Care. 2021;25(1):29.
25. Lee S, Kim SJ, Han KS, Song J, Lee SW. Comparison of the new-Poisoning Mortality Score and the Modified Early Warning Score for predicting in-hospital mortality in patients with acute poisoning. Clin Toxicol (Phila). 2024;62(1):1-9.
26. Dart RC, Hurlbut KM, Garcia R, Boren J. Validation of a severity score for the assessment of crotalid snakebite. Ann Emerg Med. 1996;27(3):321-6.
27. Kang S, Moon J, Chun B. Does the traditional snakebite severity score correctly classify envenomated patients? Clin Exp Emerg Med. 2016;3(1):34-40.
28. Senanayake N, de Silva HJ, Karalliedde L. A scale to assess severity in organophosphorus intoxication: POP scale. Hum Exp Toxicol. 1993;12:297-9.
29. Malaviya NB, Parikh R, Pancholi K, Belim OB. Assessment of the Peradeniya Organophosphorus Poisoning Scale as a severity and prognostic marker in patients with acute organophosphorus poisoning presenting to an emergency medicine department. Cureus. 2023;15(6):e40277.
30. Murali R, Bhalla A, Singh D, Singh S. Acute pesticide poisoning: 15 years experience of a large north-west Indian hospital. Clin Toxicol (Phila). 2009;47(1):35-8.
31. Pannu AK, Bhalla A, Sharma A, Sharma N. "PGI Score": a simplified three-point prognostic score for acute aluminum phosphide poisoning. Indian J Crit Care Med. 2020;24(9):790-3.
32. GOI guidelines for admission in intensive care units. [online] Available from https://nhsrcindia.org/sites/default/files/Guidelines-on-HDU_ICU.pdf.
33. Patra A, Goel V, Narang S, Aggarwal A. Reversible brain death: a rare manifestation of snake envenomation. Indian J Med Spec. 2023;14(1):50-2.
34. Bhalla A, Suri V, Sharma N, Singh S. An experience with manual ventilation in respiratory paralysis due to Indian common krait (*Bungarus caeruleus*) bite. Asia Pac J Med Toxicol. 2014;3:55-8.

1.11 Comprehensive Psychiatric Assessment in a Poisoned Patient

Shubh Mohan Singh, Eepsita Mishra

INTRODUCTION

Poisoning can be understood as the exposure to a noxious substance by means of ingestion, inhalation, inoculation, or absorption. It can be acute or chronic depending on the period of exposure and development of symptoms. Decontamination of the poisoned patient can include induced emesis, gastric lavage, single- and repeated-dose activated charcoal, whole bowel irrigation, hemoperfusion, peritoneal and hemodialysis, and alkaline diuresis, among others.[1]

According to World Health Organization (WHO) estimates, 0.3 million people die each year as a result of poisoning by various agents.[2] Of these, acute pesticide poisoning is the most common, with >300,000 cases of self-poisoning with pesticides in the Asia Pacific region alone.[3] In industrialized countries, common poisonings that may present to a critical care unit include benzodiazepines, opiates, tricyclic antidepressants, paracetamol, and carbon monoxide.[1] In the Asian region including India, insecticide poisons like aluminum phosphide ("Celphos"), paraquat, and organophosphorus compounds are more common.[4,5] Of these, aluminum phosphide is associated with the highest mortality rate.[5]

Patients with poisoning admitted to critical care unit generally carry a poorer prognosis and have a higher risk of mortality (varying between 10 and 18%) and long-term complications and higher chance for requirement of mechanical ventilation and vasopressor support—both of which carry their own risks.[6,7]

In India, the prevalence of poisoning-related deaths is estimated to be 2.4 per 100,000 population, with poisoning being the most preferred means for suicide.[8] Recent years have recorded a >6% increase in suicide rates in India.[9] Considering the wide variation in mode of poisoning, type of poison used, sociodemographic factors, and individual physiological variations, a "one-size-fits-all" approach to management is neither feasible nor wise. This is true of psychiatric aspects of poisoning as well. The approach to any patient presenting with poisoning must be carefully individualized based on history and examination. There are various aspects of poisoning that make psychiatric assessment and indeed psychiatric intervention an important aspect of the management of the poisoned patient. A psychiatrist or a mental health professional is often consulted when poisoning occurs in the context of suicide and self-harm. Therefore, this aspect will be dealt with in more detail. This chapter will provide an overview of the role of a psychiatrist in the context of the assessment and management of a poisoned patient.

POISONING SCENARIOS AND ASSOCIATED PSYCHOLOGICAL ISSUES

Deliberate Self-harm by Poisoning

Deliberate self-harm (DSH) is any act with an intention to harm or kill oneself. Ingestion of poison is often employed as a means to this end. DSH can end in the death of the affected individual, and this is called suicide by poisoning. A psychiatric consultation is usually indicated in patients with DSH. The Global Burden of Disease study estimated almost 600,000 deaths in 1990 alone to be due to self-harm.[10] Another study conducted in the same year estimated that self-harm resulted in 2 million cases of poisoning each year with 200,000 deaths.[11]

As per the National Crime Records Bureau (NCRB) data of 2021, mental illness accounts for only 8.2% of total suicide rates. The major contributors to suicide are financial bankruptcy, marital and family-related problems, and academic failure.[12] Poisoning is a common form of DSH in the developing world. While suicidal intent is often far lower than for self-immolation and hanging, the mortality rate is high due to the toxicity of the poisons used and poor medical care.[13]

The presence of a current mental disorder increases the risk of suicide with odds ratio varying from 3.1 to 19.5 as per different studies. Depression and substance use disorders—especially alcohol—in self as well as in spouse are the most common psychiatric disorders associated with an elevated suicide risk. Acute stress leading to adjustment disorders is associated with a threefold increase in suicide risk. Comorbid personality disorders are common and are associated with almost a 10-fold increased suicide risk.[14,15]

It is important to appreciate that DSH by poisoning (or any other method) is not always associated with a severe mental illness. Most DSH and suicide can be attributed to stressful life situations such as financial stress, marital discord, dysfunctional personality traits, and substance abuse.[16,17] In India, DSH is often more common in youth, females, and is associated with stressful life situations unlike the West where it is more common in older males and is associated with severe mental illness.[14] It is also important to appreciate that while a past history of DSH is common, most patients with DSH do not have a history of prior DSH and do not repeat the attempt in their lifetimes.[15,18]

Accidental Poisonings and Overdose

In the event that the poisoning is determined to be accidental, an attempt must be made to properly understand the circumstances of the poisoning. Understanding the person's cognitive functioning at the time of poisoning is essential. In cases of intellectual disability, the history will reveal below average intellectual functioning from early neurodevelopmental period and may explain the accidental event. In other cases, cognitive functioning may be transiently impaired by head injury, delirium due to other medical conditions, and, more commonly, substance abuse. Many a time, persons with acute alcohol or cannabis intoxication may accidentally ingest toxic substances not understanding the nature of the substance they are taking or the implications of the same. History taken from informants must take note of the person's usual substance use pattern; types of substances used; variations or increases in the amount, frequency, and/or potency of the substance used around the time of the poisoning; and severity of the intoxication at that time. This information would be helpful in understanding the cognitive capacity of the individual at the time of the poisoning.

Accidental poisonings can also occur in the case of overdosing with drugs that have been prescribed for some illness in self and others. These may often be misattributed as DSH especially if noted in a patient with mental illness. Psychological assessment can serve to rule out suicidality when DSH is suspected.

Homicidal Poisoning

In cases of homicidal poisoning where the victim survives the attempt (even if briefly), a detailed psychiatric examination and understanding of the circumstances of the poisoning becomes of paramount importance in view of the legal implications of the same for the victim as well as the alleged perpetrator. A psychiatric examination of the state of mind of the victim and his/her cognitive functioning is vital in order to establish the victim's testamentary capacity.

Chronic Poisoning

Chronic poisoning refers to the effects of prolonged exposure to a toxic substance and it is usually seen in the context of long-term environmental heavy metal poisoning, such as lead, mercury, and arsenic.

Chronic heavy metal poisoning generally presents with nonspecific complaints like nausea, bowel disturbances, loss of appetite, malaise, fatigue, and body aches. More advanced cases may reflect telltale signs of the particular culprit agent. A generalized neurocognitive decline including decreased performance of intellectual functioning, impairments of attention and short-term memory, visual judgment of angles and directions, psychomotor retardation, and personality changes is seen with chronic mercury poisoning. Chronic lead poisoning can mimic chronic neurological illnesses. Verbal intelligence quotient (IQ) and long-term memory can also be affected in chronic arsenic poisoning. A high index of suspicion is the key for arriving at these diagnoses. A careful environmental evaluation and comparison of levels of suspected agent in blood and environment is important in establishing the diagnosis.[19-22]

Substance Abuse and Withdrawal

Long-term substance abuse, including dependence, acute intoxication, as well as withdrawal states, adversely impacts an individual's orientation to his/her surroundings, attention, concentration, processing speed, memory, etc. Such cognitive dysfunction can be acute (e.g., alcohol withdrawal delirium, cannabis or alcohol intoxication, and opioid use) as well as chronic (e.g., chronic cannabis use, Wernicke's encephalopathy, and Korsakoff's syndrome due to alcohol dependence). Persons with substance use disorders are at an elevated risk of accidental as well as suicidal poisoning. These substances are often associated with characteristic intoxication and withdrawal syndromes that need to be assessed and identified. Examples include delirium tremens in case of alcohol withdrawal and the characteristic opioid withdrawal syndrome.

PSYCHIATRIC ASSESSMENT IN A POISONED PATIENT AS PER SCENARIOS

Once initial resuscitation and stabilization is complete, a risk assessment based on history, examination, and testing is performed, followed by formulation of a comprehensive medical and nutritional management plan and monitoring for any long-term complications.[23] A psychiatric assessment is of paramount importance in all cases of poisoning.[24,25]

Comprehensive History from Patient and Attendant/s

Once the patient is physically stable and responsive, an attempt must be made to interview the patient to understand the circumstances of the toxic exposure. The information provided must be corroborated with other reliable informants—such as family members, relatives, and friends. If the patient is not in a state to be interviewed, the role of these key informants would become even more crucial. History taking should begin with understanding the circumstances under which the poisoning occurred, with focus on suicidal intent, access to the substance, previous attempts, previous indications of self-harm, and expressions of intent to harm self. Close attention must be paid to the mood of the person at the time, whether or not he/she was under the influence of any psychoactive substance, the state of his/her sensorium, and whether the person was experiencing any delusions or hallucinations at the time.

One must explore for any past or current psychiatric illnesses, medical illnesses, trauma or injury, and past or ongoing treatments—with special focus on psychotropics as well as medications that are known to be linked with suicidality, such as isotretinoin, corticosteroids, and certain antitubercular agents.[26]

Assessment of Signs and Symptoms Associated with Agents Used in Psychiatric Practice, Substance Abuse

Mental Health Assessment

Capacity for formal assessment: A person is said to possess medical decision-making capacity if he/she can demonstrate understanding of the situation, appreciation of the consequences of his/her decision, and reasoning in his/her thought process, and if he/she can communicate his/her wishes. Capacity is assessed intuitively at every medical encounter and is usually readily apparent. However, a more formal capacity evaluation should be considered in cases of poisoning keeping in mind the legal implications of the same. If a person is determined to lack capacity for medical decision making, a surrogate decision maker should be identified and consulted.[27] Such an individual may either be a nominated representative or, more commonly, be the patient's next-of-kin or a court-appointed representative.

Furthermore, it should be noted that capacity assessment is an ongoing process and not a one-time assessment and so, serial assessments at frequent and regular intervals, as determined by the mental and physical status of the person, are recommended.[28]

Diagnostic: One of the important purposes of psychiatric assessment in a patient with poisoning is to look for and establish any pertinent psychiatric diagnoses such as affective disorders, psychoses, substance use disorders, and personality disorders, and neurodevelopmental disorders such as intellectual disability, ADHD, and autism spectrum disorders. It should be noted that more often than not, comorbidity may be the rule rather than the exception. Diagnosis of a mental illness has wide ranging implications from causation to treatment plan and prognosis.

Risk Assessment

Key areas that require clarification when assessing risk of suicidality or a repeat self-harm attempt are the following[29,30]:

- Stressors—including loss of employment, financial constraints, loss of a loved one, or recent change of residence
- Presence of hopelessness
- Nature of suicidal thinking—whether death wishes or active ideation and planning
- Impulsivity
- Substance use

Some scales that can be used for assessment include:

- Scale for Suicidal Ideation (SSI) developed in 1979 by Beck, Kovacs, and Weissman[31]
- Modified Scale for Suicidal Ideation (MSSI) developed by Miller et al.[24]
- Suicidal Intent Scale (SIS)[25]
- Suicidal Affect Behavior Cognition Scale (SABCS)[32]
- Life Orientation Inventory[26]
- Reasons for Living Inventory[33]
- Nurses' Global Assessment of Suicide Risk[34]

In case the determination is made that the person is at a high risk of suicidal attempt, high-risk measures must be put into place. These include constant surveillance of the patient by family members, caregivers, and hospital staff and not allowing any sharp objects or unattended medications to be left around the patient.[35]

Management

Acute

- Patients with a history of mental illness may be on psychotropic medication at the time of admission to critical care unit, such as antidepressants, antipsychotics, mood stabilizers, and benzodiazepines **(Table 1)**. Usually, it is advisable to minimize or stop psychotropics when the person is medically unstable so as to keep the anticholinergic load to a minimum and prevent development of delirium.[36] One may continue low-dose benzodiazepines in case of clinically significant anxiety or when one is anticipating drug discontinuation symptoms.[37] Melatonin may be preferable in isolated sleep disturbances.[38]
- Acute and chronic drug use can adversely impact course of recovery in acute resuscitative and intensive care periods. Substance abuse modifies the physiological response to injury and resuscitative and operative measures. Confusion can arise regarding depth of anesthesia which can affect selection and dosing of therapeutic agents and interpreting variations in the vital signs.[39] Initial history taking should specifically enquire about substance use and a psychiatric consultation must be sought at the earliest so as to properly assess the types and extent of substances used—including usual intake and last intake—so as to effectively predict the onset of withdrawal and manage the withdrawal state according to the substance used. Alcohol and opioid withdrawal states can be severe and complicate recovery from the poisoning. Alcohol withdrawal is managed with short-acting intravenous benzodiazepines such as lorazepam with continuous monitoring of vital signs and Alcohol withdrawal can be managed by administration of short-acting intravenous benzodiazepines such as lorazepam and continuous monitoring of vital signs with an instrument such as the Clinical Institute Withdrawal Assessment Alcohol Scale Revised (CIWA-Ar) scores.[40] Opioid withdrawal states can be managed by intravenous opioids such as tramadol or transdermal buprenorphine patches, along with symptomatic management with analgesics and clonidine.[41]

Continuation

Continuity is the key in mental health care. More often than not, patients admitted to the intensive care unit (ICU) with self-poisoning attempt may be hesitant to speak to a psychiatrist for a variety of reasons, ranging from stigma, shame, or guilt to fear of legal punitive action and fear of being labeled "mentally ill." Moreover, in critically ill cases, patients may initially be physically too

TABLE 1: Psychiatric assessment in the poisoned patient.

Scenario	*Assessment (common to all)*	*Additional assessments and special considerations*
Self-inflicted acute poisoning	• Detailed history • Physical examination • Mental state examination • Capacity assessment	History of psychiatric disorders, ongoing psychotropics, mood state and/or presence of command hallucinations at the time of self-harm, previous self-harm attempts, intent, precipitating factor, risk assessment for subsequent attempts
Accidental acute poisoning		Cognitive functioning at the time of incident, history of neurodevelopmental or neurodegenerative disorders, acute substance intoxication at the time of incident
Homicidal acute poisoning		Testamentary capacity of victim
Poisoning in the setting of a substance use disorder		Duration, frequency, and last intake of substances used, types of substances used, ongoing treatment for substance use disorders, management/prevention of acute withdrawal state, monitor for emergence of delirium, adequate pain management, and monitoring of vitals
Terminal cases of acute poisoning		Adequate pain management, end-of-life care, testamentary capacity, execution of will, pastoral care, supportive therapy, and psychiatric evaluation for family members/loved ones
Chronic poisoning		High index of suspicion, detailed neurological examination, look for telltale physical signs specific for particular poisons, environmental assessment and cognitive evaluation

unstable to participate comprehendingly in a psychiatric assessment. Hence, serial mental state examinations and documentation of the same are of vital importance. Once a basic rapport is established, bedside supportive psychotherapy may be initiated—with focus on self-harm, ideas of worthlessness, hopelessness, helplessness, guilt, and shame. Simultaneous initiation of psychoeducation regarding suicide and mental illness—for the patient as well as for the primary caregivers—is important for the reduction of stigma and removing barriers to seeking mental health care.

Maintenance

Following medical stabilization and discharge, the focus of care shifts to rehabilitation and prevention of future self-harm attempts **(Flowchart 1)**. From a psychiatric perspective, this involves:

Flowchart 1: Approach to a patient with poisoning.

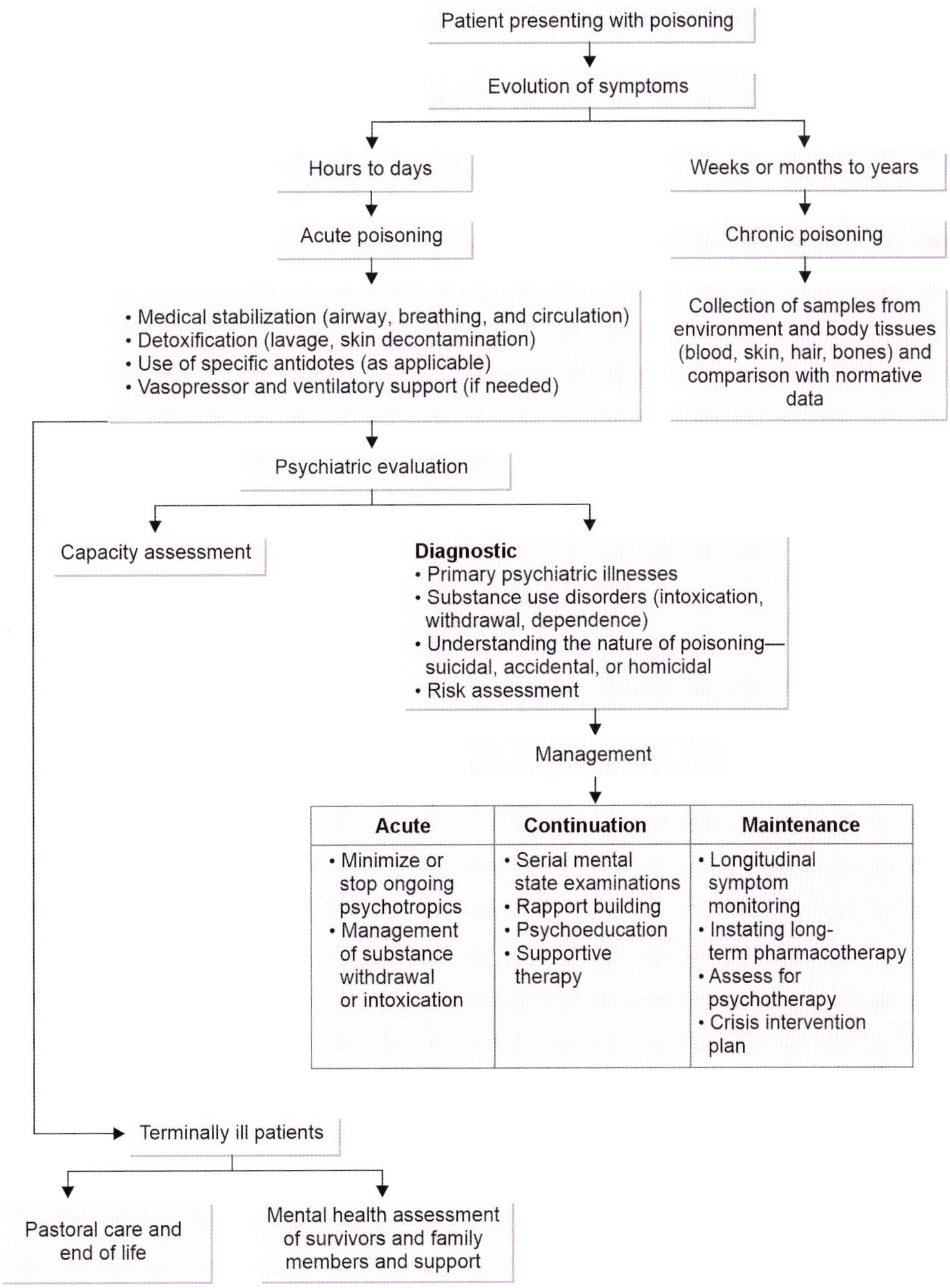

- Longitudinal monitoring of mood and anxiety symptoms, psychotic symptoms, suicidality, and substance use
- Assessment of personality and exploration of psychosocial stressors
- Pharmacological as well as nonpharmacological management of underlying mental illness, if any
- Continued psychiatric and psychological interventions and support for substance use disorders, if any
- Long-term psychotherapy, if indicated
- Formulating a crisis management plan with emphasis on seeking help without hesitation.

Pastoral Care and End of Life

Quite often, the end-organ damage and concurrent complications such as sepsis may render all efforts to save the life of the patient with poisoning fruitless. In cases where the patient is conscious and understands the terminal nature of the illness, pastoral care and supportive treatment may be helpful in aiding the person navigate the multifaceted experience of coming to terms with one's impending mortality. Pastoral caregivers provide broad spiritual care at the end of life, and discuss several matters besides spiritual issues with patients in the palliative phase, supporting them when making medical end-of-life decisions. People with or without religious beliefs can have their spiritual needs attended to by qualified personnel. Pastoral care can help mitigate anxiety and fears surrounding death, mediate communication and emotional exchange between the dying person and loved ones, and assist in decisions such as preparing a will, resuscitation, and life support.[42]

Mental Health Assessment of Survivors and Family Members and Support

Close relatives and family members of persons who succumb to poisoning go through a difficult grieving process. In the setting of a suicidal poisoning death, the already tough grief experience may be further complicated. This is due to several reasons—including feeling stigmatized and ostracized from extended family and community. Furthermore, they may experience mixed emotions. On one hand, the suicidal act may seem like an assault on or a rejection of those left behind. On the other hand, survivors may blame themselves for failing to predict the death or to have effectively intervened. In view of these unique challenges, they are at a higher risk of developing psychiatric morbidity such as depression, post-traumatic stress disorder (PTSD), and anxiety disorders, and, indeed, possibly also at a higher risk for suicide themselves. Assessment of family members and caregivers should ideally begin at the patient's bedside. Initial interactions should focus on building rapport and empathetic listening—which may later prove to be of vital importance when breaking bad news or helping them through the grieving process. Close monitoring is advisable in the immediate aftermath of loved one's death for signs of self-harm and long-term management may include grief-oriented psychotherapy along with treatment (pharmacological, nonpharmacological, and somatic) of any psychiatric disorders that may arise along the way.[43]

CONCLUSION

Poisoning is a growing concern in terms of causes of morbidity and mortality worldwide. It may be suicidal, homicidal, accidental, or undetermined. Suicidal poisoning may or may not occur in the context of a diagnosable mental illness. Psychiatric evaluation of a patient with poisoning in the critical care setting is of utmost importance and is multifaceted in nature. It spans assessment of cognitive functions and mental state, exploration for psychiatric diagnoses including substance use disorders, and determination of medical decision making and testamentary capacity in conjuncture with the legal system and primary care team. Psychiatrists form a key part of holistic treatment team catering to the needs of the patient as well as of the primary caregivers. Formulating a management plan involves addressing the mental health needs of the patient and family members, managing ongoing substance use and/or withdrawal, close monitoring of the mental and cognitive status, and planning long-term postdischarge psychiatric care in those requiring the same. Patients with terminal illness who are unlikely to survive the effects of the poison may benefit from end-of-life pastoral care. Family members and close friends and relatives of persons who die due to acute poisoning are at an elevated risk of mental health issues themselves, and so require thorough and ongoing assessment for the same, longitudinal monitoring, and close follow-up in order to effectively manage any issues that may arise.

REFERENCES

1. Jones LO. Poisoning. Anaesth Intensive Care Med. 2006;7(4):132-4.

2. Thundiyil JG, Stober J, Besbelli N, Pronczuk J. Acute pesticide poisoning: a proposed classification tool. Bull World Health Organ. 2008;86(3):205-9.
3. Konradsen F, Dawson AH, Eddleston M, Gunnell D. Pesticide self-poisoning: thinking outside the box. Lancet. 2007;369(9557):169-70.
4. Karunarathne A, Bhalla A, Sethi A, Perera U, Eddleston M. Importance of pesticides for lethal poisoning in India during 1999 to 2018: a systematic review. BMC Public Health. 2021;21(1):1441.
5. Sharma BR, Harish D, Sharma V, Vij K. Poisoning in northern India: changing trends, causes and prevention thereof. Medicine, science and the law. 2002;42(3):251-7.
6. Ahuja H, Mathai AS, Pannu A, Arora R. Acute poisonings admitted to a tertiary level intensive care unit in northern India: patient profile and outcomes. J Clin Diagn Res. 2015;9(10):UC01-4.
7. Nambiar R, Dae D, Anjali S. Burden of poisoning on a critical care unit in southern India. Natl Med J India. 2019;32(4):197-9.
8. Singh SP, Aggarwal AD, Oberoi SS, Aggarwal KK, Thind AS, Bhullar DS, et al. Study of poisoning trends in north India—a perspective in relation to world statistics. J Forensic Legal Med. 2013;20(1):14-8.
9. Singh OP. Startling suicide statistics in India: time for urgent action. Indian J Psychiatry. 2022;64(5):431-2.
10. Global health statistics: a compendium of incidence, prevalence, and mortality estimates for over 200 conditions. UQ eSpace. [online] Available from https://espace.library.uq.edu.au/view/UQ:113991 [Last accessed September, 2024].
11. Jeyaratnam J. Acute pesticide poisoning: a major global health problem. World Health Stat Q. 1990;43(3):139-44.
12. National Crime Records Bureau. Accidental deaths & suicides in India year wise. [online] Available from https://ncrb.gov.in/accidental-deaths-suicides-in-india-year-wise.html?year=2021&keyword= [Last accessed September, 2024].
13. Eddleston M. Patterns and problems of deliberate self-poisoning in the developing world. QJM. 2000;93(11):715-31.
14. Rane A, Nadkarni A. Suicide in India: a systematic review. Shanghai Arch Psychiatry. 2014;26(2):69-80.
15. Haw C, Hawton K, Houston K, Townsend E. Psychiatric and personality disorders in deliberate self-harm patients. Br J Psychiatry. 2001;178(1):48-54.
16. Bøe AS, Mehlum L, Melle I, Qin P. Clinical determinants of hospital treated deliberate self-harm repetition: a time to recurrent event analysis. Acta Psychiatr Scand. 2022;146(6):557-67.
17. Seljenes Bøe A, Mehlum L, Melle I, Qin P. Psychiatric disorders among adult deliberate self-harm patients and subsequent risk of dying by suicide, mental and behavioural disorders and other external causes. J Psychiatr Res. 2023;165:83-90.
18. Vuagnat A, Jollant F, Abbar M, Hawton K, Quantin C. Recurrence and mortality 1 year after hospital admission for non-fatal self-harm: a nationwide population-based study. Epidemiol Psychiatr Sci. 2020;29:e20.
19. Shukla V, Shukla P, Tiwari A. Lead poisoning. Indian J Med Spec. 2018;9(3):146-9.
20. Kapaj S, Peterson H, Liber K, Bhattacharya P. Human health effects from chronic arsenic poisoning—a review. J Environ Sci Health A. 2006;41(10):2399-428.
21. Butler EJ. Chronic neurological disease as a possible form of lead poisoning. J Neurol Neurosurg Psychiatry. 1952;15(2):119-28.
22. Rafati-Rahimzadeh M, Rafati-Rahimzadeh M, Kazemi S, Moghadamnia AA. Current approaches of the management of mercury poisoning: need of the hour. Daru. 2014;22(1):46.
23. Chandran J, Krishna B. Initial management of poisoned patient. Indian J Crit Care Med. 2019;23(Suppl 4):S234-40.
24. Miller IW, Norman WH, Bishop SB, Dow MG. The Modified Scale for Suicidal Ideation: reliability and validity. J Consult Clin Psychol. 1986;54(5):724-5.
25. Beck RW, Morris JB, Beck AT. Cross-validation of the Suicidal Intent Scale. Psychol Rep. 1974;34(2):445-6.
26. Range LM, Knott EC. Twenty suicide assessment instruments: evaluation and recommendations. Death Stud. 1997;21(1):25-58.
27. Barstow C, Shahan B, Roberts M. Evaluating medical decision-making capacity in practice. Am Fam Physician. 2018;98(1):40-6.
28. Sessums LL, Zembrzuska H, Jackson JL. Does this patient have medical decision-making capacity? JAMA. 2011;306(4):420-7.
29. Gelder MG, Mayou R, Geddes J. Psychiatry. Oxford: Oxford University Press; 2005. 333 pp.
30. Seaward BL. Managing Stress. Massachusetts: Jones & Bartlett Learning; 2017. 609 pp.
31. Beck AT, Kovacs M, Weissman A. Assessment of suicidal intention: the Scale for Suicide Ideation. Consult Clin Psychol. 1979;47(2):343-52.
32. Harris KM, Syu JJ, Lello OD, Chew YLE, Willcox CH, Ho RHM. The ABC's of suicide risk assessment: applying a tripartite approach to individual evaluations. PLoS One. 2015;10(6):e0127442.
33. Linehan MM, Goodstein JL, Nielsen SL, Chiles JA. Reasons for staying alive when you are thinking of killing yourself: the reasons for living inventory. J Consult Clin Psychol. 1983;51(2):276-86.
34. Cutcliffe JR, Barker P. The Nurses' Global Assessment of Suicide Risk (NGASR): developing a tool for clinical practice. J Psychiatr Ment Health Nurs. 2004;11(4):393-400.
35. Olfson M, Marcus SC, Bridge JA. Focusing suicide prevention on periods of high risk. JAMA. 2014;311(11):1107-8.
36. Shafiekhani M, Mirjalili M, Vazin A. Psychotropic drug therapy in patients in the intensive care unit—usage,

adverse effects, and drug interactions: a review. Ther Clin Risk Manage. 2018;14:1799-812.
37. Cosci F, Chouinard G. Acute and persistent withdrawal syndromes following discontinuation of psychotropic medications. Psychother Psychosom. 2020;89(5):283-306.
38. Lewis SR, Pritchard MW, Schofield-Robinson OJ, Alderson P, Smith AF. Melatonin for the promotion of sleep in adults in the intensive care unit. Cochrane Database Syst Rev. 2018;5(5):CD012455.
39. Jenkins DH. Substance abuse and withdrawal in the intensive care unit: contemporary issues. Surg Clin N Am. 2000;80(3):1033-53.
40. Ungur LA, Neuner B, John S, Wernecke K, Spies C. Prevention and therapy of alcohol withdrawal on intensive care units: systematic review of controlled trials. Alcohol Clin Exp Res. 2013;37(4):675-86.
41. Arroyo-Novoa CM, Figueroa-Ramos MI, Puntillo KA. Opioid and benzodiazepine iatrogenic withdrawal syndrome in patients in the intensive care unit. AACN Adv Crit Care. 2019;30(4):353-64.
42. Koper I, Pasman HRW, Schweitzer BPM, Kuin A, Onwuteaka-Philipsen BD. Spiritual care at the end of life in the primary care setting: experiences from spiritual caregivers—a mixed methods study. BMC Palliat Care. 2019;18(1):98.
43. Pompili M, Shrivastava A, Serafini G, Innamorati M, Milelli M, Erbuto D, et al. Bereavement after the suicide of a significant other. Indian J Psychiatry. 2013;55(3):256-63.

2

SECTION

Specific Poisons

Section Editors: *JV Peter, Ashish Bhalla, Shivakumar Sankarnarayanan Iyer*

2.1 Organophosphorus Compounds and Carbamates

Anusha Cherian, JV Peter, Michael Eddleston

INTRODUCTION

Organophosphorus (OP) is the general name given for organic derivatives of phosphorus. The OP compounds are esters, amides, or thiol derivatives of phosphoric, phosphinic, or thiophosphoric acids. Tetraethyl pyrophosphate, the first OP cholinesterase inhibitor, was synthesized in 1854.[1] Between 1934 and 1945, around 2,000 OP compounds were developed at the I.G. Farben Industries, Germany, including parathion as a pesticide and sarin, soman, and tabun as nerve gas agents. Some of these agents were used during the Iran–Iraq war (1980–88) and in the chemical terrorist attacks in Japanese subway lines (1994–95). Several compounds were also developed as insecticides. Among the earliest OP insecticides were malathion and demeton which were developed in 1950–51; others (e.g., amiton) were found to be simply too toxic for agricultural use. The popularity of OP compounds as insecticides, nematocides, and fungicides increased with the withdrawal of organochlorine compounds.

Carbamates are structurally and mechanistically similar to OP compounds. Exposure to carbamates results in a similar toxidrome to OP compounds. However, unlike OP compounds which inhibit acetylcholinesterase (AChE) persistently, carbamates bind for a short time and hence the duration of toxicity is generally less than 24 hours. Although physostigmine was isolated as an active alkaloid in 1864, synthetic aliphatic esters of carbamic acid were developed as pesticides only from the 1930s. Common agents include aldicarb, carbofuran, and carbaryl.

The increasing use of insecticides has led to an alarming increase in the number of unintentional and intentional exposures to these compounds. In 2017, it was estimated that over 200,000 deaths occurred globally due to pesticide poisoning, the majority in rural areas of Asia due to intentional ingestion. A concerted multipronged effort is required to reduce the burden of pesticide-related poisoning.

TOXICOLOGY

Organophosphorus agents used in agriculture and industries, in general, are pentavalent phosphorous compounds. The phosphorus atom is attached covalently with a double bond to either oxygen (oxons) or sulfur (phosphothionate or thions). Oxons and thions are the two clinically important subclasses. Of the remaining three positions, two are occupied by either hydrogen, alkyl, aryl and alkoxyl, or other groups. Most agents have two methyl (dimethyl) or two ethyl (diethyl) groups attached to phosphorus, while a few agents have alkyl group attached with a sulfur atom. The final fifth bond is the leaving group or the dissociable group wherein the OP compound reacts with AChE. This leaving group could be halogens, cyano, alkyl, thio, and other inorganic or organic acids, which are most susceptible to hydrolysis.

Organophosphorus compounds are also grouped by the World Health Organization (WHO) based on acute toxicity into the following hazard classes based on lethal dose for 50% of those exposed to the compound by the oral route in rats (LD_{50})[2] **(Table 1)**.[2]

Toxicokinetics

Absorption

The inhalational route has the fastest absorption, followed by ingestion. Dermal absorption can be rapid if OP is mixed with a solvent or emulsifier and can result in severe toxicity if exposure is prolonged.[3]

Distribution and Storage

Following absorption, OP compounds are rapidly accumulated into fat, liver, kidneys, and salivary glands. Lipophilic agents such as fenthion and parathion are more extensively stored in fat than hydrophilic compounds (e.g., dimethoate) and often cause prolonged intoxication. Being lipophilic, they can also cross the blood-brain barrier easily.

Metabolism and Biotransformation

Oxons, in which the phosphorus has a double bond with oxygen, are in their active form. In contrast, phosphonothioates (P = S) must undergo activation by oxidative desulfuration in cytochrome p450 to their

TABLE 1: WHO classification of OP compounds based on hazard.

WHO hazard class/ chemical composition	*Dimethyl OP*	*Diethyl OP*	*S-alkyl OP*	*LD_{50} in rats (mg/kg body weight)**
I_a Extremely hazardous	Methyl parathion	Phorate		<5
	Phosphamidon	Parathion		
I_b Highly hazardous	Oxydemeton-methyl	Triazophos	Methamidophos	5–50
	Monocrotophos			
	Dichlorvos			
II Moderately hazardous	Dimethoate	Quinalphos	Profenophos	50–2,000
	Fenthion	Chlorpyrifos		
	Phenthoate	Ethion		
III Slightly hazardous	Acephate			>2,000
	Malathion			

*LD_{50} data is mg/kg body weight in rats and is for oral administration and for solids.
†Categorized as lipophilic only if log P > 4.0
(OP: organophosphorus; WHO: World Health Organization)

corresponding oxon (P = O). This may result in delayed onset of action (e.g., fenthion); however, patients ingesting potent parathion can become very sick within 15–30 minutes despite the need for conversion from thion to oxon.

Metabolism and deactivation of oxons into less toxic products occur principally through oxidation by cytochrome p450 enzymes and catalytic hydrolysis by esterases (e.g., PON-1). Other enzymatic detoxification systems include phosphotriesterases, carboxylesterases, and glutathione-S-transferases. Variability in these enzymes may affect the duration and intensity of the toxic effects of the compound. OPs can also undergo removal by conjugation with glucuronic acid, sulfate, or glycine, or by biotransformation into other metabolites that undergo similar removal.[4]

Elimination

Most of the metabolites of OP compounds are eliminated in the urine within hours unless stored in fat tissues.

Toxicodynamics

Inhibition of AChE

Acetylcholinesterase catalyzes the hydrolysis of neurotransmitter acetylcholine (ACh) at neuromuscular junctions, thereby terminating its action.

Acetylcholinesterase is highly concentrated at the synapses, while also being found on red cell membranes. The active site of AChE is a triad of serine, histidine, and glutamate where substrates and inhibitors attach. ACh attaches at the serine residue and undergoes hydrolysis by acetylation. This reaction restores the active AChE center within a few milliseconds.[5] OP compounds phosphorylate the serine residue, mimicking ACh. However, unlike ACh-bound AChE, phosphorylated AChE is stable and inhibited. Thus, there is an excess of ACh at the synaptic cleft leading onto hyperstimulation of muscarinic and nicotinic ACh receptors causing the clinical features of OP poisoning to manifest. The reactivation of the catalytic center occurs either spontaneously by hydrolysis of the phosphoryl enzyme complex or can be potentiated by the use of nucleophiles such as oximes, which results in regeneration of active AChE.

The speed of this reactivation depends on the chemical composition of the OP compound. Dimethoxy compounds result in more rapid AChE reactivation than diethyl compounds. Carbamates, on the other hand, carbamylate AChE allowing rapid spontaneous reactivation. Dimethoxy phosphorylated AChE is regenerated in 0.7–0.86 hours while diethoxy phosphorylation takes 31–57 hours for regeneration **(Table 2)**.[6] Oximes can speed up this process. However, the phosphorylated AChE can nonenzymatically replace an alkyl moiety with a hydroxyl group, in a reaction called "aging," which leads to further stabilization of the phosphorylated AChE and the OP compound being permanently bound to the enzyme. If the rate of aging is faster than that of spontaneous reactivation, the enzyme

TABLE 2: Half-life of reactivation and aging of phosphorylated AChE depending on chemical composition.[6]

OP compound	t½ spontaneous reactivation (hours)	t½ aging (hours)
Dimethoxy phosphorylated AChE	0.7–0.86	3.7
Diethoxy phosphorylated AChE	31–57	33

(AChE: acetylcholinesterase; t½: half-life)

can no longer be reactivated by a nucleophile as the center becomes negatively charged. Normal AChE function will then only be restored when new enzymes are synthesized. Dimethoxy phosphorylated AChE ages faster than diethoxy (3.7 hours vs. 33 hours) compounds suggesting that delayed oxime administration may not be helpful in dimethoxy compounds but possibly effective in diethoxy compounds. S-alkyl OP compounds appear to age very quickly with no response to oximes **(Table 2)**.[7,8]

Though evidence supports AChE as the most important site of action of OP, OPs can also cause changes in other enzymes, neurotransmitters, and the immune system.[8]

Oxidative Stress and Inflammation

There are several articles that have postulated evidence of direct cellular injury caused by lipid peroxidation and free radical formation by OP compounds. The brain is particularly susceptible to this injury due to its high oxygen consumption, lipid composition, and low levels of antioxidants.[9] Mitochondrial dysfunction and free radical-mediated injury may cause stimulation of cholinergic and glutaminergic neurotransmission in the brain causing excitotoxicity. However, the evidence is weak at present with studies demonstrating high *inter-individual* variations in terms of results and quality, and marked variation between the OP insecticides involved. There are no human studies that support the use of antioxidants to improve outcomes in OP poisoning.[9]

Factors Affecting Toxicity, Speed of Onset, and Clinical Presentation

- Exposure to hydrophilic OPs causes rapid onset of severe symptoms while some *lipophilic compounds* (dichlofenthion and profenofos) cause relatively milder symptoms at presentation with persistence or recurrence of cholinergic symptoms and delayed onset of respiratory failure.[10]
- *Alkyl group:* Dimethyl-containing OP compounds age faster than diethyl compounds. Agents that contain s-alkyl group age AChE much faster.[2,3]
- *Rate of activation:* Phosphates are active while phosphorothioates need to convert to oxons by biotransformation.
- Relative toxicity of the compound.
- Spontaneous reactivation of phosphorylated AChE: Dimethyl phosphorylated AChE reactivates spontaneously faster than diethyl phosphorylated AChE.[11]

CLINICAL FEATURES

Exposure to high concentration of OPs results in irreversible inhibition of AChE. Patients can manifest three overlapping syndromes depending on the time from exposure.[12] As muscarinic and nicotinic receptors are present in almost all organs, the clinical features are widely manifested **(Table 3)**.

Acute Cholinergic Crisis (Usually Occurs for the First Time Within 24 hours of Exposure)

The initial manifestations are usually due to muscarinic rather than nicotinic stimulation. There is a time-specificity to the order of symptom presentation based on the type of receptors that are specific to the affected organ. This has implications for treatment and prognostication.

The onset of manifestation depends upon the route of ingestion, dose, and chemical composition of the OP compound. The order of events usually described by the classical toxidrome pattern is of increased *S*alivation, *L*acrimation, *U*rination, *D*efecation, *G*astric cramps, and *E*mesis (SLUDGE), followed by effects of nicotinic receptor stimulation, which progress from weakness to fasciculation followed by type I paralysis, and eventually to coma and seizures.[1] However, presentation is more flexible and variable in actual practice.

Early respiratory failure during acute cholinergic crisis could be attributed to a central hypercholinergic muscarinic effect on the medullary centers causing a loss of central respiratory drive, respiratory muscle weakness, or excessive secretions and bronchospasms while late failure is due to paralysis of the muscles mediated by nicotinic receptor stimulation at neuromuscular junctions.[12] If excessive secretions are not promptly controlled, pulmonary edema could result. Direct overstimulation of central receptors could thus cause death in the early period.[12]

TABLE 3: Clinical features based on receptor type.

Receptor	Subtype	Organ system	Clinical manifestations
Muscarinic	M1 and M4	Striatum, cortex, and hippocampus	Anxiety, restlessness, convulsions, tremors, coma, respiratory depression, circulatory collapse, ataxia, and convulsions
	M2	Forebrain, thalamus, and spinal cord	
	M3	Brain and hypothalamus	
	M5	Dopaminergic neurons, brain vasculature, and basal ganglia	
	M2	Heart, conduction system, and peripheral arteries	• Bradycardia, hypotension • QT prolongation, and ST changes
	M3	Pupils	Constriction and miosis
		Respiratory	Bronchorrhea, bronchospasm, and rhinorrhea
		Gastrointestinal tract	Diarrhea, salivation, vomiting, fecal incontinence, and abdominal pain
		Renal	Urinary incontinence
Nicotinic	N1 (Nm)	Neuromuscular junction	Type I acute paralysis, weakness, fasciculation, and Type II paralysis (intermediate syndrome)
		Respiratory system	Diaphragmatic paralysis causing hypercarbia (hypercapnia) and respiratory failure
	N2 (Nn)	Adrenal medulla and autonomic ganglia	Tachycardia and hypertension

Muscarinic effects on the cardiovascular system present with bradycardia and hypotension. There is increased vagal stimulation leading to an increase in the refractory period of the sinus and atrioventricular nodes. Sometimes, the nicotinic effect on the adrenal medulla and autonomic ganglia may cause tachycardia and hypertension. Early death can occur due to persistent arrhythmias, refractory shock, vasodilatory state (more common), and endocardial ischemia (less common). QT prolongation and fatal late-onset tachyarrhythmias have also been described, especially in hypoxic patients who have not received atropine. Most often, the autonomic control of the heart rate and blood pressure (BP) is restored to normal levels after acute poisoning.

Neuromuscular effects occur acutely when AChE activity as measured in the blood reduces to <10%. This correlation between neuromuscular effects and AChE activity is not consistent across all OP compounds, such as in S-alkyl compounds wherein severe AChE inhibition may coexist with only mild cholinergic symptoms.[13] Severe muscle fasciculations could result in rhabdomyolysis and myopathy, and local ischemia may develop due to decreased perfusion. Acute central nervous system (CNS) symptoms are characterized by decrease in sensorium and rarely seizures if significant ingestion has occurred. Anoxia, usually a complication from the prehospital setting, is one of the main causes of long-term neurological sequelae and hence needs to be controlled early.

Delayed Effects (24 Hours to 2 Weeks Following Ingestion)

Intermediate syndrome occurs after 24–96 hours of acute poisoning and can last up to 3 weeks. However, 20% of patients can present outside this window period warranting the need for continuous monitoring. Delayed intermediate syndrome can also occur in the context of mixed OP-pyrethroid poisoning.

Intermediate syndrome is characterized by paralysis of proximal muscles, cranial nerves, and respiratory muscles. Progressive respiratory failure can occur due to paralysis of diaphragm and respiratory muscles requiring continued ventilatory support and introducing possible complications associated with prolonged ventilation and immobility. Importantly, this could also be an initial presentation in some patients and may be fatal if unrecognized.[14] Bilateral laryngeal nerve paralysis can occur as an isolated presentation that manifests as stridor or failed extubation.

Delayed organophosphorus encephalopathy (DOPE), characterized by coma and absent brain stem reflexes, mimicking brain death, can occur in a subset of patients. Unlike classical brain death, these patients have miotic pupils and other muscarinic symptoms.[15] This syndrome is likely due to leaching, redistribution, and conversion to active oxon forms of lipid-soluble OP from fat, slow regeneration of AChE. Delayed onset of extrapyramidal symptoms like cog-wheel rigidity and chorea athetosis is described, which recovers spontaneously in 1–4 weeks.[12]

Late-onset Symptoms (beyond 2 Weeks)

Organophosphorus-induced-delayed polyneuropathy (OPIDN) occurs due to prolonged nerve damage secondary to nicotinic cholinergic stimulation. It is a symmetrical sensory-motor axonopathy predominantly involving the lower limbs.[12] Symptoms are present in one-third of the patients in the form of cramping pain and paresthesia followed by weakness. On pathology, evidence of axonal degeneration and secondary demyelination is reported. Recovery is often complete. Other manifestations include delayed-onset extrapyramidal syndrome and ataxia.

DIAGNOSIS AND RISK STRATIFICATION

This includes (1) confirmation and identification of the compound, (2) assessing severity of poisoning, and (3) assessing risk of poor outcome.

Identifying the Compound

Diagnosis is based on the clinical presentation of the classic toxidrome. Identification of the particular OP insecticide involved is not essential but can be helpful for prediction of progression. In the absence of clearcut clinical indicators, a first gastric aspirate can be sent for toxicological assessment, but the result will arrive too late to guide clinical management. Confirmation of significant exposure is based on estimation of AChE activity. Compound identification is generally based on the container brought by the patient or the family member, which can be accurate for around 80% of cases when care is taken. Although plasma or urine can be sent for identification of the compound, this is generally done only in research settings.[13]

Assessment of Severity

Laboratory Tests

Plasma pseudocholinesterase or butyrylcholinesterase (BuChE) activity is used to confirm exposure to OP compounds. When there is significant exposure, cholinesterase activity is usually < 2,500 IU/mL (reference range 4,000–8,000 IU/mL) although there is marked variation between different OP insecticides.[16] After acute poisoning and elimination of the OP insecticide, recovery of the enzyme occurs at a steady rate of 7% per day. There are several limitations for these assays. Standardization of these assays is difficult as they are affected by temperature, pH, and substrate levels.[13] Low levels could be due to genetic variations.

Red cell AChE assays measure the activity of AChE expressed on the RBCs. It correlates well with neuronal AChE levels and synaptic inhibition. Once AChE undergoes aging, there is no regeneration, and AChE will be replaced only by erythropoiesis. Hence, its use in guiding treatment is limited, although it is a better indicator than BuChE.

Electrophysiology: Due to an excess of ACh and alteration of the nicotinic receptors, a single electrical stimulus results in repetitive compound muscle action potentials (CMAPs) due to prolonged endplate potential. Repetitive stimuli cause decremental CMAP response. Less severe AChE inhibition results in a decrease in CMAP due to transient desensitization of the receptors. In contrast, more severe poisoning results in progressive decrement of CMAP, owing to postsynaptic nicotinic receptor desensitization.

Other laboratory investigations: Significant increases in creatinine kinase, liver transaminases, potassium, and metabolic acidosis can occur if muscle damage is severe. Serum electrolytes and blood urea nitrogen are monitored to assess for secretory volume losses.

Risk Assessment

All patients with OP poisoning must undergo risk assessment. This is based on the context of exposure, individual patient factors, type of compound, and other environmental aspects. This has a potential for influencing further management and patient outcomes.

Exposure

Exposure can be through dermal, inhalational, or ingestional routes and can be accidental or intentional. Intentional ingestional poisoning is usually associated with the highest risk of death, in part because the solvents included in the agricultural products are also ingested. Coingestion with other compounds (e.g., pyrethroids) and alcohol can worsen outcomes.[17]

Patient Factors

Increasing age and comorbidities are associated with a higher risk of death. Polymorphism of enzymes involved in the metabolism of these compounds, for example, paraoxonases, may influence outcomes.[18] However, these are not tested routinely and have not been shown to be clinically relevant in human poisoning.

Formulation of Organophosphorus Compound

Many compounds are sold as high-concentration liquid formulations, increasing the risk of morbidity and mortality. The type of solvent used, for example, cyclohexanone, has been shown to influence cardiorespiratory failure.[40]

Toxicity also varies widely among more than 100 OP compounds that are available. The bioactivation of thion OP compounds to oxons causes a variable lag of onset of toxicity. However, most OPs cause significant inhibition of AChE within 6 hours.[19] Although the LD_{50} and lethal doses have been studied in experimental animals, the correlation in humans may be variable due to the differences in physiology and detoxification processes and is not reliable in acute ingestional poisoning with class II agents.[20] LD_{50s} are calculated in animals that do not receive any treatment, reducing their relevance to the patient who survives to receive treatment and intensive care.

Scoring Systems

Various scores such as APACHE, SAPS II, International Program on Chemical Safety Poison Severity Score (IPCS PSS), and the Glasgow Coma Scale (GCS) have been described and evaluated with varying performance.[21]

Laboratory Tests

Although it has been proposed that levels of AChE inhibition can be correlated with severity and the nature of clinical manifestations **(Table 4)**,[22] they may not be reliable in the acute clinical context. Blood gases can identify the severity of respiratory and hemodynamic compromise and detect metabolic and respiratory acidemia.

TABLE 4: Correlation of degree of inhibition of acetylcholinesterase with clinical severity.[22]

AChE activity	*Muscarinic effect*	*Nicotinic*	*CNS*
50–90% Mild symptoms	Impaired vision, nausea, and salivation		Headache and dizziness
10–50% Moderate symptoms	Diarrhea, wheezes, dyspnea, urinary incontinence, vomiting, and secretions	Muscle fasciculations	Dysarthria and ataxia
<10% Severe	Miosis, bradycardia, coma, and excess secretions	Diaphragmatic paralysis, and cardiovascular collapse	Coma and convulsion

(AChE: acetylcholinesterase; CNS: central nervous system)

MANAGEMENT

Initial Assessment and Resuscitation

Recognition of severity and risk assessment mitigates risk of death and enables stratification of patients who may need higher acuity of care. The initial cholinergic crisis could lead to death due to cardiorespiratory collapse. Although guidelines suggest low risk of exposure to healthcare workers and relatives taking care of these patients, universal precautions should be followed. A comprehensive assessment and management of the airway, breathing, and circulation should be undertaken. Sicker patients should be admitted in an intensive care unit (ICU) setup and monitored.[13]

It is important to underscore the importance of atropine in the management of OP poisoning, and hence the A of the ABCs (airway, breathing, circulation) of resuscitation may be modified to include airway and atropinization, as described below.

Airway and Atropinization

Immediate rapid-sequence induction and intubation may be necessary when there is airway compromise due to excessive secretions, airway obstruction or depressed sensorium, and high risk of aspiration. Succinylcholine should be avoided as it could lead to prolongation of neuromuscular junction blockade given that it is metabolized by BuChE. Urgent and early administration of atropine in escalating doses to target atropinization may help avoid intubation by markedly reducing oropharyngeal secretions and improving conscious state.[23] Despite concerns of atropine use prior to oxygenating a hypoxic patient, early and rapid administration of atropine in this setting may be lifesaving even if oxygen is not immediately available.[24]

Rapid atropinization using an initial dose of 1–2 mg followed by doubling of the dose every 5 minutes until target atropinization is advocated.[10] Atropinization is targeted to safe heart rate (usually around 100/min on day 1 with reduced targets on subsequent days), systolic BP of >90 mm Hg, and clear chest on auscultation.[25] Pupillary size and gastric sounds are poor treatment endpoints as they are subject to individual variations and have no influence on patient outcome.

Breathing

Patients should be continuously monitored for breathing impairment leading to hypoxia and/or hypoventilation and increased work of breathing. Tachypnea, shallow breathing, bradypnea, use of accessory muscles, bronchospasm, crepitations, increased secretions, decrease in oxygen saturation levels, and cyanosis may be observed. The importance of early and urgent atropine for bronchospasm, bronchorrhea, increased secretions, and hypoxia cannot be overemphasized. Depending on the severity, supplemental oxygen, noninvasive ventilation, or invasive ventilation should be administered. Regular assessment of neck flexion strength and then measurement of tidal (or minute) volume can guide in predicting impending respiratory failure.[26]

Circulation

Patients usually present with varying degrees of bradycardia and hypotension,[19] although they may be normotensive and have a normal heart rate or rarely hypertensive and tachycardic. Intravenous access should be secured and prompt fluid resuscitation initiated to restore volume losses alongside early atropinization to sustain BP and heart rate. Conduction blocks, arrhythmias, and myocardial dysfunction have been reported and may occur and should be monitored for.[27] Atropine-resistant hypotension is associated with poor outcomes.[7]

Rapid atropinization usually improves bradycardia and hemodynamics. If there is a lack of response to these interventions, titrated doses of vasopressors such as adrenaline, noradrenalin, and vasopressin can be used.

Neurological

Frequent assessment of the GCS is important. Muscle fasciculations, weakness, and coma can be present at admission or may develop over the next hours or days. Seizures occur in a small subset of patients; they are more frequent in patients with mixed OP-pyrethroid poisoning. Airway support, optimization of breathing and circulation, seizure control with benzodiazepines, and measures to minimize secondary brain damage are the main stay of treatment **(Table 5)**.

Treatment

The principles of treatment include resuscitation with antidotes, fluids, and oxygen, followed by supportive care. Once the patient has been fully resuscitated and stabilized, it is reasonable to consider these other elements of therapy for reducing the poison load, detoxification, and enhancing elimination.

Continuing Detoxification

It involves the continued use of anticholinergic agents and consideration of physiological antagonists and oximes to reactivate AChE.

Physiological antagonists: Anticholinergic agents, the most important of which is atropine, are the mainstay of OP poison treatment. It reverses most of the muscarinic effects of OP. Once atropinization has been achieved, atropine infusion (starting at around 20% of the loading doses required for atropinization per hour) is preferred over boluses to maintain targets. Vasopressors, such as noradrenaline and vasopressin, may be considered if hemodynamics do not improve after adequate fluid resuscitation and atropine administration. Adrenaline (often at a low dose) may be considered if there is an inadequate heart rate response to high-dose atropine therapy.

Excess, nontitrated atropine therapy may be associated with adverse effects such as agitation, delirium, fever, urinary retention, gastric ileus, dehydration, rhabdomyolysis, and acute kidney injury. In such situations, atropine should be stopped for 30 minutes and the infusion regimen reassessed (started at a lower dose).

Reactivation of AChE, oxime therapy: The basis for oxime use is to restore neuromuscular transmission and limit the complications of OP poisoning in the form of muscle weakness and ventilator dependency. However, there are conflicting reports regarding their efficacy as well as evidence of potential harm with their use.[19,20,28,29]

Since oximes have the potential to reactivate the OP–AChE complex, it should be considered before AChE undergoes irreversible aging. Two oximes are frequently

TABLE 5: Initial assessment based on signs and symptoms and management.

Physiology	***Signs and symptoms***	***Management***
Airway compromise		
Increased secretions, vomitus, and blood in the airway	Noisy breathing, stridor, increased salivation, low GCS, inspect oropharynx, and seizures	Immediate RSI if indicated, avoid succinylcholine, thorough suctioning of oropharynx, prevention of pulmonary aspiration, early and rapid atropinization
Inability to protect the airway due to severe CNS depression due to direct OP effects, seizures		
Cerebral hypoperfusion due to cardiovascular collapse, coingestion of alcohol, raised ICP levels		
Breathing		
Impaired oxygenation due to excessive secretions, aspiration of vomitus, bronchorrhea, bronchospasm, and noncardiogenic pulmonary edema	Tachypnea, bradypnea, shallow breathing, use of accessory muscles, bronchospasm, crepitations, increased secretions, reduced oxygen saturation, and cyanosis	Early atropine. Regular assessment of neck flexion, single breath count to assess for respiratory failure, high-flow oxygen, noninvasive ventilation, and invasive ventilation as indicated
Hypoventilation due to CNS depression, alcohol coingestion, neuromuscular blockade due to direct toxicity or as a metabolic consequence, intermediate syndrome		
Increased work of breathing due to above factors		
Hemodynamics		
Reduced systemic vascular resistance due to Ach-induced release of NO, bradycardia and hypotension, conduction blocks, and arrhythmias	Hypotension, bradycardia, signs of shock, reduced capillary refill time, and lactic acidosis	IV access, fluid resuscitation, atropine to improve bradycardia and blood pressure, titrated dose of vasopressors if no response
Myocardial injury and dysfunction		
Hypovolemia due to increased loss of fluids and secretions		
Neurological		
Neurological impairment due to direct toxicity, reactive oxygen species, disruption of blood–brain barrier, delayed-onset coma and encephalopathy, neuromuscular blockade due to direct effect, and intermittent syndrome	Impaired consciousness, agitation, confusion, muscle weakness, fasciculations, coma, seizures (rarely), extrapyramidal signs, ophthalmoplegia, bowel, and bladder incontinence	Support of airway, breathing, and circulation to minimize secondary brain damage, and atropine, benzodiazepines for seizure control

(ACh: acetylcholine; CNS: central nervous system; GCS: Glasgow Coma Scale; ICP: intracranial pressure; NO: nitric oxide; RSI: rapid-sequence induction and intubation)

used, the more commonly available pralidoxime and the more potent obidoxime. Although in vitro and in vivo animal and human studies have shown enzyme reactivation with oximes, multiple studies in the clinical setting of acute OP poisoning have failed to demonstrate unequivocal benefit with oximes compared to no oximes.[21,30,31]

Several reasons have been postulated for the lack of benefit with oximes and include poor CNS penetration limiting their action to the peripheries, rapid re-inhibition of oxime-reactivated AChE by circulating OP in mega-dose intoxications, increased oxidative stress, hepatotoxicity and nephrotoxicity with oximes, and inadequate dose for insufficient duration.[1]

Therefore, the current role of pralidoxime remains controversial. It may be considered in a subset of patients who present early, probably within 6 hours of poisoning with a diethyl compound, with moderate poisoning. Treatment should be given in an ICU setting with very careful observation of the patient. The risk versus benefit as well as cost should be considered prior to administration. In patients with diethyl poisoning, a dose of 1 g every 6 hours may reactivate the enzyme. There is no evidence for oximes in delayed presentations (>12 hours) especially after poisoning with dimethyl compounds.

Reducing the Poison Load

Although there is a physiological basis for prompt and early dermal and gastric decontamination, there is limited data to support these interventions. Dermal decontamination is done by washing with soap and water. Oral-activated charcoal can be administered in an awake, conscious, cooperative patient if presenting within 1–2 hours of ingestion. However, a large randomized controlled trial (RCT) comparing single- to multidose charcoal did not demonstrate a benefit.[41] Gastric lavage can be done if presentation is early and airway is protected. The risk versus benefit must be considered for gastric decontamination.

Other Supportive Therapies

These therapies include monitoring and treatment of complications.

Continuous monitoring: For respiratory failure, cardiovascular monitoring should be done in sicker patients. Relevant investigations should be sent to evaluate for complications **(Table 6)**.

Seizures: Benzodiazepines are preferred since they are allosteric modulators of gamma-aminobutyric acid (GABA) and reduce the action of glutamate and the excitotoxic effects of glutamine.[32] This may prevent neuronal injury associated with central cholinergic stimulation. Currently, it is recommended for control of seizures and reducing anxiety and agitation.[25,33]

Aspiration pneumonitis: Care should be taken to prevent aspiration. Appropriate antibiotics should be started in case of pneumonia.

Nutrition: It should be started as soon as the patient is clinically stable and does not have vomiting or high gastric aspirates.

TABLE 6: Monitoring in OP poisoning patients.

Abnormality	*Causes*
Hypokalemia	Diarrhea, vomiting, and high urine output
High BUN and creatinine (AKI)	Dehydration, increased secretions, and OP effect
High liver transaminases	Muscle injury and OP toxicity[4]
Respiratory and metabolic acidosis	Inadequate ventilation, decreased cardiac output
Lipases and amylases	OP-induced pancreatitis
Hyperglycemia	Stress hyperglycemia and OP induced

(AKI: acute kidney injury; BUN: blood urea nitrogen; OP: organophosphorus)

Enhanced Elimination

Enhanced elimination of the OP compound may be achieved with extracorporeal removal, bioscavenging, and alkalinization.

Extracorporeal removal: Extracorporeal removal of the compound by hemoperfusion with activated charcoal is an attractive option as OP compounds have low molecular weight. However, a large volume of distribution precludes its use with the majority of OP insecticides which are lipophilic. There may be possible benefit if given early enough for hydrophilic compounds such as dichlorvos. Animal studies have demonstrated an increase in AChE levels without mortality benefit. One human study showed reduced mortality, ICU stay, need for intubation, and duration of coma in patients receiving early hemoperfusion with charcoal.[42] However, there were design flaws in this study. Extracorporeal removal is still experimental and not recommended in the routine management.

Bioscavengers: These are enzymes that break down the OP compound before it reaches its target site. There are several classes of enzymes that can remove OP by different reactions. The most studied among these is BuChE. Fresh frozen plasma (FFP) contains several scavengers including albumin and BuChE. FFP is used as the source for BuCHE since purified human BuChE is not available for clinical use. Studies demonstrated an improvement in the levels of AChE with FFP, although clinical outcomes did not vary. However, these studies were too small to be conclusive.[34]

Paraoxonases: These are enzymes that hydrolyze some particular chiral forms of OP compounds. Only animal studies exist currently in the context of nerve gas OP compounds.

Alkalinization: This has several postulated benefits including enhanced removal of OP compounds by enzymatic and nonenzymatic hydrolysis, volume expansion, and improved oxime therapy. However, a systematic review of five trials failed to show a clinically meaningful outcome.[35]

Other therapies Other therapies that have been attempted in small studies are summarized in **Table 7**.

CONCLUSION

The management of OP poisoning has evolved over the years with better understanding of the mechanism of manifestations and course in hospital. Although the

TABLE 7: Other drugs used to counteract physiological effects of OP poisoning.

Drug	*Mechanism of action*	*Evidence*	*Recommendations*
Magnesium[36]	Decreases AChE release by blocking ligand-gated presynaptic calcium channels, reverses decrease in CMAP	Pooled data from eight clinical studies, did not find any difference for need for intubation and mortality[37]	Insufficient evidence to recommended
Clonidine[38,39]	Alpha 2 receptor agonist, decreases presynaptic release of AChE and descending sympathetic transmission	Two phase II trials did not show any clinical outcome benefit	Side effects of hypotension, bradycardia noted, hence not recommended

(AChE: acetylcholinesterase; CMAP: compound muscle action potential)

mortality rate in OP poisoning has come down significantly over the last few decades with legislation banning most toxic compounds and significant improvements in ICU care, OP poisoning is still associated with considerable morbidity and high case fatality. Future directions should be toward banning all highly toxic OP insecticides, prompt identification and treatment at the first responder hospital, and a multipronged treatment approach that involves effective resuscitation and atropinization, excellent nursing care, and evidence-based interventions to reduce and eliminate toxins.

REFERENCES

1. Balali-Mood M, Abdollahi M (Eds). Basic and Clinical Toxicology of Organophosphorus Compounds. London: Springer London; 2014.
2. World Health Organization. (2019). The WHO Recommended Classification of Pesticides by Hazard and Guidelines to Classification. [online] Available from https://iris.who.int/bitstream/handle/10665/332193/9789240005662-eng.pdf?sequence=1 [Last accessed September, 2024].
3. Kwong TC. Organophosphate pesticides: Biochemistry and clinical toxicology. Ther Drug Monit. 2002;24(1):144-9.
4. Balali-Mood M, Saber H. Recent advances in the treatment of organophosphorous poisonings. Iran J Med Sci. 2012;37(2):74-91.
5. Tsai YH, Lein PJ. Mechanisms of organophosphate neurotoxicity. Curr Opin Toxicol. 2021;26:49-60.
6. Eyer P. The role of oximes in the management of organophosphorus pesticide poisoning. Toxicol Rev. 2003;22(3):165-90.
7. Eddleston M, Szinicz L, Eyer P, Buckley N. Oximes in acute organophosphorus pesticide poisoning: A systematic review of clinical trials. QJM Mon J Assoc Physicians. 2002;95(5):275-83.
8. Casida JE, Quistad GB. Organophosphate toxicology: Safety aspects of nonacetylcholinesterase secondary targets. Chem Res Toxicol. 2004;17(8):983-98.
9. Rambabu L, Megson IL, Eddleston M. Does oxidative stress contribute to toxicity in acute organophosphorus poisoning? - A systematic review of the evidence. Clin Toxicol Phila Pa. 2020;58(6):437-52.
10. Eddleston M. Novel clinical toxicology and pharmacology of organophosphorus insecticide self-poisoning. Annu Rev Pharmacol Toxicol. 2019;59:341-60.
11. Jokanović M, Prostran M. Pyridinium oximes as cholinesterase reactivators. Structure-activity relationship and efficacy in the treatment of poisoning with organophosphorus compounds. Curr Med Chem. 2009;16(17):2177-88.
12. Peter JV, Sudarsan TI, Moran JL. Clinical features of organophosphate poisoning: A review of different classification systems and approaches. Indian J Crit Care Med. 2014;18(11):735-45.
13. Eddleston M, Buckley NA, Eyer P, Dawson AH. Management of acute organophosphorus pesticide poisoning. Lancet. 2008;371(9612):597-607.
14. Wadia RS, Sadagopan C, Amin RB, Sardesai HV. Neurological manifestations of organophosphorous insecticide poisoning. J Neurol Neurosurg Psychiatry. 1974;37(7):841-7.
15. Peter J. Delayed-onset encephalopathy and coma in acute organophosphate poisoning in humans. Neurotoxicology. 2008;29(2):335-42.
16. Eddleston M, Worek F, Eyer P, Thiermann H, Von Meyer L, Jeganathan K, et al. Poisoning with the S-Alkyl organophosphorus insecticides profenofos and prothiofos. QJM. 2009;102(11):785-92.
17. Eddleston M, Gunnell D, von Meyer L, Eyer P. Relationship between blood alcohol concentration on admission and outcome in dimethoate organophosphorus self-poisoning. Br J Clin Pharmacol. 2009;68(6):916-9.
18. Costa LG, Cole TB, Vitalone A, Furlong CE. Measurement of paraoxonase (PON1) status as a potential biomarker of susceptibility to organophosphate toxicity. Clin Chim Acta Int J Clin Chem. 2005;352(1-2):37-47.
19. Eddleston M, Eyer P, Worek F, Mohamed F, Senarathna L, von Meyer L, et al. Differences between organophosphorus

insecticides in human self-poisoning: A prospective cohort study. Lancet. 2005;366(9495):1452-9.
20. Dawson AH, Eddleston M, Senarathna L, Mohamed F, Gawarammana I, Bowe SJ, et al. Acute human lethal toxicity of agricultural pesticides: A prospective cohort study. PLoS Med. 2010;7(10):e1000357.
21. Akdur O, Durukan P, Ozkan S, Avsarogullari L, Vardar A, Kavalci C, et al. Poisoning severity score, Glasgow coma scale, corrected QT interval in acute organophosphate poisoning. Hum Exp Toxicol. 2010;29(5):419-25.
22. Thiermann H, Szinicz L, Eyer P, Zilker T, Worek F. Correlation between red blood cell acetylcholinesterase activity and neuromuscular transmission in organophosphate poisoning. Chem Biol Interact. 2005;157-158:345-7.
23. Abedin MJ, Sayeed AA, Basher A, Maude RJ, Hoque G, Faiz MA. Open-label randomized clinical trial of atropine bolus injection versus incremental boluses plus infusion for organophosphate poisoning in Bangladesh. J Med Toxicol Off J Am Coll Med Toxicol. 2012;8(2):108-17.
24. Konickx LA, Bingham K, Eddleston M. Is oxygen required before atropine administration in organophosphorus or carbamate pesticide poisoning? - A cohort study. Clin Toxicol Phila Pa. 2014;52(5):531-7.
25. Eddleston M, Buckley NA, Checketts H, Senarathna L, Mohamed F, Sheriff MHR, et al. Speed of initial atropinisation in significant organophosphorus pesticide poisoning – A systematic comparison of recommended regimens. J Toxicol Clin Toxicol. 2004;42(6):865-75.
26. Eddleston M, Mohamed F, Davies JOJ, Eyer P, Worek F, Sheriff MHR, et al. Respiratory failure in acute organophosphorus pesticide self-poisoning. QJM. 2006;99(8):513-22.
27. Lotti M. Clinical toxicology of anticholinesterase agents in humans. In: Kireger R (Ed). Hayes' Handbook of Pesticide Toxicology. Philadelphia: Elsevier; 2010. pp. 1543-89. [online] Available from https://linkinghub.elsevier.com/retrieve/pii/B9780123743671000720. [Last accessed September, 2024].
28. Buckley NA, Eddleston M, Szinicz L. Oximes for acute organophosphate pesticide poisoning. Cochrane Database Syst Rev. 2005;(1):CD005085.
29. Peter JV, Moran JL, Graham P. Oxime therapy and outcomes in human organophosphate poisoning: An evaluation using meta-analytic techniques. Crit Care Med. 2006;34(2):502-10.
30. Blumenberg A, Benabbas R, deSouza IS, Conigliaro A, Paladino L, Warman E, et al. Utility of 2-pyridine aldoxime methyl chloride (2-PAM) for acute organophosphate poisoning: A systematic review and meta-analysis. J Med Toxicol Off J Am Coll Med Toxicol. 2018;14(1):91-8.
31. Cherian AM, Peter JV, Samuel J, Jaydevan R, Peter S, Joel S, et al. Effectiveness of P2AM (PAM- pralidoxime) in the treatment of organophosphorus poisoning (OPP): A randomised, double blind placebo controlled trial. J Assoc Physicians India. 1997;45:22-4.
32. Marrs TC. Diazepam in the treatment of organophosphorus ester pesticide poisoning. Toxicol Rev. 2003;22(2):75-81.
33. Dickson EW, Bird SB, Gaspari RJ, Boyer EW, Ferris CF. Diazepam inhibits organophosphate-induced central respiratory depression. Acad Emerg Med Off J Soc Acad Emerg Med. 2003;10(12):1303-6.
34. Pichamuthu K, Jerobin J, Nair A, John G, Kamalesh J, Thomas K, et al. Bioscavenger therapy for organophosphate poisoning - an open-labeled pilot randomized trial comparing fresh frozen plasma or albumin with saline in acute organophosphate poisoning in humans. Clin Toxicol Phila Pa. 2010;48(8):813-9.
35. Roberts D, Buckley NA. Alkalinisation for organophosphorus pesticide poisoning. Cochrane Database Syst Rev. 2005;2005(1):CD004897.
36. Basher A, Rahman SH, Ghose A, Arif SM, Faiz MA, Dawson AH. Phase II study of magnesium sulfate in acute organophosphate pesticide poisoning. Clin Toxicol Phila Pa. 2013;51(1):35-40.
37. Brvar M, Chan MY, Dawson AH, Ribchester RR, Eddleston M. Magnesium sulfate and calcium channel blocking drugs as antidotes for acute organophosphorus insecticide poisoning - A systematic review and meta-analysis. Clin Toxicol Phila Pa. 2018;56(8):725-36.
38. Perera PMS, Jayamanna SF, Hettiarachchi R, Abeysinghe C, Karunatilake H, Dawson AH, et al. A phase II clinical trial to assess the safety of clonidine in acute organophosphorus pesticide poisoning. Trials. 2009;10:73.
39. El-Ebiary AA, Gad SA, Wahdan AA, El-Mehallawi IH. Clonidine as an adjuvant in the management of acute poisoning by anticholinesterase pesticides. Hum Exp Toxicol. 2016;35(4):371-6.
40. Eddleston M, Street JM, Self I, Thompson A, King T, Williams N, et al. A role for solvents in the toxicity of agricultural organophosphorus pesticides. Toxicology. 2012;294(2-3):94-103. doi: 10.1016/j.tox.2012.02.005.
41. Eddleston M, Juszczak E, Buckley NA, Senarathna L, Mohamed F, Dissanayake W, et al.; Ox-Col Poisoning Study collaborators. Multiple-dose activated charcoal in acute self-poisoning: a randomised controlled trial. Lancet. 2008;371(9612):579-87. doi: 10.1016/S0140-6736(08)60270-6. PMID: 18280328; PMCID: PMC2430417.
42. Peng A, Meng FQ, Sun LF, Ji ZS, Li YH. Therapeutic efficacy of charcoal hemoperfusion in patients with acute severe dichlorvos poisoning. Acta Pharmacol Sin. 2004;25(1):15-21. PMID: 14704117.

2.2 Clinical Presentation and Management of Organochlorine Poisoning

JS Thakur, Stuti Pramod

INTRODUCTION

Organochlorines (OCs) are a group of chlorinated compounds that are commonly used as pesticides. They have high persistence in the environment and are thus classified as persistent organic pollutants (POPs).

History and Epidemiology

Until the 1940s, highly toxic elements like arsenic, mercury, lead, and sulfur were used as the commonly available pesticides. In the early 1940s, Swiss chemist Paul Müller demonstrated the insecticidal properties of dichlorodiphenyltrichloroethane (DDT), an OC, thus introducing a new class of pesticides.[1] They were inexpensive to produce and had relatively low acute toxicity compared to the previously available pesticides. They were widely used in modern agriculture, structural protection from termites, and soil treatments until the late 1970s. DDT also had medical and public health applications in controlling typhus and mosquito vectors.[2] By 1953, DDT was estimated to have saved 50 million lives and prevented one billion cases of human disease, due to which it was credited as the single most important factor in the population explosion between 1950 and 1970.[3] It is still considered an effective control measure for malaria-control programs and is also used for indoor residual spraying in endemic regions of Africa.[4]

Classification

It is important to remember that pesticides are inherently acutely toxic to humans. Therefore, the World Health Organization (WHO) has developed a hazard classification system for all pesticides. This system is based on the LD_{50} value in rats, which is the dose of a substance lethal to 50% of the experimental animals involved **(Table 1)**.

TABLE 1: Classification of pesticides by hazard as per WHO.[5]

Class		*LD_50 for the rat (mg/kg body weight)*			
		Oral		*Dermal*	
		Solids	*Liquids*	*Solids*	*Liquids*
Ia	Extremely hazardous	≤5	≤20	≤10	≤40
Ib	Highly hazardous	5–50	20–200	10–100	40–400
II	Moderately hazardous	50–500	200–2,000	100–1,000	400–4,000
III	Slightly hazardous	>500	>2,000	>1,000	>4,000
III+	Unlikely to present hazard in normal use	>2,000	>3,000	–	–

(WHO: World Health Organization)

Organochlorine pesticides can be grouped into four categories based on the similarities in chemical structures and other properties: (1) DDT and its related analog, (2) cyclodienes (the related isomers aldrin, dieldrin, and endrin; heptachlor, and endosulfan) and related compounds (toxaphene and dienochlor), (3) hexachlorocyclohexane (HCH) (commonly known as lindane), and (4) mirex and chlordecone **(Table 2)**. The signs and symptoms of toxicity in humans are largely similar within each group.

Uses and Regulation

Uses

Organochlorine compounds have a variety of uses. The following are the most notable applications:

- *Vinyl chloride:* The production of vinyl chloride is the largest application of OC chemistry.
- *Chloromethanes:* Most low-molecular-weight chlorinated hydrocarbons, such as chloroform, dichloromethane, dichloroethane, and trichloroethane, are useful solvents.
- *Pesticides:* Many pesticides contain chlorine. Notable examples include DDT, dicofol, heptachlor, endosulfan, chlordane, aldrin, dieldrin, endrin, mirex, and pentachlorophenol.
- *Insulators:* Polychlorinated biphenyls (PCBs) were once commonly used electrical insulators and heat transfer agents. Their use has generally been phased out due to health concerns.

TABLE 2: Classification and properties of organochlorine pesticides.

Class	Compounds	Acute oral toxicity (man)	Dermal absorption	Lipid storage	Persistence in environment	WHO classification	Specific characteristics
DDT and its related analogs	DDT	Low to moderate	Low	Highest	High; half-life of 2–15 years	II	Tremors, CNS excitation, and odorless
	Methoxychlor	Low	Low	Moderate	High; half-life of <120 days	III+	Less toxic DDT substitute
Cyclodienes and related compounds	Aldrin	High	High	High	Moderate; half-life of 4–7 years	Ib	Rapidly metabolized to dieldrin; mild "chemical" odor
	Dieldrin	High	High	High	High; half-life of 9 months	Ib	Stereoisomer of endrin; early and late seizures; odorless
	Endrin	Highest	High	None	Moderate; half-life of 1 day to 12 years	Ib	Most toxic organic chlorine; rapid-onset seizures, status epilepticus
	Chlordane	Moderate	High	High	High; half-life of 10 years	II	Early and late seizures
	Endosulfan	High	High	Low	Moderate; half-life of 15 months	Ib	Strong sulfur odor
	Heptachlor	Moderate	High	High	High; half-life of 2 years	Ib-II	Toxic metabolite heptachlor epoxide; camphor odor
HCH	Lindane	Moderate	High	Low	High; half-life of 15 months	II	Topical scabicide; seizures; CNS excitation; musty odor
Chlordecone and mirex	Chlordecone	Moderate	High	High	Moderate; half-life of 63–148 days	II	"Kepone shakes"; structurally similar to mirex
	Mirex	Low	High	High	High; half-life of 10 years	III+	Metabolized to chlordecone; similar toxicity

(CNS: central nervous system; DDT: dichlorodiphenyltrichloroethane; HCH: hexachlorocyclohexanes; WHO: World Health Organization)

The use of OCs as pesticides poses the largest threat to human health. High levels of exposure are seen among agricultural workers from developing countries due to the lack of proper legislation, improper market regulations, and lack of awareness of the ill effects.[6] Studies have shown that nearly 40% of all pesticides used belong to the OC class of chemicals.[7]

Regulation

In 2001, the Stockholm Convention on Persistent Organic Pollutants (SCPOPs) identified 12 POPs as the "dirty dozen," which included OCs such as DDT, HCH, aldrin, dieldrin, endrin, chlordane, hexachlorobenzene, mirex, heptachlor, and toxaphene.[8] In 2009, nine more industrial chemicals, known as the "Nasty Nine", were added during the fourth meeting of the SCPOPs, which included pentabromodiphenyl ether, octabromodiphenyl ether, chlordecone, lindane, α-HCH, β-HCH, perfluorooctane sulfonate, hexabromobiphenyl, and pentachlorobenzene.[9]

In India, DDT and endosulfan are the most produced pesticides. The ban on OCs resulted in a significant decline in their consumption between 2001 and 2010. The total production of pesticides also decreased after

2020. Currently, 293 pesticides are registered in India, and 104 are still in use, despite being banned or restricted worldwide.[10]

In the United States, only dicofol and endosulfan are registered as pesticides. Lindane is sold as a second-line treatment agent for lice and scabies but is not recommended by the American Academy of Pediatrics and is also banned in several states due to acute neurological toxicity.[11,12] The most frequently reported serious or fatal events are often due to endosulfan.[13,14]

TOXICOKINETICS

Chemical Structure and Properties

An OC is an organic compound containing at least one covalently bonded chlorine atom. They are often complex, cyclic, and nonvolatile solids at room temperature. They have a molecular weight in the range of 300–550 Daltons. All OCs share the basic characteristics of low polarity, low aqueous solubility, and high lipid solubility. They also show environmental persistence, which is defined as a half-life of greater than 2 months in water or 6 months in soil.[15]

Absorption

All OC pesticides are well absorbed orally and by inhalation. Dermal absorption is variable depending on the compound. As they are not water-soluble, they are usually dissolved in an organic solvent or sold as powders for dusting.[16] DDT and its analogs have very poor dermal absorption. They also have limited volatility, and hence have low air concentrations, making toxicity by the respiratory route unlikely. All of the cyclodienes and lindane are well absorbed dermally. Chlordecone and mirex are absorbed efficiently via the skin, by inhalation, and orally.

Distribution

All OCs are lipophilic, which facilitates penetration into the central nervous system. They are then redistributed to fatty tissues via the bloodstream, which may account for the rapid central nervous system (CNS) recovery despite persistent substantial total body burden.[17]

Metabolism

Most OCs are metabolized in the liver by the cytochrome P450 enzyme systems by dichlorination and oxidation, with subsequent conjugation. The high solubility and slow metabolization of DDT, dieldrin, heptachlor, chlordane, mirex, and chlordecone cause significant storage in the adipose tissues. OCs such as endrin, endosulfan, lindane, methoxychlor, dicofol, and toxaphene are rapidly metabolized and eliminated and therefore have less persistence in bodily tissues despite being highly lipid-soluble.[18]

Elimination

All OCs are primarily excreted through bile, but most also have detectable urinary metabolites. All lipophilic compounds are also partially excreted in maternal milk.[19]

Mechanisms of Toxicity

Organochlorines primarily act on the CNS by altering the movement of ions across the nerve cell membranes, thus changing the ability of the nerve to fire. Electrophysiological studies have shown that OCs act by either interfering with repolarization, prolonging depolarization, or impairing the maintenance of the polarized state of the neurons. This results in hyperexcitability of the nervous system and repetitive neuronal discharges.[3] This hyperexcitability leads to convulsions and other signs of neurological toxicity, such as myoclonic jerking, paresthesia, tremors, ataxia, and hyperreflexia.[17] Convulsions may also lead to the alteration of pulmonary gas exchange, causing pulmonary acidosis. High tissue concentrations of OCs also increase myocardial irritability, predisposing to cardiac arrhythmias. When tissue concentrations drop below the threshold levels, recovery is seen.

Action of Specific Organochlorines

- *DDT:* It acts by interfering with the sodium channels in the axonal membrane. It has little to no effect on the resting potential or action potential. However, it greatly prolongs the depolarizing afterpotential of the action potential, which produces a period of increased neuronal excitability immediately after the spike phase. This, in turn, enhances the repetitive firing of action potentials. DDT and methoxychlor generally tend to produce less severe side effects.[1]
- *Other classes, including cyclodienes, lindane, and mirex:* Cyclodienes and lindane act as gamma-aminobutyric acid (GABA) antagonists. They inhibit GABA binding at the GABA-A receptor–chloride ionophore complex in the CNS by interacting at the picrotoxin-binding site.[20,21]

They are also associated with more severe seizures and fatalities.[1]

Drug Interactions

As OCs undergo metabolism in the liver by induction of the cytochrome enzyme systems, theoretically, it may have consequences such as enhanced metabolism of therapeutic drugs and/or reduced efficacy. However, reports suggest that such effects probably occur only following extended and substantial exposures to OCs , which is rare. There are no definitive reports of human-enhanced metabolism of therapeutic drugs or adverse reactions due to the induction of microsomal enzymes.[16]

CLINICAL PRESENTATION

Signs and Symptoms of Toxicity

In humans, the earliest symptom of poisoning by DDT is hyperesthesia of the mouth and lower part of the face, followed by paresthesia of the same area and the tongue. This is often followed by dizziness, the development of fine tremors in the extremities which then progress to coarse tremors, and eventually tonic-clonic convulsions. Other symptoms like confusion, vomiting, and hypersensitivity to external stimuli, such as light, touch, and sound, may be present. Symptoms usually appear several hours after exposure, and death, usually due to respiratory failure, may occur after 24–72 hours.[1]

The first manifestation following exposure to cyclodienes, lindane, and toxaphene is a generalized seizure. Cyclodienes have a propensity to cause seizures that may recur for several days following acute exposure. If seizures are brief and hypoxia does not set in, recovery is usually complete. Electroencephalographic (EEG) abnormalities are noted before, during, and following seizures.[22] Hyperthermia secondary to central mechanisms, increased muscle activity, and aspiration pneumonitis are also common.[1]

Seizures related to dermal application of 1% lindane for the treatment of lice or scabies may occur following a single inappropriate application or, more commonly, after repetitive prolonged exposures.[23]

Acute Versus Chronic Poisoning

Acute Exposure

In sufficient doses, OCs lower the seizure threshold or remove inhibitory influences to produce CNS stimulation with resultant seizures and respiratory failure, eventually leading to death. In the case of DDT, seizures only occur after exposure to a massive dose, typically 10 mg/kg or more.[3]

Chronic Exposure

Chlordecone, commercially known as Kepone, has a characteristic effect due to its long persistence in the body. A study was conducted among 133 factory workers in Hopewell, Virginia, from 1974 to 1975. Due to the poor industrial hygiene practices in this makeshift chlordecone factory, they developed a clinical syndrome known as the "Hopewell epidemic," which consisted of tremors in the hands, a fine tremor of the head, and trembling of the entire body, known as "Kepone shakes." Other findings were weakness of the body, ataxia, mental status changes, rash, weight loss, and elevated liver enzymes. Idiopathic intracranial hypertension, oligospermia, and decreased sperm motility were also seen in some of these workers.[24]

A study on 70 cancer patients also demonstrated high concentrations of methoxychlor, DDT, hexachlorobenzene, and chlordane in tumor-affected tissues when compared to adjacent normal tissue. A possible association between high tissue levels of OCs and the resultant molecular dysfunction in specimens of breast cancer has been proposed but requires further research to elucidate other possible mechanisms leading to carcinogenesis.[25]

DIAGNOSIS

Diagnostic Information

The history of exposure to an OC compound is the most important clue to diagnosis, as incidental exposure is otherwise rare. The patient may present with an unusual odor in the mouth, vomitus, or skin. Specific OCs have a characteristic odor, such as a mild turpentine-like odor in the case of toxaphene or a "rotten egg" sulfur-like odor in endosulfan **(*see* Table 2)**.

Laboratory Testing

In most cases, if the patient's history and clinical presentation are obvious, then laboratory evaluation is unnecessary as it does not alter the course of management, and the investigations for the detection of OCs are often not available on an emergent basis. Currently, no data is available to show the correlation between the clinical management of the health effects and the tissue concentrations. Routine surveillance in cases of occupational exposure is not advocated at present as the analytical methods are complex and not likely to detect the amounts of metabolites generated by minimal exposure.[26,27] If confirmation is indicated clinically or for documentation, it may be necessary to measure the concentration of the OCs .

Organochlorines and/or their metabolites can be identified in blood, serum, adipose tissue, or urine by gas-liquid chromatography in samples serially collected over a few days of significant pesticide exposure. Some OCs and their metabolites such as DDT, dieldrin, mirex, heptachlor, and chlordecone persist in tissues and blood for weeks or even months after absorption. Others may be excreted within a few days and may not be detected by chromatographic methods. Blood or serum levels are more telling in cases of acute toxicity, while examination of adipose tissue or breast milk holds more significance in chronic exposure. As chromatographic methods are highly sensitive, positive results may be obtained even after exposure to levels lower than those required to produce toxicity. Therefore, a positive blood or serum detection may not always be indicative of acute toxicity.

MANAGEMENT

After triaging and initial assessment of the patient, the following measures should be instituted.

General Measures[28]

- Observe the person for sensory disturbances, incoordination, speech slurring, mental confusion, and involuntary movements that precede convulsions.
- If altered mental status is observed, administration of dextrose and thiamine should be considered in adults.
- The skin should be decontaminated thoroughly with soap and water, especially in cases of topical lindane exposure.
- The clothing of the patient should be removed and placed in a plastic bag and disposed of appropriately as per the principles of biomedical waste management.
- Healthcare providers should wear appropriate personal protective equipment including gloves and aprons.
- Since OCs are mostly liquids, a nasogastric tube can be used for suction and lavage if the patient presents within an hour of exposure. Activated charcoal can be administered after nasogastric suction and lavage, or if the patient presents beyond one hour of initial exposure.
- Oil-based cathartics should never be used, as OCs are lipophilic and their absorption may be facilitated.
- Hyperthermia should be managed with external cooling.
- As OCs are neurotoxins, the risk of seizures and their associated complications outweighs the risk of gastrointestinal contamination. Therefore, if the patient is convulsing, it is almost always necessary to first control the seizures before attempting gastric decontamination.

Management of Convulsions

- If convulsions occur, place the patient in the left lateral decubitus position with the head facing down. Move away any physical obstructions such as furniture which may cause mechanical injury.
- If jaw movements are violent, place padded tongue blades and remove dentures, if any.
- Aspirate oral and pharyngeal secretions and secure an oropharyngeal airway, if available.
- Seizures caused due to OCs are often prolonged and difficult to control. Therefore, if status epilepticus occurs or patients do not respond to first-line anticonvulsants, they should be referred to a higher center immediately.
- Initial therapy with benzodiazepines should be started. Although lorazepam is generally used as the drug of choice for status epilepticus, it has little to no role in the management of seizures caused due to OCs.
- Treatment should be initiated with benzodiazepines:
  - *Adults:* Diazepam 5–10 mg IV and repeat every 5–10 minutes to achieve a maximum dose of 30 mg.
  - *Children:* Diazepam 0.2–0.5 mg/kg (or lorazepam equivalent dose) every 5 minutes, up to a maximum dose of 5 mg in children aged 5 years or under and 10 mg in those over 5 years.
- Cases that do not respond to diazepam may require a propofol infusion or even a pentobarbital-induced coma and should, therefore, be referred to a higher center for management in intensive care.

Use of Cholestyramine Resin[28]

Cholestyramine resin is a nonabsorbable, bile acid-binding anion exchange resin. It acts by accelerating the biliary-fecal excretion of the more slowly eliminated OC compounds and raising both the convulsive and the lethal dose. It may be administered in selected cases of exposure to chlordecone and other highly persistent compounds. It should never be given in its dry form and must always be administered with water or other liquids. The clinical experience of using this agent in OC poisoning is limited; therefore, it is still not considered as standard of care for OC poisoning.

Dosage of cholestyramine resin

- *Adults:* 4 g doses, 4 times a day, before meals and at bedtime
- *Children:* 240 mg/kg/day, in three divided doses administered 8 h

Management of Other Complications

- Large doses of OC may cause respiratory failure. Administer oxygen by mask and maintain pulmonary gas exchange by mechanically assisted ventilation whenever respiration is depressed.
- Continuous ECG monitoring is required to monitor cardiac status in cases of severe poisoning and the occurrence of cardiac arrhythmia.
- Do not give epinephrine, other adrenergic amines, or atropine unless absolutely necessary.
- During the phase of convalescence, parenteral therapy should be considered to increase the intake of carbohydrates and proteins.

CONCLUSION

Organochlorines are a group of chlorinated compounds commonly used as pesticides, known for their persistence in the environment. They include DDT and its analogs, cyclodienes (e.g., aldrin, dieldrin), HCH (e.g., lindane), and chlordecone/mirex. They are used in agriculture and vector control but pose significant health risks. They are banned or restricted in many countries, notably under the SCPOPs . OCs are well absorbed orally and by inhalation.[29] The lipophilic nature of OCs facilitates their penetration into the CNS. They are metabolized in the liver and excreted via bile and urine. OCs alter ion movement across nerve cell membranes, leading to hyperexcitability and seizures. They can also cause hyperesthesia, dizziness, confusion, and potential carcinogenesis. Diagnosis is often made by a history of exposure and with a characteristic odor. Gas chromatography may be indicated for documentation in selected cases. Management includes decontamination and seizure management using diazepam and, in severe cases, propofol or pentobarbital-induced coma. Cholestyramine resin may be administered to accelerate excretion. Respiratory support and ECG monitoring may be required.

REFERENCES

1. Echobichon D. Toxic effects of pesticides. In: Klaasen CD (Ed). Casarett and Doull's Toxicology: The Basic Science of Poisons, 5th edition. New York: MacMillan; 1996. pp. 643-69.
2. Costa LG. Basic toxicology of pesticides. Occup Med. 1997;12(2):251-68.
3. Ecobichon DJ, Joy RM. Pesticides and Neurological Diseases, 2nd edition. Boca Raton: CRC Press; 1993. p. 400.
4. Sadasivaiah S, Tozan Y, Breman JG. Dichloro-diphenyltrichloroethane (DDT) for indoor residual spraying in Africa: How can it be used for malaria control? In: Breman JG, Alilio MS, White NJ (Eds). Defining and Defeating the Intolerable Burden of Malaria III: Progress and Perspectives: Supplement to Volume 77(6) of American Journal of Tropical Medicine and Hygiene. [online] Am Soc Trop Med Hygiene; 2007. Available from https://www.ncbi.nlm.nih.gov/books/NBK1724/ [Last accessed September, 2024].
5. The WHO Recommended Classification of Pesticides by Hazard and Guidelines to Classification 2019.
6. Kim JH, Smith A. Distribution of organochlorine pesticides in soils from South Korea. Chemosphere. 2001;43(2):137-40.
7. Gupta PK. Pesticide exposure—Indian scene. Toxicology. 2004;198(1-3):83-90.
8. Reis TH. Stockholm convention on persistent organic pollutants. In: Elgar Encyclopedia of Environmental Law. Cheltenham: Edward Elgar Publishing; 2017. pp. 354-63.
9. United Nations Environment Program. Report of the Conference of the Parties of the Stockholm Convention on Persistent Organic Pollutants. 2009. Report No.: 4/38.
10. Statistical Database. Directorate of plant protection, quarantine and storage, Government of India. [online] Available from https://ppqs.gov.in/statistical-database [Last accessed September, 2024].
11. CDC. Unintentional topical lindane ingestions—United States, 1998–2003. [online] Available from https://www.cdc.gov/mmwr/preview/mmwrhtml/mm5421a2.htm [Last accessed March 2024].
12. Fischer TF. Lindane toxicity in a 24-year-old woman. Ann Emerg Med. 1994;24(5):972-4.
13. Brandt VA, Moon S, Ehlers J, Methner MM, Struttmann T. Exposure to endosulfan in farmers: Two case studies. Am J Ind Med. 2001;39(6):643-9.
14. Kucuker H, Sahin O, Yavuz Y, Yürümez Y. Fatal acute endosulfan toxicity: A case report. Basic Clin Pharma Tox. 2009;104(1):49-51.

15. Wauchope RD, Buttler TM, Hornsby AG, Augustijn-Beckers PW, Burt JP. The SCS/ARS/CES pesticide properties database for environmental decision-making. Rev Environ Contam Toxicol. 1992;123:1-155.
16. US EPA O. (2013). Recognition and management of pesticide poisonings. [online]. Available from https://www.epa.gov/pesticide-worker-safety/recognition-and-management-pesticide-poisonings [Last accessed September, 2024].
17. ScienceDirect Topics. Organochlorine pesticide - an overview [online]. Available from https://www.sciencedirect.com/topics/pharmacology-toxicology-and-pharmaceutical-science/organochlorine-pesticide [Last accessed September, 2024].
18. Femina Carolin C, Kamalesh T, Senthil Kumar P, Rangasamy G. An insights of organochlorine pesticides categories, properties, eco-toxicity and new developments in bioremediation process. Environ Pollut. 2023;333:122114.
19. Qi SY, Xu XL, Ma WZ, Deng SL, Lian ZX, Yu K. Effects of organochlorine pesticide residues in maternal body on infants. Front Endocrinol. 2022;13:890307.
20. Islam R, Lynch JW. Mechanism of action of the insecticides, lindane and fipronil, on glycine receptor chloride channels. Br J Pharmacology. 2012;165(8):2707-20.
21. Crowder L. Mode of Action of Cyclodiene Insecticides: The Nervous System Influenced by Toxaphene. Washington, DC: U.S. Environmental Protection Agency; 2004. [online]. Available from https://cfpub.epa.gov/si/si_public_record_Report.cfm?Lab=ORD&dirEntryId=49095 [Last accessed September, 2024].
22. Klaassen CD. Non-metallic environmental toxicants. In: Hardman JG, Limbird LE, Molinoff PB, Ruddon RW (Eds). Goodman and Gilman's the Pharmacologic Basis of Therapeutics, 9th edition. New York: McGraw-Hill; 1996. pp. 1684-99.
23. Wooltorton E. Concerns over lindane treatment for scabies and lice. CMAJ. 2003;168(11):1447-8.
24. Reich MR, Spong JK. Kepone: A chemical disaster in Hopewell, Virginia. Int J Health Serv. 1983;13(2): 227-46.
25. Eldakroory S, Morsi DE, Abdel-Rahman R, Roshdy S, Gouida M, Khashaba E. Correlation between toxic organochlorine pesticides and breast cancer. Hum Exp Toxicol. 2017;36(12):1326-34.
26. Fard NJH, Fard MP, Haghighipur S, Fard ES, Jorfi S. Monitoring and risk assessment of exposure to organochlorine pesticides through the water supply system, case of Karkheh River in southwest Iran. J Environ Health Sci Engineer. 2022;20(2):881-8.
27. Casarett LJ, Doull J, Klaassen CD (Eds). Casarett and Doull's Toxicology: The Basic Science of Poisons, 7th edition. New York: McGraw-Hill; 2008. 1310 p.
28. Nelson L, Goldfrank LR (Eds). Goldfrank's Toxicologic Emergencies, 9th edition. New York: McGraw-Hill Medical; 2011. 1940 p.
29. Bonvoisin T, Utyasheva L, Knipe D, Gunnell D, Eddleston M. Suicide by pesticide poisoning in India: A review of pesticide regulations and their impact on suicide trends. BMC Public Health. 2020;20(1):251.

2.3 Pyrethroid Poisoning

Ramya Iyadurai

INTRODUCTION

Pyrethroids are insecticides that have a wide variety of uses in agriculture, forestry, textile, furniture industry, medicine, and veterinary medicine. Pyrethroids have been recommended by the World Health Organization (WHO) for personal protection against malaria and zika virus.[1] According to the WHO classification, the pyrethroids are the fourth class of insecticides. As per data available, pyrethroids are the most common insecticides used worldwide.

Pyrethroid was originally extracted from *Tanacetum cinerariifolium* (previously genus *Chrysanthemum*). But the early pyrethroids were unstable with poor insecticidal activity; hence, more potent type 1 and type 2 pyrethroids were synthesized which were more powerful and stable.[2]

Some of the pyrethroids available for commercial use in India include permethrin cream—Permeva, Perilice; deltamethrin—DEL-28, Deltaflow; cypermethrin—Baygon spray, Laxman Rekha, Cyper 25, Cyper Gold; and transfluthrin—Goodknight mosquito repellent, All Out repellent (All Out also contains citronellol and kerosene); some common home-use pesticides can be a combination of pyrethroids, e.g., HIT—imiprothrin + cypermethrin.

Pyrethroids are available in various forms as liquid formulations, aerosol sprays, and chalk form. The chalk form usually contains cypermethrin (Laxman Rekha, Nok lines, and cockroach killer) or occasionally deltamethrin (Deltarin).

MECHANISM OF TOXICITY

On entry into the human body, pyrethroids mainly act on the sodium and the chloride channels.

The pyrethroids bond to the alpha subunit of the voltage-gated sodium channels, causing them to open and it also prevents the channel from closing. This causes sodium influx (called the tail current) and permanent depolarization of the nerve cells. This effect on the sodium channels depends on the structure of the pyrethroid rather than the tissue concentration. Hence, type 1 pyrethroids hold the channel open for a shorter time compared with type 2 pyrethroids. This action on the sodium channels is probably responsible for the clinical effects such as paresthesia and proarrhythmogenic potential of the pyrethroids.[3]

Pyrethroids, especially the type 2 pyrethroids, also reduce the chloride channel currents in the brain, peripheral nerves, muscles, and salivary glands. This results in clinical presentation with excess salivation and myotonia.[4]

At high concentrations, pyrethroids can act on gamma-aminobutyric acid chloride channels; this is probably responsible for seizures that are seen with severe pyrethroid poisoning.[5]

TOXOKINETICS

Pyrethroids are easily and extensively absorbed in the gastrointestinal tract and the respiratory tract, but only slightly across intact skin. Once absorbed, pyrethroids are degraded in the liver by hydrolysis into inert products. Extensive liver metabolism is one of the major reasons for low toxicity of pyrethroids in mammals.[6]

Studies on human volunteers with cypermethrin have shown that 43% of the metabolite (free cyclopropane carboxylic acid) is excreted within the first 24 hours. Half-life of pyrethroids is in the order of tens of hours; for example, the half-life of permethrin is 8.7 hours and deltamethrin is 5.5 hours in blood which may be shortened due to fat distribution. The short half-life is the reason most patients recover completely from pyrethroid poisoning within 48 hours of ingestion.[3]

Modes of Pyrethroid Poisoning

Oral Ingestion

Oral ingestion is the most common mode of poisoning among the Indian patients as shown in a case series of 379 patients from India in this cohort. All of the patients had taken the toxin orally in an attempt of deliberate self-harm (DSH). Patients who have ingested pyrethroid present with drowsiness, excess salivation, and vomiting; seizures in severe poisoning; and a small proportion can present with diarrhea.[7] Pyrethroids also have direct irritant action on the gastrointestinal mucosa and patients who have orally ingested pyrethroids can develop esophageal ulceration, esophagitis, sometimes gastritis even with hematemesis, and gastric and duodenal ulceration.[8]

Inhalation

Pyrethroid inhalation is associated with acute pneumonitis, especially when inhaled in a closed environment and there are repeated exposures. Patients present with acute-onset cough and dyspnea without fever. Patients will progress to developing type 1 respiratory failure. Chest radiograph and computed tomography will show bilateral ground-glass opacities **(Figs. 1A to D)**. Pyrethroid lung is a diagnosis of exclusion, a clue to diagnosis is repeated exposure to air-borne pyrethroid sprays within the last 1 week. Inflammatory markers can be mildly elevated but screen for viruses and bacteria are negative.

Pyrethroids act on the inward sodium transporter channels present in the type 1 and type 2 pneumocytes. They disrupt the osmotic gradients in these cells leading to bronchial and epithelial mucosal edema. At high doses, pyrethroids can overwhelm the cytochrome P450 enzymes leading to cell destruction due to oxidative stress and cytotoxicity. Clinicians need a high index of suspicion to identify inhalational pyrethroid poisoning.[9,10]

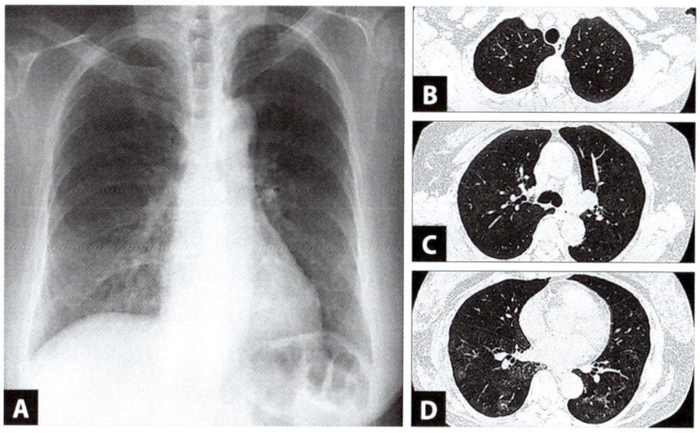

Figs. 1A to D: Chest radiograph (A) ground glass opacities in the bilateral lower lung fields, computed tomography (B to D) showing diffuse centrilobar ground glass opacities with mosaic attenuation and areas of consolidation in lower lobes of both lungs. ©Copyright Toyoshi Yanagihara.

Injection

There have been case reports of patients who have injected pyrethroid intramuscularly as an attempt of DSH. Pyrethroids are absorbed when injected intramuscularly and symptoms vary depending on the dose and the type of pyrethroid. In a case report from India, the patient developed respiratory symptoms similar to inhalational poisoning with type 1 respiratory failure after injecting prallethrin 5–7 mL (112 mg) in her thigh. In another report from China, a patient injected 20 mL of esfenvalerate intramuscularly and the patient only had local symptoms with swelling, pain, and paresthesia over the injection site.[11,12]

Toxidrome

Oral Ingestion

Clinical presentation of pyrethroid poisoning may depend on the type of pyrethroid ingested. Classically, patients with type 1 pyrethroid poisoning present with tremors and those with type 2 pyrethroid poisoning present with choreoathetosis, salivation, and in severe cases seizures. Nausea and vomiting can occur in both type 1 and type 2 pyrethroid poisoning. Studies have shown that paresthesia, hypersalivation, and seizures occur exclusively in patients with type 2 pyrethroid poisoning.

Some studies have classified pyrethroid poisoning as mild, moderate and severe. The clinical features include:

- *Mild poisoning:* Patients have only headache, nausea, vomiting, and dizziness with oral ingestion with skin application. Patients will have paresthesia and with the inhalational route they present with fatigue.
- *Moderate poisoning:* Increased salivation, increased tone, hyperexcitability, tremors (especially type 2 pyrethroids), and central nervous system (CNS) depression.[13]
- *Severe poisoning:* Seizures, coma, pulmonary edema, and respiratory failure[14]

Severe symptoms of pyrethroid poisoning such as seizures and coma can occur within 20 minutes of pyrethroid poisoning, and these effects can persist for weeks.

Recent reports have shown that the clinical presentation of pyrethroid poisoning may vary. Sometimes, patients can present with pneumonia and acute kidney injury. Atypical presentations such as respiratory failure, low Glasgow Coma Scale (GCS), and hypotension are more common in the older age group of >60 years and with higher quantities of pyrethroid consumed of >300 mL.[15]

Other Routes

Patients with inhalational poisoning will present with respiratory symptoms such as dyspnea and respiratory failure and those with injection pyrethroid poisoning will present with both respiratory and local symptoms of swelling, pain, and paresthesia.

MANAGEMENT

Investigations

Most of the routine investigations are noncontributory. Some studies have shown that patients with pyrethroid poisoning can have leukocytosis and metabolic acidosis in patients with severe poisoning. High serum lactate was seen in patients with severe toxicity.[15]

Electrocardiogram findings are most often reveals only sinus tachycardia; but patients can rarely have ventricular ectopics and sinus bradycardia.[8,16]

One study has shown that hyperglycemia indicative of increased adrenergic activity is associated with poor outcomes in patients with pyrethroid poisoning. Presence of hyperglycemia was associated with complications of respiratory failure, acidosis, and hypotension.[17]

All patients with pure pyrethroid poisoning have a normal serum cholinesterase level.[18]

In all patients with pyrethroid poisoning, acetylcholinesterase (AChE) levels must be sent to rule out additional organophosphorus (OP) toxicity.

Diagnosis

Diagnosis of pyrethroid poisoning is mainly done with the clinical presentation and the identification of the insecticide container brought by the patient. As a good practice measure, it is better to retake history and reidentify the insecticide container once the patient has reached the critical care unit. To avoid missing OP + pyrethroid pesticide combination poisoning.

Along with the routine tests, it is important to check the serum AChE level in all patients with insecticide poisoning. A normal serum acetylcholine (ACh) level will categorically rule out OP poisoning.[18]

Nonquantitative pyrethroid assays are available to prove pyrethroid exposure; these are ELISA (enzyme-linked immunosorbent assays) based assays that detect pyrethroid metabolites in urine—3PBA. They are currently used in field trials in patients with chronic pyrethroid exposures.[19]

Laboratories can identify pyrethroid in blood with high-performance liquid chromatography (HPLC). Standardization for HPLC is difficult, and assay standards are available only for a few pyrethroids.[13]

> Pyrethroid poisoning diagnosis:
>
> Good history + examination of the poison container + normal serum Ach level, if available HPLC for toxin analysis.

Treatment

Decontamination

Gastric lavage: This must be avoided as there are studies that prove that it increases the risk of aspiration pneumonia and hence prolonged hospitalization. As we have seen in the preceding text, pyrethroids have local corrosive action. It is better that gastric lavage is completely avoided in patients with pyrethroid poisoning.[3]

Forced emesis: This is widely practiced by the family members before the patients are brought to the hospital. This practice must be strongly discouraged as it increases complications and has no proven efficacy.

Activated charcoal: Single dose-activated charcoal can be used for gastric decontamination in patients who do not have features of corrosive injury due to pyrethroids. If a patient has severe oral pain, retrosternal chest pain, or epigastric pain suggestive of esophagitis and gastritis, then it is better to avoid activated charcoal in this group of patients.

Skin decontamination: In patients with dermal exposure, immediate decontamination with soap and water is recommended as it is safe but there is no evidence that it reduces toxicity.[3]

Antidotes

Atropine can be used in the management of hypersalivation and bradycardia. But it is essential to titrate the dose of atropine carefully and avoid atropine intoxication. A single dose of 0.6–1.2 mg of atropine will be enough to reduce hypersalivation.[14]

Animal studies have shown that ivermectin can be used to reduce salivation and mephenesin to reduce the cardiovascular and motor effects of deltamethrin poisoning, but there are no human trials that have proven the efficacy of these drugs.[20,21] Topical application of vitamin E is effective in reducing paresthesia due to pyrethroid poisoning.[22]

Intensive Care Management

Management is mainly supportive; in critically ill patients securing the airway, maintaining the breathing and circulation is vital.

Seizures must be adequately controlled with antiepileptics; although benzodiazepines are usually effective, phenytoin and valproate are found to be equally effective in reducing pyrethroid-induced sodium currents in animal models. Patients who develop resistant status epilepticus can be managed with thiopental in an intensive care setting after securing the airway and breathing.[23]

Acute inhalational toxicity: Along with supportive management, securing the airway and breathing, intravenous pulse methylprednisolone 500 mg once a day for 5 days has shown to improve patient outcomes and aid in early weaning off the ventilator as seen in case reports of patients with acute inhalational pyrethroid poisoning.

Patients can sometimes develop injection abscesses over the site of pyrethroid injections and this must be managed with incision and drainage.

Outcomes and Prognosis

The overall outcomes in pure pyrethroid poisoning are good, with mortality being a rare outcome. Most patients recover within 6 days.[14]

Pyrethroid Poisoning and Additives

Pyrethroid and Piperonyl Butoxide

Piperonyl butoxide inhibits the metabolism of pyrethroid. This becomes significant when large doses of a combination of pyrethroid and piperonyl are ingested for DSH. Pyrethroid toxicity is potentiated since piperonyl is a cytochrome P450 inhibitor that reduces the metabolism of pyrethroid and enhances toxicity.[24] Hence, patients with a combination of pyrethroid and piperonyl butoxide poisoning present with features of severe pyrethroid poisoning **(Table 1)**.

Combination Organophosphorus and Pyrethroid

Organophosphorus compounds, when ingested in combination with pyrethroid, bind and inhibit the esterases and monooxygenases that are responsible for degradation

TABLE 1: Isolated pyrethroid versus combination poisoning: Clinical features, identification, and outcomes.

Features	*Pyrethroid*	*Pyrethroid + piperonyl*	*Pyrethroid + organophosphorus*
Absorption	Cutaneous absorption is low Oral absorption up to 50%	Cutaneous absorption increased up to 8%	Increased oral absorption
Metabolism	Rapidly hydrolyzed by the liver	Due to CYP inhibition, reduced degradation	Reduced degradation due to carboxylesterase inhibition
Clinical features	Usually mild to moderate toxicity	Severe pyrethroid toxicity	Severe pyrethroid or OP toxicity
Diagnosis	History + toxin identification	History + toxin identification	Low ACh levels
Management	Supportive, antiepileptics for seizures	Look out for severe pyrethroid poisoning Antiepileptics for seizures	Look out and treat for severe OP poisoning/severe pyrethroid poisoning
Outcomes	Good	Mostly good	Those with severe OP manifestation have poorer outcomes

(ACh: acetylcholine; OP: organophosphorus)

of pyrethroids, and hence addition of OP to pyrethroid enhances pyrethroid toxicity. Hence, patients who have ingested this combination present with severe pyrethroid toxicity. In a case series of such patients from Nepal, all of them presented with severe pulmonary edema and seizure (10–15 per day) but with supportive treatment such as diuretics, ventilation, and benzodiazepines, patients were quickly weaned off the ventilator with 48 hours indicating predominantly severe pyrethroid toxicity.[25-27]

In a case series and reports from India, patients had ingested some combinations of pyrethroid and OP which have excess high concentration of OP (>50%) in comparison to the quantity of pyrethroid. These patients presented with severe prolonged OP poisoning as pyrethroids inhibit degradation of OP compounds.[18] Some such available combinations include cypermethrin (2%) + chlorpyriphos (50%), deltamethrin (1%) + triazophos (35%), and deltamethrin (1.25%) + chlorpyriphos (50%).

Hence, the patients who have ingested a combination of OP and pyrethroid can present with severe OP or severe pyrethroid poisoning depending on the type of combination they have ingested. Reading the container label will alert the astute intensivist regarding the complications that he should be ready for the management of such patients.[18]

We have to be aware of both of these clinical presentations in patients with a combination of OP and pyrethroid poisoning. ACh will be low in both these patients, but clinical presentations are quite different and outcomes are also different. Patients with predominantly pyrethroid poisoning have better outcomes than those with predominantly OP poisoning.

CONCLUSION

- Pyrethroid poisoning is common in medical practice, pyrethroids are available in varied forms, chalk, aerosols and liquid formulations.
- Pyrethroids are absorbed extensively from the gastrointestinal and respiratory tract, less via intact skin; they have a short half life and are mostly eliminated from the body within 48 hours.
- Pyrethroid lung occurs post recent inhalational exposure pyrethroids and is a diagnosis of exclusion, management is supportive and IV pulse Methylprednisolone 500 mg once a day for 5 days.
- Patients with pyrethroid poisoning via injection route can develop localized abscess and rarely respiratory failure.
- The pyrethroid toxidrome can be mild with headache, nausea, vomiting and fatigue, moderate with hyperexcitablity, salivation, tremors and severe with Seizures, coma, pulmonary edema, and respiratory failure.
- Diagnosis of pyrethroid poisoning is with good history, clinical examination and identification of the toxin from the container.
- Acetyl cholinesterase levels must be checked in all patients to rule out OP + pyrethroid combination poisoning.
- Treatment is decontamination with single dose activated charcoal avoid gastric lavage and forced emesis.
- Atropine single dose 0.6–1.2 mg is enough to reduce hypersalivation, seizures can be controlled with

benzodiazepines and Thiopentol can be used in the intensive care setting for resistant status epilepticus.

- Pyrethroid poisoning has good outcomes with mortality being rare and most patients will recover within 6 days.
- Combination pesticide poisonings are common and the intensivist must be aware this in routine practice.

REFERENCES

1. Zaim M/WHOPES (Eds). (2005). Safety of pyrethroids for public health use.[online] Available from https://www.who.int/publications/i/item/WHO.PCS.RA.2005.1 [Last accessed September, 2024].
2. Proudfoot AT. Poisoning due to pyrethrins. Toxicol Rev. 2005;24(2):107-13.
3. Bradberry SM, Cage SA, Proudfoot AT, Vale JA. Poisoning due to pyrethroids. Toxicol Rev. 2005;24(2):93-106.
4. Forshaw PJ, Lister T, Ray DE. The role of voltage-gated chloride channels in type II pyrethroid insecticide poisoning. Toxicol Appl Pharmacol. 2000;163(1):1-8.
5. Bloomquist JR, Adams PM, Soderlund DM. Inhibition of gamma-aminobutyric acid-stimulated chloride flux in mouse brain vesicles by polychlorocycloalkane and pyrethroid insecticides. Neurotoxicology. 1986;7(3): 11-20.
6. Hutson DH. The metabolic fate of synthetic pyrethroid insecticides in mammals. In: Bridges JW, Chasseaud LF (Eds). Progress in Drug Metabolism. New York: Wiley; 1979; pp. 215-52.
7. Iyadurai R, Peter JV, Lenin A, Yadav B, Reginald A, Abhilash KPP, et al. Pyrethroid poisoning: Insecticide with mild human toxicity. Med J Armed Forces of India. [online] Available from https://doi.org/10.1016/j.mjafi.2023.09.009. [Last accessed September, 2024].
8. Yang P-Y, Lin J-L, Hall AH, Tsao TCY, Chern M-S. Acute ingestion poisoning with insecticide formulations containing the pyrethroid permethrin, xylene, and surfactant: A review of 48 cases. J Toxicol Clin Toxicol. 2002;40:107-13.
9. Vorselaars ADM, van den Berg PM, Drent M. Severe pulmonary toxicity associated with inhalation of pyrethroid-based domestic insecticides (Bop/Sapolio): A case series and literature review. Curr Opin Pulm Med. 2021;27(4):271-7.
10. Yanagihara T, Nakagawa T, Fukushima T, Moriuchi Y, Ogata H, Ishimatsu A, et al. Acute pneumonitis associated with the inhalation of pyrethroid-based domestic insecticides. Cureus. 2023;15(8):e43200.
11. Ramachandran P, Devaraj U, D'souza G. A rare poisoning with pyrethroid by an uncommon route of self-injection. Emerg Med. 2014;4:208.
12. Li J, Tang GM, Xiang SZ, Yang MY, Yang L. A case of poisoning caused by intramuscular injection of esfenvalerate. Chin J Ind Hyg Occup Dis. 2023;41(3):225-7.
13. Jacob MS, Iyyadurai R, Jose A, Fleming JJ, Rebekah G, Zachariah A, et al. Clinical presentation of type 1 and type 2 pyrethroid poisoning in humans. Clin Toxicol (Phila). 2022;60(4):464-71.
14. He F, Wang S, Liu L, Chen S, Zhang Z, Sun J. Clinical manifestations and diagnosis of acute pyrethroid poisoning. Arch Toxicol. 1989;63(1):54-8.
15. Cha YS, Kim H, Cho NH, Jung WJ, Kim YW, Kim TH, et al. Pyrethroid poisoning: Features and predictors of atypical presentations. Emerg Med J. 2014;31(11):899-903.
16. Bhaskar EM, Moorthy S, Ganeshwala G, Abraham G. Cardiac conduction disturbance due to prallethrin (pyrethroid) poisoning. J Med Toxicol. 2010;6(1):27-30.
17. Kim D, Moon J, Chun B. The initial hyperglycemia in acute type II pyrethroid poisoning. J Korean Med Sci. 2015;30(4):365-70.
18. Iyyadurai R, Peter JV, Immanuel S, Begum A, Zachariah A, Jasmine S, et al. Organophosphate-pyrethroid combination pesticides may be associated with increased toxicity in human poisoning compared to either pesticide alone. Clin Toxicol (Phila). 2014;52(5):538-41.
19. Tremongkoltip A, Pengpumkiat S, Kongtip P, Nankongnab N, Siri S, Woskie S. Urinary cypermethrin metabolites among conventional and organic farmers in Thailand. Toxics. 2023;11(6):507.
20. Forshaw PJ, Ray DE. Development of therapy for type II pyrethroid insecticide poisoning [abstract]. Hum Exp Toxicol. 1997;16:382.
21. Bradbury JE, Gray AJ, Forshaw P. Protection against pyrethroid toxicity in rats with mephenesin. Toxicol Appl Pharmacol 1981;60(2):382-4.
22. Ramchandra AM, Chacko B, Victor PJ. Pyrethroid poisoning. Indian J Crit Care Med. 2019;23(Suppl 4):S267-71.
23. Beasley M, Temple W. Pyrethroid toxicity and its management. [online] Available from https://bpac.org.nz/BPJ/2013/December/docs/BPJ57-pyrethroid.pdf [Last accessed September, 2024].
24. Hodgson E, Levi PE. Interactions of piperonyl butoxide with cytochrome P450. In Glynne Jones D (Ed). Piperonyl Butoxide. London: Academic Press; 1999; pp. 41-53.
25. Wu YJ, Chang SS, Chen HY, Tsai KF, Lee WC, Wang IK, et al. Human poisoning with chlorpyrifos and cypermethrin pesticide mixture: Assessment of clinical outcome of cases admitted in a tertiary care hospital in Taiwan. Int J Gen Med. 2023;16:4795-804.
26. Tripathi M, Pandey R, Ambesh SP, Pandey M. A mixture of organophosphate and pyrethroid intoxication requiring intensive care unit admission: A diagnostic dilemma and therapeutic approach. Anesth Analg. 2006;103(2):410-2.
27. Uys F, O'Neill M, Farina Z, Belford J. Case report. S Afr Med J. 2023;113(2):57-60.

2.4 Neonicotinoids Poisoning

Karthik Gunasekaran, Angel Miraclin T, KPP Abhilash

INTRODUCTION

The word "neonicotinoids" is coined from a new nicotine-like-insecticide, a neuro-active synthetic insecticide developed with nicotine being the backbone in 1970.[1,2] The discovery marked a breakthrough in agrochemical research since it substituted organophosphates and carbamates. Neonicotinoids (NENIs) are preferred insecticides as they can be used in various forms, including aerosols, sprays, and seed treatments.[1-3] They are broad spectrum and demonstrate high potency against insects with favorable environmental toxicity and less potency for aquatic animals and mammals (nontarget organisms).[2-4] NENIs are approved in about 120 countries, primarily targeting chewing insects like thrips, plant hoppers, and other micro-Lepidoptera. The first recognized toxicity to the ecosystem was reported in Germany in 2008, when honeybees were mass killed, prompting an immediate ban on these compounds in the European Union.[5,6] Given their extensive use, the adverse effects are gradually being recognized and reported, especially with new evidence on their acute and chronic toxicities in humans and the various components of the food chain. Extensive use of the same is being continued in the developing nations because of rising population and threat to food security.[1,2] Awareness regarding these compounds and toxicities is mandatory for healthcare professionals to screen high-risk individuals and for environmentalists to monitor the direct and indirect effects on the food chain and the components of the ecosystem. This chapter aims to summarize the classification, mechanism of action, potential environmental and human health hazards, and diagnosis and management principles.

CLASSIFICATION AND ENVIRONMENTAL CONTAMINATION

There have been seven NENIs being marketed since 1995, and recently, three NENI-like compounds with similar mechanisms of action have been manufactured[1,2,4,7,8] **(Table 1)**. The following compounds are approved for usage in India: Imidacloprid, Thiamethoxam, Thiacloprid, Acetamiprid, Dinotefuran, and Clothianidin. In the environment, they have a very long half-life in the soil, are highly soluble in water, and have low soil absorption. NENIs are commonly used in seed treatment along with other fungicides, where less than 10% is absorbed by the plant, and the remaining stays with the soil.[1] Repeated application leads to a cumulative increase in soil concentrations and is further disseminated with dust clouds mixed with underground water through leaching during rains.[1,2] Since it is highly water-soluble, it is detected in the groundwater and surface water. However, these compounds are light-sensitive and prone to photodegradation. Hence, lower concentrations are noted in tropical regions. Freshwater sampling has reported increased concentrations of NENIs in China, the United States, Europe, and Canada.[4,8] Significant translocation of these compounds has been noted in pollen, vegetables, and fruits; despite thorough washing, small quantities persist in the produce.[9] In the market-basket study in Massachusetts, US, most fresh vegetables and fruits tested positive for NENIs, commonly imidacloprid.[10] According to the World Health Organization (WHO), 10–200 μg/kg of NENIs are acceptable without human health risks.

TABLE 1: Classification of neonicotinoids.

Classification	*Compounds*	*Year*
First generation	Imidacloprid Thiacloprid Acetamiprid Nitenpyram	1991 2001 1995 1995
Second generation	Clothianidin Thiamethoxam	2001 1998
Third generation	Dinotefuran	2002
Fourth generation	Cycloxaprid Guadipyr Imidaclothiz Paichongding	After 2005
Neo-nicotinoid-like compounds	Nithiazine Flonicamid Flupyradifurone Sulfoxaflor	1995–2015

MECHANISM OF ACTION

Neonicotinoids primarily act on the nicotinic acetylcholine receptors (nAchR) and irreversibly block these receptors at the postsynaptic membrane.[1,7,11-13] The nAchR is distributed in the central and peripheral nervous systems and has a vital role in learning, memory, and neuronal transmission.[14,15] NENIs have a selective predilection to the $\alpha 4\beta 2$ subunit of acetylcholine receptor, and pathology in these receptors has been described in many neurological disorders like Alzheimer's disease, Parkinson's disease, and psychiatric disorders including depression and schizophrenia.[11,12,16] These receptors also involve neuronal signaling and migration in the developing brain. The compounds are more toxic to insects than mammals since these receptors are high in the insect's central nervous system (CNS) and demonstrate higher affinity than the mammalian receptors, and insects have no blood–brain barrier, leading to efficient CNS penetration.[3] NENIs has a prominent action in the central and peripheral nervous systems, where they cause an initial stimulation of the NA^+/K^+ channels, leading to depolarization.[2,7] The prolonged depolarization leads to permanent inactivation of these channels, leading to a "depolarization block" in neurotransmission, causing paralysis and death. The best-studied compound with humans is imidacloprid. Inhalational and absorption (dermal exposure) risks of NENIs are negligible and have not been quantified in human studies.

Toxicokinetics

The toxicokinetics of imidacloprid have been best studied. It is metabolized through two distinct pathways by human cytochrome P450 (CYP450) isoenzymes.[17] The first pathway involves imidazolidine hydroxylation followed by desaturation to produce olefins and 5-hydroxyimidaclopride. The other pathway is through nitroimine reduction and cleavage to give the nitrosamine (IMI-NO), DN-IMI, and urea derivatives. Imidacloprid undergoes oxidative metabolism by cytochromes such as CYP3A4 and CYP2C19. Despite the relative safety profile of imidacloprid, the metabolite DNIMI demonstrates 300 times higher affinity to mammalian nAchR [vertebrate $\alpha 4\beta 2$, 50% inhibitory concentration (IC_{50}) = 8.2 nM for DNIMI and 2,600 nM for IMI] which results in higher toxicity to mammals.[17-19] The metabolism produces reactive oxygen species, leading to oxidation stress and cell damage. There is no selective accumulation/distribution of fat, and the body eliminates it in 48 hours.

CLINICAL FEATURES

The first report of human toxicity by ingestion was in 2001 when consumption of imidacloprid resulted in drowsiness, disorientation, and hemorrhagic gastritis.[20] The most common manifestations include nausea, vomiting, oropharyngeal irritation, headache, diarrhea, and drowsiness.[11,21-36] Most have mild symptoms, with less than 5% of the reported cases requiring intensive care and management. There is no specific toxidrome for NENI poisoning; hence, it is mandatory to identify the compound that will guide management. The mortality in all published series is 0–2%. The available literature based on large case series is summarized in **Table 2**. System-specific manifestations are as follows:

- *Gastrointestinal manifestations:* Nausea, vomiting, oral/pharyngeal erythema, oral ulceration, and hemorrhagic gastritis
- *Neurological manifestations:* Myalgia, fasciculations, weakness, fatigue, headache, tremors, vertigo, ataxia, drowsiness, obtundation, seizures, and rhabdomyolysis
- *Cardiovascular manifestations:* Tachycardia, hypertension, hypotension, arrhythmias (ventricular tachycardia, ventricular fibrillation, atrial flutter), myocardial dysfunction, cardiogenic shock
- *Pulmonary manifestations:* Dyspnea, bronchospasm, dry cough, respiratory depression
- *Hematological manifestations:* Anemia, leukopenia, thrombocytopenia, methemoglobinemia
- *Skin:* Erythema, dermatitis, ocular irritation and redness.

Lin et al., in their published case report and review of the literature up to 2012, reported a total of 152 cases, among which 22 were severe.[24] In a recently hospitalized cohort with NENI toxicity through deliberate consumption, 28% required intensive care but with no fatalities.[37] The majority of fatalities is due to respiratory depression, seizures, and rhabdomyolysis.[28,38,39] Cholinergic symptoms are not very prominent, like organo-phosphorus poisoning. Cases of severe acute liver injury have been reported.[40] The severity of toxicity is possibly proportional to the amount consumed; however, available studies have not found any correlation.[41]

DIAGNOSIS

A thorough history and clinical examination are mandatory to identify NENI toxicity clues. Inadvertent

TABLE 2: Review of published large cohorts on neonicotinoid toxicity.

Author	*No. of patients and compounds*	*Clinical symptoms*	*Mortality*
Forrester[36]	1,142 cases Imidacloprid (77%) Dinotefuran (17%)	Oral and ocular irritations, rash, nausea, vomiting, and headache	0
Boels and Chataigner (2014)[44]	482 cases Imidacloprid	Nausea, oral and ocular irritation, headache	0
Phua et al.[29]	70 cases Imidacloprid (91%) Acetamiprid (5%) Clothianidin (4%)	GI symptoms, cholinergic crisis Acute renal failure Respiratory depression Eight patients had severe toxicity	2.8%
Mohamed et al.[22]	68 cases Imidacloprid	Nausea, vomiting, headache, diarrhea Two patients required ICU care	0
Kim et al.[25]	24 cases	Nausea, vomiting, headache, and GI symptoms Four patients required ICU care	4.2%
Sriapha et al.[23]	128 cases	Nausea, vomiting, GI symptoms Four patients developed acute liver injury	1.6%
Perananthan et al.[34]	123 cases	Nausea, vomiting, epigastric pain and headache Seven patients developed severe toxicity	3%
Sanga et al.[37]	28 cases	Nausea, vomiting, weakness 28.6%—severe toxicity	0

(GI: gastrointestinal; ICU: intensive care unit)

exposures are common in agricultural workers' children, the majority being either inhalational or ingestional. Deliberate self-harm is common in countries like India and Sri Lanka, where often the history of consumption is apparent).[37-39,42] Since the majority of them present with vague symptoms, it is essential to identify the compound consumed. In the presence of oropharyngeal ulceration, it is mandatory to study the solvent composition since it causes corrosive injuries. In the absence of a history of definite consumption/unknown poisoning, the presence of obtundation, muscle fasciculations, muscle pains, and features of mild cholinergic symptoms should increase the suspicion of NENI toxicity.

Imidacloprid, nitenpyram, thiacloprid, and acetamiprid have a common chloropyridinyl chemical structure, further breaking into 6-chloronicotinic acid. Thiamethoxam and clothianidin have an achlorothiazole structure, which is metabolized into 2-chloro-1,3-thiazole-5-carboxylic acid. Dinotefuran is metabolized into 3-furoic acid. They follow the metabolism. They are conjugated with glycine or glucuronic acid and excreted in the urine. These metabolites have been observed in mouse and human urine.[35,43] Hence, human studies are warranted to study the diagnostic utility of measuring these compounds in serum and urine and further use it for diagnosis and surveillance in areas where these compounds are being increasingly used.

MANAGEMENT

Management of acute NENI poisoning is mainly supportive and symptomatic.[23-25,30,39,41]

Supportive Measures

Maintenance of the airway, ventilation, IV access, and fluids is an early priority, as patients can develop respiratory depression secondary to neuromuscular weakness or obtundation. The correction of acid-base disturbance and electrolyte abnormality is essential. The need for intensive care, assisted ventilation, and hemodynamic support is required in patients presenting with low sensorium, respiratory distress, and shock.

Mucosal Decontamination

Dermal and mucosal decontamination and removal of contaminated clothes should be done immediately, as these compounds undergo absorption by the dermal and inhalational routes.

Gastrointestinal Decontamination

In patients presenting within 1–2 hours of consumption, gastric lavage followed by oral activated charcoal should be given, especially if they have ingested a high volume of the compound. Activated charcoal absorbs the toxin from the GI tract and reduces its absorption into the bloodstream. The use of gastric lavage and activated charcoal is contraindicated if corrosive damage to the orogastric mucosa is suspected due to the solvent. Hemofiltration is ineffective in elimination as severity is independent of plasma concentrations. There is no role for intralipid administration since this compound has poor affinity to fatty tissues.

Antidote

There is no specific antidote for this class of insecticides. Even in the presence of muscarinic symptoms, the use of oximes is not advised as they have weak acetylcholine esterase inhibiting activity, which could cause tachycardia, hypertension, and other nicotinic symptoms. The use of atropine in severe life-threatening conditions like bronchorrhea or severe bradycardia is recommended.

FUTURE DIRECTIONS AND RESEARCH

Since these compounds are being increasingly used, surveillance studies are required to study their concentrations in humans and their health hazards. The affected patients must be followed up for longer since the evidence is still in evolution regarding the toxicity and effects on health. Long-term effects also need quantification through observational studies.

CONCLUSION

NENIs, are newer generation pesticides, currently in use for its high potency in developing countries. Knowledge on the toxicity profile has to be enhanced in the regions where it is being used, in order to recognize the toxidrome earlier for optimal management. Supportive care is adequate with majority recovering without major sequelae. Further research is warranted on the long-term effects through environmental exposure.

REFERENCES

1. Zhang X, Huang Y, Chen WJ, Wu S, Lei Q, Zhou Z, et al. Environmental occurrence, toxicity concerns, and biodegradation of neonicotinoid insecticides. Environ Res. 2023;218:114953.
2. Thompson DA, Lehmler HJ, Kolpin DW, Hladik ML, Vargo JD, Schilling KE, et al. A critical review on the potential impacts of neonicotinoid insecticide use: Current knowledge of environmental fate, toxicity, and implications for human health. Environ Sci Process Impacts. 2020;22(6): 1315-46.
3. Singh A, Leppanen C. Known target and nontarget effects of the novel neonicotinoid cycloxaprid to arthropods: A systematic review. Integr Environ Assess Manag. 2020;16(6):831-40.
4. Pietrzak D, Kania J, Kmiecik E, Malina G, Wątor K. Fate of selected neonicotinoid insecticides in soil-water systems: Current state of the art and knowledge gaps. Chemosphere. 2020;255:126981.
5. Zhao GP, Yang FW, Li JW, Xing HZ, Ren FZ, Pang GF, et al. Toxicities of Neonicotinoid-containing pesticide mixtures on nontarget organisms. Environ Toxicol Chem. 2020;39(10):1884-93.
6. EFSA. (2015). Peer review of the pesticide risk assessment of the active substance imidacloprid. [online] Available from https://www.efsa.europa.eu/en/efsajournal/pub/4211 [Last accessed September, 2024].
7. Houchat JN, Cartereau A, Le Mauff A, Taillebois E, Thany SH. An overview on the effect of neonicotinoid insecticides on mammalian cholinergic functions through the activation of neuronal nicotinic acetylcholine receptors. Int J Environ Res Public Health. 2020;17(9):3222.
8. Wang J, Yin R, Liu Y, Wang B, Wang N, Xiao P, et al. Meta-analysis of neonicotinoid insecticides in global surface waters. Environ Sci Pollut Res Int. 2023;30(1):1039-47.
9. Trends in neonicotinoid pesticide residues in food and water in the United States, 1999–2015. Environ Health. 2019;18:7.
10. Center for Food Safety and Applied Nutrition. (2014). Nutrition C for FS and A. Pesticide residue monitoring 2014 report and data. [online] Available from https://wayback.archive-it.org/7993/20170722164635/https://www.fda.gov/Food/FoodborneIllnessContaminants/Pesticides/ucm546327.htm. [Last accessed September, 2024].
11. Han W, Tian Y, Shen X. Human exposure to neonicotinoid insecticides and the evaluation of their potential toxicity: An overview. Chemosphere. 2018;192:59-65.
12. Cartereau A, Martin C, Thany SH. Neonicotinoid insecticides differently modulate acetycholine-induced currents on mammalian α7 nicotinic acetylcholine receptors. Br J Pharmacol. 2018;175(11):1987-98.
13. Taillebois E, Cartereau A, Jones AK, Thany SH. Neonicotinoid insecticides mode of action on insect nicotinic acetylcholine receptors using binding studies. Pestic Biochem Physiol. 2018;151:59-66.
14. Malhotra N, Chen KHC, Huang JC, Lai HT, Uapipatanakul B, Roldan MJM, et al. Physiological effects of neonicotinoid insecticides on non-target aquatic animals-an updated review. Int J Mol Sci. 2021;22(17):9591.

15. Tasman K, Hidalgo S, Zhu B, Rands SA, Hodge JJL. Neonicotinoids disrupt memory, circadian behaviour and sleep. Sci Rep. 2021;11:2061.
16. Zhang D, Lu S. Human exposure to neonicotinoids and the associated health risks: A review. Environ Int. 2022;163:107201.
17. Schulz-Jander DA, Casida JE. Imidacloprid insecticide metabolism: Human cytochrome P450 isozymes differ in selectivity for imidazolidine oxidation versus nitroimine reduction. Toxicol Lett. 2002;132(1):65-70.
18. Tomizawa M, Casida JE. Neonicotinoid insecticide toxicology: Mechanisms of selective action. Annual Rev Pharmacol Toxicol. 2005;45:247-68.
19. Schulz-Jander DA, Leimkuehler WM, Casida JE. Neonicotinoid insecticides: Reduction and cleavage of imidacloprid nitroimine substituent by liver microsomal and cytosolic enzymes. Chem Res Toxicol. 2002;15(9):1158-65.
20. Wu IW, Lin JL, Cheng ET. Acute poisoning with the neonicotinoid insecticide imidacloprid in N-methyl pyrrolidone. J Toxicol Clin Toxicol. 2001;39(6):617-21.
21. Vinod KV, Srikant S, Thiruvikramaprakash G, Dutta TK. A fatal case of thiacloprid poisoning. Am J Emerg Med. 2015;33(2):310.e5-6.
22. Mohamed F, Gawarammana I, Robertson TA, Roberts MS, Palangasinghe C, Zawahir S, et al. Acute human self-poisoning with imidacloprid compound: A neonicotinoid insecticide. PLoS One. 2009;4(4):e5127.
23. Sriapha C, Trakulsrichai S, Tongpoo A, Pradoo A, Rittilert P, Wananukul W. Acute imidacloprid poisoning in Thailand. Ther Clin Risk Manag. 2020;16:1081-8.
24. Lin PC, Lin HJ, Liao YY, Guo HR, Chen KT. Acute poisoning with neonicotinoid insecticides: A case report and literature review. Basic Clin Pharmacol Toxicol. 2013;112(4):282-6.
25. Kim JC, So BH, Kim HJ, Kim HM, Park JH, Choi SM, et al. Clinical characteristics of patients with neonicotinoid insecticide poisoning. J Korean Soc Clin Toxicol. 2010;24-9.
26. Viradiya K, Mishra A. Imidacloprid poisoning. J Assoc Physicians India. 2011;59:594-5.
27. Bhatta OP, Chand S, Chand H, Poudel RC, Lamichhane RP, Singh AK, et al. Imidacloprid poisoning in a young female: A case report. J Med Case Reports. 2023;17(1):43.
28. Iyyadurai R, George IA, Peter JV. Imidacloprid poisoning—newer insecticide and fatal toxicity. J Med Toxicol. 2010;6(1):77-8.
29. Phua DH, Lin CC, Wu ML, Deng JF, Yang CC. Neonicotinoid insecticides: An emerging cause of acute pesticide poisoning. Clin Toxicol Phila Pa. 2009;47(4):336-41.
30. Vikhe VB, Faruqi AA, Reddy A, Khandol D, Kore TA. Pyrethroid and neonicotinoid poisoning: A good prognosis. Cureus. 2023;15(10):e47016.
31. Zhang Q, Li Z, Chang CH, Lou JL, Zhao MR, Lu C. Potential human exposures to neonicotinoid insecticides: A review. Environ Pollut Barking Essex 1987. 2018;236:71-81.
32. Naveen A, Sahu MR, Padhi KS, Maharik SS. Self-poisoning with safer insecticide: A case series on imidacloprid poisoning. Am J Forensic Med Pathol. 2022;43(1):66-8.
33. Agarwal R, Srinivas R. Severe neuropsychiatric manifestations and rhabdomyolysis in a patient with imidacloprid poisoning. Am J Emerg Med. 2007;25(7): 844-5.
34. Perananthan V, Mohamed F, Shahmy S, Gawarammana I, Dawson A, Buckley N. The clinical toxicity of imidacloprid self-poisoning following the introduction of newer formulations. Clin Toxicol Phila Pa. 2021;59(4): 347-50.
35. Proença P, Teixeira H, Castanheira F, Pinheiro J, Monsanto PV, Marques EP, et al. Two fatal intoxication cases with imidacloprid: LC/MS analysis. Forensic Sci Int. 2005;153(1):75-80.
36. Forrester MB. Neonicotinoid insecticide exposures reported to six poison centers in Texas. Hum Exp Toxicol. 2014;33(6):568-73.
37. Sanga L, Jacob A, Jayakaran JAJ, Iyadurai R. Clinical profile and predictors of intensive care admission in neonicotinoid poisoning in a tertiary care hospital in South India. Indian J Crit Care Med. 2023;28(1):66-9.
38. Sivanandan A, Abel S, Sanjay M, Chandran J, Gunasekaran K, Abhilash KPP. Profile and outcome of patients presenting with agrochemical poisoning to the emergency department. J Fam Med Prim Care. 2020;9(3):1589-93.
39. Selvam V, Srinivasan S. Neonicotinoid poisoning and management. Indian J Crit Care Med Peer-Rev Off Publ Indian Soc Crit Care Med. 2019;23(Suppl 4):S260-2.
40. Sriapha C, Trakulsrichai S, Intaraprasong P, Wongvisawakorn S, Tongpoo A, Schimmel J, et al. Imidacloprid poisoning case series: Potential for liver injury. Clin Toxicol Phila Pa. 2020;58(2):136-8.
41. Cimino AM, Boyles AL, Thayer KA, Perry MJ. Effects of neonicotinoid pesticide exposure on human health: A systematic review. Environ Health Perspect. 2017;125(2):155-62.
42. Abhilash KPP, Murugan S, Rabbi NAS, Pradeeptha S, Kumar S, Selvaraj B, et al. Deliberate self-poisoning and harm: A meticulous quest of methods in vogue. J Fam Med Prim Care. 2022;11(1):233-9.
43. David D, George IA, Peter JV. Toxicology of the newer neonicotinoid insecticides: Imidacloprid poisoning in a human. Clin Toxicol. 2007;45(5):485-6.
44. Pulce DC, Lyon C, Viriot D, Boels D, Angers C, Langrand J, et al. Rapporteurs: David Boels, CAPTV d'Angers Dominique Chataigner, CAPTV de Paris.

2.5 Herbicides

Saurabh Chaturvedi, S Raghunathan, Mohan Gurjar

INTRODUCTION

Herbicides are a class of pesticides designed to selectively kill or damage unwanted plants. *Herbs* and *Caedo* in Latin stand for plant killer, herbicides.[1] Herbicides are a type of pesticide that target and eliminate unwanted vegetation (weeds). They are widely applied in agriculture to enhance crop productivity and quality. Herbicides are used in agricultural and wildland ecosystems to reduce the density of weeds by disrupting the metabolism and thus promote the growth of desirable species. They act by interfering with various biochemical pathways in the plant cells, such as photosynthesis, amino acid synthesis, or hormone regulation. However, excessive or improper use of herbicides can have adverse effects on crop, environment, and human health. Therefore, careful selection and application of herbicides are essential for sustainable weed management.[2]

Asia contributes to more than half of the pesticides' usage in the world. India, now being the most populous country in the world, stands 12th in pesticide use globally and 3rd in Asia, and share only 1% pesticide use.[3] Despite the efforts of international bodies adopting a number of resolutions and programs, global pesticide use has continued to grow steadily to 4.1 million tons per year, a staggering increase of nearly 81%, between 1990 and 2017.[4] Between 1994 and 1995, the usage of pesticides reported in India was 80,000 metric tons (MT).[4] According to the data and statistical analysis, India's biopesticide usage has increased steadily over the years, reaching 9,321 MT in 2021–22 from 7,203 MT in 2018–19. However, there was a significant decline in 2022–23, when the consumption dropped to 7,248 MT.[5]

The health of humans has long been endangered by poisoning from pesticides.[6] According to the World Health Organization (WHO), poisoning causes about 250,000 deaths worldwide each year and pesticides are responsible for 150,000 of them.[7] Plant poisoning in India is well documented with deaths occurring from suicide, homicide, and unintentional poisoning.[8] Lower- and middle-income countries (LMICs) have the highest rates of death from poisoning.[9] An estimated 14 million people have died of pesticides poisoning by pesticides since the advent of the Green Revolution.[9] The data show that pesticide self-poisoning killed about 110,000 people each year from 2010 to 2014, accounting for 13.7% of all global suicides. This estimate increased to 168,000 deaths per year, or 19.7% of global suicides, when a sensitivity analysis considered the under-reporting of suicides poisoning attributed to pesticides in India. Pesticide self-poisoning caused different proportions of suicides in LMICs of Europe and Western Pacific, ranging from 0.9 to 48.3%, respectively.[10]

HERBICIDES CLASSIFICATION

Herbicides form a diverse group of compounds which kill plants selectively or broadly. They have been categorized in various ways like based on translocation, based on the time of application, and based on the method of application.

Based on Translocation

Systemic or Translocation

Translocation in the plant, crop, or weeds occurs through its vascular system, from the site of absorption to the site of action. Herbicides are more effective on perennial weeds but require longer time (days or even weeks). *Examples:* Glyphosate and Glufosinate.

Nonsystemic or Contact

These types of herbicides kill only the portion of plant, crop, or weed that is in contact. They are less effective on perennial weeds. They are fast acting, but repeated application is required to kill the regrowth of underground parts. *Examples:* Bromoxynil and bentazon.

Based on Time of Application

Preplant

These are nonselective herbicides applied to soil before planting and gets incorporated into the soil which prevent dissipation through photodecomposition and/or volatility. *Example:* Dazomet.

Preemergence

These herbicides are applied before the plant, crop, or weed seedlings emerge through the soil surface. They kill the weeds by affecting the cellular division in the emerging plant/crop/weed seedling. *Example:* Pendimethalin.

Postemergence

These herbicides are applied after plant, crop, or weed seedlings have emerged. They require more than one-time application. These herbicides can be foliar or root absorbed, selective or nonselective, and contact or systemic. *Example:* 2, 4D.

Based on Method of Application

Soil Applied

These are herbicides that are being applied to the soil, taken up by the root or shoot of the emerging plant, crop, or weed seedlings, and are used as preplant or preemergence treatment. Positioning is very important. Photodecomposition and/or volatility reduce their availability. *Example:* Dinitroanilines (Pendimethalin).

Foliar Applied

These herbicides are applied to a portion of the plant that is above the ground and is absorbed by exposed tissues. These are generally postemergence herbicides and can either be translocated (systemic) throughout the plant or remain at a specific site (contact). *Example:* Glyphosate and 2, 4D.

Based on Specificity

Selective

When herbicide controls or suppresses plants, weeds, or crops without affecting the growth of other plants species, it is known as selective herbicide. Selectivity can be attributed to translocation, differential absorption, morphological, or physiological differences between the applied species. *Example:* 2, 4D.

Nonselective

Herbicides are not specific in acting against certain plant species and kill all with which they come in contact. These herbicides are used to clear industrial sites, waste ground, railways, and embankments. *Examples:* Glufosinate, glyphosate, paraquat (PQ), and diquat.

HERBICIDE POISONING

Site and Mechanism of Action

- *Acetyl coenzyme A carboxylase (ACCase) inhibitor:* Increased level of free radical, oxidative stress, cell membrane injury, and apoptosis
  Example: Diclofop
- *Acetolactate synthase (ALS)/acetohydroxyacid synthase (AHAS) inhibitor*
  Examples: Imazethapyr and Metsulfuron
- *Microtubule assembly inhibitor*
  Example: Pendimethalin
- *Synthetic auxin*
  Example: 2, 4D
- *Photosynthesis inhibitor at photosystem II site a, site B*
  - Oxidative stress, affects apoptosis and autophagy, site A
    Example: Atrazine
  - Uncoupled oxidative phosphorylation, induced oxidative stress, inflammation
    Example: Bromoxynil
- *Photosynthesis inhibitor at photosystem II site a, different binding behavior from group 5*: Reactive oxygen species and p53 increased
  Example: Diuron
- *Lipid synthesis inhibitor, not ACCase inhibition*
  Example: EPTC (S-Ethyl dipropylthiocarbamate)

Toxic Doses and Clinical Features

Poisoning due to herbicides is less understood and poorly described. ***Table 1*** *mentions an overview of the available information regarding toxic doses and clinical features in humans.*[11-32]

Paraquat (PQ) is the most commonly used herbicide in India with highest case fatality and is a significant public health threat. In fact, PQ is registered for use in over 120 developed and developing countries. It is not metabolized in the body and excreted only through the kidneys. At the same time, it is rapidly distributed in the tissues. It accumulates in alveolar cells of lungs and also gets secreted in the proximal convoluted tubules of the kidney resulting in redox cycling and generation of toxic reactive oxygen species.[30] This leads to pulmonary hemorrhage, pulmonary edema, pulmonary fibrosis, and liver and kidney damage.[33] The toxicity of PQ is dose-dependent and consumption of >20 mL of 20% PQ can lead to death.

After ingestion, PQ causes mucosal erosion and bleeding of the oral cavity and tongue within the first few

TABLE 1: Toxic dose of various herbicides and clinical features due to their poisoning.

Herbicide	*Toxic dose*	*Clinical features*	*References*
Glufosinate	LD_{50} for rats was 1,660 mg/kg/body weight	• CNS toxicities such as coma, seizure, stupor, drowsiness, and amnesia Gastrointestinal effects such as sore throat/oral ulcers, nausea/vomiting, diarrhea • Respiratory effects such as dyspnea, aspiration pneumonia • Cardiovascular effects such as hypo-/hypertension and brady/tachycardia	11–13
2,4-D	Acute lethal levels in human plasma between 447 and 826 mg/L LD_{50} for mice was 138 mg/kg; in rats, from 639 to 1,646 mg/kg (oral administration); rabbits, for dermal exposure, 1,829 to higher than 2,000 mg/kg	Cardiotoxicity, CNS toxicities, hepatotoxicity, renal toxicity, endocrine disorders, damage to the respiratory tract, neuromuscular toxicity, and myotonia	11, 14-16
Bromoxynil	LC_{50} for rats was 0.15 mg/L	Hepatotoxicity, hyperthermia, carcinogenic (hepatocellular adenoma and carcinoma), disruption of reproductive systems, and thyroid toxicity	11, 17, 18
Bentazon	686–1,764 mg/kg of body weight in blood is lethal range in humans (oral or dermal administration), LD_{50} for rats—1,100 mg/kg and for pheasants—2,918 mg/kg	Upper and lower gastrointestinal irritation, drowsiness, agitation, loss of consciousness, hyperpyrexia, cardiovascular (increased heart rate, tachypnea), musculoskeletal (muscle rigidity)	11, 19–22
Dazomet	LD_{50} for rats, 415 mg/kg and >2,000 mg/kg of body weight, LC_{50} for rats 8,400 mg/m^3	Acute dermatitis and fever	11, 23–25
Pendimethalin	Acute oral and dermal toxicity in humans, LD_{50} >5 g/kg of body weight, LD_{50} for rats, 5,000 g/kg of body weight	Headache, nausea, vomiting, sore throat, retching, hematemesis, epigastric pain, corrosive gastroduodenal injury, and carcinogenic	11, 26–28
Paraquat	Acute toxicity in humans, paraquat consumption >40 mg/kg of body weight, LD_{50} in humans, 3–5 mg/kg	Acute respiratory distress syndrome, renal failure, hepatotoxicity, pulmonary fibrosis, corrosion of the gastrointestinal tract, mediastinitis, and pneumomediastinum	11, 29–32
Diquat	–	Less common than paraquat poisoning CNS toxicities such as nervousness, irritability, combativeness, disorientation, and diminished reflexes	31, 32

(CNS: central nervous system)

days and is called "paraquat tongue." It can also cause esophageal ulceration and may progress to perforation, mediastinitis, and pneumo-mediastinum.[34] Other routes of exposure to PQ include inhalation and topical exposure (less common). They generally manifest as local irritation and superficial burns. Severity of PQ poisoning can be classified on the basis of doses as well as clinical characteristics **(Table 2)**.[35]

The best predictor of survival can be calculated as SIPP (Severity Index of Paraqaut Poisoning) score. This index is calculated by multiplying the time from PQ ingestion to intensive treatment and serum PQ levels at admission. The index is interpreted as follows: Values of <10 h/mg/L predict a good chance of survival, values between 10 and 50 h/mg/L predict a high chance of mortality because of interstitial pulmonary fibrosis, and those with values >50 h/mg/L die quickly due to circulatory collapse. This method is believed to be useful in planning treatment and determining the prognosis, comparing therapeutic results at different stages of treatment, evaluating new therapeutic methods and also study in the pathology of acute PQ poisoning.[36,37] Acidosis is also an important

TABLE 2: Severity of paraquat poisoning after ingestion.

Severity	*Mild/Subacute poisoning*	*Moderate/Severe poisoning*	*Acute fulminant/Hyperacute poisoning*
Doses	<20 mg/kg body weight	20–40 mg/kg body weight	>40 mg/kg body weight
Clinical characteristics	• Usually asymptomatic • Mild gastrointestinal symptoms • Minimal pulmonary/renal involvement	• Immediate—vomiting • Hours—diarrhea, abdominal pain, and oral ulcers • Days—renal failure, hepatic impairment, and hypotension/tachycardia • Weeks—alveolitis and pulmonary fibrosis	• Immediate—vomiting • Hours to days—diarrhea, abdominal pain, renal failure, hepatic impairment, gastrointestinal ulceration, pancreatitis, myocarditis, refractory hypotension/coma
Recovery	Complete recovery	• Survival possible • Death within 2–3 weeks (predominantly due to deteriorating lung function)	Survival difficult Death within 1–4 days (predominantly multiorgan failure)

(GI: gastrointestinal)

FLOWCHART 1: Overview of management for herbicide poisoning.

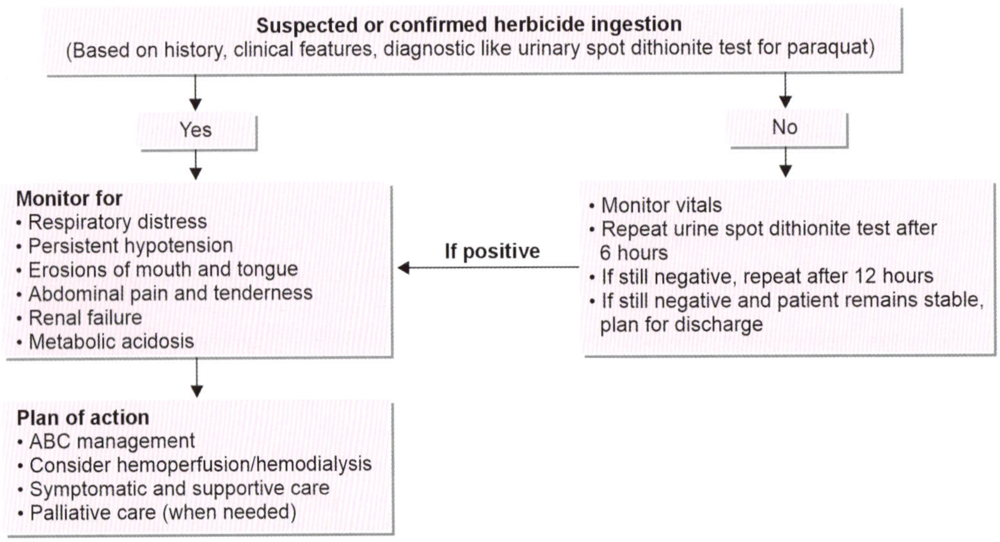

prognostic indicator of acute PQ poisoning, particularly the concentration of serum lactic acid.

DIAGNOSIS

Diagnosis of herbicide poisoning is often made on circumstantial evidence including:

- History from the patient themselves or other observers
- Look for the presence of evidence of ingestion by the victim like empty container, residue, or suicidal notes, etc.
- Clinical signs (usually nonspecific) like intractable vomiting, ulceration of oral mucous membrane, etc.
- Analytical techniques in detection and quantification in human body fluids are not available easily.

MANAGEMENT

Managing a case of herbicide poisoning is challenging due to less available information. Overall, management is mainly supportive in nature **Flowchart 1**.

Immediate Management

- Access and ensure airway, breathing, and circulation.
- Avoid ongoing exposure or contact with the poison.
- Control vomiting

    - 5HT3 antagonists, e.g., ondansetron 8 mg (5 mg/m^2 in children) by slow IV injection or IV infusion over 15 minutes, or
    - Phenothiazine antiemetics, e.g., prochlorperazine; dopamine antagonists such as metoclopramide should be avoided as they may impair therapy for renal support with dopamine.
- *Activated charcoal*
    - To be considered in case of recent ingestion of the herbicide
    - Airway protection should be ensured
    - 100 g for adults or 2 g/kg body weight in children or, Fuller's earth—15% solution; 1 L for adults or 15 mL/kg body weight in children. Normally, the use of gastric lavage without administration of an adsorbent has not shown any clinical benefit.
- Sometime in case of ingestion, a purgative could be considered, e.g., mannitol or magnesium sulfate
- *Consider doing routine investigations:* Complete blood count, blood grouping and typing, liver function test (LFT) renal function test (RFT) function test including electrolytes, arterial blood gas, electrocardiogram (ECG), X-ray chest, and ultrasonogram of abdomen.

Early Management

- Continue keeping under observation with monitoring of vitals.
- Serial monitoring of laboratory tests like LFT and RFT
- Can consider other ingestions, if clinically appropriate, including high-resolution computed tomography (HRCT) chest and echocardiogram
- Maintain adequate hydration.
- Mouth care for ulceration and inflammation
- Adequate and appropriate analgesics to be considered in case of pain
- Blistering and potentially full-thickness burns which usually develop 1–3 days after exposure
- Patients should be kept nil by mouth if there is a suspicion of oropharyngeal or esophageal injury

Specific Management

- Usually, organ-specific supportive management is to be continued as there is none or very less information available for specific antidote.[38]
- Avoid supplemental oxygen, especially in PQ toxicity, unless significant hypoxia exists (SpO_2 <90%), as oxygen enhances PQ toxicity
- *Hemofiltration/hemoperfusion:* This could be considered within 4 hours of PQ ingestion and has been found to be useful in mild to moderate poisoning and has improved 90-day survival rates.[39,40]
- *Immunosuppressants:* They include methylprednisolone, dexamethasone, and cyclophosphamide.[41] Further research is needed on their efficacy.
- *Antioxidants:* As PQ poisoning depletes antioxidants by promoting release of free oxygen radicals, antioxidants like N-acetyl cysteine (increases intracellular glutathione), high-dose vitamin C and vitamin E are being tried.
- *Free radical scavengers:* Desferrioxamine scavenges hydroxyl radicals by chelating iron. Salicylic acid supplements scavenge hydroxyl radicals as well as are found to supplement antioxidant effects. Dracone, a recently introduced free radical scavenger, was also found to have antiapoptotic, antinecrotic, and anti-inflammatory effects.[42]
- *Lung transplantation:* Patients with moderate PQ toxicity, who do not die early, often develop progressive pulmonary fibrosis. This leads to respiratory failure and death within a few weeks. In these patients, lung transplantation could be explored if facility and expertise are available.
- *Long-term follow-up and rehabilitation:* This is required among survivors of severe toxicity. PQ can cause parkinsonism by its action on substantia nigra and pars compacta due to free oxygen radical-induced damage.[43]

CONCLUSION

Herbicides toxicity in humans are not uncommon as herbicides are easily available and less expensive. In general, the ingestion route is more dangerous than other routes of exposure like inhalation and topical exposure. Managing patients with herbicides' toxicity poses a challenge to clinicians due to various reasons including delayed presentation, diagnostic dilemmas, and nonavailability of specific antidotes; supportive care remains the mainstay for the clinical treatment. However, many options are being tried, like antioxidants and hemofiltration/hemoperfusion, to improve the survival of the patients; in future, evidence-based clinical trials have to be conducted in hospitals where many patients are being managed. This will help to formulate a standard protocol. However, till then patients have to be managed with available options.

REFERENCES

1. Manno M. Herbicides. In: Descotes J (Ed). Human toxicology. Netherlands: Elsevier; 1996. pp. 551-60.
2. Bagale S. (2023). Modes of herbicide action. New insights in herbicide science. IntechOpen. [online] Available from http://dx.doi.org/10.5772/intechopen.105356. [Last accessed September, 2024].
3. Nayak P, Solanki H. Pesticides and Indian agriculture: A review. Int. J Res 2021;9(5):250-63.
4. FAOSTAT. (2018). Pesticide use data. [online] Available from http://www.fao.org/faostat/en/#data/RP. [Last accessed September, 2024].
5. Statistical Database, Directorate of Plant Protection, Quarantine and Storage, Department of Agriculture and Farmers Welfare, Ministry of Agriculture and Farmers Welfare, Government of India. Consumption of bio pesticides formulations in various states during 2018-19 to 2022-23. [online] Available from https://www.ppqs.gov.in/statistical-database. [Last accessed September, 2024].
6. Boedeker W, Watts M, Clausing P, Marquez E. The global distribution of acute unintentional pesticide poisoning: Estimations based on a systematic review. BMC Public Health. 2020;20(1):1875.
7. World Health Organization (WHO). (2020). Guidelines for establishing a poison centre. [online] Available from https://www.who.int/news/item/18-01-2021-who-guidelines-for-establishing-a-poison-centre. [Last accessed September, 2024].
8. Karunarathne A, Bhalla A, Sethi A, Perera U, Eddleston M. Importance of pesticides for lethal poisoning in India during 1999 to 2018: A systematic review. BMC Public Health. 2021;21(1):1441.
9. Karunarathne A, Gunnell D, Konradsen F, Eddleston M. How many premature deaths from pesticide suicide have occurred since the agricultural green revolution? Clin Toxicol (Phila). 2020;58(4):227-32.
10. Mew EJ, Padmanathan P, Konradsen F, Eddleston M, Chang S-S, Phillips MR, et al. The global burden of fatal self-poisoning with pesticides 2006-15: Systematic review. J Affect Disord. 2017;219:93-104.
11. Vats S. Herbicides: History, classification and genetic manipulation of plants for herbicide resistance. In: Lichtfouse E (Ed). Sustainable Agriculture Reviews. Germany: Springer; 2015. pp. 153-92.
12. Mao YC, Hung DZ, Wu ML, Tsai W-J, Wang L-M, Ger J, et al. Acute human glufosinate-containing herbicide poisoning. Clin Toxicol (Phila). 2012;50(5):396-402.
13. Lluís M, Nogué S, Miró O. Severe acute poisoning due to a glufosinate containing preparation without mitochondrial involvement. Hum Exp Toxicol. 2008;27(6):519-24.
14. Bradberry SM, Watt BE, Proudfoot AT, Vale JA. Mechanisms of toxicity, clinical features, and management of acute chlorophenoxy herbicide poisoning: A review. J Toxicol Clin Toxicol. 2000;38(2):111-22.
15. Tu P, Gao B, Chi L, Lai Y, Bian X, Ru H. et al. Subchronic low-dose 2,4-D exposure changed plasma acylcarnitine levels and induced gut microbiome perturbations in mice. Sci Rep. 2019;9(1):4363.
16. Kumar N. 2,4-D ethyl ester poisoning: A case report. Indian J Crit Care Med. 2019;23(9):432-3.
17. European Food Safety Authority (EFSA), Arena M, Auteri D, Barmaz S, Bellisai G, Brancato A, et al. Peer review of the pesticide risk assessment of the active substance bromoxynil (variant evaluated bromoxynil octanoate). EFSA J. 2017;15(6):e04790.
18. El-Nagar MMF, Elsisi AE. Exposure to bromoxynil octanoate herbicide induces oxidative stress, inflammation, and apoptosis in testicular tissue via modulating NF-κB pathway. Food Chem Toxicol. 2023;180:114008.
19. Bradberry SM, Proudfoot AT, Vale JA. Glyphosate poisoning. Toxicol Rev. 2004;23(3):159-67.
20. Škavić P, Duraković Z, Nestić M. Lethal bentazone intoxication - A report of two cases. J Forensic Sci. 2018;63(1):321-5.
21. Müller IB, Petersen HW, Johansen SS, Theilade P. Fatal overdose of the herbicide bentazone. Forensic Sci Int. 2003;135(3):235-6.
22. Lee K. A fatal case of acute bentazone overdose despite cricothyroidotomy during cardiopulmonary resuscitation. Clin Exp Emerg Med. 2017;4(4):254-7.
23. NRA special review of Metham Sodium, Dazomet and Methylisothiocyanate (MITC) by the Chemical Review Section National Registration Authority, Canberra, Australia. https://www.apvma.gov.au/sites/default/files/methamsodium-phase-8-special-review-1.pdf
24. Horiuchi N, Oguchi S, Nagami H, Nishigaki Y. Pesticide-related dermatitis in Saku district, Japan, 1975-2000. Int J Occup Environ Health. 2008;14(1):25-34.
25. Rong J, Xu M, Zhang Z, Zou Q, Xu D, Zhong J, et al. Determination of dazomet and its metabolite methyl isothiocyanate residues in plant-derived foods by gas chromatography-triple quadrupole mass spectrometry. Se Pu. 2022;40(7):661-8.
26. Kumar A, Verma A. Emergence of new poisons: A case of pendimethalin poisoning from rural India. Clin Toxicol (Phila). 2013;51(5):458-9.
27. Gad MF, Mossa AH, Refaie AA, Ibrahim NE, Mohafrash SMM. Benchmark dose and the adverse effects of exposure to pendimethalin at low dose in female rats. Basic Clin Pharmacol Toxicol. 2022;130(2):301-19.
28. Singh R, Dhaduk B, Dhalani J. A rapid quantification method for simultaneous determination of pendimethalin and metribuzin contents in suspoemulsion formulation. Results Chem. 2023;5:100779.
29. Ravichandran R, Amalnath D, Shaha KK, Srinivas BH. Paraquat poisoning: A retrospective study of 55 patients from a tertiary care center in Southern India. Indian J Crit Care Med. 2020;24(3):155-9.

30. Sukumar CA, Shanbhag V, Shastry AB. Paraquat: The poison potion. Indian J Crit Care Med. 2019;23(Suppl 4):S263-6.
31. Sha O, Cui B, Chen X, Liu H, Yao J, Zhu Y. Separation and determination of paraquat and diquat in human plasma and urine by magnetic dispersive solid phase extraction coupled with high-performance liquid chromatography. J Anal Methods Chem. 2020;2020:7359582.
32. U.S. Environmental Protection Agency. (2013). Recognition and management of pesticides poisoning. 6th edition. [online] Available from https://www.epa.gov/sites/default/files/2015-01/documents/rmpp_6thed_final_lowresopt.pdf. [Last accessed September, 2024].
33. Dinis-Oliveira RJ, Duarte JA, Sánchez-Navarro A, Remião F, Bastos ML, Carvalho F. Paraquat poisonings: Mechanisms of lung toxicity, clinical features, and treatment. Crit Rev Toxicol. 2008;38(1):13-71.
34. Honore P, Hantson P, Fauville JP, Peeters A, Manieu P. Paraquat poisoning "state of the art". Acta Clin Belg. 1994;49(5):220-8.
35. Lock EA, Wilks MF. Diquat. In: Krieger RI, (Eds) Handbook of Pesticide Toxicology, 2nd edition. San Diego: Academic Press; 2001. p. 1605.
36. Xu S, Hu H, Jian Z, Tang S, Zhou Y, Sheng J, et al. APACHE score, severity index of paraquat poisoning, and serum lactic acid concentration in the prognosis of paraquat poisoning of Chinese patients. Pediatr Emerg Care. 2015;31(2):117-21.
37. Senarathna L, Eddleston M, Wilks MF, Woollen BH, Tomenson JA, Roberts DM, et al. Prediction of outcome after paraquat poisoning by measurement of the plasma paraquat concentration. QJM. 2009;102:251-9.
38. Roberts DM. Herbicides. In: Hoffman RS, Howland M, Lewin NA, Nelson LS, Goldfrank LR (Eds). Goldfrank's Toxicologic Emergencies, 10th edition. New York: McGraw-Hill Education; 2015.
39. Hampson EC, Pond SM. Failure of hemoperfusion and hemodialysis to prevent death in paraquat poisoning - a retrospective review of 42 patients. Med Toxicol Adv Drug Exp. 1988;3(1):64-71.
40. Li C, Hu D, Xue W, Li X, Wang Z, Ai Z, et al. Treatment outcome of combined continuous venovenous hemofiltration and hemoperfusion in acute paraquat poisoning: A prospective controlled trial. Crit Care Med. 2018;46(1):100-7.
41. Gawarammana IB, Buckley NA, Mohamed F, Naser KA, Jeganathan K, Munasinghe A, et al. A randomised controlled trial of high-dose immunosuppression in paraquat poisoning. Clin Toxicol. 2012;50(4):278.
42. Yi R, Zhizhou Y, Zhaorui S, Wei Z, Xin C, Shinan N. Retrospective study of clinical features and prognosis of edaravone in the treatment of paraquat poisoning. Medicine. 2019;98(19):e15441.
43. Berry C, La Vecchia C, Nicotera P, Paraquat and Parkinson's disease. Cell Death Differ. 2010;17:1115-25.

2.6 Rodenticide Poisoning

Amarnath P, Chanaveerappa Bammigatti, Ashish Bhalla

INTRODUCTION

India, being an agricultural nation, has an increased demand for rodenticides, as rodents are one of the preliminary targets to prevent the destruction of crops. Thus, the agricultural population has easy access to rodenticides. Since the rodents have developed resistance to the initially developed rodenticides, compounds of higher virulence and toxicity are now synthesized to overcome this resistance. However, the same has proven to be a double-edged sword in terms of their toxicity on humans.

CLASSIFICATION

Rodenticides are classified based on their active compounds and mechanisms of toxicity **(Table 1)**, severity of toxicity[1] **(Table 2)**, or chemical structure among anticogulants[2] **(Table 3)**. Metal phosphides are commonly used as rodenticides and also as grain fumigants, to control insects/pests in the storage containers/silos. On the other hand, phosphorus-based rodenticides and superwarfarin are only used to contain/eliminate larger rodents like rats/mice, etc.; white/yellow phosphorus is also used in the manufacture of matches, fireworks, and fertilizers.

EPIDEMIOLOGY

The prevalence varies from region to region. There is no single consensus calculating the entire prevalence of rodenticide poisoning all through India. Multiple studies done at different sites covering the entire nation have

TABLE 1: Rodenticide classification based on active compound or mechanism of toxicity United States Environmental Protection Agency (USEPA).

Categories of rodenticides	*Active compounds*	*Mechanism of toxicity*
First-generation anticoagulants	Warfarin, chlorophacinone, diphacinone	Bleeding diathesis
Second-generation anticoagulants	Brodifacoum, bromadiolone, difenacoum, difethialone	Bleeding diathesis
Nonanticoagulants (neurotoxic)	Bromethalin, strychnine, tetramine*	Neurotoxin
Nonanticoagulant (cardiotoxic)	• Cholecalciferol* • Barium carbonate* • Red Squill*	• Hypercalcemia • Severe hypokalemia • Cardiac glycoside
Protoplasmic poisons	• Thallium,* arsenic* Metal phosphides (zinc, aluminum) • Bromethalin	• Disrupt Kreb's cycle • Mitochondrial toxins • Uncouples oxidative phosphorylation

*Not routinely used.

TABLE 2: Rodenticide classification based on toxicity.

Toxicity grading	*Active compound*
Highly toxic	Zinc phosphide, aluminum phosphide, yellow phosphorus, and strychnine
Moderately toxic	• Cholecalciferol • *Barium carbonate* • *Tetramine*
Low toxic	• Anticoagulant rodenticides • *Thallium, arsenic*

TABLE 3: Rodenticide classification based on chemical structure (among anticoagulants).

Chemical structure	*Agents*
4-Hydroxycoumarins	Warfarin, coumatetralyl, bromadiolone, brodifacoum, difenacoum, difethialone, flocoumafen
Indandione	Pindone, chlorophacinone, diphacinone

found rodenticides to be important agents implicated for self-harm. The metal phosphides are the common compound implicated for deliberate self-harm in the northern part of India and is associated with very significant case fatality.[3] On the other hand, phosphorus-based rodenticides are commonly implicated agents used for self-harm in the southern part of India.[3] This divide is, however, arbitrary with more and more cases of acute yellow phosphorus poisoning being reported from North and Western India. Metal phosphides and superwarfarin have also been reported now from other countries like Iran, Gulf nations, Morocco, and Egypt. Most importantly, the South East Asian/Indian subcontinent diaspora is responsible for metal phosphide-related incidences in middle eastern countries. Thallium and arsenic were used as rodenticides in the past, but they are no longer available, whereas barium sulfate, cholecalciferol, and tetramine are least toxic to humans but are not very popular **(Table 1)**.

The most common, clinically relevant rodenticides are metal phosphides, yellow phosphorus, and warfarin derivatives.

MODE OF POISONING

A commonly seen method of intoxication is ingestion. This is also the most toxic of the exposure routes. For phosphorus-based compounds and superwarfarin, ingestion is the only route implicated. Inhalation exposure has been reported with metal phosphide compounds releasing phosphine gas. This has been noted as accidental exposure mostly, whenever metal phosphide compounds are being used for pest control as fumigants in enclosed spaces like buildings, offices, and flats. Cutaneous or dermal exposure is rarely reported.

Recently, it has been noted that metal phosphide rodenticides poisoning-related fatalities are not only dependent on the dose but also on the formulation (tablets/granules/powder). It is also important to note that the way the metal phosphides are ingested (taken directly orally or mixed with water, juice, etc.) also influences the toxicity and fatality related to them. Whenever a fresh tablet/powder is ingested directly, the chances of severe toxicity increase, whereas mixing the powder/granules in liquids will actually cause phosphine gas to escape from the mixing container, thereby limiting the severity of the poisoning. The use of an old/exposed formulation of metal phosphides for self-harm, with most of the phosphine already escaping/used up, leads to relatively milder systemic symptoms.

YELLOW/WHITE/ELEMENTAL PHOSPHOROUS POISONING

It is one of the commonly used compounds as rodenticide which is widely available in a paste form. Its use is mostly prevalent in southern, central, and western India. It has a garlic-like odor. It needs to be mixed with food items/grain flour to make it attractive/palatable for the rodents; however, direct consumption of the paste is the favorable mode used for self-harm purpose. It is commonly available as a paste containing 2–5% of yellow phosphorus.

Mechanism of Toxicity

Yellow phosphorous causes multisystem affection. It is absorbed slowly through the gastrointestinal (GI) tract and respiratory mucosa. It is a protoplasmic toxin, known to affect ribosomal function and protein synthesis. It leads to impaired glucose homeostasis and impaired lipoprotein and triglyceride metabolism leading to fatty degeneration of the liver, kidney, and brain.

Lethal dose—1 mg/kg and fulminant poisoning is seen with doses >1–2 g.[4]

Clinical Features (Table 4)[5]

On the initial day of ingestion, patients present with mild GI symptoms such as nausea and vomiting. This can be labeled *as stage 1 or the GI stage of poisoning. Sudden death has been reported during this stage of poisoning.*[4] The most important cause of death during this period is cardiac arrhythmia due to electrolyte abnormalities. It is very important to monitor patients for metabolic abnormalities during this stage.

TABLE 4: Chronology of clinical manifestations of yellow phosphorous poisoning.

Day of illness	*Symptoms*
First day (Stage 1)	Gastrointestinal symptoms
Second and third day (Stage 2)	Asymptomatic
Fourth day and later (Stage 3)	• Liver injury (transaminitis to acute liver failure) • Vascular (hypotension) • Cardiac arrhythmias • Acute kidney injury • CNS symptoms

(CNS: central nervous system)

The *second or the asymptomatic stage* occurs during the second to fourth day of illness. Patients may remain asymptomatic during this stage. There may be a steady rise in bilirubin levels and liver enzymes at this stage. Clinically, asymptomatic but ongoing biochemical injury occurs to the liver and other organs during this stage. Since the patient appears asymptomatic, many times the clinician may think about discharging these patients; however, a close watch of liver and kidney functions is needed during this period.

The *third stage* is the most important stage usually seen between day 4 and day 7 of exposure. During this period, the symptoms return. The clinical manifestations of acute liver injury (ranging from mild transaminitis to deep jaundice with fulminant liver failure) are seen. Acute-onset alteration in sensorium, confusion, coma, and bleeding are indicators of severely impaired liver functions. Cardiac involvement will manifest as hypotension, cardiac arrhythmias, and acute kidney injury manifesting with metabolic acidosis and oligo-anuria. Central nervous system involvement manifests as confusion, psychosis, hallucinations, and coma.[6] Due to the chemical properties of yellow phosphorus, hollow viscus injury and rarely perforation have also been reported following ingestion. GI hemorrhage has also been reported. During all the clinical stages, luminescent feces and vomitus, with or without a garlic-like odor, have been noted in some patients. Death is predominantly due to cardiac arrhythmias or complications of acute liver failure.

Management (Box 1)

Treatment is mainly supportive.[7] Multiple studies show a good survival response when medical management is started at an earlier stage. Gastric lavage with a 1:1,000 potassium permanganate solution is no longer indicated.[4] Whole-bowel irrigation with strict monitoring of the electrolytes and cardiac function may be tried, but it is

BOX 1: Treatment of yellow phosphorous poisoning.

- *Gastric lavage:* 1:1,000 potassium permanganate solution or normal saline (within 1–2 hour)
- *Whole bowel irrigation:* With Polyethylene glycol if presents within 12 hour (R/O bowel perforation)
- *N-acetyl cysteine:* 150 mg/kg body weight in 250 mL of 5% dextrose over 1 hour followed by 50 mg/kg over 4 hours and 100 mg/kg over 16 hours
- Plasma exchange
- Liver transplantation

important to rule out any overt/occult GI perforation before that. Daily monitoring of liver and renal function along with electrolytes and coagulation parameters is more important.

N-acetyl cysteine is used in all cases of poisonings causing acute liver failure.[8] Acute yellow phosphorus poisoning is no exception. There are numerous case reports and case series emphasizing the benefit but there are still no randomized trials for the same. Since N-acetyl cystine is a relatively well-tolerated antidote, therefore it is being used; however, there is no convincing evidence for its benefit. Vitamin K can be given as an adjunct because of severe coagulopathy in acute liver failure along with fresh frozen plasma. Another indication for prescribing vitamin K is contamination with warfarin like agents in all types of rodenticides. Liver transplantation is the definitive treatment for acute fulminant liver failure and has been helpful in acute liver failure due to yellow phosphorus poisoning.[9] Plasma exchange has been tried with variable success in multiple trials.[10]

There are studies indicating transplant-free improvement and survival in patients undergoing therapeutic plasma exchange. There is no clear consensus on the indications, dosage, frequency, and timing of plasma exchange therapy, but standard volume plasma exchange is being tried in multiple centers. The details of plasmapheresis for hepatotoxic poisons have been discussed in another chapter of this book.

Corticosteroids are not beneficial and may be detrimental.[11] Therefore, it is best to avoid them in severe toxicity. Patients should be shifted and managed in the intensive care unit (ICU) whenever there is worsening acute liver injury, severe coagulopathy [international normalized ratio (INR) >6, model for end-stage liver disease (MELD) score ≥36], persistent lactic acidosis, and any evidence of encephalopathy.

Patients who have not developed acute liver injury can be discharged from the hospital after 5 days of observation. It is important to document no worsening in biochemical parameters during observation in the wards. Patients who develop acute liver injury can be discharged once the parameters of acute liver injury start to improve. Serial documentation of liver enzymes and coagulation parameters along with clinical signs of liver cell failure is a must in all patients. Once discharged, these patients should be followed twice weekly in the outpatient department until complete resolution of biochemical parameters of liver injury.[12]

Liver Transplantation in Yellow Phosphorous Poisoning

In patients not responding to medical management, emergency liver transplantation can be considered as one of the treatment options.[12,13] The King's College Criteria routinely used in patients with acute liver failure cannot be used in this situation for selecting candidates for a liver transplant because of multiple reasons—as patients usually fall in the mid-age (between age of 20 and 40 years), INR and bilirubin may not have reached to its peak in patients being treated with therapeutic plasma exchange. One of the main indications for liver transplantation is hepatic encephalopathy of grade 2 and above (West Haven grading). Irreversible neurological damage is considered an absolute contraindication for doing liver transplantation.

METAL PHOSPHIDES: ALUMINUM AND ZINC PHOSPHIDE POISONING

Metal phosphides are the most common agent responsible for rodenticide poisoning in India. They are popular rodenticides as they are highly potent, generally inexpensive, and do not leave toxic residue on grains. They are available as aluminum, zinc, magnesium, or calcium salts in the form of tablets, pellets, or discs. Aluminum phosphide is available as dark yellow or dark gray tablets/granules/crystals, while zinc phosphide is a gray crystalline powder. In developing countries, aluminum phosphide is used extensively as a grain fumigant and as a rodenticide. Aluminum phosphide toxicity is particularly dangerous when consumed from a freshly opened or recently packed container. The mortality due to metal phosphide poisoning ranges anywhere between 37% and 100%.[14]

Mechanism of Action

Metal phosphides react with moisture in the air to release phosphine that is an active pesticide by itself. Phosphine is a highly toxic agent and is a potent mitochondrial poison.[14] Phosphine is readily absorbed from the mucosal surfaces and diffuses in the cells rapidly.

Phosphine acts like cyanide (protoplasmic poison) and disrupts the electron transport chain in mitochondria.[15] This results in an inability of the cell to utilize delivered oxygen causing cellular/tissue hypoxia in the presence of normal oxygen-carrying capacity of the blood. The organs having very high oxygen demand for normal functioning get affected. Among them, the heart and brain are important.[16] Cardiac myocyte hypoxia/dysfunction results in left ventricular dysfunction leading to low cardiac output, compromising renal perfusion.[15] Cerebral hypoxia results in alteration in the sensorium. The hallmark of toxicity is severe lactic acidosis/metabolic acidosis due to cellular hypoxia and changes in cellular metabolism from aerobic to anaerobic.[16] Renal injury adds to the metabolic derangements/acidosis. The hallmark of metal phosphide poisoning is severe metabolic acidosis and fluid refractory hypotension.[15,16]

Pathological changes in the organs are mostly in the form of hypoxic neuronal injury in the brain, myocytolysis in the heart muscles (with minimal inflammation), centrilobular necrosis in the liver due to shock, and tubular injury in the kidney.[17]

Metal phosphides are also known to cause significant oxidative damage due to the generation of reactive oxygen species. In many studies, oxidative damage has been documented in the heart, lung, kidney and to some extent in the brain.[18]

Clinical Features

The symptoms start developing within 30 minutes of exposure. Initial symptoms are GI such as epigastric pain, nausea, and vomiting due to direct irritation of GI mucosa due to the compound. Phosphine gas produced from these metal phosphides results in a garlic odor in the breath of such patients.[15,16] The large-sized tablet traversing through esophagus may cause local ulceration due to exothermic reaction or pressure necrosis due to impaction. This may lead to hematemesis.

Cardiovascular manifestations include myocarditis, pericarditis, and congestive heart failure. Nonspecific ST-T changes or arrhythmias and global hypokinesia can be seen in electrocardiogram and echocardiogram, respectively. Severe myocarditis may result in life-threatening cardiac arrhythmia.[19] Acute renal failure, acute liver failure, and disseminated intravascular coagulation are also known to occur and are likely due to shock.[15] Metabolic fluctuation in the magnesium and blood sugar levels has been documented, which may worsen arrhythmia or organ dysfunction.

Phosphine inhalation injury is being increasingly reported from Gulf/Middle East countries.[20] This happens when a large amount of gas piles up in an enclosed space. Patients who present with inhalation of phosphine gas released from metal phosphides can develop chest tightness, headache, giddiness, lethargy, nausea, and vomiting. Severe exposure may lead to convulsions and delirium.[20] These patients should be observed as symptom onset may be delayed. Hypokalemia and hypoglycemia have also been reported to occur frequently post exposure and may affect mortality adversely.[21]

The diagnosis is clinical. It should be suspected whenever a patient presents with unexplained metabolic acidosis with hypotension.[15,16] APACHE II (acute physiology and chronic health evaluation II), SAPS (simplified acute physiology score), and SOFA (sequential organ failure assessment), scores can be used as general predictors of outcome in all critically ill patients and have been studied extensively. A new simplified score consisting of three variables—pH <7.25, Glasgow Coma Scale (GCS) <13, and impaired systolic blood pressure (SBP) <90 mm Hg—is an important development. With a score of 1 point for each parameter, the score can range from 0 (none positive) to 3 (all 3 positive). A score of 0 is associated with 100% survival whereas higher scores indicate severe poisoning correlating with mortality.[22]

Treatment

Management is supportive. Owing to its predilection for multiorgan failure and associated high mortality, these patients are best managed in an ICU. **Flowchart 1** demonstrates the proposed treatment algorithm for acute aluminum phosphide toxicity based on the prognostic index (PGI) score.[22]

Decontamination with gastric lavage is debatable as it can increase the rate of disintegration of the phosphides and increase toxicity.[14] Phosphine release curtailment by vegetable oils has been used in many studies, but its use is debatable.[15,23] The basic hypothesis is that coating of the tablet/granules with oil is likely to prevent contact with hydrochloric acid in the stomach. Most of the patients present after considerable delay with florid clinical manifestation, thereby negating the effect of vegetable oil/ghee as a preventive measure. Moreover, administration of any oil/ghee to a patient already vomiting will exponentially increase the risk of aspiration and lipoid pneumonia. Due to all these risks, administration of vegetable oil/liquid paraffin/ghee cannot be recommended as standard of care in metal phosphide ingestion.[15]

Several reports have suggested the use of potassium permanganate for gastric lavage, although the evidence to

Flowchart 1: Proposed treatment algorithm for acute aluminum phosphide toxicity.

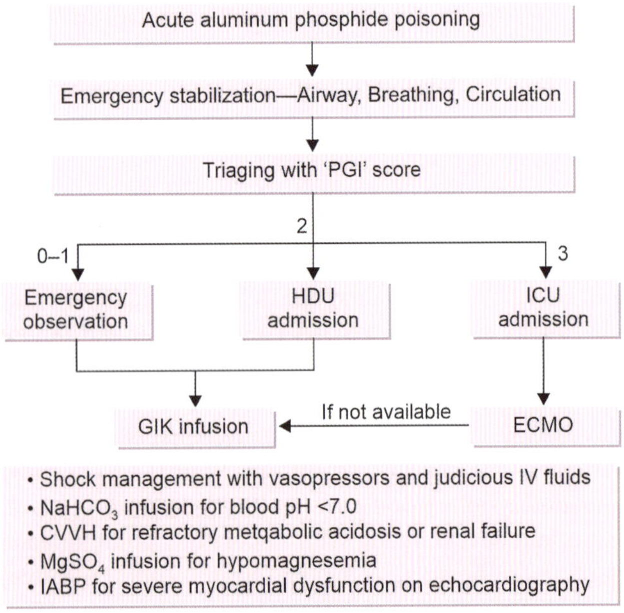

(CVVH: continuous veno-venous hemofiltration; ECMO: extracorporeal membrane oxygenation; HDU: high-dependency unit; IABP: intra-aortic balloon counter-pulsation; ICU: intensive care unit; PGI: prognostic index).

Notes: Prognostic index score—point 1 each for pH <7.25, Glasgow Coma Scale score <13, and impaired systolic blood pressure <90 mm Hg.

back its use is lacking; therefore, it is not recommended. Activated charcoal may be beneficial to reduce toxicity due to metal phosphide ingestion by adsorbing phosphine present in the stomach; however, its role is not clearly established and it may be avoided.

If inhalational is suspected, removal of victims from the site of exposure, oxygen supplementation, and meticulous observation for 6–12 hours is recommended.[20] These patients should be monitored in an ICU as they might require ventilator and organ support.

N-acetyl cysteine has been used as an antioxidant with variable results but is not recommended as a standard of care.[24] Glucose-insulin-potassium infusion pump has been tried in multiple studies in acute aluminum phosphide poisoning and found to be effective.[25] The exact mechanism of the action is not completely understood. It has been proposed that insulin shifts the cardiac myocyte energy source from free fatty acids to glucose, thereby improving cardiac function. It was found to improve blood pressure and reduce the requirement of mechanical ventilator.[25] Multiple protocols are being followed in various institutes in the dosing of insulin infusion. The common dosing of insulin and potassium is titrated such that sugars are between 70 and 200 mg/dL and potassium levels are maintained in the normal range.[25]

Extracorporeal membrane oxygenation (ECMO) has been used to tide over the acute phase of poisoning. The basic hypothesis is to support the failing left ventricle and maintain tissue perfusion till the time the body gets rid of the phosphine from the tissue, especially cardiac myocytes.[26] Since ECMO is widely available in many tertiary centers, it should be offered/tried whenever possible. The limited availability, lack of expertise, and high cost are deterrents. ECMO reduces mortality significantly when instituted earlier.[26] There are other supportive therapies like left ventricular assist devices and continuous renal replacement therapy that have been tried either alone or along with ECMO, with variable success.[20] The details have been discussed in chapters on cardiac support and ECMO.

In survivors, esophageal strictures and perforation have been reported as an important morbidity. Surgery (for perforation) or serial stricture dilatation may be needed as is done in strictures due to corrosive poisoning. A recent study has shown that poison-related factors, formulation, and mode of consumption influence the outcome greatly.[27]

SUPERWARFARIN POISONING

Superwarfarin is a long-acting, vitamin K antagonist anticoagulant rodenticide derived from warfarin (developed from dicoumarol). Compared with warfarin, superwarfarin has very long half-lives and is much more potent in terms of its anticoagulant effects. Warfarin resistance identified in many species of rats and mice leads to the birth of superwarfarin which comprises difenacoum, brodifacoum, and bromadiolone.

Discovery of Warfarin and Its Congeners

Sweet clover is grown as a green manure and hay crop in the US and Canada. Its coumarin content gives its distinctive odor (like vanilla). In the early 20th century, there was an epidemic of bleeding disease in the cattle when the sweet clover hay had been found to be infected with molds. Later, it was found that these molds metabolize the coumarin into dicoumarol. Cattle or sheep consuming the spoiled hay thus developed bleeding diathesis. Karl Link with Wisconsin Alumni Research members identified dicoumarol as the cause of bleeding and thus further led to the discovery of warfarin and its congeners.[28] The same action is being exploited when superwarfarins are used as rodenticides. A small amount of lethal dose is added to grain flour or other food items to attract rodents. Once it is consumed, severe coagulopathy and bleeding result, leading to fatality.

Mechanism of Action (Fig. 1)[29]

Vitamin K epoxide reductase helps in converting vitamin K to its reduced form which is helpful in activating clotting factors (II, VII, IX, and X) through gamma-glutamyl transferase. Warfarin and its congeners act by inhibiting vitamin K epoxide reductase, thus leading to impaired coagulation, spontaneous bleeding, and various bleeding manifestations.

When to Suspect

Clinically evident spontaneous bleeding without any evidence of fever, acute or chronic liver failure, or a hematological condition (thrombocytopenia, leukemia, or drug toxicity) should raise a suspicion of poisoning with agents causing coagulopathy. Aspirin or other nonsteroidal anti-inflammatory drugs (NSAIDs) can cause toxicity but do not lead to spontaneous bleeding due to platelet dysfunction. Superwarfarin poisoning should be considered in the differential diagnosis of a patient presenting with signs and symptoms of coagulopathy related to vitamin K deficiency without any explanation/ proven clinical condition, even if a clear exposure history is missing. Uncorrectable coagulation dysfunction with usual doses of vitamin K is another clue.

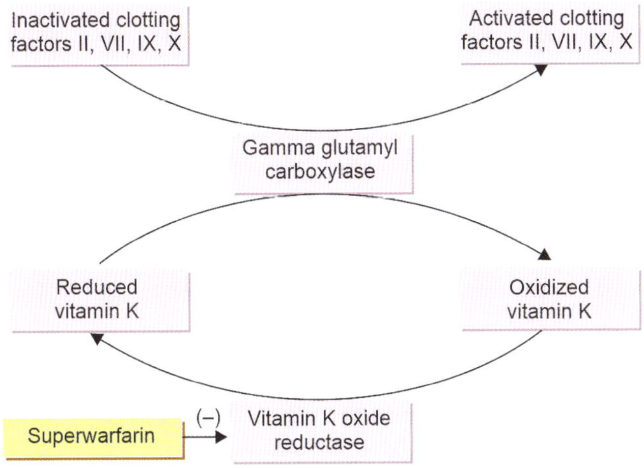

Fig. 1: Mechanism of superwarfarin toxicity.

Clinical Presentation

Patients may present with a myriad of manifestations. Nonspecific symptoms including abdominal pain, flank pain, and headache are reported.[29,30] Patients with significant consumption commonly present with unprovoked/spontaneous bleeding diathesis such as gross hematuria, mucosal bleeding, GI bleeding, soft-tissue bleeding, menorrhagia, and hemoptysis. These bleeding manifestations start occurring on the second day of ingestion, as the drug needs time to act and coagulation factors start depleting to less than 30% of the normal levels by 48 hours **(Table 5)**.[30] Rarely patients may present with clinical features of thrombosis due to protein C and S deficiency in the initial phase as opposed to bleeding as protein C and S are vitamin K-dependent factors.[30] Unusual sites of both venous and arterial thrombi, later followed by hemorrhage, may give clinicians a clue.

Laboratory Testing

Prothrombin time and INR are the investigations of choice which are deranged usually 48 hour post ingestion.[30,31] Other prolongation of vitamin k-dependent clotting factors (II, VII, IX, and X) can also be assessed. Quantitative analysis of superwarfarins is the test of choice for confirmation of superwarfarin poisoning but is not readily available, and hence not routinely done. Liquid chromatography-tandem mass spectrometry (LC-MS/MS) is the preferred technique.[32]

Treatment

Early in the course of illness (within the first 6 hours of exposure), activated charcoal may be tried; once the bleeding is established, gastric decontamination has little role.[30] The treatment of superwarfarin poisoning in a bleeding patient includes vitamin K1 therapy which addresses the underlying vitamin K antagonism, and early and rapid correction of coagulopathy to treat uncontrolled hemorrhage.[30]

TABLE 5: Plasma half-life of clotting factors.

Coagulation factor	*Mean half-life (hour)*[21]
II	41
VII	6.2
IX	13.9
X	16.5

Fresh frozen plasma and prothrombin complex concentrates are used in case of active bleeding episodes.[33] There is no obvious consensus on the optimal dose and frequency of vitamin K1 for patients with superwarfarin poisoning in the literature. The optimal frequency of administration was suggested to be every 6–8 hours. The initial dose of vitamin K used has varied from 0.1 to 3 mg/kg/day and doses as high as 500–800 mg/day have also been used.[30] The patient should be daily followed up with prothrombin time (PT) and activated partial thromboplastin time (aPTT). There are no established guidelines for the termination of vitamin K1 therapy in patients with known superwarfarin poisoning.

Termination of therapy based on a normal clotting profile obtained while the poisoned patient is still on vitamin K1 can be dangerous.[30] Poor adherence to vitamin K therapy has been seen in patients who presented with intake of superwarfarin poisoning by deliberate self-harm.

The quantitative analysis of superwarfarins in serum can be done in these patients. This will help in identifying vitamin K-dependent coagulopathy, to find out re-exposure, and most importantly can be beneficial in the termination of treatment without exposing the patient to bleeding risks which might arise from early stopping of vitamin K1. Therapeutic plasma exchange has been studied in superwarfarin poisoning with variable results.[34]

CONCLUSION

Rodenticide poisoning is a common mode of self-harm in India due to easy access to these compounds in agricultural population. Metal phosphides such as aluminum and zinc phosphide, yellow phosphorus, and warfarin derivatives are most common and clinically relevant. Metal phosphide and yellow phosphorus poisoning can present with multi-organ dysfunction. Treatment is mainly supportive. Warfarin derivative poisoning usually presents with bleeding diathesis and can be treated with vitamin K, fresh frozen plasma and prothrombin complex concentrate.

REFERENCES

1. D'Silva C, Krishna B. Rodenticide poisoning. Indian J Crit Care Med. 2019;23:S272-7.
2. ScienceDirect Topics. 4 Hydroxycoumarin derivative: an overview. [online] Available from https://www.sciencedirect.com/topics/medicine-and-dentistry/4-hydroxycoumarin-derivative. [Last accessed September, 2024].
3. Peshin SS, Srivastava A, Halder N, Gupta YK. Pesticide poisoning trend analysis of 13 years: A retrospective study based on telephone calls at the National Poisons Information Center, All India Institute of Medical Sciences, New Delhi. J Forensic Leg Med. 2014;22:57-61.
4. Winek CL, Collom WD, Fusia EP. Yellow phosphorus ingestion–Three fatal poisonings. Clin Toxicol. 1973;6:541-5.
5. Rubitsky HJ, Myerson RM. Acute phosphorus poisoning. Arch Intern Med (Chic). 1949;83:164-78.
6. Mishra AK, Devakiruba NS, Jasmine S, Sathyendra S, Zachariah A, Iyadurai R. Clinical spectrum of yellow phosphorous poisoning in a tertiary care center in South India: A case series. Trop Doct. 2017;47:245-9.
7. Santos O, Restrepo JC, Velásquez L, Castaño J, Correa G, Sepúlveda E, et al. Acute liver failure due to white phosphorus ingestion. Ann Hepatol. 2009;8:162-5.
8. Nabi T, Nabi S, Rafiq N, Shah A. Role of N-acetylcysteine treatment in non-acetaminophen-induced acute liver failure: A prospective study. Saudi J Gastroenterol. 2017;23:169-75.
9. Pahari H, Raj A, Sonavane A, Sawant A, Gupta DK, Gharat A, et al. Liver transplantation for acute liver failure due to yellow phosphorus poisoning: A comprehensive review. Transplant Proc. 2023;55:2450-5.
10. Stahl K, Hadem J, Schneider A, Manns MP, Wiesner O, Schmidt BMW, et al. Therapeutic plasma exchange in acute liver failure. J Clin Apher. 2019;34:589-97.
11. Marin GA, Montoya CA, Sierra JL, Senior JR. Evaluation of corticosteroid and exchange-transfusion treatment of acute yellow-phosphorus intoxication. N Engl J Med. 1971;284:125-8.
12. Reddy MS, Rajakumar A, Mathew JS, Venkatakrishnan L, Jothimani D, Sudhindran S, et al. Liver transplantation society of India guidelines for the management of acute liver injury secondary to yellow phosphorus-containing rodenticide poisoning using the modified Delphi technique of consensus development. J Clin Exp Hepatol. 2021;11:475-83.
13. Saraf V, Pande S, Gopalakrishnan U, Balakrishnan D, Menon RN, Sudheer OV, et al. Acute liver failure due to zinc phosphide containing rodenticide poisoning: Clinical features and prognostic indicators of need for liver transplantation. Indian J Gastroenterol. 2015;34:325-9.
14. Proudfoot AT. Aluminum and zinc phosphide poisoning. Clin Toxicol (Phila). 2009;47:89-100.
15. Singh S, Bhalla A. Aluminum phosphide poisoning. J Mahatma Gandhi Inst Med Sci. 2015;20:15-9.
16. Sivvach SB, Yadav DR, Arora BB, Dalal S, Jagdish. Acute aluminum phosphide poisoning. An epidemiological, clinical and histopathological study. J Assoc Phys India. 1988;36:594-6.
17. Mehrpour O, Dolati M, Soltaninejad K, Shadnia S, Nazparvar B. Evaluation of histopathological changes in fatal aluminum phosphide poisoning. Indian J Forensic Med Toxicol. 2008;2:34-6.
18. Anand R, Kumari P, Kaushal A, Bal A, Wani WY, Sunkaria A, et al. Effect of aluminum phosphide exposure on rats:

A biochemical and histological correlation. Toxicol Lett. 2012;215(1):62-9.
19. Katira R, Elhence GP, Mehrotra ML, Srivastava SS, Mitra A, Agarwala R, et al. A study of aluminum phosphide (AlP) poisoning with special reference to electrocardiographic changes. J Assoc Physicians India. 1990;38:471-3.
20. Mehrpour O, Jafarzadeh M, Abdollahi M. A systematic review of aluminum phosphide poisoning. Arh Hig Rada Toksikol. 2012;63:61-73.
21. Doğan E, Güzel A, Çiftçi T, Aycan İ, Çelik F, Çetin B, et al. Zinc phosphide poisoning. Case Rep Crit Care. 2014;2014:589712.
22. Pannu AK, Jhuria L, Bhalla A, Sharma N. PGI score: Prospective validation and correlation with SOFA, SAPS-II, and APACHE-II scores for predicting outcomes in acute aluminum phosphide poisoning. Toxicol Res (Camb). 2022;11:361-6.
23. Shadnia S, Rahimi M, Pajoumand A, Rasouli M-H, Abdollahi M. Successful treatment of acute aluminum phosphide poisoning: Possible benefit of coconut oil. Hum Exp Toxicol. 2005;24(4):215-8.
24. Bhalla A, Jyothinath P, Singh S. Antioxidant therapy in patients with severe aluminum phosphide poisoning: A pilot study. Indian J Crit Care Med. 2017;21(12):836-40.
25. Pannu AK, Bhalla A, Gantala J, Sharma N, Kumar S, Dhibar DP. Glucose-insulin-potassium infusion for the treatment of acute aluminum phosphide poisoning: An open-label pilot study. Clin Toxicol (Phila). 2020;58:1004-9.
26. Mohan B, Gupta V, Ralhan S, Gupta D, Puri S, Mahajan R, et al. Impact of extra-corporeal membrane oxygenation on outcome of aluminum phosphide poisoning complicated with myocardial dysfunction. Clin Toxicology. 2019;57(11):1095-102.
27. Anbalagan LC, Pannu AK, Bhalla A, Dhibar DP, Sharma N. Prognostic significance of poison-related factors and consumption patterns in acute aluminum phosphide poisoning. Turk J Emerg Med. 2023;23:88-95.
28. Lim GB. Milestone 2: Warfarin: From rat poison to clinical use. Nat Rev Cardiol. 2017. DOI: 10.1038/nrcardio.2017.172
29. de Genover Gil A, Gonzalez Suarez GM, Moret Puig C, Hurtado Ganoza A. Superwarfarin poisoning: Challenges still remain. BMJ Case Rep. 2022;15:e248385.
30. King N, Tran MH. Long-acting anticoagulant rodenticide (superwarfarin) poisoning: A review of its historical development, epidemiology, and clinical management. Transfus Med Rev. 2015;29:250-8.
31. Semantic Scholar. Survival time of prothrombin and factors VII, IX, and X after completely synthesis blocking doses of coumarin derivatives. [online] Available from https://www.semanticscholar.org/paper/Survival-Time-of-Prothrombin-and-Factors-VII%2C-IX-X-Hellemans-Vorlat/b2dedea538d6fb8cb6e5cb40326612930bfda382. [Last accessed September, 2024].
32. Ye L, Wang Z, Zhang H, Guo H, Guo Y, Chen L. Application of a new established system for toxic doses in children with 4-hydroxycoumarin rodenticide intoxication. Front Pediatr. 2018;6:141.
33. Haesloop O, Tillick A, Nichol G, Strote J. Superwarfarin ingestion treated successfully with prothrombin complex concentrate. Am J Emerg Med. 2016;34:116.e1-2.
34. Deng Y, Qiu L. Therapeutic plasma exchange: A second-line treatment for brodifacoum poisoning following an anaphylactoid reaction to vitamin K. Clin Case Rep. 2017;5:35-8.

2.7 Prescription Drug Poisoning (Paracetamol, Beta-blockers, Calcium Channel Blockers, Antiepileptics, Antihistamine Drugs, Antidiabetic Drugs)

Ashish Kumar Kakkar, Ashish Thomas George

INTRODUCTION

Prescription drug poisoning is a significant public health concern, encompassing a variety of medications with diverse mechanisms of toxicity. This chapter focuses on common agents implicated in overdose, including paracetamol (PCM) (acetaminophen), known for its hepatotoxicity; beta-blockers, which can cause severe cardiovascular effects; calcium channel blockers (CCBs), associated with profound hypotension and bradycardia; antiepileptics, which present neurological and systemic toxicities; and antihistamines, often leading to anticholinergic syndrome. Understanding the clinical manifestations and management strategies for poisoning by these agents is crucial for effective patient care and prevention of morbidity and mortality.

PARACETAMOL

Paracetamol (acetaminophen) is commonly implicated in both intentional and unintentional poisonings, often used alone or with other medications. Available as both immediate-release and extended-release formulations, the therapeutic dose ranges from 325 to 1,000 mg in adults administered every 4–6 hours with a maximum daily dose of 4 g. For children, the dose is 10–15 mg/kg with a maximum daily dose of 80 mg/kg. Although toxic doses may vary individually, acute consumption of >150–200 mg/kg in children or 7 g in total for adults is considered potentially harmful because it leads to the production of a highly hepatotoxic metabolite in the liver—N-acetyl-p-benzoquinone imine (NAPQI).[1] The plasma half-life of IV PCM is 8 minutes, whereas oral PCM has a half-life of 1.9–2.5 hours. Within 4.5–5.5 hours, PCM is completely eliminated from the body. The toxicity may occur if a large single dose of PCM is orally ingested or if repeated small doses are frequently being taken with a cumulative dose exceeding 6–7 g within 24 hours (staggered overdose). This happens when PCM is frequently taken for control of fever or body aches. The toxicity of PCM is further accentuated by preexisting liver dysfunction, as seen in patients with cirrhosis of liver. The potential for toxicity also increases exponentially if the fever-causing organisms have a predilection for liver leading to hepatitis. The classic examples are dengue, malaria, scrub typhus, and leptospirosis. One should be careful regarding liver toxicity in acute febrile illness.

At therapeutic doses, PCM is metabolized in the liver to form glucuronide and sulfate conjugates that undergo urinary excretion. Normally, a small proportion of the drug is converted to a highly reactive NAPQI that is toxic to both liver and kidneys. NAPQI readily reacts with the sulfhydryl group of hepatic glutathione (GSH) rendering it harmless. However, at toxic doses, the conjugation pathways are saturated, and more of the drug is diverted to form NAPQI. During an overdose, the levels of GSH are depleted, leading to the binding of the NAPQI metabolite to cellular proteins causing enzymatic, structural, and metabolic disruption. Further, GSH depletion predisposes hepatocytes to oxidative injury and apoptosis. Additionally, renal tubular necrosis, hypoglycemia, and encephalopathy may manifest.[2]

The clinical manifestations of PCM toxicity are typically divided into four stages[3]:

Stage I: Clinical features are usually nonspecific including nausea, vomiting, malaise, pallor, and sweating. These symptoms may be mild and often do not reliably predict the severity of subsequent hepatotoxicity. Laboratory studies are usually within the normal range.

Stage II: It presents the onset of hepatic toxicity with or without renal involvement. Aspartate aminotransferase (AST) is the most sensitive measure, and elevation begins within 24 hours of consumption and is seen by 36 hours in nearly all patients. Alanine aminotransferase (ALT) elevation is noted shortly after the AST and the latter falls earlier than the former. Hence, AST is recommended as the preferred marker for detecting hepatic toxicity as well as recovery.

Stage III: This is the stage of maximal hepatic toxicity with liver function test (LFT) abnormalities peaking between 72 and 96 hours of PCM ingestion. Clinically, this manifests as jaundice, markedly elevated liver enzymes (ALT/AST >10,000 IU/L), encephalopathy, coma, and occasionally hemorrhage. Derangements of prothrombin time (PT), international normalized ratio (INR), lactic acidosis, hypoglycemia, and creatinine are critical determinants of patient prognosis. Renal function abnormalities are seen in nearly one-quarter of patients with severe hepatotoxicity and more than half of patients with fulminant hepatic failure. Mortality is seen most often in this stage of PCM toxicity.

Stage IV: This represents recovery occurring in survivors of acute overdose. Laboratory abnormalities—AST, PT/INR, and lactic acidosis—are the first to normalize. Clinical recovery precedes histologic recovery and may be prolonged in cases of severe poisoning. However, the hepatic recovery is usually complete with no residual chronic liver dysfunction.

Hepatic necrosis, which is the most severe and potentially deadly immediate adverse consequence of PCM overdose, can be caused by this metabolite. It occurs when acetaminophen is converted into the harmful metabolite NAPQI, which is quickly removed by combining with GSH. It is then further metabolized into mercapturic acid and expelled in the urine. In adults, hepatotoxicity may arise after a single dose of 10–15 g (150–250 mg/kg), and in children, it occurs with doses >150 mg/kg. Doses of 20–25 g or more are potentially fatal.

Conditions such as chronic heavy alcohol consumption or GSH depletion due to fasting or malnutrition increase liver vulnerability to damage. This has been observed, though rarely, with doses within the therapeutic range. Plasma transaminases begin to rise, sometimes significantly, between 12 and 36 hours after ingestion. Initial symptoms of acute poisoning appear within the first 2 days and are indicative of gastrointestinal distress, such as nausea, abdominal pain, and anorexia, which may not accurately reflect the seriousness of the poisoning. The clinical manifestations of liver damage become apparent 2–4 days after consuming toxic amounts. These manifestations include pain in the upper right part of the abdomen, a swollen and painful liver, yellowing of the skin and eyes (jaundice), and abnormal blood clotting (coagulopathy). Renal dysfunction or complete renal failure may also manifest. Liver enzyme abnormalities usually reach their highest levels between 72 and 96 hours after consuming a substance, and this may be accompanied by hepatic encephalopathy.[2]

Management of Paracetamol Overdose

Patients with plasma concentrations of acetaminophen exceeding 300 µg/mL at 4 hours or 45 µg/mL at 15 hours after ingestion will encounter serious liver damage in 90% of cases. Administering activated charcoal within 4 hours after administration can significantly reduce acetaminophen absorption. It is recommended to offer activated charcoal if the swallowed amount exceeds 7.5 g or 150 mg/kg in a dose of 1 g/kg up to 50 g orally. Gastric lavage and induced emesis are usually not recommended in these patients.

N-acetylcysteine (NAC) is the cornerstone of management in patients with PCM overdose and is recommended for individuals who are susceptible to liver damage. NAC functions in multiple ways by acting as a precursor for the synthesis of GSH and by neutralizing the NAPQI metabolite through direct binding.[4] When given within a time frame of 8–16 hours following an overdose, the mortality rate significantly decreases to <1%. Indications for NAC therapy include cases where serum PCM levels drawn within 4–24 hours lie in the toxic range as per the Rumack–Matthew nomogram,[5] in cases where the ingested amount exceeds 150 mg/kg or 7.5 g and serum levels are unavailable, serum levels in excess of 10 µg/mL with unknown time of ingestion, and where there is ingestion with any evidence of hepatic injury. Both oral and IV NAC preparations are available, and the latter is preferred in case of pregnant women, in cases with hepatic failure and in those with intractable vomiting.[3] The usual oral regimen consists of a loading dose of 140 mg/kg. This is followed by 17 maintenance doses of 70 mg/kg over a period of 72 hours. Any dose vomited within 1 hour needs to be repeated orally or IV. For the IV route, 150 mg/kg is the recommended loading dose given over 60 minutes, followed by 50 mg/kg over 4 hours and 100 mg/kg over the next 16 hours.[6] All infusions are prepared in 5% dextrose. NAC may be continued beyond this period in case PCM levels remain detectable, AST is significantly elevated, or where there is evidence of hepatic failure. IV NAC can be continued at 6.25 mg/kg/h. Additionally, it is imperative to provide active supportive care, which entails addressing hepatic and renal failure, performing intubation when indicated, and closely monitoring plasma glucose levels due to the potential for hypoglycemia resulting from liver failure.[1,2]

■ BETA-BLOCKERS

Beta-blockers are a widely used class of medications for various cardiovascular conditions, including hypertension, ischemic heart disease, and arrhythmias. However, their overdose can lead to significant morbidity and mortality, necessitating a comprehensive understanding of their adverse effects and appropriate management strategies.

Clinical features of beta-blocker toxicity depend upon the pharmacology of the ingested agent including beta receptor selectivity, intrinsic sympathomimetic activity, and membrane stabilizing properties. Clinical symptoms generally appear within hours of overdose; for example, propranolol overdose leads to rapid development of hypoglycemia, seizures, coma, and arrhythmias. In general, bradycardia and hypotension are the most common manifestations. Beta-blockers can cause severe cardiac failure in susceptible individuals due to their ability to reduce myocardial contractility and excitability. In patients with compromised cardiac function, the heart's ability to pump blood can depend on sympathetic stimulation. By blocking this stimulation, beta-blockers can result in cardiac decompensation. Impairment of sinoatrial (SA) and atrioventricular (AV) node functions leads to sinus bradycardia, sinus arrest, prolongation of PR interval, and AV block. Propranolol, due to its high lipid solubility and sodium channel-blocking effects, is particularly toxic. It can enter the central nervous system

(CNS) and cause seizures and wide QRS complex cardiac conduction block.[3,7]

Management of beta-blocker overdose involves several strategies. General supportive care is crucial, including maintaining airway, breathing, and circulation. Although initial treatment consists of IV fluid bolus and atropine, these measures are likely to be inadequate in severe toxicity. Gastrointestinal decontamination with orogastric lavage may be attempted in patients with severe ingestions, provided the drug is expected to be lying unabsorbed within the timeframe, which is followed by activated charcoal. The latter may be attempted alone in patients with ingestion of water-soluble agents and those with minor symptoms. In cases of ingestion involving sustained-release tablets, whole-bowel irrigation following multidose-activated charcoal may be considered. Seizures may be managed with benzodiazepines (BZD) or barbiturates or propofol in cases where BZDs are ineffective. Symptomatic hypoglycemia may be treated with an IV bolus of 50% dextrose in water.[8]

The antidote for beta-blocker overdose is glucagon. It raises intracellular cyclic adenosine monophosphate (cAMP) in cardiac cells independent of beta receptors, improving heart rate and blood pressure.[1] High doses of glucagon (5–10 mg IV) are typically required although it is prudent to start with a lower dose of 3–5 mg over 5–10 minutes to minimize nausea and vomiting. In case the patient responds with an increase in blood pressure, infusion at the rate of 2–5 mg/h is started.[3] Calcium salts given IV have also demonstrated efficacy in beta-blocker poisonings. Calcium gluconate can be employed IV at a dose of 3 g of 10% solution. The same dose may be repeated every 10–20 minutes up to a total dose of 9 g. High-dose insulin and glucose may be administered in patients who fail to respond to IV fluids, atropine, and glucagon. The bolus IV dose consists of regular insulin 1 U/kg along with dextrose 0.5 g/kg. The latter may be omitted when blood glucose exceeds 300 mg/dL. The maintenance infusion is typically dosed at regular insulin 1 U/kg/h (up-titrated to up to 10 U/kg/h in case cardiac function remains depressed) along with dextrose 0.5 g/kg/h and requires regular monitoring of blood glucose and electrolytes. (Details are given in the chapter on insulin as antidote.) Use of catecholamines—epinephrine or isoproterenol—may be required in refractory cases with the choice of agent usually guided by hemodynamic monitoring. Epinephrine may be used initially; however, discontinuation may be indicated in case of worsening of hypotension or acute cardiac failure develops due to excessive alpha stimulation. IV lipid emulsions have also been used in patients not responding to usual treatments, especially in cases of poisoning with lipid-soluble agents, but at the present, the evidence available is preliminary and insufficient to recommend them conclusively.[8,9]

CALCIUM CHANNEL BLOCKERS

Calcium channel blockers are commonly prescribed to manage hypertension, angina, arrhythmias, and other cardiovascular conditions. The primary hazardous consequences of overdose of CCBs are a direct result of their pharmacologic action. They are broadly classified into two groups: (1) Dihydropyridines (e.g., nifedipine and amlodipine) that preferentially block L-type calcium channels in the blood vessels and (2) nondihydropyridines (verapamil and diltiazem) that have a greater affinity for the channels in the myocardium. Therefore, while the former are potent vasodilators, the latter primarily depress the conduction and contractility of the heart. However, this selectivity may be lost at higher doses in case of poisoning.

The key clinical features of CCB toxicity are bradycardia and hypotension. Negative inotropic effects and cardiac conduction abnormalities predominate in nondihydropyridine CCB poisoning, while hypotension results from bradycardia, reduced inotropy, and peripheral vasodilation. Mild-to-moderate cases of dihydropyridine CCB poisoning may present with reflex tachycardia, however, severe cases typically exhibit bradycardia on account of loss of selectivity.[1] Electrocardiogram (ECG) shows PR interval prolongation, and hyperglycemia may be present owing to loss of calcium-mediated insulin release. CNS hypoperfusion results in dizziness and fatigue initially in the affected patients, while severe cases present with syncope and coma. Acute respiratory distress syndrome may result from precapillary vasodilation in severe toxicity.

Management of CCB overdose begins with providing general supportive care. It is imperative to intervene promptly to hinder complete absorption from the gastrointestinal tract (GIT), especially in the case of sustained-release preparations. To get optimal results, it is crucial to commence whole-bowel irrigation with polyethylene glycol (1–2 L/h oral) and deliver oral activated charcoal (1 g/kg) prior to the onset of ileus in these patients. In cases with symptomatic bradycardia, atropine is often administered although its effectiveness in this case is limited. The usual dose is 0.5–1 mg IV every 2–3 minutes up to a maximum of 3 mg. Administering IV calcium as either calcium chloride (10–20 mL of 10% solution) or gluconate (30–60 mL of 10% solution) may counteract reduced blood pressure although the clinical efficacy is limited and usually transient. Glucagon can be used to increase heart rate and contractility independent of β-adrenergic receptors through elevated cAMP levels, offering another treatment option in severe cases of CCB overdose. High doses of glucagon are typically required although it is prudent to start with a lower dose of 3–5 mg over 5 minutes which may be followed by 4–10 mg after 5 minutes in case of no response. Additional treatment approaches include administering high-dose regular insulin therapy beginning with a bolus dose of 1 U/kg. This is followed by a continuous insulin infusion of 1–2 U/kg/h that may be increased to up to 10 U/kg/h if required. Since hyperglycemia is often encountered in CCB toxicity, supplemental dextrose 0.5 g/kg is indicated only if blood glucose exceeds 300 mg/dL. Additionally, lipid emulsion therapy has shown promise in severe verapamil overdose cases.[3,9,10]

ANTIEPILEPTIC DRUGS

Antiepileptic drugs (AEDs) are crucial for treating seizure disorders, but overdosing can pose substantial medical problems because of their varied modes of action and potential for severe toxicity. Phenytoin, sodium valproate, carbamazepine, and phenobarbital are frequently involved in cases of overdose with antiepileptic drugs. Each of these medications can result in unique clinical symptoms that necessitate various treatment approaches.[11]

Phenytoin and Fosphenytoin

Phenytoin poisoning predominantly impacts the CNS and cardiovascular system (CVS). Common signs include nystagmus, ataxia, slurred speech, and, in severe cases, seizures and coma. IV overdose produces similar symptoms to oral route with additional CVS manifestations—hypotension and arrhythmias. When administered rapidly for the management of status epilepticus, fosphenytoin may produce cardiac arrhythmias, hypotension, and CNS depression. Intravenous administration can cause "purple glove syndrome" due to propylene glycol, leading to edema, pain, and skin discoloration. Severe cases may be associated with necrosis requiring amputation. Fosphenytoin being water soluble is less commonly associated with these symptoms. Management includes supportive care, such as stabilization of airway, breathing, and circulation, and administration of multidose-activated charcoal to limit drug absorption. In severe cases, hemodialysis may be necessary.[11-13]

Sodium Valproate

Valproate overdose is characterized by ataxia and lethargy with severe cases manifesting hypotension, respiratory depression, and coma. It can lead to hyperammonemia encephalopathy, cerebral edema, and, rarely, fulminant hepatic failure. General supportive care, including airway management, is essential and activated charcoal may be used for initial treatment. Hyperammonemia is managed with carnitine supplementation, which helps mitigate ammonia buildup and fulminant hepatitis. An IV loading dose of 100 mg/kg (max 6 g) over 30 minutes is recommended followed by 15 mg/kg over 10–30 minutes every 4 hours until clinical improvement is seen.[3]

Carbamazepine

Carbamazepine overdose presents with CNS symptoms such as dizziness, drowsiness, nystagmus, ataxia, and, in severe cases, seizures and coma.[13] Cardiac toxicity, including hypotension, arrhythmias, and occasionally widened QRS complexes and QT prolongation, is also common. Hyponatremia has also been seen in overdose cases. Activated charcoal is recommended for gastrointestinal decontamination, with multiple doses being more effective in significant overdoses. Sodium bicarbonate is administered to treat cardiac toxicity, particularly in the presence of widened QRS complexes, while seizures can be managed with BZDs. Hemodialysis may be utilized in severe cases presenting with intractable convulsions or arrhythmias.[14]

Phenobarbitone

Phenobarbitone overdose results in CNS depression, respiratory depression, and hypotension. Symptoms include sedation, ataxia, and, in extreme cases, coma and respiratory failure. Management focuses on supportive care, with particular attention to respiratory function. Endotracheal intubation may be necessary for patients with severe respiratory depression. Activated charcoal can reduce drug absorption, and repeated doses may be required. Urinary alkalinization with sodium bicarbonate can aid in enhanced elimination. Extracorporeal methods such as hemodialysis are indicated for removing phenobarbital in severe cases of poisoning.[11,15,16]

ANTIHISTAMINES

Antihistamines widely used to treat allergic conditions are commonly encountered in overdose scenarios due to their extensive availability. Overdose management of these drugs, particularly the sedating types, necessitates a comprehensive understanding of their pharmacological effects and appropriate medical interventions. This section will focus on the toxicity of H1 antihistamines.

Antihistamines can be broadly categorized into sedating and nonsedating types. Sedating antihistamines, such as promethazine, hydroxyzine, cyclizine, and diphenhydramine, are characterized by their lipid solubility, allowing rapid penetration of the CNS. This results in pronounced anticholinergic effects which are central to their toxicity profile. In contrast, nonsedating antihistamines like loratadine and cetirizine are less likely to cross the blood–brain barrier, making them generally safer in overdose situations.[17]

Sedation is commonly seen in overdose which may be worsened by other concomitant CNS depressants. Hallucinations, ataxia, incoordination, fixed dilated pupils, sinus tachycardia, dry mouth, fever, and urinary retention are the primary clinical features ascribed to anticholinergic effects. Although nonsedating antihistamines are generally less hazardous, they can nevertheless induce tachycardia, drowsiness, gastrointestinal disorders, and headache when consumed in excessive amounts. Nonsedating antihistamines have been associated with rare cases of arrhythmias.[17,18]

Management of antihistamine overdose begins with the administration of activated charcoal, especially if the patient presents early. General supportive care is paramount, focusing on monitoring the patient's consciousness and respiratory status. In cases of severe CNS depression, endotracheal intubation may be necessary to secure the airway. Cardiovascular monitoring is critical due to the risk of tachycardia and potential arrhythmias. An ECG should be performed to monitor heart rhythm, with continuous ECG monitoring indicated for patients exhibiting signs of toxicity or abnormal initial ECG results. Intravenous fluids are administered to manage hypotension, and intravenous sodium bicarbonate is utilized to treat severe QRS widening associated with sodium channel blockade. For convulsions, BZD such as diazepam or lorazepam are employed. These agents are also beneficial in managing agitation and delirium in overdose patients. Physostigmine may also be used cautiously in these patients provided the cardiovascular concerns have been ruled out. Correction of metabolic abnormalities, including hypoxia, acidosis, and electrolyte imbalances, is essential to prevent complications like torsade de pointes or other ventricular arrhythmias.[3,17]

ORAL ANTIDIABETIC AGENTS

A plethora of oral antidiabetic drugs are available to treat diabetes. Each one of them has the potential to cause severe metabolic derangements if taken in overdose for self-harm purposes. Some of the long-acting oral antidiabetic drugs with renal elimination may cause symptoms of overdose in the presence of new-onset renal failure with conventional doses.

Overdose of oral hypoglycemic agents can result in a drop in blood sugar level that affects the normal function of the body's organs. Symptoms include:

- Agitation; sometimes patients may become violent
- Nervousness, anxiety
- Tremor, shaking
- Apathy (lack of desire to do anything)
- Coma (decreased level of consciousness and lack of responsiveness)
- Confusion
- Convulsions (seizures, especially in infants and children)
- Increased appetite
- Some patients may present with focal neurological deficits as well.

The diagnosis of the overdose is clinical and is substantiated by transient or complete improvement with oral or intravenous administration of exogenous glucose **(Table 1)**.

Metformin is a biguanide and its action/toxicity is different from other oral hypoglycemic agents. Metformin acts by increasing cellular insulin sensitivity and increasing glucose uptake by muscles. Its action is mainly antihyperglycemic rather than hypoglycemic. Therefore, overdose of metformin does not cause severe hypoglycemia. Overdose of this drug is generally associated with severe lactic acidosis. Development of lactic acidosis, a potentially lethal complication following metformin overdose, does not follow a well-defined dose–response

TABLE 1: Antidiabetic drugs and their toxicity.

Drug class	*Drug name*	*Toxicity*	*Management/antidote*
Sulfonylureas	Glibenclamide Glipizide, Glimepiride	Hypoglycemia, rash, jaundice, bone marrow suppression	Dextrose, octreotide
Biguanides	Metformin	Lactic acidosis	• Dialysis • Supportive care
Meglitinides	• Repaglinide • Nateglinide	Hypoglycemia, diarrhea	• Glucagon (1 mg) • Dextrose
GLP 1 agonists	• Liraglutide • Exenatide • Semaglutide • Dulaglutide	• Hypoglycemia • Nausea, vomiting, pancreatitis	• Dextrose • Glucagon
DPP-4 inhibitors	• Sitagliptin Saxagliptin • Linagliptin • Vildagliptin • Teneligliptin	• Hypoglycemia, anaphylaxis, angioedema • Stevens-Johnson syndrome	• Dextrose • Hemodialysis
Thiazolidinediones	Pioglitazone	Nausea, vomiting	Supportive therapy
Dual PPAR agonists	Saroglitazar	Nausea, vomiting, diarrhea	Supportive therapy
Alpha glucosidase inhibitors	• Acarbose • Miglitol • Voglibose	• Abdominal pain/distention • Diarrhea	• Supportive therapy • Intravenous glucose in case of combination therapy-induced hypoglycemia
SGLT-2 inhibitors	• Dapagliflozin • Empagliflozin • Canagliflozin	• Hypoglycemia, hypotension • Ketoacidosis	Supportive therapy

(DPP-4: dipeptidyl peptidase-4 inhibitor; GLP 1: glucagon-like peptide-1; PPAR: peroxisome proliferator-activated receptor; SGLT-2: sodium-glucose cotransporter 2)

relationship. It is difficult to predict the severity based on the dosage consumed and presentation may also differ based on the type of formulation consumed (regular vs. sustained release).[19] The toxicity also depends on the renal function and would depend on the amount of drug consumed as overdose or renal impairment.[20]

The management principles remain the same—stopping the exposure, reducing the absorption by elimination, and enhancing the elimination of drugs/metabolites/toxic metabolic by-products. Orogastric lavage may be considered but may be ineffective if there is a bezoar formation in the stomach.[21] Some of the oral antidiabetic drugs (metformin) have a tendency to form bezoars. In such situations, upper gastrointestinal endoscopy will help. Activated charcoal (single large dose or multidose) may be tried, especially for sustained-release preparations. Whole-bowel irrigation may be considered for sustained-release preparation, but it has to be done after ruling out intestinal obstruction/perforation. Urgent hemodialysis is indicated where severe worsening lactic acidosis develops following metformin overdose as it enhances the elimination of metformin and rapidly corrects the profound lactic acidosis.[19]

Dextrose is a specific antidote for sulfonylurea poisoning and, as discussed in the preceding text, is central to the resuscitation of the sulfonylurea-poisoned patient. However, attempts to maintain euglycemia by continued infusion of concentrated dextrose are problematic, as administration of glucose stimulates further insulin release and rebound hypoglycemia.[22] Octreotide, a synthetic octapeptide analog of somatostatin, is fairly readily available and used frequently to control acute gastrointestinal bleeding; it is an effective antidote for long-acting sulfonylurea overdose.[23] Used in the dose of 50 μg every 12 hours, it effectively suppresses insulin secretion from the pancreas by blocking calcium influx into beta cells and has a relatively benign adverse effect profile.[23]

CONCLUSION

Prescription drug overdose is a growing concern, especially in developing countries. Early recognition and prompt management are crucial. Activated charcoal, whole-bowel irrigation, and specific antidotes can limit toxicity. Supportive therapy remains the cornerstone of treatment, emphasizing the need for preventive strategies, regulatory control, and increased public awareness.

REFERENCES

1. Smollin C, Petrou S. Management of the poisoned patient. In: Vanderah TW, (Ed). Katzung's Basic and Clinical Pharmacology, 16th edition. New York: McGraw-Hill Education; 2024.
2. Grosser T, Ricciotti E, FitzGerald GA. Pharmacotherapy of inflammation, fever, pain, and gout. In: Brunton LL, Knollmann BC (Eds). Goodman & Gilman's: The Pharmacological Basis of Therapeutics, 14th edition. New York: McGraw-Hill Education; 2023.
3. Goldfrank's Clinical Manual of Toxicologic Emergencies, 2nd edition. New York: McGraw-Hill Education. [online]. Available from https://www.mhprofessional.com/goldfrank-s-clinical-manual-of-toxicologic-emergencies-second-edition-9781260474992-usa [Last accessed September, 2024].
4. Lauterburg BH, Corcoran GB, Mitchell JR. Mechanism of action of N-acetylcysteine in the protection against the hepatotoxicity of acetaminophen in rats in vivo. J Clin Invest. 1983;71(4):980-91.
5. Rumack BH, Matthew H. Acetaminophen poisoning and toxicity. Pediatrics. 1975;55(6):871-6.
6. Hodgman MJ, Garrard AR. A review of acetaminophen poisoning. Crit Care Clin. 2012;28(4):499-516.
7. Tilley DG, Houser SR, Koch WJ. Adrenergic agonists and antagonists. In: Brunton LL, Knollmann BC (Eds). Goodman & Gilman's: The Pharmacological Basis of Therapeutics, 14th edition. New York: McGraw-Hill Education; 2023.
8. Rotella JA, Greene SL, Koutsogiannis Z, Graudins A, Hung Leang Y, Kuan K, et al. Treatment for beta-blocker poisoning: A systematic review. Clin Toxicol. 2020;58(10):943-83.
9. Cole JB, Arens AM, Laes JR, Klein LR, Bangh SA, Olives TD. High dose insulin for beta-blocker and calcium channel-blocker poisoning. Am J Emerg Med. 2018;36(10):1817-24.
10. Graudins A, Lee HM, Druda D. Calcium channel antagonist and beta-blocker overdose: Antidotes and adjunct therapies. Br J Clin Pharmacol. 2016;81(3):453-61.
11. Murty S. Antiepileptic overdose. Indian J Crit Care Med. 2019;23(Suppl 4):S290-5.
12. Rogawski MA. Antiseizure medications. In: Vanderah TW (Ed). Katzung's Basic & Clinical Pharmacology, 16th edition. New York: McGraw-Hill Education; 2024.
13. Metcalf CS, Smith MD, Wilcox KS. Pharmacotherapy of the epilepsies. In: Brunton LL, Knollmann BC (Ed). Goodman & Gilman's: The Pharmacological Basis of Therapeutics, 14th edition. New York: McGraw-Hill Education; 2023.
14. Karaman K, Türkdoğan KA, Deniz AT, Çanakçı SE. Which is the best in carbamazepine overdose? Clin Case Rep. 2017;5(10):1612-5.
15. Mactier R, Laliberté M, Mardini J, Ghannoum M, Lavergne V, Gosselin S, et al. Extracorporeal treatment for barbiturate poisoning: Recommendations from the EXTRIP workgroup. Am J Kidney Dis. 2014;64(3):347-58.
16. Ghannoum M, Gosselin S. Enhanced poison elimination in critical care. Adv. Chronic Kidney Dis. 2013;20(1):94-101.
17. Thomas SHL. Antihistamine poisoning. Medicine. 2016;44(3):141-2.
18. Zuraw BL, Christiansen SC. Histamine, bradykinin, and their antagonists. In: Brunton LL, Knollmann BC (Ed). Goodman & Gilman's: The Pharmacological Basis of Therapeutics, 14th edition. New York: McGraw-Hill Education; 2023.
19. Gjedde S, Christiansen A, Pedersen SB, Rungby J. Survival following a metformin overdose of 63 g: A case report. Pharmacol Toxicol. 2003;93(2):98-9.
20. Teale KF, Devine A, Stewart H, Harper NJ. The management of metformin overdose. Anaesthesia. 1998;53(7):698-701.
21. Daly FFS, Little M, Murray L. A risk assessment based approach to the management of acute poisoning. Emerg Med J. 2006;23(5):396.
22. McLaughlin SA, Crandall CS, McKinney PE. Octreotide: An antidote for sulfonylurea-induced hypoglycemia. Ann Emerg Med. 2000;36(2):133-8.
23. Krentz AJ, Boyle PJ, Justice KM, Wright AD, Schade DS. Successful treatment of severe refractory sulfonylurea-induced hypoglycemia with octreotide. Diabetes Care. 1993;16(1):184-6.

2.8 Recreational Drug Poisoning

Manu Ayyan, Ezhilkugan Ganessane, Anas Mohammed Muthanikkatt

INTRODUCTION

Recreational drug use is the use of one or more psychoactive substances to induce altered levels of consciousness, either for pleasure or as an intoxicating effect. The recreational use of psychoactive substances has emerged as an important public health problem in the last decade. Acute drug toxicity that can occur immediately or for a short time after the uptake of one or more drugs is the leading cause of admission to the intensive care unit (ICU). Over the last years, exponential growth of new psychoactive substances (NPS) has occurred. High-risk drug use results in a considerable burden of mortality and morbidity. These drugs are often taken in combination with other drugs, contributing to the severity of toxicity. Classical drug presentations are more common. Toxicological laboratory tests to determine toxic agents are not very helpful in treatment. Management is based on clinical features. Treatment must be initiated before any blood tests are available. Supportive care remains the mainstay of treatment for substances with no specific antidote.

HISTORY

Humans have used psychoactive plants and substances for millennia, initially often for religious or spiritual purposes. Some of the earliest known drugs include alcohol, opium, cannabis, and psychedelics like peyote. In the 19th century, drugs morphine, heroin, and cocaine became available and were first utilized medically before their addictive potential was recognized, leading to rapid growth in recreational use.[1]

The early 20th century ushered in the first drug prohibition laws, such as the 1912 International Opium Convention. The United States passed the 1914 Harrison Narcotics Tax Act regulating opioids and cocaine. Despite prohibition efforts, recreational drug use escalated through the 1960s counterculture, which embraced psychedelics like lysergic acid diethylamide (LSD) and stimulants like amphetamines, sparking the "War on Drugs" policies.

The 1970s through 1990s saw an explosion in the popularity of drugs like heroin, crack cocaine, and club drugs like 3,4-methylenedioxymethamphetamine (MDMA), creating major public health crises which met with tough criminal penalties. Gamma hydroxybutyrate (GHB) acid and gamma butyrolactone (GBL) acid, used initially as anesthetics in the 1960s–70s and later as bodybuilding supplements in the 1980s–90s, also emerged as club scene drugs, sometimes implicated in drug-facilitated sexual assaults during this era.

Today, cannabis is becoming legally available recreationally and medically in many regions.[2] However, illegal opioids like heroin and fentanyl are driving overdose epidemic levels, prompting shifts toward harm-reduction policy approaches. The use of mind-altering substances has persisted throughout history, propelled by curiosity, cultural influences, and the challenge of addiction. The global surge in recreational drug use poses significant challenges for healthcare professionals, particularly in emergency settings where acute poisonings are frequent.

EPIDEMIOLOGY

Data on club drugs in India is limited, with minimal systematic efforts to gather comprehensive information. Various studies and surveys indicate that metropolitan cities serve as hubs for synthetic drug consumption in the country, often occurring around rave parties held in tourist destinations like Goa and Kullu, where both domestic and international attendees may consume club drugs.[3-5] Regarding the opioid burden, approximately 2.1% of India's population uses opioids, with significant variation across states; Uttar Pradesh has the highest number of users, while Mizoram and Nagaland exhibit the highest prevalence rates.[6] Unlike the United States, India's opioid epidemic is primarily driven by heroin addiction rather than prescription opioids, with opioids for people who inject drugs originating from informal markets rather than medical prescriptions. Statistical data on drug-related deaths in Mizoram from 1984 to 2023 indicates an increasing trend, with the highest number of 139 deaths reported in 2000 and heroin appearing as the most commonly involved substance based on the "h + y" (heroin or any type of drug) column displaying the highest figures across most years.[7]

The top 10 drugs/substances of misuse involved in telephonic inquiries and Toxbase online accesses are:

1. Cocaine
2. Cannabis
3. Synthetic cannabinoids
4. Diazepam
5. MDMA
6. Methadone
7. Heroin
8. Amphetamine
9. Ketamine
10. Nitrous oxide

WHAT ARE NOVEL RECREATIONAL DRUGS?

Novel recreational drugs are also known as new psychoactive substances. These are synthetic substances with minor structural modifications of existing drugs. Before the Psychoactive Substances Act of 2016, drugs were described as sufficient to take outside legal control and insufficient to change pharmacology/desired effects significantly.[8] Fifty-two drugs were reported in 2021. Currently, 880 drugs are being monitored under the European Union (EU) warning system.

CLASSIFICATION OF RECREATIONAL DRUGS

Recreational drugs are typically classified based on their chemical structure, effects on the body and mind, and potential for abuse and addiction. An overview of common classifications is as follows:

- *Depressants:* These drugs slow down brain activity and can induce sleep or cause a calming effect. Examples include alcohol, benzodiazepines (BZDs), barbiturates, and certain opioids.
- *Stimulants:* These drugs increase brain activity, alertness, and energy levels. Examples include cocaine, methamphetamine, amphetamines, and prescription medications used to treat attention-deficit hyperactivity disorder (ADHD).
- *Hallucinogens:* These drugs can cause hallucinations, distort perceptions of reality, and produce other psychoactive effects. Examples include LSD, psilocybin mushrooms, and mescaline.
- *Opioids:* These drugs derived from the opium poppy plant or synthetic alternatives can relieve pain and produce a sense of euphoria. Examples include heroin, morphine, oxycodone, and fentanyl.
- *Cannabinoids:* These drugs are derived from the cannabis plant and can produce relaxation, altered perception, and other psychoactive effects. Examples include marijuana [tetrahydrocannabinol (THC)] and synthetic cannabinoids like K2 or Spice.
- *Dissociative anesthetics:* These drugs can cause a feeling of detachment from reality and distort sensory perceptions. Examples include phencyclidine, ketamine, and dextromethorphan (DXM).

GENERAL APPROACH TO THE INTOXICATED PATIENT

For any patient who has suffered from a recreational drug overdose/poisoning, the most crucial first step is to resuscitate. Once their condition has been stabilized, a thorough risk evaluation should be conducted to determine if they require an antidote, decontamination procedures, or techniques to accelerate the elimination of the toxin from their body. However, for most recreational drug overdose/poisoning cases, simply providing supportive care and monitoring the patient in an appropriate medical setting for a period of time are sufficient.[9]

If a patient who has overdosed on recreational drugs goes into cardiac arrest, the standard advanced cardiac life support protocols should be followed but with the addition of interventions that may be beneficial specifically for cardiac arrest induced by toxic substances.[10] Prolonged resuscitation efforts are generally warranted, as recreational drug overdose/poisoning victims are often young individuals without preexisting comorbidities.

In all patients, the initial priorities are stabilizing the airway, breathing, and circulation. If the patient's airway is compromised or their respiratory drive is diminished, it is crucial to establish a mechanical airway and provide assisted ventilation. For hypotension, the first-line treatment is an intravenous bolus of crystalloid fluids (10–20 mL/kg). A specific antidote may be beneficial if hypotension persists despite adequate fluid resuscitation. Otherwise, cautious administration of an inotropic agent is indicated to improve cardiac contractility. The choice of inotrope should be guided by understanding the toxicodynamic properties of the specific drug involved and assessing whether the patient is experiencing cardiogenic or vasodilatory shock. In cases of cardiovascular failure that do not respond to other treatments, extracorporeal membrane oxygenation (ECMO) should be considered to provide cardiac and respiratory support.[11]

While proper use of antidotes is essential, only a few, like naloxone for opioids, are indicated before stabilizing cardiopulmonary function. Hypoglycemia should be treated with intravenous dextrose, and those at risk of Wernicke's encephalopathy will also need thiamine, though dextrose can be given first.[12] In cases of altered mental status, it is common to empirically administer a "cocktail" of supplemental oxygen, thiamine, glucose, and naloxone. This works in most of the patients and may be administered; however, a "coma cocktail" containing flumazenil is to be avoided. At the same time, efforts are made to obtain a diagnosis of the ingested drug (clinical + biochemical) to guide antidote use.

Toxin-induced cardiac arrhythmias generally respond better to correcting hypoxia and metabolic derangements and administering antidotes rather than using antiarrhythmic medications, which can be proarrhythmic. Wide QRS complex tachyarrhythmias from stimulant toxicity may improve with sodium bicarbonate, and overdrive pacing can help terminate ventricular tachyarrhythmias.[13]

For seizures caused by toxin exposure, BZDs are the first-line treatment. Hypoglycemia and hyponatremia must also be ruled out as metabolic causes. Second-line agents are propofol and barbiturates, but phenytoin has no role.[14,15]

Agitated patients should receive titrated doses of BZDs. While antipsychotics are sometimes used as second-line therapy, they carry risks of adverse anticholinergic and extrapyramidal effects.[16,17] Any temperature >41°C requires aggressive active cooling measures to prevent complications. Severe hyperthermia may necessitate sedation, paralysis, and intubation. Specific toxidromes causing hyperthermia are treated with additional pharmaceutical agents **(Table 1)**. Conversely, temperatures <32°C indicate a need for active rewarming of the patient.

ASSESSMENT

Following initial treatment and stabilization of a patient with suspected recreational drug toxicity, an assessment should be done to predict the likely clinical course, interventions needed, and whether the patient requires admission or can be discharged. This risk assessment is based on the patient's history, physical examination findings, and any relevant test results. However, acute drug toxicity is a dynamic process, so the risk assessment may change over time and require ongoing re-evaluation.

Obtaining an accurate history can be challenging, as patients may not provide clear information due to altered mental status from drug exposure, psychiatric issues, or fear of legal repercussions. Details like the specific substance(s) used, amounts, and route of exposure are critical. Collateral information should be sought from family, friends, medical records, and prehospital providers. Scene details like empty containers or chemical odors can provide clues.

The physical examination may reveal signs suggesting the class of drug involved, such as pupil size, vital signs, and other toxidrome findings. However, toxidrome recognition can be difficult, especially with polysubstance use.

Diagnostic testing is generally focused on identifying potentially life-threatening toxins and evaluating for end-organ injuries. Tests may include routine blood investigations, including creatine kinase, arterial blood gas (ABG), electrocardiogram (ECG), drug/toxin levels, and urine toxicology screens. However, urine drug screens often have limitations and may not significantly impact management.

Decontamination has a scarce part in recreational drug poisoning as most of them would have already been absorbed. Removing/washing off any remaining drug residue is important, especially for dermal exposures. Gastrointestinal decontamination with activated charcoal can bind the remaining drug in the gut if given soon after ingestion and is indicated in cocaine poisoning. Whole-bowel irrigation may be used for some types of body-packing to expel ingested drug containers.

The radiological investigation includes chest X-ray for aspiration pneumonitis and verifying endotracheal tube position. Noncontrast computerized tomography (NCCT) of the brain is indicated when any of the following exists:

- History or evidence of head injury
- Focal neurological deficit
- Recurrent seizures
- Prolonged reduced consciousness

Alternatively, one can follow the local protocol also for radiological investigations.

Overall, managing recreational drug toxicity requires a careful risk assessment weighing the potential severity against the risks of interventions like decontamination procedures. Close monitoring is required as the clinical picture can evolve rapidly.

TABLE 1: Toxicological differentials to consider in a patient with hyperthermia.

Condition	*Medication history*	*Symptom onset period*	*Vital signs*	*Pupils*	*Mucosa*	*Skin*	*Bowel sounds*	*Neuromuscular tone*	*Reflexes*	*Mental status*
Serotonin syndrome	Pro-serotonergic **(Box 2)**	<12 hours	Hypertension, tachycardia, tachypnea, hyperthermia (41.1°C)	Mydriasis sialorrhea	Sialorrhea	Diaphoresis	Hyperactive	Increased	Hyper-reflexia, clonus	Agitation, coma
Anticholinergic toxidrome	Anticholinergic	<12 hours	Hypertension, tachycardia, tachypnea, hyperthermia (typically 38.8°C or less)	Mydriasis	Dry	Erythema, dry, hot	Decreased or absent	Normal	Normal	Agitation, delirium
Neuroleptic syndrome	Dopamine antagonist	1–3 days	Hypertension, tachycardia, tachypnea, hyperthermia (41.1°C)	Normal	Sialorrhea	Pallor, diaphoresis	Normal or decreased	Lead pipe-like rigidity	Bradyreflexia	Stupor, mutism, coma
Malignant hyperthermia	Inhalational anesthesia	30 minutes to 24 hours	Hypertension, tachycardia, tachypnea, hyperthermia (46.0°C)	Normal	Normal	Decreased	Decreased	Rigor mortis-like rigidity	Hyporeflexia	Agitated

Approaches to individual classes are discussed in the following text.

STIMULANT OVERDOSE

Clinical Presentation

Stimulant drugs such as cocaine, amphetamines, methamphetamine, cathinone, and MDMA elicit sympathomimetic effects, resulting in agitation, hypertension, tachycardia, and hyperthermia.[18] These can also cause serotonin syndrome **(Table 1)**. Severe cases may progress to seizures, acute myocardial infarction, and cerebrovascular accidents.

Diagnosis

Diagnosis primarily relies on clinical presentation and patient history. Toxicological screening may assist in confirming exposure but is not typically required for initial management.

Management Strategies

Immediate management focuses on stabilizing the patient through airway management, cardiovascular support, and targeted treatment for hyperthermia and seizures. Activated charcoal is rarely indicated due to the route of administration (e.g., intranasal, inhalation, or injection). If a stimulant has been ingested, the greatest benefit of activated charcoal is within 1–2 hours of ingestion. BZDs are the cornerstone of treatment for agitation and seizure control. If there is no response with BZDs, the choice of antipsychotic in an agitated patient should be driven by the local protocol. Haloperidol may be considered. No specific antidotes exist for stimulant poisoning, making supportive care paramount.

Consider aggressive external cooling in patients with significant hyperthermia (>41°C). Rapid cooling measures should be implemented in such cases. Comparative rates of cooling are as follows:

- *Packing in ice*: 0.20°/min
- *Helicopter downdraft*: 0.11°/min
- *Spraying with water*: 0.05°/min
- *Endovascular cooling*: 0.004°/min

The following can be used for external cooling in resource-poor settings:

- Ice packs
- Water and fan

Monitor core body temperature and shivering. Antipyretics have no role as increased body temperature arises from muscular activity rather than an alteration in the hypothalamic temperature set point. Consider cold IV fluids in immediate resuscitation for hyperthermia. The endpoint of cooling is the core body temperature of <38.5°C.[19] Rule out other causes of fever (hyperthermia). In case of a shivering response and core body temperature which is not coming down, sedate and paralyze the patient.[20] Prefer nondepolarizing paralytic agents, as succinylcholine is relatively contraindicated because of the risk of rhabdomyolysis from severe methamphetamine intoxication, which may result in a sudden increase in serum potassium. Paralyzed patients at risk for seizures should receive continuous bedside electroencephalography.[21]

Treat regular wide complex tachycardia with bicarbonate administration.[22,23] If ineffective, administer lidocaine or amiodarone if all other electrolyte abnormalities have been corrected. In case of hypertension due to stimulant overdose, administer BZDs.[24] If blood pressure is not controlled with BZDs, nitrates are the preferred agent. Beta-blockers should not be used.[25] A neurological examination is performed in patients with severe headaches and any neurological deficit, and a CT scan should be obtained per local guidelines.

COCAINE OVERDOSE

Cocaine abuse produces dose-dependent toxicity, leading to multisystem involvement, predominantly affecting the cardiovascular system and central nervous system (CNS).

Clinical Presentation

Cardiovascular system: Cocaine increases heart rate and blood pressure, raising the myocardial oxygen demand. It causes coronary vasoconstriction and accelerates atherosclerosis, potentially leading to myocardial ischemia and acute coronary syndrome in about 5% of cases.[26,27] It can trigger tachyarrhythmias (supraventricular and ventricular) or conduction blocks due to ischemia or direct myocardial toxicity. Rarely, it has been associated with aortic dissection and rupture.[28]

Central nervous system effects: Cocaine is a stimulant that increases arousal, alertness, vigilance, and euphoria. Intoxication can cause headaches, psychomotor agitation, hallucinations, seizures, coma, intracranial bleeds, and focal neurological deficits.[29] Seizures occur in 3–4% of cases.[30] Intracerebral hemorrhages are more common than ischemic strokes.

Respiratory effects: Inhalation can cause pneumothorax, pneumomediastinum, bronchospasm, and exacerbation of existing airway diseases.[31,32] Heated fumes from smoking crack cocaine can lead to pharyngeal and laryngeal burns. Pulmonary infarction and "crack lung" (acute respiratory distress syndrome) are rare but serious complications.

Gastrointestinal effects: Cocaine increases gastric acid production, leading to peptic ulcers and gastrointestinal perforations. It can cause local ischemia, resulting in intestinal infarction and ischemic colitis.

Body packer syndrome: "Body packers" swallow large quantities of prepackaged drugs for smuggling purposes, while "body stuffers" swallow smaller quantities.

Ocular Effects

Cocaine causes pupillary dilatation due to sympathetic stimulation while preserving the pupillary light reflex. It can lead to vision loss and precipitate acute angle-closure glaucoma.[34]

Effects of Adulterants

Levamisole, a common adulterant, can cause agranulocytosis, leukoencephalopathy, cutaneous vasculitis, and necrosis.[35,36] Clenbuterol, another adulterant, has beta-agonistic activity and can cause tachycardia, palpitations, arrhythmias, hyperglycemia, and hypokalemia.[37] Fentanyl is increasingly found as an adulterant of cocaine and crack cocaine, leading to symptoms of opioid poisoning such as miosis, respiratory depression, and altered consciousness.

Pregnancy Effects

Cocaine readily crosses the placenta and is secreted in breast milk. It can lead to fetal malformations, developmental delays, mental retardation, and potential neonatal drug dependence.[38] It increases the risk of abruptio placenta and subsequent antepartum hemorrhage.

Diagnosis

Cocaine and its metabolite, benzoylecgonine, can be detected in various body fluids like urine, blood, saliva, and hair.[39] Rapid urine tests can detect cocaine metabolites for up to 10 days, but they only confirm cocaine abuse, not acute toxicity. Blood levels of cocaine and metabolites can be detected for 12–48 hours after intoxication but do not correlate well with symptom severity.

Routine urine/blood toxicological screening is not recommended. Any patient presenting to the emergency room (ER) with symptoms like tachycardia, hypertension, hyperthermia, and a history of sympathomimetic toxidrome should be evaluated for possible cocaine intoxication, regardless of toxicology results.

Management Strategies

Maintain airway patency and support breathing and circulation. Airway management is important in acute intoxication as these patients will have poor sensorium due to intoxication or a sedative agent administered by a physician for agitation. Consider intubation in those at risk of aspiration, hypoventilation, or oversedation.

Hyperthermia

Hyperthermia is common and has a high mortality rate of 30%.[33] It results from agitation and peripheral vasoconstriction, increasing heat production and inadequate heat loss. Severe cases may present with rhabdomyolysis, electrolyte imbalances, acidosis, and acute kidney injury. Cocaine intoxication can cause serotonin syndrome **(Table 1)**.

Cocaine-associated Chest Pain

At the time of acute presentation, in case of severe chest pain with cocaine overdose suggestive of acute coronary syndrome, administer BZDs if the patient is anxious, agitated, hypertensive, or tachycardic. Diazepam (5 mg IV every 3–5 minutes) or lorazepam (1 mg IV every 5–10 minutes) can be given until sedation is achieved. Administer oxygen if necessary to maintain SpO_2 ≥93%. In case of hypertension, administer BZDs. If blood pressure is not controlled with BZDs, nitrates are the preferred agent. Nitroglycerin 0.4 mg sublingual every 5 minutes as needed for a maximum of three doses. If additional nitroglycerin is needed, an infusion can be started. Beta-blockers should not be used to control blood pressure as they can lead to unopposed alpha-adrenergic stimulation, which can cause hypertension and coronary arterial vasoconstriction, further exacerbating myocardial ischemia and infarction.[40] Chest pain or hypertension that is refractory to BZDs and nitrates can be treated with phentolamine.[41] It is given as an IV bolus of 1–2.5 mg every 5–15 minutes. Aspirin can be given if there is no suspicion of aortic dissection, and consult cardiology. Treat regular wide complex tachycardia with bicarbonate administration. The optimal dose is unclear, but a 1-2 mEq/kg bolus is usually given, followed by intermittent boluses or as an infusion.[42] There is no fixed duration of therapy. If ineffective, administer lidocaine or amiodarone if all other electrolyte abnormalities have been corrected.

Neuropsychiatric Effects

Benzodiazepines are the drugs of choice for cocaine-induced psychomotor agitation. BZDs can lead to respiratory depression and hypotension, and patients need to be monitored closely. Midazolam (1-2 mg), diazepam (5-10 mg IV every 3-5 minutes), or lorazepam (1 mg every 3-5 minutes) can be administered. In patients with severe headaches and any neurological deficit, perform a neurological examination and obtain CT per local guidelines.

Hyperthermia Management

Aggressive external cooling measures should be initiated promptly for significant hyperthermia (core temperature exceeding 41°C). These include the application of ice packs and the use of water mist or fan. Continuous monitoring of core body temperature and observation for shivering response are crucial. Administration of cold intravenous fluids can aid in immediate resuscitation. The primary objective is to lower the core temperature below 38.5°C. The underlying causes of fever or hyperthermia must be evaluated and ruled out. In cases where shivering persists despite cooling efforts, sedation and paralytic agents may be considered under close medical supervision to facilitate the cooling process.

OPIOID OVERDOSE

Clinical Presentation

It is characterized by a triad of respiratory depression, pinpoint pupils, and reduced consciousness. Severe cases may involve apnea, circulatory collapse, and death. Pethidine, dextropropoxyphene, and tramadol overdose will not have miosis. Seizures can be seen in tramadol, pethidine, and dextropropoxyphene overdose.[43-45] Dysrhythmias can be seen in mixed drug overdose.[46-49] ECG should be done in all patients with opioid overdose to look for QTc prolongation and arrhythmias.

Diagnosis

Clinical assessment is key, with naloxone administration serving both a therapeutic and diagnostic role.

Management Strategies

Naloxone, administered via IV, IM, or intranasal routes, is the antidote for opioid poisoning. The effect of naloxone is short-lived than many opioids, so repeated doses or continuous infusion may be necessary. Management also includes support for respiratory and cardiovascular function and monitoring for withdrawal symptoms.

The duration of observation in opioid poisoning is dictated by the properties of the opioids involved and the patient's response to naloxone treatment. Observe patients with heroin poisoning post naloxone for 1-2 hours and discharge if the following criteria are met: (1) ambulation without assistance, (2) oxygen saturation >92%, (3) respiratory rate >10/minute, and (4) heart rate >50/minute. Extend observation to 4-6 hours for nonheroin opioids, 12-24 hours for methadone due to its longer half-life, and at least 24 hours for tramadol poisoning. Frequent monitoring of vitals and cardiac and metabolic parameters should be done. The frequency of monitoring depends on the severity of toxicity. If a patient needs a second dose of naloxone, he should be admitted to the ICU.

Naloxone

Naloxone is a medication that acts as an opioid antagonist, binding to and blocking the effects of opioids at all opioid receptor types, especially the mu receptor. By doing so, naloxone can rapidly reverse the respiratory depression, sedation, pupillary constriction, and analgesia caused by opioid overdose.

Naloxone has a relatively short half-life of 60-90 minutes, but its duration of action can be as brief as 20 minutes if a large amount of opioid is present that needs to be displaced from the receptors. It is not effectively absorbed orally but can be given intravenously, intramuscularly, subcutaneously, via inhalation, or intranasally.

The ideal naloxone dose depends on the clinical situation. For opioid-dependent patients with mild-to-moderate respiratory depression, a low starting dose of 0.04 mg IV is preferred to avoid precipitating acute withdrawal. For nonopioid-dependent patients or severe respiratory failure, higher initial doses like 0.4-2 mg IV are given, with repeated dosing every 2-3 minutes until reversal occurs.

Exposures to potent synthetic opioids like fentanyl, sustained-release opioid formulations, or overdoses from ingested drug packets may require naloxone doses up to 10 mg or more. Continuous naloxone infusions are sometimes required for longer-acting opioids.

While precipitating withdrawal can cause unpleasant symptoms like nausea and anxiety, naloxone has an overall very safe profile when used properly. Serious complications are rare. Careful, incremental dosing can minimize the withdrawal risk in opioid-dependent patients when possible.

CANNABIS OVERDOSE

Clinical Presentation

Symptoms range from euphoria, altered perception, and mild tachycardia to anxiety, psychosis, and, in severe cases, cardiovascular instability. Children are more susceptible to cannabis toxicity, and severe toxicity can happen due to accidental exposure in small children as a result of the increased availability of edible products.[50] Cannabis use disorder has a wide spectrum of clinical manifestations, predominantly neuropsychiatric features, and cardiac arrest, though rare, occurs mostly due to coronary ischemic events and/or dysrhythmias. Severe CNS depression from cannabis exposure is unique to the pediatric population and can present with profound depression, lethargy, and coma.[51-53]

Diagnosis

Diagnosis is based largely on clinical presentation and history. Toxicological tests have limited immediate clinical utility but may be used for confirmation.

Management Strategies

Management is primarily supportive, focusing on hydration, sedation for significant agitation, and monitoring for complications. There is no specific antidote for cannabis poisoning.

Anxiety and dysphoria in cannabis toxicity can be managed with reassurance and short-acting BZDs (e.g., oral lorazepam or diazepam). Agitation, psychosis, and seizures in natural cannabis toxicity can be managed as outlined below:[54]

- Placing the patient in a dimly lit space, reassuring them, and decreasing stimulation. In most cases, the intoxication would fade in a few hours.
- The patient may be given BZD orally if the patient is accepting the medication orally. Clonazepam 0.5 mg or lorazepam 1 mg can be given in such a situation.
- If the patient is agitated or violent, then appropriate measures should be taken for the management of agitation or violence. This may include the use of antipsychotics [like haloperidol 5 mg with promethazine (Phenergan) 25 mg, given intravenously or intramuscularly] or cautious and limited use of restraints.
- In cases of chest pain, the patient should be evaluated for cardiac or pulmonary etiological causes. These may focus on myocardial infarction, angina, arrhythmia, pneumothorax, pneumomediastinum, or exacerbation of asthma. ECG or X-rays coupled with referral to cardiologists/pulmonologists or medicine specialists would be useful.
- Once the patient recovers from cannabis intoxication, they should be debriefed and offered counseling, providing information about the harms associated with cannabis use. If a cannabis use disorder is identified (harmful use or dependence), then the patient should be suitably referred for further treatment of substance use disorder.

BENZODIAZEPINE OVERDOSE

Clinical Presentation

Symptoms include drowsiness, confusion, diminished reflexes, and, in severe cases, coma. Respiratory depression may occur, particularly with IV use or co-ingestion of other CNS depressants. Minimal/moderate overdose can present with initial feelings of relaxation, mild euphoria, motor in-coordination, ataxia (isolated ataxia in children), blurred vision, slurred speech, slowed reflexes, impaired perception of time and space, and reduced pain sensitivity.

Diagnosis

This is suspected based on clinical presentation and history of exposure. Toxicological screening can confirm exposure but is not essential for initial management.

Management Strategies

Besides the standard ABCDE (airway, breathing, circulation, disability, exposure) management approach, flumazenil can be used as an antidote. Flumazenil has the potential to reverse the effects of BZDs, but its use should be carefully considered due to the risk of inducing seizures. It is contraindicated in cases of mixed drug overdoses and in patients with a history of epilepsy or seizure disorders.[55,56] Supportive care, such as maintaining an open airway and monitoring vital signs, is essential in managing these situations.

Flumazenil

Flumazenil is a medication that acts as a selective antagonist to reverse the CNS effects of BZDs. Its potential uses include reversing coma from BZD overdose or oversedation during procedures using BZDs. In some cases, reversing the effect of BZDs may avoid the need for intubation and ventilatory support.

However, the utility of flumazenil in the emergency department setting is controversial. Some argue that it is mainly useful for reversing short-acting BZDs used procedurally, as the effects can often be safely waited out otherwise. A key issue is that flumazenil's duration of action is relatively short (elimination half-life ~1 hour), so recurrence of BZD toxicity can happen once it wears off, especially with longer-acting BZDs.

There are important precautions with flumazenil use. Contraindications of flumazenil are given in **Box 1**.[57]

Flumazenil administration can precipitate acute BZD withdrawal, including seizures, in patients chronically taking BZDs or those coingesting seizure-provoking agents like cyclic antidepressants. Seizures from withdrawal may require treatment with antiseizure medications like phenobarbital or propofol.

Flumazenil should also be avoided if the depressed mental status could be from a condition that increases intracranial pressure, as it can adversely affect cerebral hemodynamics. Additionally, nonspecific side effects like agitation and vomiting are more common when given empirically to unconscious overdose patients.

The typical dosing is initially 0.2 mg IV, which can be repeated every 1 minute up to a total of 3 mg and then titrated to clinical response. Very careful monitoring is required, as some patients may experience recurrent toxicity, seizures, or other complications from flumazenil use.

BOX 1: Contraindications to flumazenil.

- Overdose of unknown agents
- Suspected or known physical dependence on benzodiazepines
- Suspected cyclic antidepressant overdose
- Coingestion of seizure-inducing agents
- Known seizure disorder
- Suspected increased intracranial pressure

GAMMA HYDROXYBUTYRATE POISONING

Clinical Presentation

Suspect GHB poisoning when a patient presents with a reduced level of consciousness or coma with preserved airway reflexes. Patients show agitation in mild poisoning or when recovering from the poisoning. In addition to the above symptoms, myoclonus, hypothermia, bradycardia, and hypotension are also seen in GHB poisoning. Symptoms typically last for 2–5 hours, with complete recovery in 3–8 hours. Abrupt onset and offset of symptoms are typically seen in acute GHB intoxication.

Diagnosis

Clinical diagnosis is supported by history of exposure. Laboratory tests have limited immediate clinical relevance.

Management Strategies

Supportive care is the mainstay concerning airway management and cardiovascular support. No specific antidote exists for GHB poisoning.

LYSERGIC ACID DIETHYLAMIDE OVERDOSE

Clinical Presentation

Patients with LSD overdose are marked by profound perceptual disturbances, confusion, agitation, and visual hallucinations. Sympathomimetic symptoms such as tachycardia may also be present.

Diagnosis

Diagnosis is predominantly clinical, based on symptomatology and exposure history.

Management Strategies

Supportive care ensures safety and addresses specific symptoms. BZDs may be beneficial for significant agitation or anxiety.

DEXTROMETHORPHAN POISONING

Clinical Presentation

Dextromethorphan poisoning can present with a wide range of symptoms, including altered mental status, such as agitation, delirium, or psychosis. Patients may also experience nystagmus, ataxia, dilated pupils, tachycardia, and hypertension. Even at a regular daily dosage, DXM may cause a potentially fatal serotonin syndrome when combined with monoamine oxidase inhibitors or other serotonergic drugs (such as cocaine, meperidine, and serotonin-specific reuptake inhibitors).

Complications of Dextromethorphan Poisoning from Coingestants

Over-the-counter cough formulations often contain additional pharmaceutical agents like chlorpheniramine or other antihistamines, acetaminophen, and pseudoephedrine, which can complicate DXM poisoning.

- *Antihistamines (e.g., chlorpheniramine):*
  Anticholinergic poisoning symptoms: Tachycardia, hypertension, hyperthermia, flushing, warm and dry skin, sluggishly reactive pupils, delirium, agitation, seizures, and rhabdomyolysis
  Management: Treat agitation and delirium with BZDs (lorazepam). In severe cases, consider physostigmine.
- *Alpha-1 adrenergic agonist decongestants (e.g., phenylephrine, pseudoephedrine)*
  Symptoms: Tachycardia or reflex bradycardia, hypertension, headache, agitation, hypertensive emergencies
  Management: Severe hypertension may require IV antihypertensive medication like phentolamine.
- *Acetaminophen*
  Symptoms: Rare immediate symptoms but high potential for severe delayed hepatotoxicity, hepatic failure, and death
  Management: Measure acetaminophen concentration in all patients with significant DXM exposure. Treat those with toxic levels using N-acetylcysteine, following the Rumack–Matthew nomogram guidelines.

Diagnosis

Routine toxicology screens may not detect DXM levels. Urine screening tests can show false positives for morphine and PCP after DXM ingestion.[58] A thorough history and physical examination, along with findings of empty cough syrup bottles or DXM tablets, can raise suspicion of DXM poisoning.[59] An ABG may show a low anion gap with falsely elevated chloride levels due to bromide present in some formulations.[59]

Management

There is no specific antidote for DXM poisoning. However, naloxone (0.1 mg/kg, maximum 2 mg, which can be repeated up to a total of 10 mg) can be tried in cases where an opioid toxidrome is present, as DXM also acts on opioid receptors.[59] Supportive care is the mainstay of treatment for DXM poisoning. It involves maintaining the patient's airway, breathing, and circulation and monitoring temperature, heart rate, and blood pressure. Sedation with BZDs may be provided if needed. Temperature-control measures such as administering cold fluids, aeration, and cooled-inspired air can help manage hyperthermia. Rarely, complications of serotonin syndrome **(Table 1)** may arise, requiring sedation, prevention of hyperthermia, and administration of antiseizure medications. Even if symptoms resolve after receiving naloxone, patients still need to be admitted to the hospital and closely monitored for recurrence of symptoms.

KETAMINE OVERDOSE

Clinical Presentation

Ketamine poisoning is suspected when patients present with a behavior change and are in a dissociative state. Impaired consciousness is the most common presentation. They may also exhibit mood swings, irritability, and nystagmus. Severe overdose can cause respiratory depression or apnea. Laryngospasm and heavy salivation may occur with intravenous use. Laryngospasm is rare but more frequent in infants. Apart from these symptoms, they can also have mydriasis (dilated pupils), hypertension, and tachycardia. These effects are due to ketamine's inhibitory action on N-methyl-D-aspartate (NMDA) receptors and stimulatory action on serotonergic receptors.

Diagnosis

No routine testing is recommended for confirming ketamine poisoning. Laboratory tests are not routinely available, so the diagnosis is based on the history and clinical presentation. Urine dipstick tests may help to detect ketamine use.

Management

There is no specific antidote for ketamine poisoning. The management is primarily supportive care since the effects of ketamine usually last from 15 minutes to a few hours, and long admission is seldom needed.[60] Agitated patients may be given BZDs like intravenous lorazepam (2 mg) every 10 minutes, and in case of status epilepticus, barbiturates or phenytoin is advised. Laryngospasm and respiratory depression typically resolve with noninvasive support (bag-mask ventilation and supplemental oxygen). Endotracheal intubation is rarely required. Treat hypersalivation with glycopyrrolate or atropine. Patients with uncomplicated ketamine toxicity may be discharged after approximately 6 hours of observation, provided they remain asymptomatic.

SYNTHETIC CANNABINOIDS

Clinical Features

Synthetic cannabinoid receptor agonists (SCRAs) can cause a range of concerning clinical manifestations. Neuropsychiatric effects are common, including acute psychosis, agitation, anxiety, and paranoia. Cardiovascular complications like tachycardia and hypertension frequently occur. More recent SCRAs have been associated with life-threatening respiratory depression and coma. Other potential complications include seizures, convulsions, acute kidney injury, and cardiac toxicity.

Diagnosis

Diagnosing SCRA toxicity involves taking a thorough history and looking for the use of synthetic cannabinoid products sold under names like "Spice" or "K2." The clinical presentation, with neuropsychiatric, cardiovascular, respiratory, or renal manifestations, can point to SCRA exposure. Toxicology screening, if available, may detect the presence of specific SCRAs, although these tests have limitations.

BOX 2: Agents causing serotonin syndrome.[61,62]

- *Monoamine oxidase (MAO) inhibitors*: Tranylcypromine, isocarboxazid, rasagiline, selegiline
- *Selective serotonin reuptake inhibitors (SSRIs)*: Fluoxetine, paroxetine, fluvoxamine, sertraline, citalopram, escitalopram
- *Serotonin/norepinephrine reuptake inhibitors (SNRIs)*: Venlafaxine, desvenlafaxine, duloxetine
- *Cyclic antidepressants*: Amitriptyline, nortriptyline, imipramine, clomipramine, desipramine, doxepin
- *Atypical antidepressants*: Trazodone, vilazodone
- *Other drugs*: Cocaine, amphetamine, methamphetamine, MDMA (ecstasy), LSD, psilocybin (magic mushroom), mescaline

(LSD: lysergic acid diethylamide; MDMA: 3,4-methylenedioxy methamphetamine)

Management

The management of SCRA toxicity is largely supportive. Airway management and ventilatory support are critical if respiratory depression is present. Agitation, seizures, hypertension, and tachycardia should be treated according to established protocols. Monitoring and treating acute kidney injury and cardiac complications are important aspects of care. In recent ingestions, decontamination measures like gastric lavage may be considered. BZDs can be used for sedation and to control agitation and seizures. Involvement of toxicology and addiction services is recommended for comprehensive care. Early recognition and prompt supportive treatment are crucial, as SCRA toxicity can rapidly become life-threatening.

CONCLUSION

Recreational drug toxicity presents a significant challenge requiring early recognition of toxidromes and prompt supportive care for airway, breathing, and hemodynamics. Antidotes should be used judiciously when available. Close monitoring is crucial as presentations can rapidly evolve, with severe cases potentially needing advanced measures like extracorporeal support. A high index of suspicion is needed for novel psychoactive substances. A summary of recreational drug poisoning is provided in **Table 2**. Addressing this public health issue demands a multidisciplinary approach involving healthcare, law enforcement, community outreach, and expanded

TABLE 2: Summary of recreational drug poisoning.

Category	*Substances*	*Mechanism of action*	*Clinical presentation*	*Diagnosis*	*Management*
Stimulants	Amphetamines, methamphetamine, cocaine, MDMA, nicotine, caffeine	Increases neurotransmitter levels (dopamine, norepinephrine, serotonin)	Hyperactivity, tachycardia, hypertension, hyperthermia, paranoia, seizures	Urine toxicology, blood tests (electrolytes, renal/ liver function), ECG, imaging for cerebral complications	Supportive care, BZDs for agitation, cooling measures, antihypertensives, antiarrhythmics

Contd...

Contd…

Category	Substances	Mechanism of action	Clinical presentation	Diagnosis	Management
Depressants	Barbiturates, BZDs, GHB, antihistamines	Enhance GABA activity (CNS depressants)	CNS depression, respiratory depression, hypotension, hypothermia, coma	Blood toxicology, urine tests, ABGs, electrolyte levels, serum levels, ECG	Supportive care, specific antidotes (flumazenil for BZDs), activated charcoal, vasopressors, seizure management
Hallucinogens	LSD, mescaline, psilocybin (mushrooms), DXM	Act on serotonin receptors (5-HT2A), NMDA receptor antagonist (DXM)	Visual/auditory hallucinations, altered perception, anxiety, paranoia, psychosis, nausea	Urine toxicology, blood tests (electrolytes, renal function)	Supportive care, BZDs for agitation, antipsychotics for severe psychosis, cardiovascular support, cooling measures
Dissociative anesthetics	Ketamine, PCP	NMDA receptor antagonists, additional effects on other receptors (opioid, monoamine transporters)	Dissociation, hallucinations, euphoria, violent behavior, nystagmus, hypertension, rhabdomyolysis, seizures	Urine toxicology, blood tests (electrolytes, renal function, creatine kinase), serum levels, ECG	Supportive care, benzodiazepines for agitation, antipsychotics for psychosis, cooling measures, antihypertensives
Cannabinoids	Ganja, Hashish, Marijuana (pot, grass, weed, Mary Jane)	Act on cannabinoid receptors (CB1, CB2)	Euphoria, relaxation, altered perception, increased appetite, tachycardia, anxiety, paranoia	Urine toxicology, blood tests for THC levels	Supportive care, benzodiazepines for anxiety, antiemetics for hyperemesis, cardiovascular support
Opiates	Opium, heroin, morphine, fentanyl, codeine, oxycodone, tramadol	Act on opioid receptors (mu, delta, kappa)	Respiratory depression, pinpoint pupils, unconsciousness, hypotension, bradycardia	Urine toxicology, blood tests (opioid levels, ABGs, electrolytes), serum levels, ECG	Supportive care, naloxone for overdose, respiratory support, withdrawal management (methadone, buprenorphine)
Inhalants	Acetone, aerosol sprays, paint thinner, nitrous oxide, glue, amyl nitrite, gasoline, Iodex, pen ink, marker, room deodorizers	Depress the CNS	Euphoria, dizziness, headache, slurred speech, disorientation, hallucinations, cardiac arrhythmias, sudden sniffing death syndrome	Blood tests (electrolytes, renal/liver function), specific toxicology screens, clinical diagnosis based on history and presentation	Supportive care, respiratory support, cardiovascular support, BZDs for seizures, psychiatric evaluation
Others	Alcohol, anabolic steroids	Alcohol: Enhances GABA, inhibits glutamate; Anabolic steroids: Act on androgen receptors	Alcohol: Euphoria, sedation, respiratory depression; Steroids: Aggression, hypertension, liver damage	Blood alcohol concentration, liver/renal function tests, serum testosterone, hormone panel, ECG	Alcohol: Supportive care, thiamine, benzodiazepines for withdrawal; Steroids: Discontinuation, hormonal therapy, psychiatric support

(ABG: arterial blood gas; BZD: benzodiazepines; CNS: central nervous system; DXM: dextromethorphan; ECG: electrocardiogram; GABA: gamma-aminobutyric acid; GHB: gamma hydroxybutyrate; LSD: lysergic acid diethylamide; MDMA: 3,4-methylenedioxymethamphetamine; NMDA: N-methyl-D-aspartate; PCP: phencyclidine; THC: tetrahydrocannabinol) addiction services. Given the increasing burden, ongoing research in improved antidotes and management strategies is warranted.

REFERENCES

1. Crocq MA. Historical and cultural aspects of man's relationship with addictive drugs. Dialogues Clin Neurosci. 2007;9:355-61.
2. Pacula RL, Smart R. Medical marijuana and marijuana legalization. Annu Rev Clin Psychol. 2017;13:397-419.
3. Chakraborty K, Neogi R, Basu D. Club drugs: Review of the 'rave' with a note of concern for the Indian scenario. Indian J Med Res. 2011;133:594-604.
4. Saldanha A. Trance and visibility at dawn: Racial dynamics in Goa's rave scene. Soc Cult Geogr. 2005;6:707-21.
5. Saldanha AS. Vision and viscosity in Goa's psychedelic trance scene Arun Saldanha. ACME: Int J Crit Geogr. 2005;4:172-93.
6. Singh B, Rao R. Is there an opioid epidemic in India? J Public Health. 2021;43:ii43-50.
7. Drug related death. [online]. Available from https://excise.mizoram.gov.in/uploads/attachments/ed7e80ee307acaf936752204264983c9/drug-related-deathyear-wise-upto-11th-october-2019.pdf [Last accessed September, 2024].
8. Hill RG. Understanding the UK psychoactive substances act. Br J Clin Pharmacol. 2020;86:499-504.
9. Chandran J, Krishna B. Initial management of poisoned patient. Indian J Crit Care Med. 2019;23:S234-40.
10. Gunja N, Graudins A. Management of cardiac arrest following poisoning. Emerg Med Australas. 2011;23:16-22.
11. Wang GS, Levitan R, Wiegand TJ, Lowry J, Schult RF, Yin S, et al. Extracorporeal membrane oxygenation (ECMO) for severe toxicological exposures: Review of the toxicology investigators consortium (ToxIC). J Med Toxicol. 2016;12:95-9.
12. Schabelman E, Kuo D. Glucose before thiamine for Wernicke encephalopathy: A literature review. J Emerg Med. 2012;42:488-94.
13. Greene S. General management of poisoned patients. In: Tintinalli JE, Ma OJ, Yealy DM, Meckler GD, Stapczynski JS, Cline DM, et al. (Eds). Tintinalli's Emergency Medicine: A Comprehensive Study Guide, 9th edition. New York: McGraw-Hill Education; 2020. [online]. Available from https://accessmedicine.mhmedical.com/content.aspx?aid=1174959920 [Last accessed September, 2024].
14. Shah ASV, Eddleston M. Should phenytoin or barbiturates be used as second-line anticonvulsant therapy for toxicological seizures? Clin Toxicol (Phila). 2010;48:800-5.
15. Chen HY, Albertson TE, Olson KR. Treatment of drug-induced seizures. Br J Clin Pharmacol. 2016;81:412-9.
16. Greene SL, Dargan PI, Jones AL. Acute poisoning: Understanding 90% of cases in a nutshell. Postgrad Med J. 2005;81:204-16.
17. Calver L, Page CB, Downes MA, Chan B, Kinnear F, Wheatley L, et al. The safety and effectiveness of droperidol for sedation of acute behavioral disturbance in the Emergency Department. Ann Emerg Med. 2015;66:230-238.e1.
18. Yin S. Adolescents and drug abuse: 21st Century synthetic substances. Clin Pediatric Emerg Med. 2019;20:17-24.
19. Tek D, Olshaker JS. Heat illness. Emerg Med Clin North Am. 1992;10:299-310.
20. Callaway CW, Clark RF. Hyperthermia in psychostimulant overdose. Ann Emerg Med. 1994;24:68-76.
21. Lee WG, Huh SY, Lee JH, Yoo BG, Kim MK. Status epilepticus as an unusual manifestation of heat stroke. J Epilepsy Res. 2017;7:121-5.
22. Winecoff AP, Hariman RJ, Grawe JJ, Wang Y, Bauman JL. Reversal of the electrocardiographic effects of cocaine by lidocaine. Part 1. Comparison with sodium bicarbonate and quinidine. Pharmacotherapy. 1994;14:698-703.
23. Beckman KJ, Parker RB, Hariman RJ, Gallastegui JL, Javaid JI, Bauman JL. Hemodynamic and electrophysiological actions of cocaine. Effects of sodium bicarbonate as an antidote in dogs. Circulation. 1991;83:1799-807.
24. Richards JR, Garber D, Laurin EG, Albertson TE, Derlet RW, Amsterdam EA, et al. Treatment of cocaine cardiovascular toxicity: A systematic review. Clin Toxicol (Phila). 2016;54:345-64.
25. Ramoska E, Sacchetti AD. Propranolol-induced hypertension in treatment of cocaine intoxication. Ann Emerg Med. 1985;14:1112-3.
26. Afonso L, Mohammad T, Thatai D. Crack whips the heart: A review of the cardiovascular toxicity of cocaine. Am J Cardiol. 2007;100:1040-3.
27. Lange RA, Cigarroa RG, Yancy CW, Willard JE, Popma JJ, Sills MN, et al. Cocaine-induced coronary-artery vasoconstriction. N Engl J Med. 1989;321:1557-62.
28. Eagle KA, Isselbacher EM, DeSanctis RW; International Registry for Aortic Dissection (IRAD) Investigators. Cocaine-related aortic dissection in perspective. Circulation. 2002;105:1529-30.
29. Smith JA, Mo Q, Guo H, Kunko PM, Robinson SE. Cocaine increases extraneuronal levels of aspartate and glutamate in the nucleus accumbens. Brain Res. 1995;683:264-9.
30. Koppel BS, Samkoff L, Daras M. Relation of cocaine use to seizures and epilepsy. Epilepsia. 1996;37:875-8.
31. Kloss BT, Broton CE, Rodriguez E. Pneumomediastinum from nasal insufflation of cocaine. Int J Emerg Med. 2010;3:435-7.
32. Maeder M, Ullmer E. Pneumomediastinum and bilateral pneumothorax as a complication of cocaine smoking. Respiration. 2003;70:407.
33. Marzuk PM, Tardiff K, Leon AC, Hirsch CS, Portera L, Iqbal MI, et al. Ambient temperature and mortality from unintentional cocaine overdose. JAMA. 1998;279:1795-800.
34. Hoffman RS, Reimer BI. "Crack" cocaine-induced bilateral amblyopia. Am J Emerg Med. 1993;11:35-7.

35. Gross RL, Brucker J, Bahce-Altuntas A, Abadi MA, Lipoff J, Kotlyar D, et al. A novel cutaneous vasculitis syndrome induced by levamisole-contaminated cocaine. Clin Rheumatol. 2011;30:1385-92.
36. Chang A, Osterloh J, Thomas J. Levamisole: A dangerous new cocaine adulterant. Clin Pharmacol Ther. 2010;88:408-11.
37. Centers for Disease Control and Prevention (CDC). Atypical reactions associated with heroin use—five states, January-April 2005. MMWR Morb Mortal Wkly Rep. 2005;54:793-6.
38. Addis A, Moretti ME, Ahmed Syed F, Einarson TR, Koren G. Fetal effects of cocaine: An updated meta-analysis. Reprod Toxicol. 2001;15:341-69.
39. Verstraete AG. Detection times of drugs of abuse in blood, urine, and oral fluid. Ther Drug Monit. 2004;26:200-5.
40. Richards JR, Hollander JE, Ramoska EA, Fareed FN, Sand IC, Izquierdo Gómez MM, et al. β-blockers, cocaine, and the unopposed α-stimulation phenomenon. J Cardiovasc Pharmacol Ther. 2017;22:239-49.
41. Lange RA, Hillis LD. Cardiovascular complications of cocaine use. N Engl J Med. 2001;345:351-8.
42. Hoffman RS. Treatment of patients with cocaine-induced arrhythmias: Bringing the bench to the bedside. Br J Clin Pharmacol. 2010;69:448-57.
43. Schlick KH, Hemmen TM, Lyden PD. Seizures and meperidine: Overstated and underutilized. Ther Hypothermia Temp Manag. 2015;5:223.
44. Basu D, Banerjee A, Harish T, Mattoo SK. Disproportionately high rate of epileptic seizure in patients abusing dextropropoxyphene. Am J Addict. 2009;18:417-21.
45. Nakhaee S, Amirabadizadeh A, Brent J, Miri-Moghaddam E, Foadoddini M, Farrokhfall K, et al. Tramadol and the occurrence of seizures: A systematic review and meta-analysis. Crit Rev Toxicol. 2019;49:710-23.
46. Ehret GB, Voide C, Gex-Fabry M, Chabert J, Shah D, Broers B, et al. Drug-induced long QT syndrome in injection drug users receiving methadone: High frequency in hospitalized patients and risk factors. Arch Intern Med. 2006;166:1280-7.
47. Soroosh D, Neamatshahi M, Zarmehri B, Nakhaee S, Mehrpour O. Drug-induced prolonged corrected QT interval in patients with methadone and opium overdose. Subst Abuse Treat Prev Policy. 2019;14:8.
48. Sheibani M, Zamani N, Hassanian-Moghaddam H. Electrocardiographic findings in mortalities due to pure methadone toxicity. Cardiovasc Toxicol. 2019;19:62-71.
49. Berling I, Whyte IM, Isbister GK. Oxycodone overdose causes naloxone responsive coma and QT prolongation. QJM. 2013;106:35-41.
50. Vo KT, Horng H, Li K, Ho RY, Wu AHB, Lynch KL, et al. Cannabis intoxication case series: The dangers of edibles containing tetrahydrocannabinol. Ann Emerg Med. 2018;71:306-13.
51. Noble MJ, Hedberg K, Hendrickson RG. Acute cannabis toxicity. Clin Toxicol (Phila). 2019;57:735-42.
52. Onders B, Casavant MJ, Spiller HA, Chounthirath T, Smith GA. Marijuana exposure among children younger than six years in the United States. Clin Pediatr (Phila). 2016;55:428-36.
53. Thomas AA, Moser E, Dickerson-Young T, Mazor S. A Review of pediatric marijuana exposure in the setting of increasing legalization. Clin Pediatric Emerg Med. 2017;18:159-62.
54. Sarkar S, Bhatia G, Dhawan A. Clinical practice guidelines for assessment and management of patients with substance intoxication presenting to the Emergency Department. Indian J Psychiatry. 2023;65:196-211.
55. Spivey WH. Flumazenil and seizures: Analysis of 43 cases. Clin Ther. 1992;14:292-305.
56. Seger DL. Flumazenil--treatment or toxin. J Toxicol Clin Toxicol. 2004;42:209-16.
57. Quan D. Benzodiazepines. In: Tintinalli JE, Ma OJ, Yealy DM, Meckler GD, Stapczynski JS, Cline DM, et al. (Eds). Tintinalli's Emergency Medicine: A Comprehensive Study Guide, 9th edition. New York, NY: McGraw-Hill Education; 2020. [online]. Available from https://accessmedicine.mhmedical.com/content.aspx?aid=1166599923. [Last accessed September, 2024].
58. Omoto N, Kanzawa Y, Ishimaru N, Kinami S. Serotonin syndrome after an overdose of over-the-counter medicine containing dextromethorphan. J Gen Fam Med. 2021;23:38-40.
59. Chyka PA, Erdman AR, Manoguerra AS, Christianson G, Booze LL, Nelson LS, et al. Dextromethorphan poisoning: An evidence-based consensus guideline for out-of-hospital management. Clin Toxicol (Phila). 2007;45:662-77.
60. Cichon J, Wasilczuk AZ, Looger LL, Contreras D, Kelz MB, Proekt A. Ketamine triggers a switch in excitatory neuronal activity across neocortex. Nat Neurosci. 2023;26:39-52.
61. UpToDate. Serotonin syndrome agents–. [online]. Available from https://www.uptodate.com/contents/image/print?imageKey = EM/64604&topicKey = 301&search = serotonin [Last accessed September, 2024].
62. LoVecchio F, Mattison EG. Atypical and serotonergic antidepressants. In: Tintinalli JE, Ma OJ, Yealy DM, Meckler GD, Stapczynski JS, Cline DM, et al. (Eds). Tintinalli's Emergency Medicine: A Comprehensive Study Guide, 9th edition. New York, NY: McGraw-Hill Education; 2020. [online]. Available from https://accessmedicine.mhmedical.com/content.aspx?aid=1173991542 [Last accessed September, 2024].

2.9 Heavy Metal Poisoning

Nayer Jamshed, Karthikeyan A

INTRODUCTION

Acute and chronic heavy metals and metalloids toxicity can lead to significant morbidity and mortality. These metals mainly affect various enzymatic systems of the body leading to significant cardiovascular, neurological, gastrointestinal (GI), renal, hematological, endocrine, and genitourinary complications. High index of suspicion, detailed history that includes demography, food intake, and occupation, along with meticulous physical examination will help in early recognition and treatment. In 2021, the American Association of Poison Control Centers (AAPCC) reported 8,884 single exposures to heavy metals.[1] Data from other regions of the world is sparse; however, pollution, poor quality of ground water, and increased used of heavy metals in industries have increased the risk of heavy or toxic metal poisoning worldwide.

ARSENIC

Epidemiology

Arsenic toxicity is most associated with inorganic forms. Other forms of arsenic include the organic, gaseous (highly toxic arsine gas), and the elemental forms. The major source of acquiring toxicity includes contaminated water, soil, and food. In India, the highest prevalence of chronic toxicity is found in areas of West Bengal, where contaminated groundwater serves as sources of inorganic arsenic.[2]

Pharmacology/Pathophysiology

Inorganic arsenic exists in two forms, trivalent (arsenite) and pentavalent (arsenate). Arsenite forms primarily act by inhibition of the pyruvate dehydrogenase (PDH) complex which results in oxygen-free radical production and hypoglycemia (via reduced gluconeogenesis). Other effects result in dysrhythmias, anemia, arterial thrombosis (from increased platelet aggregation), and pigmentary changes (secondary to increased melanin production). Chronic exposure may cause noncirrhotic portal fibrosis and is even considered to be a carcinogen.

Pentavalent forms can get converted into trivalent forms and result in toxicity. These forms resemble phosphate molecule structurally and chemically and can cause competitive reactions, one such reaction causing uncoupling reactions which leads to decreased adenosine triphosphate (ATP) production. The detailed mechanism behind each of these processes is beyond the scope of discussion in this chapter.

Pharmacokinetics

The usual routes of absorption include GI tract, respiratory tracts, and mucosal or intravenous routes. Inorganic arsenic is tasteless and odorless. Organic forms are more absorbed from the GI tract compared to inorganic forms. Systemic absorption through lungs depends on the particle size, compound, and solubility.

Upon systemic absorption, arsenic is rapidly cleared from plasma and is distributed to skin, liver, kidney, and muscle, and over time, distributes evenly to all tissues. Hence, blood testing in arsenic poisoning holds value only in acute poisoning.

Compounds undergo methylation in liver and the metabolites are more toxic than parent compounds. Major excretion occurs through kidney. Arsenic also crosses the placenta and is secreted in breast milk.

Clinical Features

Manifestations depend on whether poisoning was acute or chronic. In acute toxicity, the typical early presentation includes GI symptoms of watery diarrhea, abdominal pain, nausea, and vomiting. Rice watery stools seen with cholera closely resemble these symptoms and should be considered as a strong differential diagnosis. Certain clinical points favoring arsenic poisoning over cholera include early onset of symptoms (as early as 10 minutes postexposure) and metallic taste or oropharyngeal irritation. Significant fluid deficits can cause tachycardia and hypotension. Myocardial dysfunction has also shown to contribute to this. Fever can also be present making sepsis as a differential diagnosis. QTc prolongation can occur over 4 days to weeks and lead to dysrhythmias.

Acute encephalopathy can also occur secondary to cerebral edema and microhemorrhages and can present with delirium, coma, or seizures. Other less common symptoms include acute lung injury (ALI), hepatitis, acute kidney injury (AKI), hemolytic anemia, nerve palsies, pancreatitis, pericarditis, and pleuritis.

Peripheral neuropathy (sensory > motor) can occur and takes 1–3 weeks to develop. A differential diagnosis of atypical Guillain–Barré syndrome (GBS) is considered in this context. (Lead poisoning causes painful, rapidly progressive ascending peripheral neuropathy with more motor involvement and mercury poisoning causes characteristic central intention tremor and mixed sensorimotor neuropathy.) Dermatologic lesions are also seen and include alopecia (also seen in thallium poisoning), Mees' lines (uncommon), nonspecific rashes, and desquamation. Nephropathy is also seen with subacute toxicity.

Most common central nervous system (CNS) findings of chronic toxicity include encephalopathy and peripheral neuropathy.

Chronic toxicity can lead to diabetes mellitus, hypertension, peripheral vascular disease, and skin lesions. Skin lesions include hyperpigmentation (hypopigmentation less commonly) and hyperkeratosis that can even lead on squamous cell carcinoma, basal cell carcinoma, and Bowen's disease. Certain lung, bladder, and liver malignancies are also attributed to chronic arsenic exposure.

Investigations

The 24-hour urine levels >50 μg/L or 100 μg/g creatinine or total 100 μg confirms diagnosis.[3] There is good correlation between spot *U* values and 24-hour urinary values.

Blood pictures show initial leukocytosis followed by leukopenia (associated with agranulocytosis) with relative eosinophilia. Thrombocytopenia and hemolytic anemia picture can also be seen. Basophilic stippling is also seen (nonspecific). Basic renal function test (RFT), liver function test (LFT), and urea test (URE) may demonstrate increased creatinine values, elevation of liver enzymes, bilirubin levels and proteinuria, hematuria, and pyuria.

Electrocardiogram (ECG) changes include QTc prolongation, QRS widening, and nonspecific ST-T changes. Abdominal X-ray may be done to look for any radio-opaque material.

Hair and nail testing may be done as an ancillary testing. Nerve conduction studies may demonstrate the specific neuropathic changes.

Management

General Management

The first and foremost is to prevent further contamination. Arsenic can be removed from skin with the use of soap and water. Maintain adequate fluid balance as chances of cerebral and pulmonary edema are present. Drugs that prolong QTc interval should be avoided. IV fluids with dextrose should be given to counteract the hypoglycemia episodes.

Arsenic poorly adsorbs to activate charcoal. If radio-opaque material is seen on abdominal X-ray, then whole bowel irrigation can be administered. Arsenic gets resecreted in the gastric and biliary tract; hence, continuous nasogastric drain helps.

Chelation Therapy

British anti-Lewisite (BAL) and succimer are the first-line agents for chelation. The usual dose with common adverse drug reactions is given in **Table 1**. Indications for chelation depend on the clinical condition of the patient as well as the laboratory results in urine, hair, or nails. Any severely ill patient if suspecting acute arsenic poisoning should be chelated immediately. BAL is the chelator of choice in acute arsenic poisoning, whereas succimer is preferred in

TABLE 1: Chelation for as arsenic poisoning.

Name	*Dose*	*Adverse effects*
British anti-Lewisite (aka dimercaprol)	3–5 mg/kg every 4–6 hourly	Febrile reactions, diaphoresis, headache, GI symptoms including excessive secretions, pain and sterile abscess formation at the injection site, hemolysis in G6PD-deficient patients
Succimer (2,3-dimercaptosuccinic acid)	10 mg/kg/dose every 8 hours for 5 days and then 10 mg/kg/dose every 12 hourly	GI symptoms, transiently deranged liver function tests, pruritus, sore throat, rhinorrhea, thrombocytosis, eosinophilia

(G6PD: glucose-6-phosphate dehydrogenase; GI: gastrointestinal)

subacute and chronic toxicity. Liver function tests should be monitored in patients requiring prolonged therapy.

Hemodialysis

Arsenic is poorly dialyzable; hence, it is not currently recommended in the management of acute or chronic poisoning.

Summary

Arsenic poisoning should be considered as a differential when rice watery stools are present and not responding to the initial management. An atypical GBS-like picture can also be another presentation. Chronic poisoning presents with encephalopathy. Apart from general management, chelators with BAL and succimer is associated with better outcome.

LEAD

Epidemiology

The usual population where lead poisoning is seen is young infants who are exposed to lead paints on toys and working population who are exposed to lead as part of occupational exposure. Manufacturing workers of western Maharashtra have been shown to have toxicity.[4] In a recent study,[5] higher blood lead levels were seen in Indian children with a habit of frequently consuming roadside food and proximity of residence to vehicular traffic.

Pharmacology/Pathophysiology

Lead has no physiological role in the body. It exists in the metallic form, and is available as inorganic and organic compounds. Lead forms complexes with many groups of which binding to sulfhydryl groups is associated with most toxicity. In CNS, Schwann cell destruction results in peripheral neuropathy. In acute lead toxicity, cerebral edema is seen. In blood, it inhibits certain enzymes of the heme biosynthesis pathway. Renal dysfunction is caused resulting in decreased erythropoietin production. Both these factors together can lead to anemia in the patient. Renal dysfunction can sometimes manifest in acute toxicity as Fanconi syndrome as well. Spasmodic contractions of the smooth walls of intestine can result in abdominal pain.

Chronic toxicity is associated with hypertension, gout (aka saturnine gout), progressive interstitial fibrosis, adverse effects on the reproductive system, hypothyroidism, hypopituitarism, and stunted growth in children.

Pharmacokinetics

Routes of absorption include respiratory, GI, and skin. In inorganic poisoning, the absorption rate from inhaled forms is 30–40% and that from the GI tract is much less (10–15%, which gets increased with diet that are deficient in iron, calcium, and zinc). Almost all of the lead is absorbed on to the red blood cells (RBCs). From blood is distributed to soft tissues and bones. Lead is excreted from urine (65%) and bile (35%).

Organic forms (tetra ethyl lead) get more distributed to lipophilic tissues in the brain. It gets metabolized to triethyl lead which accounts for its toxicity. It can also get metabolized into inorganic forms over time.

Clinical Features

Clinical features depend on whether the presentation was acute or chronic. Acute lead encephalopathy presents as altered mental status, coma, seizures, and signs of raised intracranial tension such as vomiting, headache, papilledema, and cranial nerve palsies. Recurrent abdominal pain, vomiting, and constipation can be seen 2–7 days prior to encephalopathic changes. A patient presenting with anemia, abdominal pain, and any neurological manifestations such as even irritability should be suspected of having lead toxicity. Any child presenting with iron deficiency anemia, encephalopathy, lead toxicity should be considered as a differential diagnosis. Other manifestations include hepatitis, pancreatitis, and hemolytic anemia.

Chronic toxicity presents with CNS manifestations. Earliest changes can include increased tiredness at the end of the day, irritability, etc.

Organic lead toxicity is associated with increased deep tendon reflexes (DTR) compared to inorganic forms where DTR are decreased. Also, hematologic manifestation is not seen here.

Investigations

Blood lead levels are a measure of recent and remote exposure and not diagnostic of toxicity. Hair and urine levels have little clinical use. Serum erythrocyte protoporphyrin levels reflect inhibition of the heme synthesis pathway and can be used to monitor treatment.

The X-ray of bones reveals dense metaphyseal bands which is a nonspecific finding. There are other methods as well, including atomic absorption spectrometry to identify the type of lead compounds.

Basic investigations include complete blood count (CBC) which can show basophilic stippling and anemia. Urine electrolytes, serum electrolytes, and RFTs can demonstrate renal tubular acidosis with loss of all electrolytes (Fanconi syndrome).

Management

General Management

For X-ray positive patients, whole-bowel irrigation can be considered. If large objects are seen, endoscopic removal may also be considered. Proton-pump inhibitors and prokinetic therapy have been recommended for gastric foreign bodies. Diet rich in iron and calcium may decrease iron absorption. Vitamin C may enhance renal lead excretion. Careful hydration with IV fluids is recommended. Calcium carbonate therapy has been recommended to reduce breast milk lead content (1,200 mg/day).

Chelation Therapy

British anti-Lewisite, CaNa2EDTA, and succimer have been used for chelation purposes. The doses, route, and common adverse drug reactions (ADR) are summarized in **Table 2**. It must be noted that there are no proven human studies showing that chelation is effective in clinical outcome.

TABLE 2: Chelation therapy for lead poisoning.

Clinical symptoms/BLL	*Drugs and dose*
Encephalopathy	• Dimercaprol 75 mg/m^2 IM every 4 h × 5 days • Edetate calcium disodium 1,500 mg/m^2 day in 2–4 divided doses × 5 days (should be started 4 hours after dimercaprol)
Symptomatic: • Adults BLL >100 µg/dL • Children BLL >70 µg/dL	• The above regimen OR • Edetate calcium disodium alone OR • Succimer 350 mg/m^2 PO Q8h × 5 days followed by • Succimer 350 mg/m^2 PO Q12h × 5 days
Asymptomatic: • Adults BLL = 70–100 µg/dL • Children BLL = 45–69 µg/dL	Succimer

(BLL: blood lead level)

Summary

Encephalopathy or iron deficiency anemia in children should be investigated for lead poisoning. Any patient presenting with abdominal pain, anemia, and mild neurological dysfunction should also be given a differential diagnosis of lead poisoning. Apart from general measures, chelation is advised. Iron, calcium, and vitamin supplementation may help, so does calcium carbonate therapy in feeding mothers.

CADMIUM

Epidemiology

Cadmium toxicity is usually associated with contamination of food grown in cadmium-contaminated areas (mining areas). Smokers are noted to have higher cadmium levels, due to soil contamination. Occupational exposure by inhalation of fumes has also been seen to cause poisoning, In India, groundwater contamination with cadmium is seen in western parts of Uttar Pradesh.[6]

Pharmacology/Pathophysiology

Cadmium is not an essential metal; that is, it has no biological value in humans. Cadmium concentrates in proximal tubules of kidney and causes nephrotoxicity (proteinuria and hypercalciuria), which in turn can lead to bone lesions. Cadmium ions bind to sulfhydryl groups and make the cell vulnerable to oxidative stress. GI hemorrhage, necrosis, and perforation occur secondary to irritant effect. Inhalation injury can cause bilateral infiltrates on chest X-rays.

Pharmacokinetics

Absorption occurs by routes of GI and inhalation routes with bioavailability of 5–40% and 7–40%, respectively.[7] After absorption, cadmium gets bound to albumin and gets preferentially redistributed to liver and kidney.

Liver and kidney produce a protein called metallothionein which complexes with cadmium (Cd-MT), which acts as a natural chelator and is then secreted into blood.

Clinical Features

Clinical features depend on whether exposure is acute or chronic and mode of absorption. Acute inhalational injury presents within 6–12 hours with mild complaints of fever, chills, and cough. Initial physical examination findings may also be within normal limits. However, over time, ALI sets in, and patient symptoms worsen, and death usually occurs within 3–5 days. One important consideration here is the differential diagnosis of metal fume fever when the patient presents early, which is usually a self-limiting condition. Oral poisoning with cadmium salts is exceedingly rare and results in hemorrhagic GI injury.

Chronic poisoning presents with irreversible nephrotoxicity (proteinuria). Lung carcinogenesis has been implicated. Other uncommon presentations include neurotoxicity (olfactory disturbances, Parkinson syndrome), hepatotoxicity, and musculoskeletal toxicity.

Investigations

Urinary cadmium levels are a better reflection of the total body burden than serum levels in chronic toxicity. Urinary cadmium concentrations ≥0.5 μg/g Cr is associated with renal damage and levels >2 μg/g Cr may cause extensive damage.[8]

Routine investigation includes CBC, renal and liver function tests, and urine analysis.

Management

General Management

Lowest oral cadmium salt lethal dose is 5 g. Gastric lavage may be done if the patient presents acutely and has no emesis. Other routine supportive measures may be implemented as required.

Chelation Therapy

Succimer as a chelating agent has been shown to be beneficial only in animal studies. There is no role for chelation in inhalational injury. No studies have demonstrated efficacy with steroids for the same.

Summary

Cadmium toxicity usually occurs from inhalational injury and presents with respiratory symptoms which gradually progresses over 3–5 days and results in death despite best aggressive supportive management. Chronic toxicity most commonly presents with irreversibly proteinuria.

■ CHROMIUM

Epidemiology

Chromium is found in ores combined with other metals. It usually exists in the trivalent or hexavalent forms, with the hexavalent forms being more toxic. Most exposures occur as a part of occupational reasons among people who are working in chromate production, chromium pigment manufacturing, and chrome plating and welding. General populations are usually exposed to chromium from contaminated drinking water and food and from cigarettes. Dermal exposure is rare and can occur from tanned leather products. The Sukinda Valley of Jajpur district, Odisha, is where majority of chromite reserves is found in India and around 1.8 lakh people are getting affected by chromium poisoning.[9]

Pharmacology/Pathophysiology

Chromium is an essential element which is involved in glucose metabolism, and its efficiency can lead to diabetes mellitus and atherosclerosis over time. It is also present in implants and has been implicated to cause immunosuppression causing implant-related infections. Toxicity depends on the valency and solubility of the compounds. The reduction of hexavalent chromium to trivalent forms results in toxicity. Detailed discussions regarding the exact mechanisms are beyond the scope of this chapter.

Pharmacokinetics

The usual routes of absorption include inhalational (usually chronic), GI (usually acute), and rarely dermal exposure. Oral absorption is less for both the forms, with Cr^{6+} showing better absorption rates (secondary to structural similarity to phosphate and sulfate molecules). Greatest harm comes from inhalation. The hexavalent forms get immediately reduced in the GI tract and RBCs and get distributed principally to kidney and liver. Chromium is maximally eliminated by the renal system (80%).[10]

Clinical Features

Clinical presentation can vary depending on whether exposure was acute or chronic. Acute exposure results in GI hemorrhage and causes multiorgan dysfunction syndrome with AKI, disseminated intravascular coagulation (DIC), metabolic acidosis with elevated lactates, and ALI. Hexavalent forms can act as a corrosive on the skin and can lead to inflammation and ulcerations which in turn can lead to more systemic absorption.

Chronic exposures cause continuous inflammation which can lead to a spectrum of symptoms ranging from mild cough to occupational lung disorders (pneumoconiosis) to lung cancers. Nasal septum perforation is also a finding that can be seen with chronic exposures. Contact dermatitis (type 4 hypersensitivity reaction) can occur after acute exposure. Blackjack disease and chrome holes are some other skin manifestations of chronic toxicity.

Investigations

Serum chromium levels are indicative of exposure rather than toxicity or severity. No clear correlation has been found between serum/blood levels and clinical symptoms. No clearcut values for chromium toxicity have been defined. 24-hour urine samples are reflective of the acute absorption. Estimation of chromium from hair and nails is not reliable and does not add to diagnostic value.

Ancillary tests include CBC, renal and liver function tests, urine analysis, and DIC profile with serial monitoring.

Management

Orogastric lavage can be considered in hexavalent chromium poisoning if the patient presents early and does not have vomiting. Activated charcoal is a reasonable option if coingestion is strongly suspected.

Chelation therapy has not shown to have any benefits. N-acetyl cysteine (NAC) administration has shown some benefits in animal models. Similarly, no studies have shown any benefit with extracorporeal methods, although it may be reasonable to consider hemodialysis in patients with AKI or chronic kidney disease.

Summary

Acute chromium toxicity presents with GI hemorrhage and multiple organ dysfunction syndrome (MODS). whereas chronic toxicity primarily presents with pulmonary symptoms ranging from mild cough to cancer. Treatment is supportive with no clear benefits with chelation therapy or hemodialysis. NAC has shown to have some benefits.

MERCURY

Epidemiology

Mercury occurs in the elemental form (quicksilver), inorganic salts (divalent mercuric and univalent mercurous forms), and organic compounds (methyl mercury). Mercury-contaminated seafood and mercury-based preservatives (thiomersal) can cause toxic exposures in the general population. It can also occur as an occupational hazard. Certain ayurvedic medications are associated with inorganic mercuric poisoning. The Sonbhadra district of Uttar Pradesh contains many coal mines and thermal power plants and serves as an area of mercury poisoning in India.[11]

Pharmacology/Pathophysiology

Mercury has no role in human physiology. It covalently binds to sulfur groups (also reacts with other groups) and causes widespread cellular dysfunction of a variety of proteins. It causes direct oxidative damage which is responsible for GI necrosis and proximal renal tubular dysfunction. Immune mechanisms cause membranous glomerulonephritis and acrodynia. Brain atrophy is more commonly seen in children and neonates and is most prominent in the cerebrum and cerebellum resulting in ataxia, sensory neuropathy, and visual field constriction.

Pharmacokinetics

Elemental mercury causes toxicity by the inhalation route and is nontoxic by ingestion. It is distributed primarily to kidney, liver, spleen, and CNS. Elemental mercury gets converted to cations over time and causes retention in local tissues and symptoms resembling inorganic toxicity. Majority of the elimination takes place through urine and feces with a half-life of 30–60 days.[12] Intentional subcutaneous or IV injection of elemental mercury is also seen **(Fig. 1)**.

Inorganic salt toxicity appears from absorption by the GI tract with divalent forms being more readily absorbed. Absorption can also take place from skin. Inorganic mercury concentrates in the renal tubules resulting in nephrotoxicity. It has poor blood–brain barrier (BBB) penetration, but prolonged exposure can lead to toxicity as well. It can get converted to organic forms. Inorganic

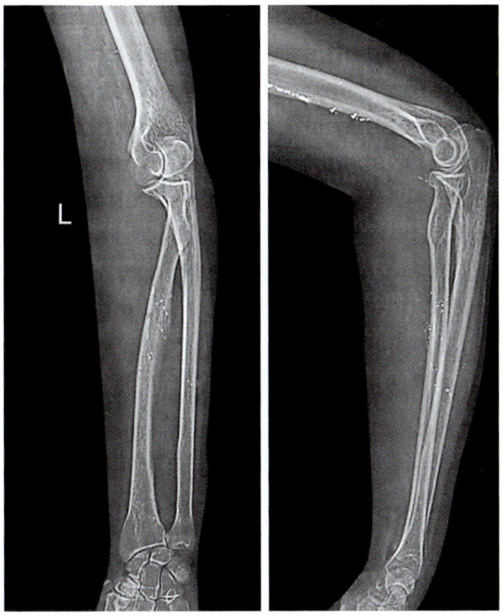

Fig. 1: Radio-opaque elemental mercury seen traversing through the vein after intentional IV injection.

forms do not cross placenta. Routes of elimination are like those of elemental mercury.

Organic forms get absorbed through the GI tract. Organic compounds in general cause fewer caustic effects on the GI tract since these compounds are readily absorbed. Organic forms are of two types: (1) Long-chain and (2) short-chain compounds. Long-chain compounds break and form inorganic mercuric forms and resemble inorganic toxicity. Short-chain compounds readily cross BBB and placenta. The greatest concentration of organic mercury is found in kidneys and liver. Elimination from body is by the fecal route with a higher half-life of 80 days owing to enterohepatic circulation.[13]

Clinical Features

Elemental mercury toxicity presents within a few hours with complaints of fever with chills and respiratory complaints of cough with shortness of breath. Nausea, vomiting, diarrhea, metallic tastes, hypersalivation, visual disturbances, headache, and weakness are some other presenting complaints. The symptoms may resolve or progress to death. Survivors can develop fibrosis and restrictive type of lung diseases.

Hallmarks of severe acute mercuric salt ingestion are hemorrhagic gastroenteritis, massive fluid loss resulting in shock, and acute tubular necrosis. Grayish discoloration of mucous membranes and metallic taste are common manifestations. Early development of oliguria is associated with poorer outcomes. Neurasthenia, erethism, and central intention tremor are neurological findings seen associated with chronic toxicity. Mixed sensorimotor neuropathy is even. Pink disease is characterized by erythematous popular rashes seen over palms, soles, and face. It is also associated with decreased DTR and tremors.

Organic mercury poisoning usually is caused by seafood contamination and results in purely neurological symptoms and is usually permanent. Infants are more prone. Clinical manifestations occur after weeks to months following exposure. Acute GI symptoms and dermatitis may occur. Tremors and paresthesia involving lips, nose, and distal extremities are seen.

Investigations

Urine 24-hour levels and blood levels for mercury are usually used for diagnosis.

Blood and urine concentrations <10 and 20 µg/L, respectively, are generally considered to be normal.[14] In inorganic toxicity, urine concentration of mercury roughly correlates with exposure and neurological symptoms. Urinary levels also have a role in monitoring the efficacy of chelation. Whole blood levels may reflect acute inorganic exposure but become less reliable in a chronic setting. Whole blood concentration, however, reflects total body methyl mercury burden. Cold atomic absorption spectrometry is a rapid and sensitive test used to confirm diagnosis. Hair analysis is not reliable.

Ancillary tests include CBC, renal and liver function tests, urine analysis, chest, and abdominal X-rays to look for radio-opaque material **(Figs. 1 to 3)**. ECGs show nonspecific ST-T changes.

Management

General Management

In elemental mercury poisoning, cardiopulmonary resuscitation is the priority. In organic salt poisoning, fluid resuscitation is the priority. Activated charcoal adsorbs inorganic salts and can be considered if the patient presents early. Whole bowel irrigation with polyethylene glycol can be attempted if radio opaque material is seen on x-rays and these can be used to monitoring elimination as well. Role of GI decontamination is limited. In organic poisoning since most patients present late.

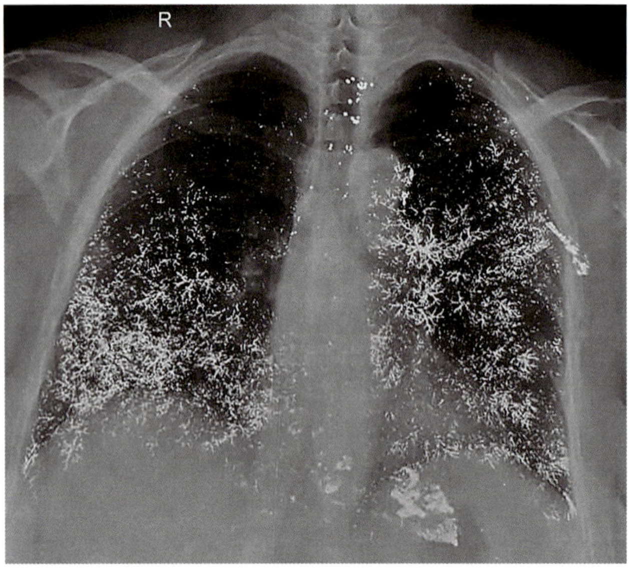

Fig. 2: Radio-opaque elemental mercury seen on chest X-ray of a patient after intentional IV injection through the peripheral vein.

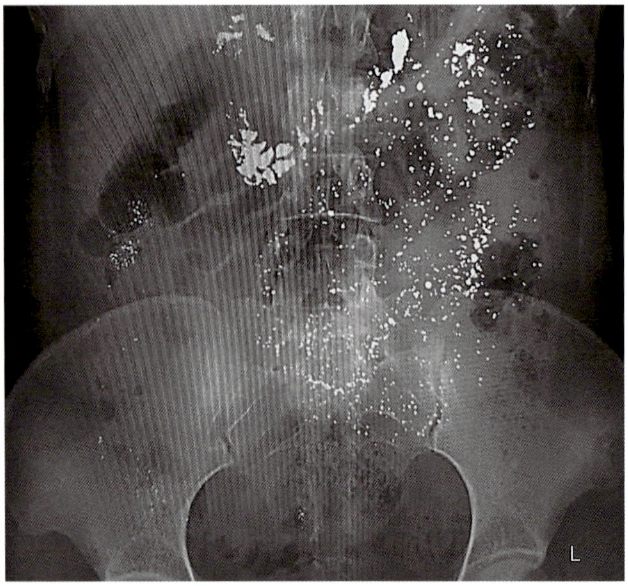

Fig. 3: X-ray abdomen showing radio-opaque substance (mercury).

Chelation Therapy

Chelation has been found to minimize or prevent effects of poisoning. It tends to increase urinary elimination. Usual dose, route of administration, and common adverse effect are given in **Table 3**. Organic mercury toxicity is in general resistant to treatment. Use of succimer may be beneficial with the current limited evidence.

TABLE 3: Chelation therapy for mercury poisoning.

Elemental and inorganic forms	
Severe acute poisoning	• Dimercaprol 75 mg/m^2 IM Q4h × 2 days f/b • 2.5 mg/kg IM Q6h × 2 days f/b • 2.5 mg/kg IM Q12–24h till clinical improvement occurs or able to switch to oral succimer therapy, total 10 days
Mild acute poisoning or chronic poisoning	Succimer 10 mg/kg PO Q8h × 5 days; then Q12h × 14 days
Organic forms	
Severe acute poisoning	Succimer (above dose)

(f/b: followed by)

Summary

Elemental mercury toxicity causes pulmonary toxicity, inorganic toxicity causes GI symptoms followed by nephrotoxicity while organic compounds principally produce neurological toxicity. Unexplained neuropsychiatric and renal abnormalities should be considered in the differential for mercury poisoning. Apart from general supportive measure, chelation has a role to play in the management of elemental and inorganic mercury toxicity. Hemodialysis can be reasonable under the setting of AKI.

THALLIUM

Epidemiology

Thallium salts (univalent thallous salts and trivalent thallic salts) are very toxic. They are found in rodenticides. Certain herbal products and illicit drugs may contain thallium as contaminants. The prevalence of thallium poisoning to a particular area in India is unclear.

Pharmacology/Pathophysiology

Thallium is odorless and tasteless. It behaves biologically like potassium and replaces potassium in the activation of potassium-dependent enzymes and causes variable effects on these enzymes which results in failure of energy production. Thallium ions form insoluble complexes which cause impairment of energy production. Thallium has affinity for sulfhydryl groups and interferes with the formation of disulfide bonds and causes decreased keratin strength. All these mechanisms result in reduction of hair follicle formation, causing clinical alopecia.

Thallium toxicity also shows symptoms similar to thiamine deficiency. Localized areas of edema can occur in CNS and diffuse axonopathy resulting in peripheral neuropathy (sensory followed by motor symptoms). (Motor neuropathy is seen with lead poisoning while sensory neuropathy is predominantly seen with arsenic.)

Pharmacokinetics

Exposure occurs from inhalation, ingestion, and through skin absorption. Once absorbed, thallium gets initially absorbed and gets distributed to kidney, liver, and muscle and then later gets distributed to CNS. The volume of distribution (Vd) is 3.6 L/kg.[15] Elimination primarily occurs through feces and urine.

Clinical Features

The characteristic findings of thallium toxicity include delayed alopecia (also seen with arsenic) and painful ascending peripheral neuropathy.

Unlike other metal poisoning, thallium poisoning commonly causes mild GI symptoms. Almost all systems are affected. Tachycardias and hypertension frequently occur with persistent and pronounced tachycardia pointing toward poorer prognosis. CNS symptoms include confusion, seizures, headache, tremors, etc. The most affected cranial nerve is the occult motor nerve with one out of four patients having permanent optic atrophy changes. Renal symptoms include oliguric AKI which usually resolves by 10 days. Mees' lines (uncommon with arsenic poisoning) are also seen.

Investigations

Definitive clinical diagnosis is made by showing elevated thallium concentrations in body fluids/organs. The 24-hour urine sample with atomic absorption spectroscopy is the confirmatory test. Under normal conditions, thallium in urine exceeds 1 mg/g Cr.[16]

Thallium is radio-opaque; hence, X-rays of abdomen may detect thallium.

Ancillary tests include hair inspection, ideally to be done by an expert. Other tests include basic investigations like CBC, renal and liver function tests, and urine analysis. ECGs may show QTc prolongation and nonspecific ST-T segment changes.

Management

General Management

Gastric decontamination can be attempted in the patient who presents early (1–2 hours).

Specific Therapy

Prussian blue is an ion exchanger which is approved by the Food and Drug Administration (FDA) for the treatment of thallium toxicity. Mechanism of action includes interference with the enterohepatic circulation. Dose is 250 mg/kg/day in two to four divided doses. Mannitol can be used as an adjunct if constipation is also present.

Currently, no compound has been shown to have good chelating effects without significant adverse effects.

Extracorporeal Treatment

Thallium is a dialyzable drug and the indications for dialysis as per EXTRIP guidelines[17] include:

- If thallium exposure is highly suspected based on history or clinical features
- Serum thallium >1 mg/L or 4.9 μmol/L if serum values are readily available

Extracorporeal treatment should be initiated as soon as possible, ideally within 24–48 hours of exposure and it is suggested that ECTR be continued until serum thallium concentration is 0.1 mg/L or 0.5 μmol/L for a minimal duration of 72 hours.

CONCLUSION

Thallium is odorless and tasteless which make it an ideal homicidal agent. Characteristic features of thallium toxicity include alopecia and painful ascending peripheral neuropathy. Apart from general measure, specific therapy includes administration of Prussian blue. Chelation has no proven beneficial role. Hemodialysis may be attempted for selected indications.

REFERENCES

1. Gummin DD, Mowry JB, Beuhler MC, Spyker DA, Rivers LJ, Feldman R, et al. 2021 annual report of the National Poison Data System(©) (NPDS) from America's Poison Centers: 39th annual report. Clin Toxicol (Phila). 2022;60(12):1381-643.
2. Roychowdhury T. Groundwater arsenic contamination in one of the 107 arsenic-affected blocks in West Bengal, India: Status, distribution, health effects and factors

responsible for arsenic poisoning. Int J Hyg Environ Health. 2010;213(6):414-27.
3. Kuivenhoven M, Mason K. Arsenic toxicity. Treasure Island (FL): StatPearls Publishing; 2023.
4. Kshirsagar MS, Patil J, Patil A, Ghanwat G, Sontakke A, Ayachit RK. Biochemical effects of lead exposure and toxicity on battery manufacturing workers of Western Maharashtra (India): With respect to liver and kidney function tests. National Libr Med. 2015;8(12):107-14.
5. Malavika L, Goyal T, Mitra P, Saikiran G, Sharma S, Sharma P. Risk factors for lead toxicity and its effect on neurobehavior in Indian children. Indian J Clin Biochem. 2022;37(3):294-302.
6. Idrees N, Tabassum B, Allah EFA, Hashem A, Sarah R, Hashim M. Groundwater contamination with cadmium concentrations in some West U.P. Regions, India. Saudi J Biol Sci. 2018;25(7):1365-8.
7. Nordberg M, Nordberg GF. Metallothionein and cadmium toxicology—Historical review and commentary. Biomolecules. 2022;12(3):360.
8. Crinnion WJ. The benefits of pre and postchallenge urine heavy metal testing: Part 1. Altern Med Rev. 2009;14(1):3-8.
9. Mishra H, Sahu HB. Environmental scenario of chromite mining at Sukinda Valley—A review. Int J Environ Eng Manag. 2013;4(4):287-92.
10. Paustenbach DJ, Hays SM, Brien BA, Dodge DG, Kerger BD. Observation of steady state in blood and urine following human ingestion of hexavalent chromium in drinking water. J Toxicol Environ Health. 1996;49(5):453-61.
11. Sahu R, Saxena P, Johnson S, Mathur HB, Agarwal HC. Mercury pollution in the Sonbhadra district of Uttar Pradesh, India, and its health impacts. Toxicol Environ Chem. 2014;96(8):1272-83.
12. Park JD, Zheng W. Human exposure and health effects of inorganic and elemental mercury. J Prev Med Public Health. 2012;45(6):344-52.
13. Jo S, Woo HD, Kwon HJ, Oh SY, Park JD, Hong YS, et al. Estimation of the biological half-life of methylmercury using a population toxicokinetic model. Int J Environ Res Public Health. 2015;12(8):9054-67.
14. Goyer RA, Clarkson TW. Toxic effects of metals. In: Klaasen CD (Ed). Casarett and Doullis Toxicology: The Basic Science of Poisons. 6th edition, New York: McGraw-Hill Education; 2001. pp. 861-7.
15. de Groot G, van Heijst AN. Toxicokinetic aspects of thallium poisoning. Methods of treatment by toxin elimination. Sci Total Environ. 1988;71(3):411-8.
16. Karbowska B. Presence of thallium in the environment: Sources of contaminations, distribution and monitoring methods. Environ Monit Assess. 2016;188(11):640.
17. Ghannoum M, Nolin TD, Goldfarb DS, Roberts DM, Mactier R, Mowry JB, et al. Extracorporeal treatment for thallium poisoning: Recommendations from the EXTRIP Workgroup. Clin J Am Soc Nephrol. 2012;7(10):1682-90.

2.10 Toxic Gases

Meera Ekka, Soorya Suresh

INTRODUCTION

Toxic gases are those gaseous substances that interfere with one or more steps of oxygen delivery and utilization. The severity of symptoms of toxic gas exposure depends on the concentration of the agent in the inspired air, duration of exposure, toxicity of the substance, its water solubility, and individual susceptibility of the victim.[1] These can be asphyxiants, irritant gases, or knockout gases **(Table 1)**. Gases that interfere with oxygen delivery by displacing oxygen from inspired air are called simple asphyxiants [e.g., carbon dioxide (CO_2), hydrogen, nitrogen, methane, noble gases like helium]. Systemic asphyxiants are agents that alter the configuration of hemoglobin to hamper oxygen delivery [e.g., carbon monoxide (CO), nitrite, methylene chloride], or chemical asphyxiants—those agents that interfere in mitochondrial oxygen utilization [e.g., cyanide, hydrogen sulfide, phosphide]. Those agents that irritate and alter the integrity of mucosa of the respiratory tract are termed irritant gases (e.g., ammonia, chlorine, chloramine). Knockout gases are agents that on inhalation lead to immediate loss of consciousness and may even turn fatal (e.g., hydrogen sulfide, hydrogen cyanide, and phosphine). A single agent can have different mechanisms of exerting its toxicity and varying degrees of toxicity.

Indicators of a toxic gas exposure can be:
- Multiple patients with varying degrees of similar symptoms: Cough, dyspnea, headache, disorientation, and unresponsiveness
- Mass casualties with no obvious reason or visible trauma

TABLE 1: Toxic gases: Classification, mechanism of action, and examples.		
Class of agent	***Mechanism of action***	***Examples***
Asphyxiants	Agents displacing oxygen from air	Carbon dioxide, hydrogen, nitrogen, noble gases, methane, butane
	Agents that alter hemoglobin	Carbon monoxide, methylene chloride, nitrites
	Agents that hamper mitochondrial oxygen utilization	Cyanide, hydrogen sulfide, phosphine, sodium azide
Irritant gases	Agents that produce irritation and inflammation of respiratory mucosa	Ammonia, chlorine, chloramine, phosgene, hydrogen chloride, hydrogen fluoride
Knockout gases	Agents that have profound effect on consciousness	Carbon monoxide, cyanide, hydrogen sulfide

- Presence of chemical containers at the scene
- Presence of containers filled with unknown substances at the scene
- Residues around containers or at the scene

ASPHYXIANTS

Simple Asphyxiants

Pathophysiology

These agents hamper oxygen delivery by displacing oxygen from inspired air.[2] Theoretically, every gas, except oxygen, is capable of acting as a simple asphyxiant. The fraction of oxygen in inspired air (FiO_2) at ambient pressure is 21%. As the concentration of these gases increases in the inspired air, there is a decrease in the FiO_2 which in turn reduces the partial pressure of O_2 in inspired air. Agents acting as simple asphyxiants may not be pharmacologically active. Asphyxiation usually occurs in confined, poorly aerated spaces and with rapid release of these agents into the atmosphere

Systemic Asphyxiants

Agents that Alter Hemoglobin

Pathophysiology: Agents like carbon monoxide (CO) and methylene chloride, which is metabolized to CO, bind with hemoglobin to form carboxyhemoglobin (COHb) which is incapable of binding to oxygen. Certain other agents like nitrites cause the oxidation of divalent iron (Fe^{2+}) in hemoglobin to trivalent iron (Fe^{3+}). Hemoglobin with trivalent iron is called methemoglobin which is not capable of binding and transporting oxygen. Hence, even if the partial pressure of oxygen in inspired air remains normal, these agents lead to cellular hypoxia.

Chemical Asphyxiants

Pathophysiology: These are the agents that interfere with the cellular utilization of oxygen. Even though the oxygen delivery at the cellular level remains normal, these agents render the cells incapable of carrying out anaerobic metabolism by interrupting the mitochondrial electron transport chain. Agents like cyanide, hydrogen sulfide, sodium azide, and phosphine belong to this class of agents. These agents bind to the cytochrome oxidase a3 which is involved in oxidative phosphorylation, disrupts aerobic metabolism, and leads to acidosis.

Clinical Manifestations

Simple asphyxiants are generally odorless and irritant, making the identification of these agents challenging. Signs and symptoms of patients exposed to these agents would be similar to those of hypoxia due to a lack of oxygen at the cellular level.[3] Cardiovascular system and central nervous system manifestations are the predominant ones. Prolonged exposure to agents or extremely low partial pressures of oxygen may lead to multiorgan dysfunction and death.[4] Manifestations depend on the FiO_2 of the inspired air. Patients develop mild headache, euphoria, tachycardia, and tachypnea at FiO_2 of 15–17%. At a FiO_2 of 12–14%, patients develop incoordination, impaired judgment, and cyanosis. FiO_2 <10% causes severe headaches, severe in-coordination, and coma. Exposure to FiO_2 of <6% leads to seizure, coma, and death. Exposure to simple asphyxiants generally does not hinder CO_2 exchange and hence hypercapnia does not occur but if the asphyxiant is CO_2, hypercapnia is an early feature, which in itself would produce mental status changes.

Clinical features and manifestations of systemic asphyxiants are similar to those of simple asphyxiants as they ultimately lead to hypoxia. Signs and symptoms depend on the concentration of the agent in the blood and the duration of exposure. Methemoglobinemia leads to the development of cyanosis and dark chocolate-colored blood, whereas COHb turns the blood to cherry red colored. These agents can lead to lactic acidosis secondary to the anaerobic metabolism. Blood gas analysis and co-oximetry help to detect the level of these agents in blood.

Treatment

Removal of the individual from exposure is the first and foremost step in management. Since these agents are not systemic toxins, reversal of hypoxia by supplemental oxygen constitutes a mainstay of management. Other supportive care includes stabilization of the airway, breathing, and circulation depending on the clinical condition of the patient along with identification and treatment of any underlying condition that led to the exposure (trauma, burns, or cognitive decline).

Treatment specific to agents include intravenous methylene blue (1 mg/kg IV over 5 minutes) for methemoglobinemia. Clinical improvement may be observed within 20 minutes of administration. Repeat doses may be considered in patients with persistent symptoms after 1 hour of the first dose.

The antidote of choice in cases of cyanide toxicity is hydroxocobalamin [5 g reconstituted in 200 mL normal saline (NS) over 15 minutes and to be repeated if no clinical improvement].[5] Cyanide antidote kit which consists of amyl nitrite, sodium nitrite, and sodium thiosulfate can also be used in cases of cyanide toxicity. Hyperbaric oxygen therapy may be considered in patients with CO poisoning.[6]

IRRITANT GASES

Pathophysiology

Exposure to these irritant gases can damage both type I and type II pneumocytes in the lung.[7] The resultant injury leads to the release of inflammatory mediators, neutrophil influx, and disruption of capillary endothelium.[8,9] This finally leads to plasma leak and accumulation of cellular debris in the mucosa of the respiratory tract which produces a condition similar to acute respiratory distress syndrome (ARDS). The mechanisms by which different irritant gases exert their toxic effects vary, but the final pathway in the pathogenesis remains the same. Some gases dissolve in water present in the mucus to produce their toxic substance [e.g., hydrochloric acid (HCl), hydrogen fluoride (HF), and sulfur dioxide (SO_2)] while some others produce free radicals to induce damage by oxidative stress [e.g., nitric oxide (NO), nitrogen dioxide (NO_2), and ozone (O_3)].

Two types of injuries are observed with these toxic agents depending on their water solubility. Gases that rapidly dissolve in water (e.g., ammonia, chloramine, HCl, and SO_2) produce immediate symptoms, especially in the upper respiratory tract involving irritation, discomfort, and edema,[10] while those agents which are not highly water soluble (e.g., chlorine, phosgene, H_2S) may lead to delay in onset of clinical symptoms and may include tracheobronchitis, bronchiolitis, and ARDS.

Clinical Manifestations

Though the mechanisms by which these agents exert their irritant effect may vary, the clinical manifestations are largely similar. Agents like hydrogen chloride, ammonia, etc., which rapidly dissolve in water produce prompt discomfort and symptoms like burning in the throat, drooling, cough, bronchospasm, and mucosal edema.[9] In addition to these respiratory symptoms, they may also produce eye irritation, conjunctival congestion and chemosis, lacrimation, and skin irritation. The immediate discomfort on exposure caused by these agents acts as a warning signal for the victim and thus aids in the prompt escape of the victim. On the other hand, those agents that do not produce symptoms immediately after exposure would give no warning signal regarding their presence in the inspired air and thus lead to prolonged exposure to these agents. Prolonged exposure allows these gases to enter the entire tracheobronchial tree which results in tracheobronchitis, bronchiolitis, and ARDS.

The most serious manifestation associated with these agents is ARDS which severely affects oxygenation.[11,12] Patients develop cough, chest discomfort, dyspnea, hypoxemia, and crepitation on auscultation. The severity of ARDS depends on the extent of lung injury and is graded using PaO_2/FiO_2 ratio. Imaging shows bilateral heterogeneous infiltrations in the lung parenchyma.

In addition to these features, HF is capable of causing hypocalcemia. Patients may present with symptoms of hypocalcemia like paresthesia, muscle spasms, tetany, or seizures. Patients exposed to HF hence require monitoring of serum calcium levels.

Treatment

Immediate removal of the victim from the source along with supplemental humidified oxygen constitutes the immediate management of any patient exposure to irritant gases. Treatment is directed at monitoring pulmonary status irrespective of the exposed agent. Intubation and mechanical ventilation depend on the clinical condition and extent of lung injury. Patients with ARDS may require intubation and positive-pressure ventilation. Management of such patients is done in lines of ARDS due to any other cause.[12]

Supportive care constitutes the mainstay of treatment irrespective of the agent. Patients with mild symptoms or symptoms limited to the upper respiratory tract may be treated with supplemental oxygen, clearance of airway secretions, and nebulized bronchodilators.[13] Corticosteroids are shown to be of some benefit in limiting lung damage caused by the inflammatory cascade and hence improve oxygenation.[14,15] Though no robust data is available in this regard, corticosteroids form a part of the routine care of patients with ARDS secondary to irritant gas exposure.

Neutralization therapy using nebulized sodium bicarbonate (2%) has shown to be beneficial in those acid-generating agents like chlorine.[16–18] 1 mL of sodium bicarbonate (7.5% or 8.4%) diluted in 3 mL of distilled water gives approximately 2% solution which can be used for nebulization.

Patients exposed to HF require monitoring of serum calcium levels as well as electrocardiography as HF can lead to hypocalcemia. Patients with hypocalcemia require cardiac monitoring along with administration of calcium salts. Nebulization of calcium leads to binding of fluoride ion by calcium, thus preventing its systemic effects.[19,20] Nebulization of 2.5% calcium gluconate (1.5 mL of 10% calcium gluconate with 4.5 mL of NS) should be considered in patients exposed to HF.

KNOCKOUT GASES

Agents like CO, cyanide, and hydrogen sulfide are also called knockout gases as they have an immediate and profound effect on consciousness and can "knock down" successive people entering the room.

Carbon Monoxide

Carbon monoxide is a colorless and odorless gas. CO exposure can be accidental or suicidal. Major sources of CO are automobile exhaust, wood or coal-burning stoves, heaters, etc.[21] Methylene chloride, which is found in varnishes, is metabolized by the liver to CO which hence forms a source of CO.[22] CO has a higher binding affinity to hemoglobin, leading to the formation of COHb and hinders the formation of oxyhemoglobin. COHb shifts the oxyhemoglobin dissociation curve to the left, impairing O_2 release to tissues.[23] As a result, tissue hypoxia ensues and anaerobic metabolism takes place. It also inhibits cytochrome oxidase and increases lipid peroxidation leading to oxidative stress.

The wavelength of COHb is similar to oxyhemoglobin and hence the standard pulse oximetry fails to detect its presence.[24] About 1% of CO is found in healthy nonsmokers, and levels can go up to 10% in active smokers.[25] Blood gas analysis with co-oximetry is the only reliable method to detect the presence of CO. Since the levels can be typically high in active smokers, elevated COHb associated with a history of exposure and signs and symptoms consistent with the CO should be considered by making a clinical diagnosis. Symptoms are secondary to tissue hypoxia and may range from mild symptoms like headache, dizziness, and confusion to severe dyspnea, ataxia, seizure, and cardiac arrest. Anaerobic metabolism leads to elevated lactate levels in the body. Concomitant cyanide poisoning is a possibility that needs to be considered while managing such patients. Treatment consists of supplementation of 100% oxygen along with supportive care to stabilize the hemodynamic parameters.[26] Patients with severe symptoms like altered mental status, seizure, coma, hypotension, arrhythmias, severe metabolic acidosis, and pregnant females may be considered for hyperbaric oxygen therapy.[6,27]

Cyanide

Cyanide is a toxic gas that acts by binding to the cytochrome oxidase in mitochondria leading to disruption of oxidative phosphorylation.[28] The major sources of cyanide are the burning of wool, silk, and nylon, the fabrication of plastics, mining, vehicle exhaust, precious metal reclamation, etc. Seeds of plants like cherries, peaches, plums, and apricots are some of the natural sources of cyanide.[29] Cyanide is metabolized by the liver to thiocyanate which is renally excreted. Symptoms of toxicity depend on the route, source, concentration, duration of exposure, and time since exposure. Symptoms following inhalational exposure are immediate compared to other routes.

Symptoms range from mild headaches, anxiety, and restlessness to severe dyspnea, loss of consciousness, and death.[30,31] Severely poisoned patients typically manifest altered sensorium, tachypnea, hypotension, and bradycardia.[24,31] Cyanide toxicity does not typically produce cyanosis as it does not impair the oxygen-carrying capacity of hemoglobin. No rapid confirmatory tests are available to diagnose cyanide toxicity. History of exposure and symptoms along with severe lactic acidosis (typically >10 mmol/L), high anion gap metabolic acidosis, elevated venous oxygen saturation, and a normal pulse oximetry aid in the diagnosis.[32]

Management consists of supportive care with supplementation of 100% oxygen, vasopressors for hypotension, and administration of antidotes. The antidote of choice is hydroxocobalamin which binds cyanide to cyanocobalamin which is then excreted by the kidneys.[33,34] Hydroxocobalamin is administered as 5 g IV (70 mg/kg in children) over 15 minutes which may be repeated to a total of 10 g. The cyanide antidote kit available for use in cyanide poisoning consists of inhaled amyl nitrite, sodium nitrite (3%, 10 mL IV given over 5 minutes), and sodium thiosulfate (25%, 50 mL IV).[35,36] The administration of these nitrites induces the formation of methemoglobin which binds to cyanide with more affinity compared to cytochrome oxidase. However, nitrites may lead to excess production of methemoglobin and hypotension. Hence, hydroxocobalamin is preferred over cyanide antidote kit in the management of cyanide poisoning. Two other antidotes available against cyanide are dimethylaminophenol and dicobalt edetate, although these agents are not widely used for this purpose.[5]

Hydrogen Sulfide

Hydrogen sulfide is a colorless, flammable gas with a characteristic "rotten egg" smell. It is produced as a result of organic decomposition as in sewer or manure gas.[37] It is one of the most common causes of fatal toxic gas exposures. It acts as a chemical asphyxiant like cyanide and also has irritant properties on the respiratory mucosa. Exposure to higher concentrations leads to rapid loss of consciousness, seizure, and death. Treatment consists of removal from the source, decontamination, and supplemental oxygen. Intravenous sodium nitrate should be administered at a dose of 300 mg over 2–4 minutes for those patients with hemodynamic instability or altered sensorium.[38] It produces rapid improvement if only given within minutes of exposure. Low levels of methemoglobin that are produced by nitrites are considered to convert sulfide to less-toxic sulfmethemoglobin. The role of hyperbaric oxygen in cases of hydrogen sulfide toxicity is controversial.[39-41]

CONCLUSION

Toxic gases pose a significant threat to human health and safety, with the potential to cause widespread harm and even death. From simple asphyxiants, which deprive the body of oxygen, to more complex and highly lethal gases like carbon monoxide and cyanide, understanding their properties and effects is essential for preventing exposure and ensuring effective response measures. The importance of proper ventilation, personal protective equipments, and emergency response planning cannot be overstated. Irrespective of their varying mechanisms of action, awareness and preparedness remain critical in mitigating the dangers associated with toxic gases.

REFERENCES

1. Dries DJ, Endorf FW. Inhalation injury: Epidemiology, pathology, treatment strategies. Scand J Trauma Resusc Emerg Med. 2013;21:31.
2. Borron SW, Bebarta VS. Asphyxiants. Emerg Med Clin North Am. 2015;33(1):89-115.
3. Miller TM, Mazur PO. Oxygen deficiency hazards associated with liquefied gas systems: Derivation of a program of controls. Am Ind Hyg Assoc J. 1984;45(5):293-8.
4. DeBehnke DJ, Hilander SJ, Dobler DW, Wickman LL, Swart GL. The hemodynamic and arterial blood gas response to asphyxiation: A canine model of pulseless electrical activity. Resuscitation. 1995;30(2):169-75.
5. Borron SW, Baud FJ. Antidotes for acute cyanide poisoning. Curr Pharm Biotechnol. 2012;13(10):1940-8.
6. Mathieu D, Marroni A, Kot J. Tenth European Consensus Conference on Hyperbaric Medicine: Recommendations for accepted and nonaccepted clinical indications and practice of hyperbaric oxygen treatment. Diving Hyperb Med. 2017;47(1):24-32.
7. Laskin DL, Heck DE, Laskin JD. Role of inflammatory cytokines and nitric oxide in hepatic and pulmonary toxicity. Toxicol Lett. 1998;102-103:289-93.
8. McDonald DM, Thurston G, Baluk P. Endothelial gaps as sites for plasma leakage in inflammation. Microcirculation. 1999;6(1):7-22.
9. Reinhart PG, Bassett DJ, Bhalla DK. The influence of polymorphonuclear leukocytes on altered pulmonary epithelial permeability during ozone exposure. Toxicology. 1998;127(1-3):17-28.

10. Tanen DA, Graeme KA, Raschke R. Severe lung injury after exposure to chloramine gas from household cleaners. N Engl J Med. 1999;341(11):848-9.
11. Avecillas JF, Freire AX, Arroliga AC. Clinical epidemiology of acute lung injury and acute respiratory distress syndrome: Incidence, diagnosis, and outcomes. Clin Chest Med. 2006;27(4):549-57; abstract vii.
12. Bernard GR, Artigas A, Brigham KL, Carlet J, Falke K, Hudson L, et al. The American-European Consensus Conference on ARDS. Definitions, mechanisms, relevant outcomes, and clinical trial coordination. Am J Respir Crit Care Med. 1994;149(3 Pt 1):818-24.
13. Meduri GU, Annane D, Confalonieri M, Chrousos GP, Rochwerg B, Busby A, et al. Pharmacological principles guiding prolonged glucocorticoid treatment in ARDS. Intensive Care Med. 2020;46(12):2284-96.
14. Wang J, Zhang L, Walther SM. Administration of aerosolized terbutaline and budesonide reduces chlorine gas-induced acute lung injury. J Trauma. 2004;56(4):850-62.
15. Gunnarsson M, Walther SM, Seidal T, Lennquist S. Effects of inhalation of corticosteroids immediately after experimental chlorine gas lung injury. J Trauma. 2000;48(1):101-7.
16. Douidar SM. Nebulized sodium bicarbonate in acute chlorine inhalation. Pediatr Emerg Care. 1997;13(6):406-7.
17. Bosse GM. Nebulized sodium bicarbonate in the treatment of chlorine gas inhalation. J Toxicol Clin Toxicol. 1994;32(3):233-41.
18. Aslan S, Kandiş H, Akgun M, Cakir Z, Inandi T, Görgüner M. The effect of nebulized $NaHCO_3$ treatment on "RADS" due to chlorine gas inhalation. Inhal Toxicol. 2006;18(11):895-900.
19. Lee DC, Wiley JF, Synder JW. Treatment of inhalational exposure to hydrofluoric acid with nebulized calcium gluconate. J Occup Med Off Publ Ind Med Assoc. 1993;35(5):470.
20. Tsonis L, Hantsch-Bardsley C, Gamelli RL. Hydrofluoric acid inhalation injury. J Burn Care Res Off Publ Am Burn Assoc. 2008;29(5):852-5.
21. Hampson NB. Myth busting in carbon monoxide poisoning. Am J Emerg Med. 2016;34(2):295-7.
22. Chang YL, Yang CC, Deng JF, Ger J, Tsai WJ, Wu ML, et al. Diverse manifestations of oral methylene chloride poisoning: Report of 6 cases. J Toxicol Clin Toxicol. 1999;37(4):497-504.
23. Rose JJ, Wang L, Xu Q, McTiernan CF, Shiva S, Tejero J, et al. Carbon monoxide poisoning: Pathogenesis, management, and future directions of therapy. Am J Respir Crit Care Med. 2017;195(5):596-606.
24. Hall AH, Rumack BH. Clinical toxicology of cyanide. Ann Emerg Med. 1986;15(9):1067-74.
25. Reade MC, Davies SR, Morley PT, Dennett J, Jacobs IC, Australian Resuscitation Council. Review article: Management of cyanide poisoning. Emerg Med Australas EMA. 2012;24(3):225-38.
26. Hampson NB, Piantadosi CA, Thom SR, Weaver LK. Practice recommendations in the diagnosis, management, and prevention of carbon monoxide poisoning. Am J Respir Crit Care Med. 2012;186(11):1095-101.
27. Weaver LK. Carbon monoxide poisoning. Undersea Hyperb Med J Undersea Hyperb Med Soc Inc. 2020;47(1):151-69.
28. Beasley DM, Glass WI. Cyanide poisoning: Pathophysiology and treatment recommendations. Occup Med Oxf Engl. 1998;48(7):427-31.
29. Cliff J, Muquingue H, Nhassico D, Nzwalo H, Bradbury JH. Konzo and continuing cyanide intoxication from cassava in Mozambique. Food Chem Toxicol Int J Publ Br Ind Biol Res Assoc. 2011;49(3):631-5.
30. Sang-A-Gad P, Guharat S, Wananukul W. A mass cyanide poisoning from pickling bamboo shoots. Clin Toxicol Phila Pa. 2011;49(9):834-9.
31. Borron SW, Baud FJ. Acute cyanide poisoning: Clinical spectrum, diagnosis, and treatment. Arh Hig Rada Toksikol. 1996;47(3):307-22.
32. Parker-Cote JL, Rizer J, Vakkalanka JP, Rege SV, Holstege CP. Challenges in the diagnosis of acute cyanide poisoning. Clin Toxicol Phila Pa. 2018;56(7):609-17.
33. Hamad E, Babu K, Bebarta VS. Case files of the University of Massachusetts Toxicology Fellowship: Does this smoke inhalation victim require treatment with cyanide antidote? J Med Toxicol Off J Am Coll Med Toxicol. 2016;12(2):192-8.
34. Borron SW, Baud FJ, Barriot P, Imbert M, Bismuth C. Prospective study of hydroxocobalamin for acute cyanide poisoning in smoke inhalation. Ann Emerg Med. 2007;49(6):794-801, 801.e1-2.
35. Chen KK, Rose CL. Nitrite and thiosulfate therapy in cyanide poisoning. J Am Med Assoc. 1952;149(2):113-9.
36. Streitz MJ, Bebarta VS, Borys DJ, Morgan DL. Patterns of cyanide antidote use since regulatory approval of hydroxocobalamin in the United States. Am J Ther. 2014;21(4):244-9.
37. Barbera N, Montana A, Indorato F, Arbouche N, Romano G. Domino effect: An unusual case of six fatal hydrogen sulfide poisonings in quick succession. Forensic Sci Int. 2016;260:e7-10.
38. Yalamanchili C, Smith MD. Acute hydrogen sulfide toxicity due to sewer gas exposure. Am J Emerg Med. 2008;26(4):518.e5-7.
39. Tomaszewski CA, Thom SR. Use of hyperbaric oxygen in toxicology. Emerg Med Clin North Am. 1994;12(2):437-59.
40. Asif MJ, Exline MC. Utilization of hyperbaric oxygen therapy and induced hypothermia after hydrogen sulfide exposure. Respir Care. 2012;57(2):307-10.
41. Policastro MA, Otten EJ. Case files of the University of Cincinnati fellowship in medical toxicology: Two patients with acute lethal occupational exposure to hydrogen sulfide. J Med Toxicol Off J Am Coll Med Toxicol. 2007;3(2):73-81.

2.11 Smoke Inhalation

Mohit Kharbanda, Saswati Sinha, Anupam Kumar Singh

INTRODUCTION

Smoke inhalation is a devastating injury that affects one-third of burn injury victims and increases mortality by up to 20 times as compared to burn injury alone.[1] The most common mechanism of inhalation injury occurs from exposure to fire, but it may also happen due to chemicals, vapor, toxic fumes, gases, or smoke. The injury to the respiratory system occurs both as a result of the heat of the fire and as local and systemic effects of the toxic chemicals formed during the decomposition of materials during combustion.[2] The mainstay of therapy for smoke inhalation comprises adequate respiratory support with airway toileting, optimizing fluid resuscitation, appropriate antimicrobial therapy, and early and aggressive surgical interventions when necessary. Although several novel therapeutic modalities have been under investigation, supportive therapy still forms the cornerstone in the management of patients with inhalation injuries.

PATHOPHYSIOLOGY

Inhalation injury comprises supraglottic thermal injury, subglottic airway and alveolar insult, and systemic toxicity. The severity of the injury is determined by the ignition source, composition of smoke (size and diameter of the particles) including the solubility of gases, the temperature of inhaled smoke, and the duration of exposure.[3]

Inhalational injuries are classified based on the localization of the primary insult into (1) upper airway, (2) tracheobronchial tree, and (3) lung parenchyma **(Flowchart 1)**.[4]

Upper Airway

Upper airway primarily refers to injury above the level of the vocal cords and comprises thermal injury, leading to erythema, ulcerations, and edema. Burns to the face and neck can additionally contribute to anatomical distortion which in addition to airway edema due to fluid resuscitation

Flowchart 1: Pathophysiology of smoke inhalation injury.

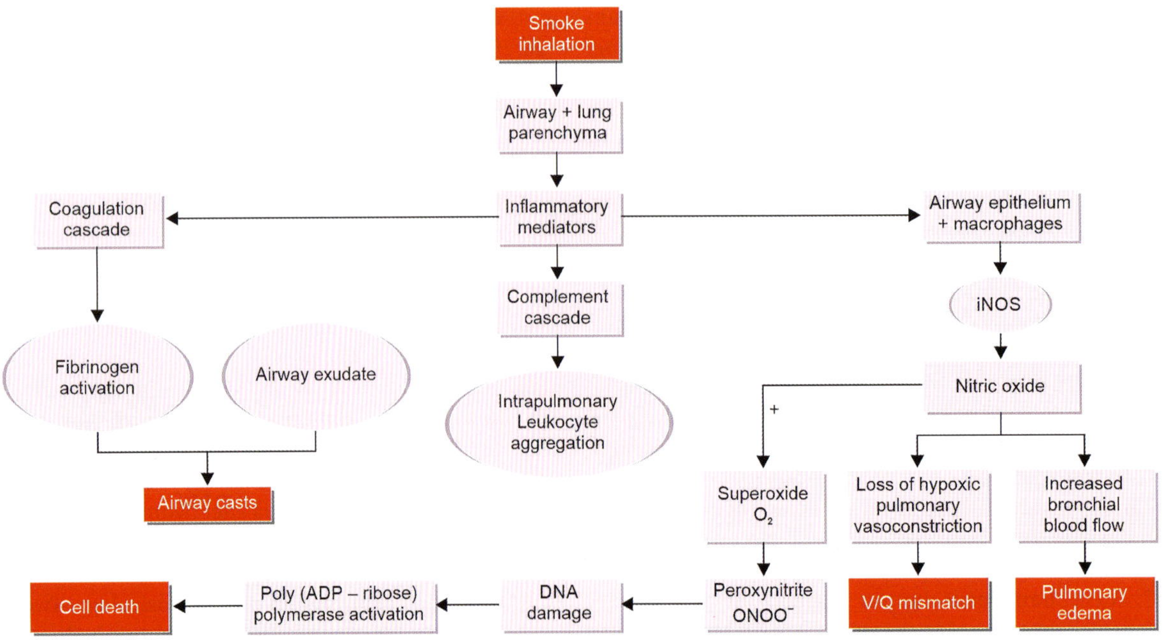

(DNA: deoxyribonucleic acid; iNOS: Inducible nitric oxide synthase; V/Q: ventilation–perfusion)

can complicate airway management.[5] Damage to the ciliary function of the airway causes impairment of the ability to clear secretions which further predisposes the patient to an increased risk of bacterial infections which can last for several weeks.

Tracheobronchial Tree

Injury to the tracheobronchial tree is predominantly caused by the chemicals in the inhaled smoke as well as noxious gases such as chlorine and liquids such as acids. The richly innervated area is stimulated to release neuropeptides which stimulate nitric oxide synthase (NOS) to generate reactive oxygen species (ROS) and induce bronchoconstriction. This leads to vasodilatation and increased vascular permeability and also impairs hypoxic pulmonary vasoconstriction leading to a marked increase in bronchial blood flow which also delivers cytokines and polymorphonuclear leukocytes compounding the host inflammatory response.[6] Damage to the bronchial epithelium along with leakage of fluid and plasma proteins into the alveoli and bronchioles leads to cast formation in the airways which leads to ventilation-perfusion (V/Q) mismatch which is the primary mechanism underlying the hypoxemia in case of inhalation injury.[7]

Lung Parenchyma

Most of the thermal injury is adsorbed in the upper airway but other components of smoke such as particulate materials, respiratory irritants, and systemic toxins descend into the lung and the subsequent cascade of events lead to pulmonary edema, bronchiolar obstruction, and V/Q mismatch.[8] The drivers of this cascade are the inflammatory mediators such as tumor necrosis factor-alpha, interleukins (IL)—IL-6, IL-8, IL-1β, and nuclear factor kappa B. Activation of the complement cascade triggers leukocyte aggregation and release of cytokines and free radicals of oxygen and nitrogen.[7] Inducible nitric oxide synthase (iNOS) leads to the production of nitric oxide (NO) which causes vasodilation, thereby markedly increasing the bronchial blood flow, and impairs the hypoxic pulmonary vasoconstriction in the poorly ventilated lung zones which further potentiates the V/Q mismatch.[9] NO combines with superoxide produced from the activated neutrophils to produce peroxynitrite peroxynitrite ($ONOO^-$) which leads to deoxyribonucleic acid (DNA) damage and cell death.[7] Parenchymal injury is characterized by atelectasis and alveolar collapse leading to edema due to transvascular fluid flux, loss of surfactant, and impaired hypoxic pulmonary vasoconstriction leading to hypoxemia. In addition, a massive impairment in alveolar hemostasis, decreased fibrinolysis, and massive deposition of fibrin in the airways accentuate the V/Q mismatch.[10] There is an increased predisposition to pneumonia due to airway obstruction and impaired mucociliary clearance which is further compounded by impaired function of polymorphonuclear leukocytes and macrophages.[11] This injured lung is also at a high risk of ventilator-induced lung injury (VILI) due to the biotrauma mediated by the chemokines released from the ventilation of the inhomogeneous lung, the normal lung being overdistended and interspersed with areas of collapse due to widespread cast formation and airway plugging.[12]

Systemic Toxicity

Systemic toxicity after inhalation injury which accounts for morbidity and mortality is usually attributed to carbon monoxide (CO) and hydrogen cyanide which are products of incomplete combustion.

Carbon Monoxide

Carbon monoxide is a colorless and odorless gas with a 200 times higher affinity for hemoglobin than that of oxygen and is one of the most frequent causes of immediate death following inhalation injury. Carboxyhemoglobin (COHb) shifts the oxygen dissociation curve to the left, thereby impairing tissue delivery of oxygen and utilization in the mitochondria leading to tissue hypoxia.[8,10]

Carbon monoxide poisoning should be suspected in all patients following inhalation injury unless a normal level of COHb by co-oximetry excludes the diagnosis. Pulse oximetry is not useful as it cannot distinguish between oxyhemoglobin and COHb since COHb absorbs approximately the same amount of 660 nm light as oxyhemoglobin. Due to the interference of high levels of COHb, life-threatening hypoxemia may be masked by a falsely reassuring pulse oximeter reading.[13] Arterial oxygen tension (PaO_2) measurements tend to be normal because PaO_2 reflects O_2 dissolved in the blood, and this process is not affected by carbon monoxide. Hence, whenever COHb is suspected, co-oximetry is recommended to estimate COHb levels.[14]

Hydrogen Cyanide

Hydrogen cyanide is the gaseous form of cyanide which has the smell of bitter almonds. Due to the high probability of its presence, cyanide poisoning should always be considered in all patients with inhalation injury.[15] Cyanide can be liberated during the combustion of carbon- and nitrogen-containing products as well as vehicular fires. It binds to the ferric ion of cytochrome oxidase a3, thereby inhibiting this final enzyme of the mitochondrial cytochrome complex causing cessation of oxidative phosphorylation. Cells are compelled to switch to anaerobic metabolism to generate ATP leading to the formation of lactic acid. Despite sufficient oxygen supply, the cells cannot utilize oxygen because the electron transport chain is damaged which predominantly hampers the cardiovascular and the central nervous system.[16] Hence, it is prudent to initiate empiric treatment in patients at risk who present with cardiac arrest, hemodynamic decompensation, or altered sensorium pending laboratory confirmation.[17]

CLINICAL FEATURES

History

Inhalation injury should be suspected based on the history of exposure to smoke, flames, and chemicals, and pertinent information should include:

- Duration of exposure
- Exposure in a closed space or not
- Loss of consciousness[1]

Usual symptoms include dizziness, nausea, and vomiting. Symptoms of upper airway injury such as shortness of breath may not be immediately obvious but may develop fast once the edema is severe enough to reduce the airway diameter. The presence of productive cough including carbonaceous sputum and shortness of breath may indicate involvement of the lower respiratory tract.

Signs and symptoms vary according to the concentration of COHb **(Table 1)**.

Physical Examination

Early clues to smoke inhalation injury include facial burns, hoarse voice, soot in the oropharynx, nasal passage, and singed nasal hair. The presence of facial or oral edema, stridor, wheezing, dyspnea, rales, and rhonchi and the use of accessory muscles point toward more severe injury also involving the lower respiratory tract and more severe damage.[18,19]

TABLE 1: Carboxyhemoglobin concentration and signs and symptoms in carbon monoxide poisoning.

Carboxyhemoglobin concentration (%)	*Signs and symptoms*
<20	Mild headache, tightness across the forehead, dilatation of blood vessels
21–40	Severe headache, vertigo, dizziness, nausea, vomiting, circulatory collapse
41–60	Same as above, high pulse and respiratory rates, intermittent seizures, syncope, coma, Cheyne–Stokes respiration, shock
61–80	Coma, intermittent seizures, weak pulses, slow breathing, death ensues within hours
>80	Death occurs within minutes

Investigations

Baseline Investigations

- Complete blood count
- Urea, creatinine, electrolytes
- Arterial blood gas (ABG) analysis
- X-ray chest—atelectasis, pulmonary edema, and consolidation may be present
- Computed tomography scan of thorax—ground-glass opacities in peribronchial distribution appear within a few hours. A normal CT scan of the thorax can rule out inhalation injury and has an ability to quantify the extent of injury to the lungs which may not be identified by fiberoptic bronchoscopy.[20]

Other Investigations

- COHb—estimation by a co-oximeter[21,22]
- Toxicology screen—for other toxins
- Blood cyanide level[22,23]

MANAGEMENT

One of the cornerstones of managing smoke inhalation is to have a high index of suspicion considering the circumstances and look out for symptoms, signs, and possible complications of inhalational injury.

The suspicion should be high in the following circumstances:

- History of closed-space entrapment
- History of syncope
- Carbonaceous sputum

- Arterial PaO_2 <60 mm Hg
- Metabolic acidosis
- COHb levels >15%
- Bronchospasm/wheezing
- Facial burns
- Central nervous system depression, lethargy, and obtundation
- Irritability, severe temporal headache, and generalized muscle weakness
- Coma

History should be obtained from emergency services, bystanders, and family members regarding where the burn occurred and whether the patient has had high-risk features.[23]

The priority in these patients as in most situations in critical care is airway, breathing, and circulation (ABC).

Airway

If the patient has features/suspicion of inhalational injury, early endotracheal intubation should be considered as the oropharyngeal, glottic, and facial edema may make endotracheal intubation very difficult/impossible later on. Repeated assessments and close monitoring of the airway will be required to reach a balance between prophylactic and unnecessary intubation versus a too-late loss of airway. Airway procedures like endotracheal intubation/tracheostomy should be performed by the most experienced person available.

It may be prudent to intubate the patient without using muscle relaxants so that even if the operator is unable to intubate the patient, the patient will continue breathing. Succinylcholine should not be used after 24 hours of burn injury considering that it can produce exaggerated hyperkalemic responses severe enough to induce cardiac arrest.[24]

Inhalation injuries frequently manifest damage to the airway and lungs after a latent period of several hours, a process influenced by concomitant injuries and the extent of fluid resuscitation necessary. Despite these considerations, continuous reassessment of airway management and the patient's oxygenation status is imperative, even in the absence of intubation. The dynamic nature of smoke inhalation injury underscores the need for frequent reevaluation to ensure optimal care.[25]

High-flow moist oxygen should be administered to all patients to decrease the COHb concentration and to prevent the development of inspissated secretions.[19]

Standard cardiopulmonary monitoring (electrocardiogram, pulse oximetry, and noninvasive blood pressure) and intravenous access should be established. It should be remembered that the presence of COHb may give falsely high oxygen saturation readings.

Breathing

Bronchospasm is a commonly observed phenomenon and inhaled bronchodilators, specifically β-2 agonists, are frequently employed to alleviate this condition. Their administration not only mitigates bronchospasm but also enhances respiratory mechanics by reducing airflow resistance and peak airway pressures in mechanically ventilated patients. Consequently, there is an improvement in dynamic compliance. Additionally, β-2 agonists exhibit anti-inflammatory properties, reducing inflammatory mediators such as histamine, leukotrienes, and tumor necrosis factor α. Moreover, the use of β-2 agonists is linked to enhanced clearance of fluid in the airspace and the stimulation of mucosal repair.[26,27]

Circulation

Burn shock encompasses both hypovolemic shock and cellular shock, presenting with distinctive hemodynamic alterations such as reduction in cardiac output, extracellular fluid volume, plasma volume, and oliguria. Similar to the approach in managing other forms of shock, the primary objective is to reinstate and maintain tissue perfusion to prevent ischemia. However, the resuscitation process in burn shock is complex due to mandatory burn edema, and the extensive transvascular fluid shifts resulting from a significant burn are exclusive to thermal trauma.[28] Smoke inhalation per se increases the fluid requirement substantially.

The amount of fluid resuscitation in burn patients with smoke inhalation is not well defined. Our practice is to start with a plan of fluid resuscitation of 2 mL/kg body weight × total body surface area (TBSA) burn to be given over 24 hours, half of which is given in the first 8 hours and the rest over 16 hours as per Advanced Trauma Life Support (ATLS) 10th edition.[29] The target is to maintain arterial pressure (MAP) >65 mm Hg, urine output 0.5–1.0 mL/kg/h, and a lactate of <2. If the planned fluids are inadequate to maintain targets, then an additional bolus of 500 mL to 1.0 L can be given intermittently.

Treatment of Carbon Monoxide Intoxication

Contemporary guidelines for treating CO poisoning commence with discontinuing exposure, promptly administering 100% oxygen, and providing supportive care. The justification for hyperbaric oxygen therapy (HBOT) lies in its capacity to swiftly displace CO from hemoglobin, thereby diminishing the duration of the hypoxemic state. The administration of 100% oxygen at 3 atmospheres decreases the CO half-life from 250 minutes when using room air to a significantly shorter duration of 30 minutes.[30,31] HBOT has been studied as a treatment for CO poisoning, but one of the major drawbacks is that the other resuscitation and care of the patient are hampered when the patient is in the hyperbaric chamber. It is not universally available either. An examination of six randomized controlled trials (RCTs) in the Cochrane database failed to demonstrate a favorable impact of HBOT compared to standard treatment concerning neurologic sequelae.[32]

Treatment of Cyanide Poisoning

Diagnosing cyanide poisoning again requires a high index of suspicion. It is very commonly present concurrently with CO poisoning. Some features that should raise suspicion are headache, drowsiness, unconsciousness, seizures and coma, bradycardia, hypotension, unexplained severe lactic acidosis despite adequate resuscitation, and high anion gap metabolic acidosis. Another typical feature is a narrowing of the venoarterial PO_2 gradient (i.e., venous hyperoxia). The tissues are not able to extract oxygen from the blood. Cyanide concentrations are not easily available, and the turnaround times are too long for it to be clinically useful.

Hydroxocobalamin, a precursor of vitamin B_{12}, incorporates a cobalt moiety that strongly binds to intracellular cyanide, surpassing the affinity of cytochrome oxidase. This binding results in the formation of cyanocobalamin, a stable molecule that is easily eliminated through urine.[33]

As hydroxocobalamin acts rapidly, is relatively safe and does not adversely affect tissue oxygenation; it is generally considered the first-line therapy for suspected cyanide poisoning. The other antidotes amyl nitrate and sodium thiosulfate are employed to oxidize hemoglobin to methemoglobin, which exhibits a preference for binding cyanide. This facilitates the dissociation of cyanide, allowing for its metabolism by liver enzymes. It is important to note, however, that these substances act as methemoglobin generators and may potentially impede oxygen transport. Therefore, their use is reserved for cases with a confirmed diagnosis, indicated by increased plasma levels of cyanide, and should be administered under continuous monitoring in an intensive care unit **(Box 1)**.

BOX 1: Management of cyanide poisoning.

General treatment:

- *Secure airway, breathing, and circulation.* Intubation is usually required. Administer high-flow oxygen and by nonrebreather face mask regardless of pulse oximetry reading
- *Do not perform mouth-to-mouth resuscitation* in case of suspected cyanide toxicity. Patients with dermal exposure must be decontaminated using proper precautions
- Give a single dose of activated charcoal if the airway is adequately protected (50 g in adults; 1 g/kg in children with a maximum dose of 50 g)
- Treat hypotension with rapid IV boluses of isotonic fluid and vasopressors as needed. Treat seizure with a benzodiazepine (e.g., diazepam 5 mg IV)

Antidotal treatment:

- Administer cyanide antidote when cyanide poisoning is clinically suspected. Hydroxocobalamin is the preferred antidote.
- If hydroxocobalamin is available, give the following:
  - Hydroxocobalamin 5 g (adults) or 70 mg/kg IV (pediatric patients, maximum 5 g)
- If hydroxocobalamin is not available, cyanide toxicity is known or strongly suspected in an adult patient, and there are no contraindications to nitrite, give the following:
  - Sodium nitrite (3% solution) 10 mL IV (300 mg) at 2.5–5 mL/min; may repeat once
  - Sodium thiosulfate (25% solution) 50 mL IV (12.5 g) immediately following sodium nitrite administration; may repeat once
- If hydroxocobalamin is not available and cyanide toxicity is possible but not certain in an adult patient, or the patient has contraindications to nitrites, give the following:
  - Sodium thiosulfate (25% solution) 50 mL IV (12.5 g) may repeat once

(IV: intravenously; PO_2: partial pressure of oxygen)
Source: Adapted from UpToDate.

Pulmonary Care

The management of inhalation injury is primarily supportive, focusing on alleviating bronchospasm, minimizing pulmonary secretions, and clearing the airways of fibrin casts, as well as sloughed and necrotic bronchial epithelium. These elements can contribute to airway obstruction and atelectasis, ultimately leading to pneumonia. Prophylactic antibiotics are not recommended in this context.

Bronchoscopy

An airway assessment by fiberoptic laryngoscopy/bronchoscopy should be undertaken to assess the severity of inhalation injury.[34] Various scoring systems exist to assess the severity of inhalation injury by bronchoscopic examination, yet none of them has been shown to be better than others in predicting outcomes **(Table 2)**. A recent prospective observational study on 99 intubated burn patients on whom bronchoscopy was done found that only inhalation injury severity score (I-ISS) was associated with survival.[35]

Inspissated secretions may form casts and lead to atelectasis; frequent therapeutic bronchoscopies may need to be done to remove the casts and open up the airways.

Mucolytics and Anticoagulants

N-acetylcysteine (NAC) can be used as a mucolytic agent in the treatment of smoke inhalation. The dosage used is 3 mL of a 20% solution every 4 hours. It may cause bronchospasm in which case a bronchodilator may be given before giving NAC.

Inhaled anticoagulants mitigate the formation of fibrin casts after inhalation injury without affecting systemic indicators of clotting and anticoagulation. Inhaled heparin at 5,000–10,000 units in 3 mL normal *saline*, every 4 hours, is used at times. Nebulized heparin or NAC has demonstrated a role in the reduction in reintubation rates, and the incidence of atelectasis and improved mortality, better lung compliance, less pulmonary edema, and less airway obstruction compared to controls decreased the duration of mechanical ventilation and increased the number of ventilator-free days in various studies.[36-39]

Mechanical Ventilation

There are no RCTs in adult burn patients with inhalation injury comparing various ventilatory modes, positive end-expiratory pressure (PEEP), and tidal volumes. The open lung concept is generally extrapolated and used in smoke inhalation injury patients as well. The acute respiratory distress syndrome (ARDS) network trial[40] recommended tidal volumes of 6 mL/kg, a plateau pressure of <30 cm of water, and the corresponding PEEP is adjusted as per the PEEP—FiO_2 table of the ARDS Network trial. Self-injurious ventilator demand and respiratory rate may be controlled by analgesia and sedation.[41] One retrospective study has reported a mortality rate of 69.7% for smoke inhalation patients developing ARDS and it is much higher than

TABLE 2: Inhalation injury scoring system.

Scoring system	*Grade 0 No injury*	*Grade 1 Mild injury*	*Grade 2 Moderate injury*	*Grade 3 Severe injury*	*Grade 4 Massive injury*
AIS	Absence of carbonaceous deposits, erythema, edema, bronchorrhea, or obstruction	Minor/patchy erythema, carbonaceous deposits in proximal of distal bronchi (any or combination)	Moderate erythema, bronchorrhea with or without compromise of bronchi (any or combination)	Severe inflammation with friability, copious carbonaceous deposits, bronchorrhea, bronchial obstruction (any or combination)	Evidence of mucosal sloughing, necrosis, endoluminal obliteration (any or combination)
MS	Normal mucosal appearance	Mild mucosal erythema	Mucosal erythema and swelling	Mucosa with pale, dry necrosis	–
I-ISS	Negative bronchoscopy	Mucosal edema and hyperemia, with or without carbon soot	Severe mucosal edema and reddening, with or without carbon soot	Ulcerations, necrosis, and absence of both cough reflex and bronchial secretion	–

(AIS: abbreviated injury score; I-ISS: inhalation injury severity score; MS: mucosal score).
Source: Adapted from reference 36.

mortality in ARDS due to cutaneous burns without smoke inhalation (54.6%).[42]

Extracorporeal Membrane Oxygenation

In severe ARDS cases with refractory hypoxemia, extracorporeal membrane oxygenation (ECMO) has been tried, and two case series—one from the USA and another from the UK have reported good survival rates in smoke inhalation-induced ARDS.[43,44]

Tracheostomy—maintaining an endotracheal tube on a burned face is a significant challenge and accidental extubation is a concern. Tracheostomy provides the advantage of requiring less sedation, facilitating earlier mobilization, and offering a more comfortable method of ventilation for patients requiring long-term care. However, the data regarding the optimum timing for tracheostomy is not definitive.[19] Septal ties are routinely employed by some centers to secure the endotracheal tubes. Tracheostomy provides the advantage of requiring less sedation, facilitating earlier mobilization, and offering a more comfortable method of ventilation for patients requiring long-term care. However, the data regarding the optimum timing for tracheostomy is not definitive. In a survey done in North America, most of the tracheostomies were done around the 2-week mark.[45] In a study done on 600 adult ICU patients by Terragni et al., although the number of ventilator days and ICU days were reduced, there was no difference in the incidence of ventilator-associated pneumonia.[46]

Extubation

As in other critically ill patients, the primary criterion for extubation/weaning from a ventilator is whether the reason for which the patient has been intubated has been taken care of. If the patient was intubated for airway edema, one needs to make sure that the airway edema has gone down or a tracheostomy has been done. We should look for audible leaks around the tube, decreased inflammation, decreased secretions, and the ability of the patient to cough out.

For weaning from ventilation, the following conventional criteria may be used:

- Vital capacity at a minimum of 15–20 mL/kg
- Spontaneous tidal volume within the range of 5–7 mL/kg
- Maximal voluntary ventilation reaching two times the minute volume
- PaO_2/FiO_2 ratio exceeding 250 mm Hg

CONCLUSION

Inhalation injury is a complex multifaceted condition with high morbidity and mortality. It is important to anticipate the complications and judiciously manage them. The basic principles remain to manage the ABC which include high-flow oxygen, judicious and timely intubation, protective mechanical ventilation, goal-directed and cautious fluid resuscitation, etc. CO and cyanide poisoning need to be identified early and managed with high-flow oxygen and hydroxocobalamin, respectively. Careful monitoring and multidisciplinary management can improve the outcomes of this devastating injury.

REFERENCES

1. Enkhbaatar P, Pruitt BA Jr, Suman O, Mlcak R, Wolf SE, Sakurai H, et al. Pathophysiology, research challenges, and clinical management of smoke inhalation injury. Lancet. 2016;388(10052):1437-46.
2. Shubert J, Shehada ER. Inhalation injury. Treasure Island (FL): StatPearls Publishing; 2018.
3. Kimura R, Traber LD, Herndon DN, Linares HA, Lubbesmeyer HJ, Traber DL. Increasing duration of smoke exposure induces more severe lung injury in sheep. J Appl Physiol (1985). 1988;64(3):1107-13.
4. Woodson LC. Diagnosis and grading of inhalation injury. J Burn Care Res. 2009;30(1):143-5.
5. Demling RH. Smoke inhalation lung injury: An update. Eplasty. 2008;8:e27.
6. Walker PF, Buehner MF, Wood LA, Boyer NL, Driscoll IR, Lundy JB, et al. Diagnosis and management of inhalation injury: An updated review. Crit Care. 2015;19:351.
7. Murakami K, Traber DL. Pathophysiological basis of smoke inhalation injury. News Physiol Sci. 2003;18:125-9.
8. Prien T, Traber DL. Toxic smoke compounds and inhalation injury: A review. Burns Incl Therm Inj. 1988;14: 451-60.
9. Westphal M, Cox RA, Traber LD, Morita N, Enkhbaatar P, Schmalstieg FC, et al. Combined burn and smoke inhalation injury impairs ovine hypoxic pulmonary vasoconstriction. Crit Care Med. 2006;34:1428-36.
10. Rehberg S, Maybauer MO, Enkhbaatar P, Maybauer DM, Yamamoto Y, Traber DL. Pathophysiology, management and treatment of smoke inhalation injury. Expert Rev Respir Med. 2009;3(3):283-97.
11. Al Ashry HS, Mansour G, Kalil AC, Walters RW, Vivekanandan R. Incidence of ventilator associated pneumonia in burn patients with inhalation injury treated with high frequency percussive ventilation versus volume control ventilation: A systematic review. Burns. 2016;42(6):1193-200.
12. Maybauer MO, Rehberg S, Traber DL, Herndon DN, Maybauer DM. Pathophysiology of acute lung injury

in severe burn and smoke inhalation injury. Anaesthesist. 2009;58:805-12.
13. Grace RF. Pulse oximetry. Gold standard or false sense of security? Med J Aust. 1994;160(10):638-44.
14. Hampson NB. Pulse oximetry in severe carbon monoxide poisoning. Chest. 1998;114(4):1036-41.
15. Walsh DW, Eckstein M. Hydrogen cyanide in fire smoke: An underappreciated threat. Emerg Med Serv. 2004;33(10):160-3.
16. Mizock BA. Lactic acidosis. Dis Mon.1989;35(4):233-300.
17. Sanders KN, Aggarwal J, Stephens JM, Michalopoulos SN, Dalton D, Lewis DE, et al. Cost impact of hydroxocobalamin in the treatment of patients with known or suspected cyanide poisoning due to smoke inhalation from closed-space fires. Burns. 2022;48(6):1325-30.
18. Ogura H, Sumi Y, Matsushima A, Tohma Y, Inoue Y, Tasaki O, et al. Smoke inhalation injury: Diagnosis and respiratory management. Nihon Geka Gakkai Zasshi. 2005;106: 740-4.
19. Toon MH, Maybauer MO, Greenwood JE, Maybauer DM, Fraser JF. Management of acute smoke inhalation injury. Crit Care Resusc. 2010;12:53-61.
20. Koljonen V, Maisniemi K, Virtanen K, Koivikko M. Multi-detector computed tomography demonstrates smoke inhalation injury at early stage. Emerg Radiol. 2007;14:113-6.
21. Rose JJ, Wang L, Xu Q, McTiernan CF, Shiva S, Tejero J, et al. Carbon monoxide poisoning: Pathogenesis, management, and future directions of therapy. Am J Respir Crit Care Med. 2017;195:596-606.
22. Lawson-Smith P, Jansen EC, Hyldegaard O. Cyanide intoxication as part of smoke inhalation – A review on diagnosis and treatment from the emergency perspective. Scand J Tray ma Resusc Emerg Med. 2011;19:14.
23. Lafferty KA, Bonhomme K, Martinez CV, Wiener SW, Serebrisky D, Dillinger R, et al. Smoke inhalation. 2008. [online] Available from http://emedicine.medscape.com/article/771194-overview [Last accessed September, 2024].
24. Tolmie JD, Joyce TH, Mitchell GD. Succinylcholine danger in the burned patient. Anesthe siology. 1967;28:467-70.
25. Parrillo JE, Dellinger RP. Critical care medicine: Principles of diagnosis and management in the adult. 5th edition. Amsterdam: Elsevier; 2018. pp. 46,733-743.e4.
26. Morina P, Herrera M, Venegas J, Mora D, Rodríguez M, Pino E. Effects of nebulized salbutamol on respiratory mechanics in adult respiratory distress syndrome. Intensive Care Med. 1997;23:58-64.
27. Zhang H, Kim YK, Govindarajan A, Baba A, Binnie M, Ranieri VM, et al. Effect of adrenoreceptors on endotoxin-induced cytokines and lipid peroxidation in lung explants. Am J Respir Crit Care Med. 1999;160:1703-10.
28. Warden GD. Burn shock resuscitation. World J Surg. 1992;16:16-23.
29. Henry S. ATLS 10th edition offers new insights into managing trauma patients. Bulletin of the American College of Surgeons. 2018. [online] Available from https://www.facs.org/for-medical-professionals/news-publications/news-and-articles/bulletin/2018/06/atls-10th-edition-offers-new-insights-into-managing-trauma-patients/ [Last accessed October, 2024]
30. Maybauer DM, Traber DL, Radermacher P, Herndon DN, Maybauer MO. Treatment strategies for acute smoke inhalation injury. Anaesthesist. 2006;55:980-2:984-8.
31. Kealey GP. Carbon monoxide toxicity. J Burn Care Res. 2009;30:146-7.
32. Juurlink DN, Buckley NA, Stanbrook MB, Isbister GK, Bennett M, McGuigan MA. Hyperbaric oxygen for carbon monoxide poisoning. Cochrane Database Syst Rev. 2005;(1):CD002041.
33. Thompson JP, Marrs TC. Hydroxocobalamin in cyanide poisoning. Clin Toxicol (Phila). 2012;50(10):875-85.
34. Endorf FW, Gamelli RL. Inhalation injury, pulmonary perturbations, and fluid resuscitation. J Burn Care Res. 2007;28:80.
35. Flinn AN, Kemp Bohan PM, Rauschendorfer C, D Le T, Rizzo JA. Inhalation injury severity score on admission predicts overall survival in burn patients, J Burn Care Res. 2023;44(6):1273-7.
36. Cha SI, Kim CH, Lee JH, Park JY, Jung TH, Choi WI, et al. Isolated smoke inhalation injuries: Acute respiratory dysfunction, clinical outcomes, and short-term evolution of pulmonary functions with the effects of steroids. Burns. 2007;33:200-8.
37. Desai MH, Mlcak R, Richardson J, Nichols R, Herndon DN. Reduction in mortality in pediatric patients with inhalation injury with aerosolized heparin/N-acetylcystine [correction of acetylcystine] therapy. J Burn Care Rehabil. 1998;19:210.
38. Miller AC, Rivero A, Ziad S, Smith DJ, Elamin EM. Influence of nebulized unfractionated heparin and N-acetylcysteine in acute lung injury after smoke inhalation injury. J Burn Care Res 2009;30:249.
39. McIntire AM, Harris SA, Whitten JA, Fritschle-Hilliard AC, Foster DR, Sood R, et al. Outcomes following the use of nebulized heparin for inhalation injury (HIHI study). J Burn Care Res. 2017;38:45.
40. Brower RG, Matthay MA, Morris A, Schoenfeld D, Thompson BT, Wheeler A, et al. Acute Respiratory Distress Syndrome Network. Ventilation with lower tidal volumes as compared with traditional tidal volumes for acute lung injury and the acute respiratory distress syndrome. N Engl J Med. 2000;342:1301-8.
41. Dries DJ, Tawfik PN. A rationale for safe ventilation with inhalation injury: An editorial review. J Burn Care Res. 43(4):787-91.
42. Lam NN, Hung TD. ARDS among cutaneous burn patients combined with inhalation injury: Early onset and bad outcome. Ann Burns Fire Disasters. 2019;32(1): 37-42.

43. Eldredge RS, Zhai Y, Cochran A. Effectiveness of ECMO for burn-related acute respiratory distress syndrome. Burns. 2019;45(2):317-21.
44. Szentgyorgyi L, Shepherd C, Dunn KW, Fawcett P, Barker JM, Exton P, et al. Extracorporeal membrane oxygenation in severe respiratory failure resulting from burns and smoke inhalation injury. Burns. 2018;44(5):1091-9.
45. Chung KK, Rhie RY, Lundy JB, Cartotto R, Henderson E, Pressman MA, et al. A survey of mechanical ventilator practices across burn centers in North America. J Burn Care Res. 2016;37(2):e131.
46. Terragni PP, Antonelli M, Fumagalli R, Faggiano C, Berardino M, Pallavicini FB, et al. Early vs late tracheotomy for prevention of pneumonia in mechanically ventilated adult ICU patients: A randomized controlled trial. JAMA. 2010;303(15):1483-9.

2.12 Caustics and Corrosives

Rakesh Kocchar

INTRODUCTION

"Corrosive" and "caustic" ingestion is a rare but devastating medical emergency. It is common in many developed as well as developing countries including India.[1] Because of the under-reporting of these events, epidemiological data is scarce. As per the 2013 annual report of the American Association of Poison Control Centers, 60,000 new cases of caustic agent exposure were reported (48,000 to bleach, 7,500 to acids, and 4,000 to alkalis), most of which occurred by ingestion.[1] The data from most of the developing countries including India is not available.

Both "corrosive" and "caustic" are used interchangeably to describe the injury through the chemical reaction. The word "corrosive" could be more commonly found in the old literature while "caustic" is a relatively new terminology. The term "corrosive" is used for both living and nonliving material while "caustic" specifically refers to the chemical damage to the organic tissue. Thus, "caustic" is more commonly used now to describe these injuries.

EPIDEMIOLOGY AND PATHOPHYSIOLOGY

Caustic ingestion has a bimodal presentation with the first peak in young children and adolescents and a second peak in young adults.[2] Among the children, the commonly affected age group includes 1–6 years which is primarily accidental while adolescents and adults aged 16–49 years commonly take these substances with suicidal intent or under the effect of alcohol.[3] Although there is no gender difference for caustic ingestion for children, among the adolescents, and adult population, caustic ingestion is equal or slightly more common among females in developed countries while males are more affected in developing countries including India. In developing countries, majority of the caustic injuries are secondary to acidic substance with alkali contributing to minority of patients (<10–20%) while in western and developed countries, the majority of cases were accounted for by alkali, i.e., household bleach, laundry detergent.[4] **Table 1** provides the details of commonly encountered acids and alkali agents.

However, both acidic and alkaline substances cause chemical injury to the gastrointestinal (GI) wall. They produce the injury through different mechanisms. Acids cause coagulation necrosis, with eschar formation, which may limit the deeper penetration of substance and thus cause injury, while alkalis combine with tissue proteins and cause liquefactive necrosis and penetrate deeper into tissues. Injury occurs quickly depending on the substance concentration and exposure time. Based on the pathophysiological sequence, alkaline substances are thought to produce more severe injury. However, this is not clinically relevant in the settings of strong acid and base ingestion where full-thickness injury can develop.

Once the caustic substance contacts the GI wall, mucosal injury begins within minutes and rapidly progresses in the initial 24 hours. Within 48 hours, the submucosa is infiltrated by the inflammatory cells and thrombosis of arteries and veins could also develop.[5] After 3–7 days of injury, mucosa sloughs and fibroblasts start

TABLE 1: Commonly ingested caustic agents.

Caustic agent	*Examples*	*Commercially available forms*
Alkali	Sodium hydroxide	• Drain cleaners • Home soap manufacturing
	Potassium hydroxide	• Oven cleaners • Washing powders • Liquid drain cleaners • Disk batteries
	Ammonia	• Household cleaners
	Sodium carbonate	• Soap manufacturing • Fruit drying on farms
Acid	Sulfuric acid	• Batteries • Industrial cleaning agents • Metal plating
	Hydrochloric acid	• Toilet and drain cleaners • Solvents • Metal cleaners • Antirust compounds
	Phosphoric	Toilet cleaner
Bleaches and other caustic	Hypochlorous acid	• Household bleach • Cleaners
	Peroxide	Mildew remover

to migrate at the site of injury and help in the formation of granulation tissue. By the end of 2–3 weeks, collagen deposition and fibroblast proliferation lead to the development of stricture.

Determinants of Injury

Substances with extreme pH (acidic substances with pH <3 and alkaline substances with pH >11) are likely to cause more severe damage.[6] It is unclear whether the nature of the substance (i.e., alkali or acid) affects the patient outcomes in cases of massive ingestion. The physical form also determines the pattern of damage. Solid form adheres to the mucosa and produces more damage to the mouth and pharynx. On the other hand, liquids transit easily and produce distal esophageal and stomach injuries. The amount of substance ingested also determines the extent and severity of injury; however, such data is sparingly available. Other factors like fasting status and contact period to the tissue also determine the severity of injury.

TABLE 2: Common presenting manifestations of acute caustic ingestion.[7,8]

Clinical features	*Percentage (%)*
Asymptomatic	41–44
Vomiting and retching	39–50.5
Throat pain	1–31.1
Hypersalivation	1.6–6
Odynophagia	1–13.1
Chest or epigastric pain	1–10.9
Dysphagia	6
Laryngeal edema	1.1

CLINICAL PRESENTATION

The clinical presentation depends on multiple factors including the type and physical form of the substance, amount ingested, and intention of ingestion. Injury to the oral cavity and pharynx presents with burning pain in the throat, hoarseness of voice, stridor, respiratory distress, and odynophagia. Esophageal involvement includes retrosternal burning, odynophagia, or dysphagia. Gastric involvement is suggested by the presence of epigastric pain, recurrent vomiting, and hematemesis. Though a significant number of patients are symptomatic, asymptomatic presentation is not uncommon and does not rule out significant injury.[7,8] **Table 2** describes the common presenting symptoms.[7,8]

ASSESSMENT OF GASTROINTESTINAL INJURY

Clinical Assessment

Studies have tried to predict the presence of esophageal and gastric injury using the presenting symptoms and signs. Most studies identify that the absence of clinical symptoms or signs does not rule out severe GI tract (GIT) injury, though few have suggested that the presence of symptoms predicts severe GI involvement.[9] Betalli et al. in a prospective study showed that the presence of three or more symptoms (oral and/or oropharyngeal lesions and vomiting, dyspnea, dysphagia, drooling, and hematemesis) is an important predictor of severe esophageal lesions.[10] Similarly, Uygun et al. developed a DROOL (drool, reluctance, oropharynx, others, leukocytosis) score and suggested that a score of ≤4 was a good predictor of esophageal stricture formation

(100% sensitivity, 96.63% specificity, 85% positive predictive value, 100% negative predictive value).[11] Other scores including PEWS (pediatric early warning score) score, Gorman score, Crain score, and Med-TU chart have also been suggested to predict the severity of the injury..[9,12-14] However, the benefit of symptoms to predict the severe lesions is not consistently shown by all the authors neither the suggested tools are validated in further studies.

Recently, Tosca et al. described a hybrid score based on the clinical, laboratory, and endoscopic parameters.[15] The score predicted the outcome with high sensitivity and specificity of 93.3 and 92.7%, respectively, and was better than endoscopy alone. Although recent studies have shown the predictive role of clinical score, the data is still limited for assessing the severity of injury. Thus, all the patients should be assessed on admission for vitals, hemodynamic instability, respiratory symptoms and signs, and any signs of mediastinitis or peritonitis. All the external surfaces and organs should also be examined to look for injury and to avoid continuous contamination.

Blood Investigations

All the patients with caustic ingestion should undergo a set of standard investigations at presentation including complete blood counts (CBC), liver and renal function tests, international normalized ratio (INR), serum lactate, and electrocardiogram (ECG) which act as a reference value for subsequent follow-up. Limited data suggested that increased leukocyte counts with neutrophilia, elevated alanine aminotransferase, and low platelet counts can predict the visceral necrosis.[16] Additionally, blood gas analysis should be obtained whenever available which can identify the life-threatening acid-base disorders at an earlier stage.[17] Initial tests may be normal and do not exclude transmural necrosis. The change in laboratory values on follow-up may be useful in guiding the management.

X-Ray Chest and Abdomen

Chest and abdominal (erect) x-rays may identify aspiration pneumonia or free intraperitoneal air secondary to viscera perforation and should be done in all patients before endoscopic evaluation.

Esophagogastroduodenoscopy

Early esophagogastroduodenoscopy (EGD) or upper GIT endoscopy has traditionally been used for the assessment of injury and remains the initial approach at most of the centers. Endoscopy helps in guiding the further treatment, prognosis, and timing of discharge. Recommendation of early endoscopy is based on the safety of the procedure in the caustic injury before the injured segment enters the weaker reparative phase with an increased risk of perforation. A large American database study showed that all clinical outcomes (death, perforation, sepsis, aspiration pneumonia, parenteral feeding, GI bleeding, and systemic complications) were less common in the early EGD (within 48 hours) group compared to the delayed EGD (after 48 hours) group.[18] Delayed EGD also had poor clinical outcomes and increased cost of hospital admissions. Thus, EGD should be done at the earliest and preferably in the initial 24–48 hours of caustic ingestion in all the patients who are stable. The principle of gentle handling during endoscopy with use of carbon dioxide insufflation and conscious sedation should be practiced. In selected cases when a patient presents late, endoscopy can be safely performed after 48 hours in expert hands to assess the extent and severity of injury.[2,19]

During the endoscopic examination of the GIT, Zargar's grading **(Figs. 1A to F and Table 3)** should be used to assess the extent and severity of injury for the esophagus, stomach, and duodenum.[19] Use of grading systems standardizes the reporting of injury and also helps in prognosis. The injury should be described using standard definitions, words, and phrases **(Table 3)**. Classification of injury in low (Grade ≤2a) and high (Grade ≥2b) grades helps in identifying the patients who can be allowed orally with early discharge from the hospital and also those who require long-term hospitalization. Kochhar et al. showed that patients with low-grade injury are less likely to develop follow-up complications and could be discharged early.[20] Patients with high-grade injury require long-term hospitalization, intensive care unit (ICU) admission, and nutritional support and are also likely to develop long-term complications.

Computed Tomography Scan

Endoscopic evaluation remains the most acceptable approach for assessment of injury; however, it has several shortcomings including invasive procedure, interobserver variability in grading injury, overprediction of injury, and inability to assess the full-thickness necrosis. These limitations have led to the utilization of computed tomography (CT) in acute caustic injury. Ryu et al.

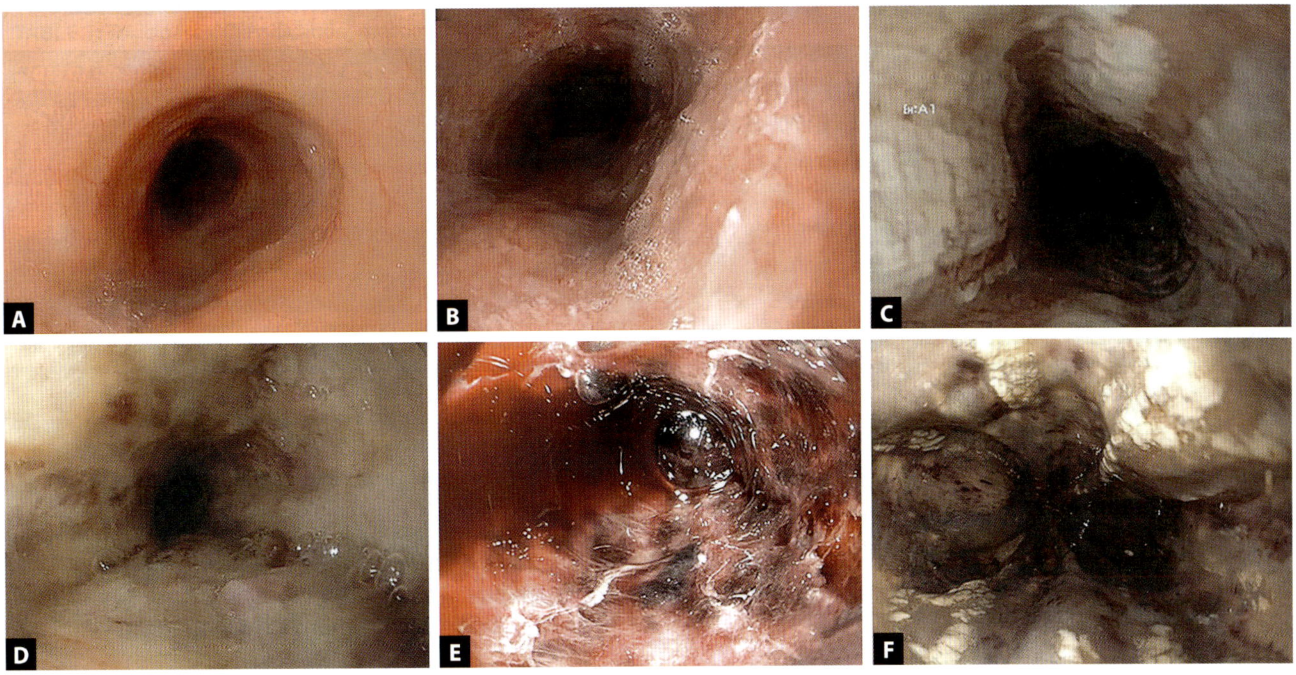

Figs. 1A to F: Zargar grades of injury on endoscopic evaluation after caustic ingestion. (A) Zargar grade 0: Normal mucosa; (B) Zargar grade 1: Edema and erythema of the mucosa; (C) Zargar grade 2: Superficial erosions whitish membranes over the mucosa; (D) Zargar grade 2b: Circumferential ulcerations involving circumferential mucosa; (E) Zargar grade 3a: Focal area of necrosis; (F) Zargar grade 3b: Extension area of necrosis involving most of the circumference.

TABLE 3: Endoscopic grading of caustic injury as per Zargar's classification.

Endoscopic grading	*Findings*
Grade 0	Normal findings
Grade 1	Edema and hyperemia of the mucosa
Grade 2a	Superficial localized ulcerations, friability, hemorrhage and blisters
Grade 2b	Deep ulcerations (either discrete or circumferential), in addition to friability, hemorrhage, and superficial ulcerations
Grade 3a	Small, scattered areas of necrosis
Grade 3b	Extensive necrosis

evaluated the role of CT in predicting the development of esophageal stricture.[21] Later, Chirica et al. studied the role of emergency CT in patients of acute caustic injury for predicting the necrosis and suggested a three-grade classification as shown in **Figures 2A to C.**[22] The studies showed that a contrast-enhanced CT scan accurately predicted the transmural necrosis of the esophagus and stomach and avoided the unnecessary esophagectomy and laparotomy in 19 and 16 patients, respectively, compared to endoscopic assessment of the injury.[16,22] Thus, a CT scan could be of particular importance in assessing the extent and severity of injury in hemodynamically unstable patients who cannot undergo endoscopic examination. Additionally, a CT scan also helps in detecting the perforations by identifying the pneumoperitoneum or pneumomediastinum and in assessing the injury to the small bowel, colon, and other abdominal organs which cannot be detected on EGD. The follow-up study for stricture prediction has also shown that emergency CT predicts the development of esophageal stricture more accurately compared to initial endoscopy.[23]

However, recent studies suggest that CT performs better than initial endoscopy. There are several limitations which need evaluation. First, the majority of patients with caustic ingestion has low-grade injury. The generalization of CT as an initial assessment modality for injury should be weighed against the risk of radiation exposure. Second, CT grading has been validated during the initial period of injury, i.e., for the initial 24–48 hours. A significant proportion of patients present late in the course and the validity of CT for their assessment of injury is not known.

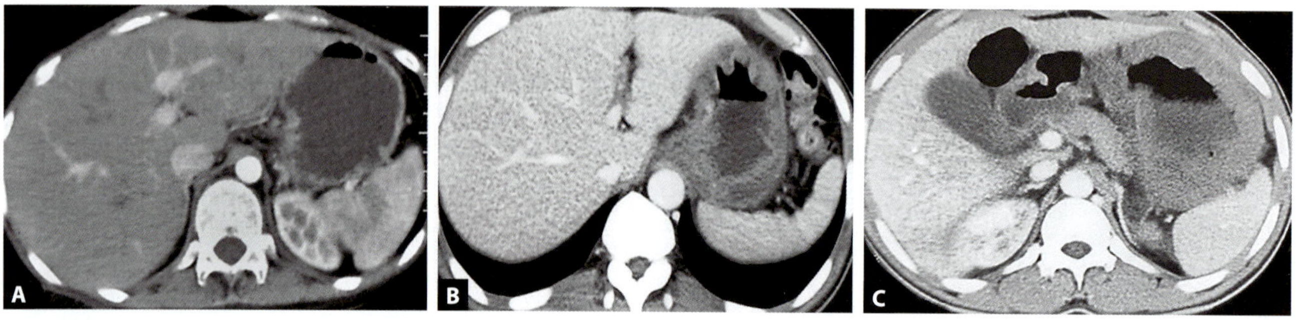

Figs. 2A to C: Grade of injuries on contrast enhanced computed tomography after caustic ingestion. (A) *Grade 1:* Normal appearing mucosa and gastrointestinal wall; (B) *Grade 2:* Hyperenhancement of mucosa with hypodence wall due to edema with enhancement of outer wall; (C) *Grade 3b:* Absence of postcontrast esophageal/gastric wall-enhancement, wall blurring, and peri-organ fat blurring.

Third, the available studies on the use of CT for caustic injury include alkali as the main damaging substance. Whether the results of CT are applicable to patients with acid injury is a matter of research.

Esophagogastroduodenoscopy versus Computed Tomography

The choice among the esophagoduodenoscopy or CT as the initial modality for injury assessment remains a topic of research. Studies have compared endoscopy (within 24 hours of ingestion) with CT chest and abdomen in the early phase of caustic ingestion with variable results. Lurie et al. in a small retrospective series of 23 patients identified that a CT scan was less sensitive and more specific than endoscopy in identifying the severe injury and need for emergency laparotomy.[24] Bahrami-Motlagh et al. also showed that the agreement rates between CT scan and endoscopy for identifying esophageal and gastric injuries were moderate to fair and the need for endoscopy cannot be precluded.[25] However, other studies have suggested that a CT scan is better than traditional endoscopy for identifying the severity and extent of the injury and triaging the patients for emergent surgery or observation.[22]

Available studies point toward the greater accuracy of CT in identifying the necrosis of GIT in acute caustic injury. However, it is not known if CT performs better than endoscopy in predicting the injury and stricture formation. Both endoscopy and CT scan have their benefits and shortcomings **(Table 4)**. Endoscopy has traditionally been utilized for assessing the severity and extent of injury. Thus, till more studies are available, endoscopy should be the initial modality for assessment of extent and severity of injury. A CT scan should be used as a complementary modality in situations (1) when high clinical suspicion or signs of mediastinitis or peritonitis are present, (2) for the assessment of the viability of the GIT in patients having high-grade injury (Zargar grade 3b), (3) for evaluation of GIT injuries in patients who cannot undergo endoscopic examination, and (4) for assessment of GIT with suspicion of injury beyond stomach.

TABLE 4: Benefits and limitation of esophagogastroduodenoscopy (EGD) and computed tomography (CT) scan in caustic injury.

Parameters	*EGD*	*CT scan*
Easy availability	✓	×
Can be used for Zargar grading for steroid therapy	✓	×
Visualization of entire GIT and other system	×	✓
Easily identifies perforation	×	✓
Identifies the candidates for emergency surgery	×	✓
Facilitates insertion of feeding tube	✓	×
Risk of radiation	No	Yes
Validity beyond 48–72 hours of ingestion	✓	×

(GIT: gastrointestinal tract)

MEDICAL MANAGEMENT

Initial Assessment, Airway Management, and Fluid Therapy

The initial measures should be focused to avoid the aggravation of injury, pain management, organ support, and management of other potential systemic complications. At presentation, hemodynamic assessment, respiratory assessment, signs of mediastinitis or peritonitis, and the presence of any organ failure should be looked at. History taking and clinical evaluation should include the details of the corrosive substance, volume, timing before admission, prehospital treatment, and cause of ingestion but should not delay the fluid resuscitation and organ support.

Airway compromise should be attended to immediately in all patients. Hoarseness of voice, stridor, or dyspnea should point toward laryngeal involvement. Management includes adrenaline nebulization every 2–4 hourly. Intravenous corticosteroids (50–100 mg every 6–8 hourly) should also be used to reduce the laryngeal edema. In case of rapid or progressive worsening of airway, endotracheal intubation or surgical tracheostomy could be considered. Patients should be looked for fluid deficiency since these patients have recurrent vomiting, dysphagia, and poor oral intake. Intravenous fluid resuscitation should be initiated as per the clinical assessment. Since the appropriate type and amount of fluid to be given are not known, the basic principles of resuscitation along with the maintenance of airway and circulation should be followed. The fluid should be chosen based on the availability, electrolyte and acid–base balance, and physician's preference.[26]

Role of Nasogastric Tube, Gastric Lavage, and pH Neutralization

It is a common practice in toxicology to perform gastric lavage by inserting a nasogastric (NG) tube. However, such acts could lead to catastrophic events. Blind insertion of a NG tube may increase the risk of esophageal and/or gastric perforation in high-grade injuries and should not be attempted.[27] Additionally, the risk of caustic substance reflux during insertion of a NG tube could also lead to more damage in the esophagus. Similarly, gastric lavage, pH neutralization, and induced emesis have no proven benefit in caustic injury and should not be avoided. Additionally, these measures may aggravate the injury of a possible exothermic reaction, re-exposure of the esophagus to the corrosive agents, and reflux vomiting and chemical pneumonitis due to high volume.

Role of Sucralfate, Proton-pump Inhibitors, Antibiotics, and Corticosteroids

Sucralfate

The rationale of its use in caustic injury is the maintenance of mucosal blood flow and the provision of a physical barrier to allow healing. Limited data suggests its role in the prevention of esophageal stricture. A randomized controlled study of 15 patients showed reduced esophageal stricture with oral sucralfate at 6 months follow-up.[28] A recent study included 60 children with corrosive injury (Zargar grade 2b) and demonstrated similar benefits in stricture prevention with oral sucralfate than the control arm.[29] The dose of sucralfate used in this study was 80 mg/kg every 2 hours for 72 hours. However, studies suggest the role of sucralfate in stricture prevention. The use of sucralfate in the initial phase of caustic ingestion is often limited by persistent dysphagia, odynophagia, and laryngeal edema with an increased risk of aspiration. Thus, until more robust data is available, sucralfate should not be used routinely after caustic ingestion.

Proton-pump Inhibitors

The role of proton-pump inhibitors (PPI) in acute caustic injury has been limited by evidence. The rationale of use of PPI includes a reduction in acid production and anti-inflammatory and anti-apoptotic effects leading to re-epithelization and mucosal healing.[30] A small open label randomized controlled trial of 20 patients of acute corrosive (Zargar grades 2b and 3a) compared the use of omeprazole with standard of care.[31] The study showed significantly lower esophageal strictures in the omeprazole group. However, the study included only a small number of patients and was underpowered for the outcome of stricture formation. Larger studies are needed to validate these findings before the use of PPI could be recommended.

Antibiotics

The routine use of antibiotics in caustic injury is not recommended. No study has evaluated the role of antibiotics for preventing infectious complications or strictures. Studies on the use of steroids in acute caustic had used antibiotics alongside. Antibiotics should only be administered in case of suspected or proven perforation, infection, aspiration, or when requiring surgical intervention. Although there is a suggestion to start antibiotics in high-grade corrosive injuries, these are not supported by any evidence.

Corticosteroids

Corticosteroids are immunosuppressives and reduce the inflammation and fibrotic process at the site of injury. Thus, the use of corticosteroids for stricture prevention after a caustic injury was hypothesized to prevent fibrosis and thus stricture. Earlier randomized studies and a recent meta-analysis have shown no role of corticosteroids in stricture prevention.[32,33] However, a randomized study in 83 children with limited injury (Zargar grade 2b) showed the benefit of high-dose intravenous corticosteroids in preventing stricture formation.[34] However, the recent small study with a similar protocol showed no benefit of corticosteroid in preventing stricture formation but helps in reducing respiratory complications.[35] Thus, routine use of corticosteroids in acute caustic injury is not recommended and should be reserved for those with airway compromise.

Nutrition

Caustic injury is a catabolic state with increased loss of nitrogen and risk of micronutrient deficiency after a severe acute caustic injury.[36] The risk of malnutrition is not limited to the acute stage of caustic injury. Stricture development in patients with high-grade injury leads to poor oral intake and increases the risk of malnutrition. Good nutritional support is quintessential for enhanced healing of mucosa and also for satisfactory postsurgery outcomes. Despite the importance of nutrition in corrosive injury management, there are no guidelines on it till date. Enteral nutrition is the preferred choice with parenteral nutrition being indicated in a small number of patients with contraindications to enteral feeding. The contraindications to enteral feeding in patients with caustic ingestion include suspected perforation with or without peritonitis and GI bleeding.

For low-grade injuries (Zargar grade ≤2a), oral feeding can be allowed once a patient can tolerate or when swallowing is adequate. High-grade injuries (Zargar ≥2b) would require a long period of nil by mouth and fluid resuscitation. The decision to start enteral versus parenteral feed should be individualized. Enteral feeding could be initiated with a NG or a nasojejunal tube or feeding jejunostomy (FJ) could be performed. Kochhar et al. compared the nasoenteral versus FJ in 96 patients of caustic injury.[37] All the patients were able to maintain weight at 8 weeks' follow-up in both the groups. However, the complication rates were lower in the nasoenteral feeding group compared to FJ. Total parenteral nutrition is required in patients when enteral feeding is not tolerable or when nutritional requirements could not be fulfilled with enteral feeding. Calorie and protein requirements should be estimated for each patient as there is significant weight loss during the course of illness.[38] The recommended daily dose of multivitamins and omega-3 fatty acids should also be kept in mind while deciding the diet plan in collaboration with a dedicated dietician. **Figure 3** summarizes the nutritional support in patients with acute caustic injury.

Psychological Evaluation and Support

A large nationwide cohort study showed that 23% of the patients presenting with caustic ingestion have underlying psychiatric disorders.[39] The identification of these disorders could help in the allocation of resources more effectively toward patients with depression, anxiety disorder, and other psychiatric disorders, thus reducing

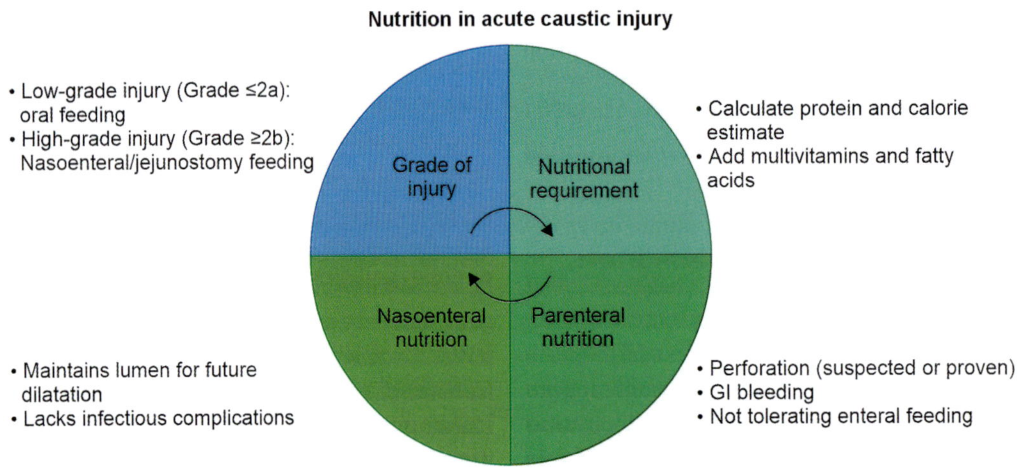

Fig. 3: Nutritional assessment and support in patients with caustic ingestions.

TABLE 5: Outcome of emergency surgery in patients with caustic injuries.

Study	*Year*	*Emergency resections (n)*	*Operative mortality (n, %)*	*Reoperation (n, %)*
Wu et al.	1993	28	5 (18%)	–
Andreoni et al.	1995	11	3 (27%)	–
Landen et al.	2000	14	7 (50%)	–
Rigo et al.	2002	11	9 (82%)	–
Ertekin et al.	2004	7	3 (43%)	–
Chou et al.	2010	71	29 (41%)	–
Zerbib et al.	2011	24	4 (17%)	2 (8%)
Javed et al.	2012	13	2 (15%)	–
Chirica et al.	2012	253	42 (17%)	51 (20%)
Wu et al.	2015	64	29 (45%)	–

the recurrence of such events. Thus, all patients of caustic ingestion with unknown or suicidal intent should be evaluated by a psychiatrist and initial evaluation should be done before discharge.

EMERGENCY SURGERY

Emergency surgery is required for complications. Complication after an acute caustic injury includes perforation leading to mediastinitis or peritonitis, peritonism suggestive of impending perforation, and massive bleeding after caustic ingestion. Few authors suggest preventive surgery in patients with transmural necrosis of the GIT to avoid penetrating complications. However, this remains a relative indication of emergency surgery. In a survey conducted by the World Society of Emergency Surgery (WSES), only 10% of respondents agreed to operate based on the transmural necrosis in the absence of peritonitis.[40] The reason for this approach is high mortality when emergency surgery is performed. The mortality varies from 15 to –82% in different series after emergency surgery for caustic injury **(Table 5)**.[41-50]

The type of surgery during an emergency procedure depends on the organ system affected. The principle of "damage control surgery" is followed. Laparotomy remains the standard approach with resection of all the transmural necrotizing injuries. The esophagus and stomach remain the most commonly involved organs, and their removal depends on the involvement. The presence of pancreaticoduodenal necrosis or extensive bowel necrosis carries high mortality and morbidity. Thus, resection of the pancreaticobiliary system and extensive bowel should be decided on a case-to-case approach.

FOLLOW-UP

Patients with low-grade injury (Zargar grade ≤2a) could be discharged early from the hospital once they start taking orally. Patients with high-grade injury (Zargar grade ≥2b) require close monitoring and should be overserved for clinical and laboratory worsening. Hospital discharge for these patients should be individualized based on the severity of injury and clinical and laboratory stability.

Regular follow-up is recommended for early detection of nutritional insufficiency and stricture detection. Strictures become symptomatic when the esophagus or antropyloric regions are severely affected. Occasionally, cicatrization of the body region of stomach could lead to symptomatic luminal obstruction. These strictures can develop at different periods of time, and thus no single time point for assessment of these strictures is available. Studies have identified that majority of these symptomatic strictures develop within 8 weeks of injury.[20,23] Thus, at the end of 8 weeks or whenever symptomatic, objective assessment of stricture could be done with imaging or endoscopy. Barium examination can provide valuable information about the number, length, and complexity of the strictures and help in deciding the appropriate management strategy **(Figs. 4A and B)**. Endoscopy can also be used to define strictures, but it may fail to provide complete information when strictures are complex and scope is not negotiable.

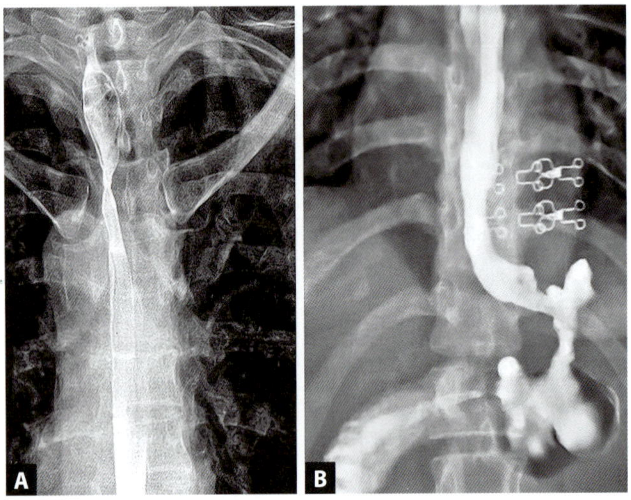

Figs. 4A and B: Barium examination showing strictures involving different segments of upper gastrointestinal tract. (A) Esophageal stricture; (B) Complex gastric stricture.

CONCLUSION

Caustic ingestion is a potentially devastating emergency worldwide. Irrespective of the presence of absence of symptom, clinical assessment should be done as a whole. A hybrid evaluation including clinical and basic laboratory parameters could be more informative. All patients should be assessed for hemodynamic instability, airway compromise, fluid status, and potential local and systemic complications. Initial management should be directed toward pain alleviation, fluid and electrolyte correction, and avoiding aggravation of injury. NG tube insertion, pH neutralization, and gastric lavage should not be done. Routine use of antibiotics, sucralfate, proton-pump inhibitors, and corticosteroids is not evidence based and should be discouraged. The extent and severity assessment of injury should be done with EGD as early as possible after initial resuscitation. Additionally, contrast-enhanced CT scan of chest and abdomen should be done as a complementary modality for assessment of the disease severity and identifying the complications. Nutrition should be taken care of in all the patients by appropriate use of oral, nasoenteral, or jejunostomy feeding. Early hospital discharge can be considered in low-grade injury (Zargar grade ≤2a) once patients start taking orally. Patients with high-grade injury (Zargar grade ≥2b) should be monitored for clinical or laboratory worsening, and discharge should be individualized once stable. Emergency surgery should be considered in case of perforation, mediastinitis or peritonitis, massive GI bleeding or clinical or laboratory worsening. Post discharge, a regular follow-up is mandatory to detect the stricture early. Barium examination of the upper GIT can identify the stricture anatomy and help in deciding the definitive management strategy.

REFERENCES

1. Mowry JB, Spyker DA, Cantilena LR Jr, McMillan N, Ford M. 2013 annual report of the American Association of Poison Control Centers' national poison data system (NPDS): 31st annual report. Clin Toxicol (Phila). 2014;52(10): 1032-283.
2. De Lusong MAA, Timbol ABG, Tuazon DJS. Management of esophageal caustic injury. World J Gastrointest Pharmacol Ther. 2017;8(2):90-8.
3. Rafeey M, Ghojazadeh M, Sheikhi S, Vahedi L. Caustic ingestion in children: A systematic review and meta-analysis. J Caring Sci. 2016;5(3):251-65.
4. Cheng HT, Cheng CL, Lin CH, Tang JH, Chu YY, Liu NJ, et al. Caustic ingestion in adults: The role of endoscopic classification in predicting outcome. BMC Gastroenterol. 2008;8:31.
5. Bosher LW Jr, Burford TH, Ackerman l. The pathology of experimentally produced lye burns and strictures of the esophagus. J Thorac Surg. 1951;21(5):483-9.
6. Keh SM, Onyekwelu N, McManus K, McGuigan J. Corrosive injury to upper gastrointestinal tract: Still a major surgical dilemma. World J Gastroenterol. 2006;12(32):5223-8.
7. Bautista Casasnovas A, Estevez Martinez E, Varela Cives R, Villanueva Jeremias A, Tojo Sierra R, Cadranel S. A retrospective analysis of ingestion of caustic substances by children. Ten-year statistics in Galicia. Eur J Pediatr. 1997;156(5):410-4.
8. Arıcı MA, Ozdemir D, Oray NC, Buyukdeligoz M, Tuncok Y, Kalkan S. Evaluation of caustics and household detergents exposures in an emergency service. Hum Exp Toxicol. 2012;31(6):533-8.
9. Crain EF, Gershel JC, Mezey AP. Caustic ingestion: Symptoms as predictors of esophageal injury. Am J Dis Child. 1984;138:863-5.
10. Betalli P, Falchetti D, Giuliani S, Pane A, Dall'Oglio L, de Angelis GL, et al. Caustic ingestion in children: Is endoscopy always indicated? The results of an Italian multicenter observational study. Gastrointest Endosc. 2008;68(3):434-9.
11. Uygun I, Aydogdu B, Okur MH, Arayici Y, Celik Y, Ozturk H, et al. Clinico-epidemiological study of caustic substance ingestion accidents in children in Anatolia: The DROOL score as a new prognostic tool. Acta Chir Belg. 2012;112(5):346-54.
12. Sharif AF, Gameel DEGE, Abdo SAE, Elgebally EI, Fayed MM. Evaluation of pediatric early warning system and drooling reluctance oropharynx others leukocytosis scores as prognostic tools for pediatric caustic ingestion:

A two-center, cross-sectional study. Environ Sci Pollut Res Int. 2022;29(4):5378-95.
13. Gorman RL, Khin-Maung-Gyi MT, Klein-Schwartz W, Oderda GM, Benson B, Litovitz T, et al. Initial symptoms as predictors of esophageal injury in alkaline corrosive ingestions. Am J Emerg Med. 1992;10(3):189-94.
14. Havanond C, Havanond P. Initial signs and symptoms as prognostic indicators of severe gastrointestinal tract injury due to corrosive ingestion. J Emerg Med. 2007;33(4):349-53.
15. Tosca J, Villagrasa R, Sanahuja A, Sanchez A, Trejo GA, Herreros B, et al. Caustic ingestion: Development and validation of a prognostic score. Endoscopy. 2021;53(8):784-91.
16. Chirica M, Resche-Rigon M, Zagdanski AM, Bruzzi M, Bouda D, Roland E, et al. Computed tomography evaluation of esophagogastric necrosis after caustic ingestion. Ann Surg. 2016;264(1):107-13.
17. Vezakis AI, Pantiora EV, Kontis EA, Sakellariou V, Theodorou D, Gkiokas G, et al. Clinical spectrum and management of caustic ingestion: A case series presenting three opposing outcomes. Am J Case Rep. 2016;17:340-6.
18. Abbas A, Brar TS, Zori A, Estores DS. Role of early endoscopic evaluation in decreasing morbidity, mortality, and cost after caustic ingestion: A retrospective nationwide database analysis. Dis Esophagus. 2017;30(6):1-11.
19. Zargar SA, Kochhar R, Mehta S, Mehta SK. The role of fiberoptic endoscopy in the management of corrosive ingestion and modified endoscopic classification of burns. Gastrointest Endosc. 1991;37(2):165-9.
20. Kochhar R, Ashat M, Reddy YR, Dhaka N, Manrai M, Sinha SK, et al. Relook endoscopy predicts the development of esophageal and antropyloric stenosis better than immediate endoscopy in patients with caustic ingestion. Endoscopy. 2017;49(7):643-50.
21. Ryu HH, Jeung KW, Lee BK, Uhm JH, Park YH, Shin MH, et al. Caustic injury: Can CT grading system enable prediction of esophageal stricture? Clin Toxicol (Phila). 2010;48(2):137-42.
22. Chirica M, Resche-Rigon M, Pariente B, Fieux F, Sabatier F, Loiseaux F, et al. Computed tomography evaluation of high-grade esophageal necrosis after corrosive ingestion to avoid unnecessary esophagectomy. Surg Endosc. 2015;29(6):1452-61.
23. Bruzzi M, Chirica M, Resche-Rigon M, Corte H, Voron T, Sarfati E, et al. Emergency computed tomography predicts caustic esophageal stricture formation. Ann Surg. 2019;270(1):109-14.
24. Lurie Y, Slotky M, Fischer D, Shreter R, Bentur Y. The role of chest and abdominal computed tomography in assessing the severity of acute corrosive ingestion. Clin Toxicol (Phila). 2013;51(9):834-7.
25. Bahrami-Motlagh H, Hadizadeh-Neisanghalb M, Peyvandi H. Diagnostic accuracy of computed tomography scan in detection of upper gastrointestinal tract injuries following caustic ingestion. Emerg (Tehran). 2017;5(1):e61.
26. Martin C, Cortegiani A, Gregoretti C, Martin-Loeches I, Ichai C, Leone M, et al. Choice of fluids in critically ill patients. BMC Anesthesiol. 2018;18(1):200.
27. Sarma MS, Tripathi PR, Arora S. Corrosive upper gastrointestinal strictures in children: Difficulties and dilemmas. World J Clin Pediatr. 2021;10(6):124-36.
28. Gümürdülü Y, Karakoç E, Kara B, Taşdoğan BE, Parsak CK, Sakman G. The efficiency of sucralfate in corrosive esophagitis: A randomized, prospective study. Turk J Gastroenterol. 2010;21(1):7-11.
29. Akhijahani RF, Farahmand F, Rahmani P, Motamed F, Eftekhari K, da Silva Magalhães EI, et al. Effectiveness of sucralfate in preventing esophageal stricture in children after ingestion of caustic agents. Eur J Pediatr. 2023;182(6):2591-6.
30. Biswas K, Bandyopadhyay U, Chattopadhyay I, Varadaraj A, Ali E, Banerjee RK. A novel antioxidant and antiapoptotic role of omeprazole to block gastric ulcer through scavenging of hydroxyl radical. J Biol Chem. 2003;278(13):10993-1001.
31. Mahawongkajit P, Tomtitchong P, Boochangkool N, Mingmalairak C, Awsakulsutthi S, Havanond C. A prospective randomized controlled trial of omeprazole for preventing esophageal stricture in grade 2b and 3a corrosive esophageal injuries. Surg Endosc. 2021;35(6):2759-64.
32. Anderson KD, Rouse TM, Randolph JG. A controlled trial of corticosteroids in children with corrosive injury of the esophagus. N Engl J Med. 1990;323(10):637-40.
33. Katibe R, Abdelgadir I, McGrogan P, Akobeng AK. Corticosteroids for preventing caustic esophageal strictures: Systematic review and meta-analysis. J Pediatr Gastroenterol Nutr. 2018;66(6):898-902.
34. Usta M, Erkan T, Cokugras FC, Urganci N, Onal Z, Gulcan M, et al. High doses of methylprednisolone in the management of caustic esophageal burns. Pediatrics. 2014;133(6):E1518-24.
35. Sheikh I, Jamshed N, Neseem A, Aggarwal P, Kedia S, Khan MA, et al. Role of high-dose methylprednisolone in Zargar Grade IIB corrosive esophageal burns: A randomized control study. Turk J Emerg Med. 2024;24(1):20-6.
36. Zabalegui A, Miján de la Torre A, Sáez-Royuela F, López Morante A, Yuguero del Moral L, Ojeda Giménez C. Lesiones gastroesofágicas graves por cáusticos: Papel del soporte nutricional [Severe gastroesophageal lesions due to caustics: The role of nutritional support]. Nutr Hosp. 1995;10(6):364-7.
37. Kochhar R, Poornachandra KS, Puri P, Dutta U, Sinha SK, Sethy PK, et al. Comparative evaluation of nasoenteral feeding and jejunostomy feeding in acute corrosive injury: A retrospective analysis. Gastrointest Endosc. 2009;70(5):874-80.
38. Chibishev A, Markoski V, Smokovski I, Shikole E, Stevcevska A. Nutritional therapy in the treatment of acute corrosive intoxication in adults. Mater Sociomed. 2016;28(1):66-70.

39. Chen CM, Chung YC, Tsai LH, Tung YC, Lee HM, Lin ML, et al. A nationwide population-based study of corrosive ingestion in Taiwan: Incidence, gender differences, and mortality. Gastroenterol Res Pract. 2016;2016:7905425.
40. Kluger Y, Ishay OB, Sartelli M, Katz A, Ansaloni L, Gomez CA, et al. Caustic ingestion management: World Society of Emergency Surgery Preliminary Survey of Expert Opinion. World J Emerg Surg. 2015;10:48.
41. Wu MH, Lai WW. Surgical management of extensive corrosive injuries of the alimentary tract. Surg Gynecol Obstet. 1993;177:12-6.
42. Andreoni B, Farina ML, Biffi R, Crosta C. Esophageal perforation and caustic injury: Emergency management of caustic ingestion. Dis Esophagus. 1997;10:95-100.
43. Landen S, Wu MH, Jeng LB, Delugeau V, Launois B. Pancreaticoduodenal necrosis due to caustic burns. Acta Chir Belg 2000;100:205-9.
44. Rigo GP, Camellini L, Azzolini F, Guazzetti S, Bedogni G, Merighi A, et al. What is the utility of selected clinical and endoscopic parameters in predicting the risk of death after caustic ingestion? Endoscopy. 2002;34:304-10.
45. Ertekin C, Alimoglu O, Akyildiz H, Guloglu R, Taviloglu K. The results of caustic ingestions. Hepatogastroenterology. 2004;51:1397-400.
46. Chou SH, Chang YT, Li HP, Huang MF, Lee CH, Lee KW. Factors predicting the hospital mortality of patients with corrosive gastrointestinal injuries receiving esophagogastrectomy in the acute stage. World J Surg. 2010;34:2383-8.
47. Zerbib P, Voisin B, Truant S, Saulnier F, Vinet A, Chambon JP, et al. The conservative management of severe caustic gastric injuries. Ann Surg. 2011;253:684-8.
48. Javed A, Pal S, Krishnan EK, Sahni P, Chattopadhyay TK. Surgical management and outcomes of severe gastrointestinal injuries due to corrosive ingestion. World J Gastrointest Surg. 2012;4:121-5.
49. Chirica M, Resche-Rigon M, Bongrand NM, Zohar S, Halimi B, Gornet JM, et al. Surgery for caustic injuries of the upper gastrointestinal tract. Ann Surg. 2012;256(6):994-1001.
50. Wu MH, Wu HY. Perioperative evaluation of patient outcomes after severe acid corrosive injury. Surg Res Pract. 2015;2015:545262.

2.13 Plant Poisons

Jasper Rathinam J, JV Peter

INTRODUCTION

Plant poisoning poses several diagnostic and management challenges. The clinical effects of plant poisoning are protean. No commercial kits are available to diagnose poisoning with specific plant toxins. In a critically ill patient, history may not be reliable and in accidental ingestion, clarity on the culprit plant and toxin may not be available. Tailored management depends on the availability of accurate information on the ingested plant. There is limited literature on the management of plant poisoning as it is less frequently encountered in clinical practice when compared with pesticides, drugs, and corrosives. Finally, no specific antidotes are available except for oleander. Hence, treatment is predominantly supportive and can be challenging in severe poisoning.

EPIDEMIOLOGY

The geographical variation in plant poisoning is determined by the nature and distribution of poisonous plants in that region as well as local beliefs and perceptions on its use as traditional medicines and as agents of deliberate self-harm (DSH). The incidence of plant poisoning in various studies varies between 1.7% and 8.2% among patients with DSH.[1-4] Among the plant poisons, oleander was the most commonly used agent in many studies despite varied geographical locations.[1,2,5] Oduvanthalai (*Cleistanthus collinus*) was the second most prevalent plant poison in a study from northern Tamil Nadu,[5] while Odollam (Glory Lily) was the most common plant poison in a coastal south Kerala district.[6] Datura was most frequently reported to the National Poisoning Centre in Delhi.[3] Accidental poisoning accounts for a minority (19.4%) of the plant poisonings, a majority of which (50%) was among children.[4]

PLANT POISONS IN INDIA

Table 1 provides a list of the common plant poisons encountered in India, their botanical names, and the common local names. Plant poisoning is categorized as cardiotoxic poisons, neurotoxic poisons, irritants, and miscellaneous. The principles of initial management and

TABLE 1: Categorization of plant poisons and their botanical and common names.

Category	Common name and botanical name	Other names/local names
Cardiotoxic	Oleander (Yellow)—*Cascabela thevetia* (or) *Thevetia peruviana*	Yellow Oleander, Karavira, Kaner, Arali, Karabi, Kadukkai, Pacha ganneru
	Oleander (Pink)—*Nerium oleander*	Rosebay, Rose Laurel, Kaner, Arali, Raktakarabi, Kabirei
	Aconite—*Aconitum ferox*	Monk's hood, Wolf's bane, Bikh, Bish, Nabhi, Mahavisha, Vatsanabha, Karunaabi
	Suicide Tree—*Cerebra odollam*	Othalam, Kattu-arali, Dabur, Chande, Pong-pong
Neurotoxic	Thorn Appl—*Datura stramonium*, D. metal	Angel's Trumpet, Devil's Apple, Jimson weed, Kanaka, Umatthai, Dhustoora
	Nux Vomica—*Strychnos nux-vomica*	Poison nut, Snake wood, Kuchila, Kanjaram, Etti, Kakrungali, Jahar
	Calotropis—*Calotropis procera, C. gigantea*	Apple of Sodom, King's crown, Giant Milkweed, Aak, Mudar, Vellai erukku
	Chickling Pea—*Lathyrus sativus*	Indian Pea, Grass pea, Lang, Khesari Dhal, Laag, Lamka,
Irritant	Castor—*Ricinus communis*	Amanakku, Erandi, Haralu, Beranda, Amudamuchettu
	Colocynth—*Citrus colocynthis*	Bitter apple, Wild Gourd, Hanjal, Indrayan, Anedri, Kattu Vellari
	Purging Croton—*Croton tiglium*	Jamalgota, Narchalam, Nepalamu, Neervalam
	Glory Lily—*Gloriosa superba*	Tiger claw, Odollam, Kalihari, Languli, Agnishike, Senganthal
	Marking Nut—*Semecarpus anacardium*	Oriental cashew, Bhilawan, Billar, Cenkottai, Theenkotta
	Himalayan Mayapple—*Podophyllum hexandrum*	Bankakri, Papra, Paadbal, Laghu Patra
	Rosary Pea—*Abrus precatorius*	Crab's eyes, Gundumani, Kunnikuru, Chanothi, Gunja
Miscellaneous	Neem—*Azadirachta indica* (Hepatotoxic)	Nimbay, Veppai, Turakabevu
	Oduvanthalai—*Cleisthanthus collinus*	Toxic gooseberry, Oduvan, Kadise, Oduku, Vadisaku, Garari, Nilappala
	Physic Nut—*Jatropa curcas*	Jamal Ghota, Maraharalu, Kattukottai, Kattamank, Nepalam, Kananeranda
	Cassava—*Cassava manioc*	Tapioca, Kappa, Maravalli Kizhangu
	Henna—*Lawsonia inermis*	Mehendi, Marudaani, Goranti, Madhurangi
	Autumn Crocus—*Colchicum autumnale*	Meadow Saffron, Gowri gedde

supportive care remain the same for plant poisons. Specific details on the individual plant poisons are discussed in the following text.

Spectrum of Clinical Manifestation

The nature and severity of manifestations would depend on the toxicity of the plant, the part that was consumed, the manner in which that part was consumed, and the quantity that was ingested. Patients may present with mild or no symptoms if the exposure is small. Severe poisoning is usually associated with a large ingestion of a highly toxic plant which is crushed and consumed in the setting of DSH or intentional recreational use.

Clinical manifestations may be broadly divided into gastrointestinal (GI), cardiac, and neurological manifestations.[7] *GI manifestations* include mucosal irritation and swelling with oral swelling or dysphagia, minor GI irritation resulting in nausea, vomiting or diarrhea, and acute gastroenteritis which usually occurs about 6 hours after consumption. Rarely, atypical symptoms like delayed gastroenteritis, hemorrhagic gastritis, rectorrhagia, and systemic toxicity may occur.[7]

Mucosal irritation is caused by chewing plants such as peace lily, rhubarb, and plants of Araceae family, which release proteolytic enzymes that cause tissue swelling and localized irritation. GI irritation leads to minor symptoms like nausea, vomiting, and diarrhea which are often self-limiting. These are commonly seen with daffodils, berries of holly, and poinsettia.[7]

Acute gastroenteritis with significant diarrhea and volume loss may be seen, sometimes with severe mucosal damage and GI bleeds. Systemic toxicity in certain plant poisons may prove fatal. Castor seed ingestion can result in renal and liver dysfunction with hemolysis, along with severe gastroenteritis. Rosary pea can be associated with central nervous system (CNS) toxicity with severe gastroenteritis. Delayed gastroenteritis with some neurological manifestations may be seen with some wild solanaceous plant consumption. Autumn crocus ingestion leads to features of colchicine toxicity which include GI toxicity with cytopenia and multiorgan failure.

Cardiac manifestations are commonly due to poisoning by plants that contain cardiac glycosides, such as oleander, odollam, and foxglove. The clinical manifestations depend on the amount of glycoside ingested. Manifestations may range from sinus bradycardia to supraventricular arrhythmia, conduction abnormalities and blocks to severe life-threatening ventricular arrhythmia and fibrillation. These agents act by inhibiting the sodium-potassium ATPase channel which maintains the resting membrane potential.[7]

Grayanotoxins, found in the pollen of some plants, affect voltage-gated sodium channels causing prolonged depolarization and bradycardia. Poisoning frequently occurs due to consumption of contaminated honey and is called mad honey disease, with few reports from Nepal.[8] Aconitine is another plant alkaloid with a similar mechanism of action and cardiotoxicity. Aconite poisoning is seen with consumption of aconitum ferox or monk's hood which is frequently used in Indian indigenous medicine. GI and neurological manifestations are also seen with aconite poisoning.[9] Other cardiac toxins are veratridine and taxines, which are not so common in India. Veratridine causes persistent opening of voltage-gated sodium channels, whereas taxines cause inhibition of sodium and calcium channels, leading to cardiotoxicity.[7]

Neurological symptoms range from anticholinergic toxidromes and seizures to encephalopathy. Anticholinergic toxidromes are due to mushroom poisoning (e.g., *Atropa belladonna*) or due to ingestion of *Datura* species. Seizures, altered behavior, and delirium could be seen. Nicotine poisoning which could be seen with tobacco ingestion or plants like poison hemlock, that have nicotinic compounds, could lead to a mixture of primary nicotinic symptoms and secondary muscarinic symptoms like cholinergic toxidrome. Seizures and status epilepticus may be seen with water hemlock poisoning. Cicutoxin, which is a neurotoxic compound, acts as a gamma-aminobutyric acid (GABA) antagonist. Encephalopathy and hypoglycemia related to litchi consumption led to high mortality among malnourished children, due to toxic compounds hypoglycin A and methylenecyclopropylglycine.[10] Hallucinations may be seen with ingestion of plants that contain lysergic acid diethylamide (LSD) or its congeners like morning glory, baby woodrose, or peyotes.

INITIAL ASSESSMENT, IDENTIFICATION OF PLANT, AND DETERMINATION OF SEVERITY

Patients who present with plant poisoning may present with three possible clinical scenarios: (1) An unconscious symptomatic patient with a possible plant poison ingestion, (2) a symptomatic patient with an unknown/known plant poison ingestion, or (3) an asymptomatic patient with a potentially poisonous plant ingestion/plant ingestion of unknown toxicity.

The initial assessment and stabilization would depend on the severity of the symptoms at presentation. Systematic management involving the *airway, breathing, circulation, disability, exposure, and elimination* (ABCDE) approach should be used as with any other poisoning. As the primary focus of management of a patient with plant poison is decontamination and supportive care, these should be initiated without any delay and further analysis into the nature of the plant poison ingested and potential toxicity should be done simultaneously.

Identification of the plant: This may be challenging, especially when the family/patient is unaware of the ingested plant. Clinical symptoms, profile, and toxidromes may help in identifying the potential plant poison. Knowledge of the local plant poison profile is also key to identifying the poison. If the plant is available or pictures of the plant/tree are available, this may be shown to help identify the incriminating agent **(Figs. 1A to H)**. If there

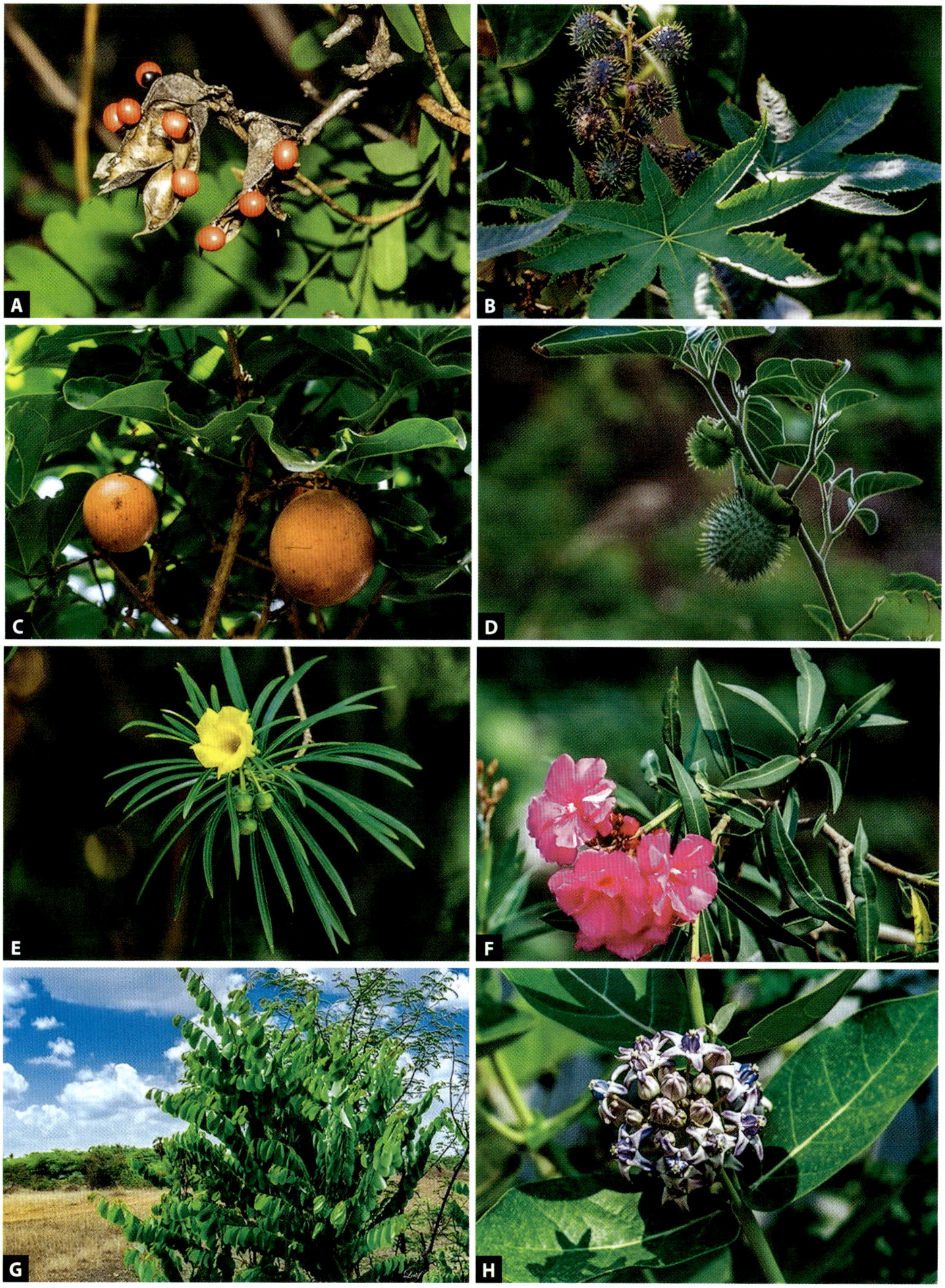

Figs. 1A to H: Common plant poisons in India. (A) Rosary Pea (*Abrus precatorius*); (B) Castor (*Ricinus communis*); (C) Strychnine (*Strychnos nux-vomica*); (D) Thorn Apple (*Datura metal*); (E) Yellow oleander (*Thevetia peruviana*); (F) Pink oleander (*Nerium oleander*); (G) Oduvanthalai (*Cleistanthus collinus*); (H) Calotropis (*Calotropis procera*).
Courtesy: Dr Latif Rajesh Johnson, Department of Forensic Medicine, CMC, Vellore.

TABLE 2: Factors that help in determining the severity of poisoning.

Plant-related factors	*Patient-related factors*	*Clinical features*
Identity of the plant	Age	Severity of symptoms
Quantum ingested	Co-morbidities	Poison severity score
Part ingested (varies between plants)	Delay in presentation	
Mode of ingestion (crushed leaves, decoction increase toxicity)	Co-ingestions	
Route of exposure (oral, skin, inhalational)		

are difficulties, it would be better to contact a regional poison center for expert advice and identification. Parts of the plant, if available, and gastric contents should be stored for further analysis or expert opinion if the identity of the plant cannot be established.

Severity assessment: This is critical in order to determine the place of admission, prognosis, and complications for symptomatic patients and the duration of observation for asymptomatic and stable patients. The key factors that can help in assessing the severity of poisoning are summarized in **Table 2** and include plant-related factors, patient-related factors, and clinical presentation. This can guide further levels of care and monitoring.

CARDIOTOXIC PLANTS

Oleander

Yellow oleander is a common poisonous plant used for DSH in rural India. Pink oleander is also widely available in India. Clinically, the presentation resembles "digoxin toxicity." It can be fatal if a large amount is ingested. The mortality is 5–6.7% for yellow oleander poisoning.[11,12] Both yellow and pink oleander were used earlier in native Indian medicine.[13] Occasionally, ingestion due to native medical management could also lead to toxicity.

Toxicology

All parts of the Oleander plants are toxic.[14] Commonly, plant seeds and leaves are consumed.[11] The toxic compounds are cardiac glycosides which have a steroid ring, sugar, and an alkyl group. Pink oleander contains oleandrin, rosagenin, digitoxigenin, folinerin, and nerin, while yellow oleander contains thevetin A, thevetin B, nerifolin, cerebrin, rutoside, and peruvoside.

The cardiac glycosides act by blocking the sodium-potassium ATPase pump.

Clinical Features

Clinical features of yellow and pink Oleander poisoning closely mimic digoxin toxicity. Initially, patients develop GI symptoms in the form of nausea, vomiting, diarrhea, and abdominal pain and occasionally numbness and burning in the mouth. This is followed by cardiac toxicity, and occasionally neurological symptoms may also be seen. Cardiac toxicity can lead to both bradycardic rhythms such as varying degrees of heart blocks, sinus bradycardia, sinus arrest, and junctional bradycardia. Tachyarrhythmias in the form of ventricular tachycardia or fibrillation, junctional tachycardia, atrial tachyarrhythmias, and occasionally atrial fibrillation can lead to hemodynamic instability or circulatory arrest.[11,14,15] CNS symptoms that may be observed are lethargy, fatigue, dizziness, and rarely convulsions and coma. The severity of symptoms depends on the amount of toxin consumed. Hyperkalemia is an indicator of severe toxicity and is associated with fatal cardiac arrhythmias and mortality.[16]

Management

Management of oleander poisoning can be approached as initial management and decontamination, management of cardiotoxicity, and definitive management.

Initial management and decontamination: These patients need continuous electrocardiographic (ECG) monitoring in a high dependency unit (HDU) or intensive care unit (ICU), particularly when there are ECG abnormalities. Decontamination can be done with gastric lavage and activated charcoal if presentation is within 1–2 hours following ingestion. Multidose-activated charcoal (MDAC) given up to 24 hours following ingestion was shown to be of benefit in a large single-center randomized controlled trial (RCT) in the early 2000s.[12] However, a subsequent large RCT, which included 36% of patients with oleander poisoning, did not show any added benefit with MDAC when compared with single-dose-activated charcoal.[17] The proposed mechanism of benefit of activated charcoal is by interrupting delayed absorption and enterohepatic circulation of the toxin. Pharmacokinetic studies have not shown added benefit with repeated doses of charcoal when compared with a single dose.[18]

Management of Cardiotoxicity: Bradycardia is managed medically with atropine and other chronotropic agents, and if refractory, a temporary pacemaker can be considered. The benefit of prophylactic pacemaker insertion is unclear with the current evidence.[15] It is suggested that high-risk patients with lethal dose ingestion, hyperkalemia, and life-threatening ECG abnormalities could be treated. Fatal ventricular arrhythmias are managed with lidocaine or phenytoin. Amiodarone is not preferred as it can decrease clearance of cardiac glycosides and further worsen the atrioventricular (AV) conduction. Calcium infusion should also be avoided in view of the possibility of intracellular calcium overload and cardiac standstill. Other extracorporeal methods for drug removal are ineffective and not recommended.

Definitive management: The only definitive therapy available is digoxin antibodies, which have reactivity to many of the oleander toxins. Both observational and RCT data show clinical efficacy of Digibind in severe cases.[19,20] A dose of 10 vials is recommended for adults. Availability and cost make the use of digoxin antibodies impractical in many resource-limited settings.

Datura Poisoning

Datura is a common Indian shrub with frequent reports of deliberate and accidental poisonings. It accounted for 3% of plant poisons in a large study from south India.[1] Another observational study from north India reported datura as the most common (65%) plant poison ingested.[3] Datura has been one of the commonly used plant poisons historically, both for self-harm and as a homicidal agent.[21] Recent reports of datura poisoning from other countries are more often accidental than deliberate.[22]

Toxicology

All parts of the plant are toxic. Flowers have the highest content of alkaloids, but the seeds are the most commonly ingested part.[14] The toxic constituents are called belladonna alkaloids which are seen in *Atropa belladona*, another toxic plant of the same *Solanaceae* family. They have antimuscarinic effects and lead to a clinical syndrome of anticholinergic toxidrome. The belladonna alkaloids include scopolamine (hyoscine), atropine, and hyoscyamine (tropane alkaloids). There are numerous other tropane and nontropane alkaloids that have been identified.[23]

Clinical Features

The clinical features could be classified as peripheral and central, with central features indicating more severity of intoxication **(Table 3)**. The peripheral features include

TABLE 3: Clinical features of datura poisoning.

Feature	***Clinical manifestation and mechanism***	***Description***
Peripheral features		
Skin	Loss of sweat, cutaneous vasodilation compensating to dissipate heat	*"Red as a beet"* *"Dry as a bone"*
Hyperthermia	Anhidrotic, due to inability to sweat	*"Hot as a hare"*
Eye	Mydriasis with loss of accommodation	*"Blind as a bat"*
Bladder	Detrusor and sphincter dysfunction	*"Full as a flask"*
Central features		
CNS stimulation	Anxiety, agitation, delirium	*"Mad as a hatter"*
Eye	Visual hallucinations, diplopia	–
Speech	Dysarthria	–
Cerebellar	Ataxia	–
Late stages	Coma, seizures	–

(CNS: central nervous system)

loss of sweating, hyperthermia, mydriasis, and detrusor and sphincter dysfunction, leading to urinary retention. Clinical features include anxiety, agitation, delirium, hallucinations, dysarthria, and ataxia and in severe intoxication, coma, seizures, and death. The clinical presentation may range from mild peripheral features to severe central features that can be life-threatening, depending upon the amount of alkaloids ingested.[22,24] Tachycardia and tachypnea could be of concern to the intensivist and rarely cardiac arrhythmias, rhabdomyolysis, and paralytic ileus may develop.

Management

Supportive care and monitoring are sufficient in most patients with peripheral symptoms. If presentation is early, gastric decontamination with gastric lavage and/or activated charcoal could be done if the airway is secure. Sinus tachycardia may not need any intervention as long as there are no major hemodynamic effects. Hyperthermia must be managed aggressively with cooling measures, to prevent the development of rhabdomyolysis and other complications.[14]

Agitation and anxiety can be managed with benzodiazepines. Typical antipsychotics like haloperidol (butyrophenones) and phenothiazines should be avoided as they have anticholinergic actions. Atypical antipsychotics have milder anticholinergic effects, but it is still better to avoid them.

In patients with severe central features unresponsive to benzodiazepines, physostigmine, which functions as an antidote, can be considered. Other cholinesterase inhibitors like neostigmine and pyridostigmine cannot be used as they do not cross the blood–brain barrier and do not reverse the CNS effects of the alkaloids. Physostigmine's clinical efficacy has been shown in trials,[25] but safety concerns and the possibility of life-threatening cholinergic crisis have not led to standard use of this agent in datura poisoning. If it is used, a dose of 0.5–1 mg every 10–15 minutes may be safer than earlier rapid protocols which used 2 mg doses every 5 minutes, which has a much higher risk of adverse reactions.[25] Rivastigmine has CNS penetration and a longer half-life but has not been studied yet for this indication.

Strychnine Poisoning

Nux Vomica is derived from Latin and means the nut that causes vomiting. It is a relatively common plant poison encountered in India, with both suicidal ingestion and accidental exposure to strychnine-based rodenticides. Strychnine accounted for 3% of plant poisons in a large observational study in south India.[1]

Toxicology

The toxic parts are the seeds, bark, and leaves.[26] The toxic compounds include strychnine, brucine, and loganin.[27] Strychnine has the maximum toxicity while brucine has a milder, similar clinical effect. They act as competitive antagonists at the postsynaptic glycine receptors and lead to loss of inhibition of the spinal interneurons, leading to uncontrolled muscle contractions and spasms. Spinal sympathetic outflow is also blocked, but it is a minor effect. The half-life of strychnine is about 12 hours with first-order kinetics.[28]

Clinical Features

The severity of symptoms depends upon the amount of the strychnine consumed; 1–2 mg/kg is considered as a lethal dose, but reports of survival at much higher doses have been reported.[27,28] Poisoning consists of an initial prodrome characterized by anxiety, hyperreflexia, mydriasis, clonus and neck and facial rigidity. Vomiting, though part of the name, is a rare manifestation. This is followed by the clinical stage, which is characterized by the classical spinal seizure, seizure-like movements with preserved consciousness. In severe cases, there may be opisthotonic posturing and facial grimacing (risus sardonicus) as a part of the spasms. Spasms may be induced by stimulation.

The other differentials which closely resemble strychnine poisoning are tetanus, meningitis, seizures, rabies, hypocalcemic tetany and also the rigidity of serotonin syndrome and neuroleptic malignant syndrome. The spasms may lead to further complications like respiratory muscle paralysis and death, rhabdomyolysis, hyperthermia, and lactic acidosis.[28-30]

Management

The mainstay of management is supportive care. There are no antidotes for strychnine poisoning. MDAC may have a theoretical benefit. Symptoms generally resolve if we manage to tide over the critical phase, without the development of fatal complications.[31] Muscle spasms are managed with benzodiazepines such as diazepam or lorazepam through GABA mimetic action on the motor neurons. Other agents that can be used are propofol and barbiturates, but the agents frequently necessitate the need for mechanical ventilation. Intubation and mechanical ventilation with sedation and muscle relaxant are indicated in uncontrollable spasms, hyperthermia, and severe metabolic acidosis. Succinylcholine must be avoided as it may worsen the spasms and to avoid fatal hyperkalemia. Rhabdomyolysis and hyperkalemia, if developed, must be managed aggressively.

Oduvanthalai Poisoning

Cleistanthus collinus is a common poisonous plant consumed in southern India. It is a deciduous toxic shrub that grows in central and south India and parts of Africa and Malaysia.[32] In a large observational study from Vellore, oduvanthalai was the second most common plant poison consumed, accounting for 30.2% of plant poisoning.[5] Numerous case reports have been reported from south India from early 1900s till date. There are a few reports from Bengal but no reports from North India.[32]

Toxicology

All parts of the plant are toxic. Leaves are commonly used in human poisoning. The toxic compounds include the *arylnaphthelene lignin lactones, diphyllin,* and *collinusin. Cleistanthin* A and B are glycoside derivatives of diphyllin. The other toxic compounds are cleistanthin C, D, and cleistanone.[33,34]

Numerous mechanisms have been proposed for the action of these toxins, such as potassium channel blockade, alpha adrenergic blockade, adenosine triphosphate (ATP) and glutathione depletion, sodium-potassium pump inhibition, DNA synthesis blockade, vacuolar ATPase inhibition, mitochondrial uncoupling, and oxidative damage. However, the exact pathophysiology of acute respiratory distress syndrome (ARDS), vasodilatory shock, and distal renal tubular acidosis is not established.[35-38]

Clinical Features

Clinical presentation is very varied, depending on the amount of toxins ingested and ranges from asymptomatic to mild GI symptoms to life-threatening arrhythmias and ARDS and refractory shock.[32]

Gastrointestinal symptoms include nausea, vomiting, abdominal pain, diarrhea, constipation, dysphagia, and ileus. Cardiorespiratory symptoms include chest pain, dyspnea, tachypnea, tachycardia, hypotension, bradycardia, and cyanosis. Neurological symptoms comprising mydriasis, altered sensorium, tremors, giddiness, dysarthria, and visual disturbances may be observed.

Laboratory abnormalities include severe hypokalemia requiring huge amounts of potassium replacement, normal anion gap metabolic acidosis, leukocytosis, elevated liver enzymes, and rarely hyponatremia, hyperbilirubinemia, coagulopathy, and elevated creatine phosphokinase.

Hypokalemia with metabolic acidosis is due to a toxin-induced renal tubular acidosis which is seen in almost two-thirds (62.5%) of patients.[35] ARDS may also develop and prove fatal. Refractory shock with vasodilation and a possible cardiogenic component is seen, which frequently proves fatal. Life-threatening conduction abnormalities and arrhythmias also lead to mortality. Mortality ranges from 12.5 to 56% among a large case series.[32] The presence of acute kidney injury (AKI), acute hypoxic respiratory failure needing mechanical ventilation, shock, and metabolic acidosis were poor prognostic markers. Hypokalemia was not associated with mortality.[39]

Management

Oduvanthalai should be considered in patients with unknown poisoning presenting with hypokalemia, metabolic acidosis, and kaliuresis. Supportive care is the mainstay as there are no antidotes available. Gastric decontamination with gastric lavage and activated charcoal could be considered if presentation is early and airway is secure, since the poisoning may prove fatal, and no antidotes are available.

Specific supportive therapy in these patients would be aggressive correction of hypokalemia and metabolic acidosis. Hypokalemia may precipitate fatal arrhythmias. If AKI worsens with oliguria setting in, renal replacement therapy (RRT) must be initiated as early as possible. For shock, fluid management and vasopressor support should be based on the dynamic assessment of volume responsiveness, cardiac function, and safety of filling due to possible co-existent ARDS and AKI. Central venous pressure (CVP)-based guidelines that were recommended earlier[32] may not be relevant anymore, given advances in the understanding of assessment of fluid responsiveness in critically ill patients.[40] ARDS should be managed with standard of care lung-protective mechanical ventilation and prone positioning, if required. QTc prolongation is common. If there are conduction abnormalities with bradycardia, prophylactic transvenous pacing can be considered. There are no practice-changing RCTs available to help us in these sensitive decision points. N-acetyl cysteine (NAC), a thiol containing compound, and

L-cysteine have been tried as antidotes with no evidence of clear benefit.[41]

Odollam Poisoning

Cerbera odollam, commonly called "suicide tree," is a poisonous plant encountered in the southern state of Kerala. It is a medium-sized tree with a fruit that resembles a mango but is highly toxic. It accounts for 50% of plant poisonings in Kerala and about 10% of all poisonings in Kerala.[42] In a large review, 30% of all poisonings were due to *Cerbera odollam*. It has a mortality rate of about 16.7%.[6]

Toxicology

The most toxic part is the kernel of the fruit.[43] The toxic compounds include cerebrin and nerifolin. The mechanism of action is like a cardiac glycoside with action on the sodium-potassium ATPase pump, causing inhibition of the pump, like digoxin.

Clinical Features

Clinical presentation of *Cerbera odollam* poisoning is similar to digoxin toxicity and oleander poisoning. Abdominal, neurological, and cardiac symptoms are seen. Thrombocytopenia has been noticed as a prominent feature in some large case series.[44] The severity of symptoms ranges from mild nausea, vomiting, and abdominal pain to severe neurological and cardiac manifestations. Common ECG abnormalities are sinus bradycardia, sinus pauses, first- and second-degree heart block, and complete heart block; fatal ventricular arrhythmias are also reported.[43,44] Headache, altered sensorium, drowsiness, and visual disturbances are the common neurological symptoms.

The severity of poisoning depends on the amount of the kernel of the fruit that is consumed. Other predictors of mortality that were noted were hyperkalemia, thrombocytopenia, hypotension, and bradycardia.[45]

Management

The management of odollam poisoning is similar to the management of oleander. The potential antidote is antidigoxin antibodies due to the similar profile of the toxin. There are reports of its benefit from case report outside India, where odollam was consumed for DSH after purchasing the seeds of the plant sold online for ornamental purposes.[43,46] Due to the cost and availability issues, Digibind has not been used yet in the reports from other countries.

Other supportive measures remain the same. If the presentation is early, then gastric decontamination may be considered. If there is a significant risk of bradyarrhythmia and signs of fatal cardiac toxicity, temporary pacemaker insertion can be done.[6] There is no evidence for prophylactic pacemaker insertion. Hyperkalemia can be managed with insulin dextrose. Calcium should be avoided for the same reason as in oleander poisoning.

Irritant Poisons

Plants that come under irritant poisons include castor,[47] colocynth,[48] glory lily,[49] marking nut,[50] and rosary pea.[51] The toxicology and the symptoms and signs are summarized in **Table 4**. Broadly, depending on the plant to which the patient was exposed or consumed, manifestations include topical skin manifestations (dermatitis, blisters, and eruptions), GI manifestations

TABLE 4: Irritant plant poisons.

Irritant	*Toxicology*	*Clinical features*
Castor[47]	Ricin—toxalbumin	• Abdominal pain, vomiting, diarrhea • Hemorrhagic gastritis • Renal failure and CNS symptoms—severe toxicity
Colocynth[48]	Saponin	• Vomiting, diarrhea, shock • Tenesmus, rectal erosions, and bleeding— rectorrhagia
Glory Lily[49]	Colchicine, Gloriosine, Superbine	• Initially gastroenteritis • Later multiorgan dysfunction and cytopenias • Long-lasting toxicity
Marking Nut[50]	Semicarpol, Bhilawanol	• Topical—dermatitis, blisters, eruptions • Ingestion—oral and throat blisters, gastroenteritis, tachycardia, dyspnea, cyanosis
Rosary Pea[51]	Abrin—toxic component inhibits protein synthesis and causes endothelial damage and leaky capillaries	• Parenteral or inhalation—fatal • Ingestion—vomiting, diarrhea, dysentery, abdominal pain, rarely renal failure, cerebral edema • Mortality—5.3%

(CNS: central nervous system)

(abdominal pain, nausea, vomiting, and diarrhea), GI bleeding, renal failure, CNS symptoms, and rarely multiorgan failure **(Table 4)**.

Management

The management principles of most of these poisons are the same. As no antidotes are available, supportive care with appropriate fluid resuscitation, management of electrolyte imbalances, and ensuring vital organ perfusion and function are the key to the management of these patients. Gastric decontamination may be useful in early presentation with no obvious upper airway or GI irritation or inflammation. Granulocyte colony-stimulating factor (G-CSF) maybe useful in glory lily poisoning with bone marrow suppression.

CONCLUSION

Plant poisoning is a common modality of DSH. Ingestions are mostly suicidal or accidental and rarely even homicidal. Supportive care is the mainstay of treatment, as antidotes are mostly not available and the only antidote that is available (Digibind) is not accessible in India. Sound knowledge of the local potential plant poisons may help in guiding appropriate supportive therapy and interventions to improve outcomes.

REFERENCES

1. Abhilash KPP, Murugan S, Rabbi NAS, Pradeeptha S, Kumar S, Selvaraj B, et al. Deliberate self-poisoning and harm: A meticulous quest of methods in vogue. J Family Med Prim Care. 2022;11(1):233.
2. Kumari M, Latha PS, Kalyanasundaram. Epidemiological and clinical profile of various plant poisons in a tertiary care center in South Tamil Nadu, India. Int J Res Med Sci. 2019;7(9):3517-21.
3. Srivastava A, Peshin SS, Kaleekal T, Gupta SK. An epidemiological study of poisoning cases reported to the National Poisons Information Centre, All India Institute of Medical Sciences, New Delhi. Hum Exp Toxicol. 2005;24(6):279-85.
4. Babu S, Chandrika D, Kulkarni M. Plant poisoning - An observational study in a tristate region emergency department. Int J Med Sci Public Health. 2016;5(10):2158.
5. Gunasekaran K, Abhilash KPP, Rabbi AS, Pradeeptha S, Pradeep R. Deliberate self-poisoning due to plant toxins: Verdant footprints of the past into the present. Indian J Crit Care Med. 2021;25(4):392-7.
6. Renymol B, Suma TK. Pattern of poisoning in a tertiary care center with special reference to odollam poisoning. J Assoc Physicians India. 2019;67(3):64-6.
7. Barbuto AF, Burns MM, Drutz JE. UpToDate; 2023. Potentially toxic plant ingestions in children: Clinical manifestations and evaluation. [online] Available from https://www.uptodate.com/ [Last accessed September, 2024].
8. Baniya A, Duwadee P, Sujata KC, Shahi M, Shrestha N, Bam PK, et al. Mad honey poisoning presenting with syncopal attack: A case report. Ann Med Surg (Lond). 2023;85(7):3649-52.
9. Tak S, Lakhotia M, Gupta A, Sagar A, Bohra G, Bajari R. Aconite poisoning with arrhythmia and shock. Indian Heart J. 2016;68:S207-9.
10. Shrivastava A, Kumar A, Thomas JD, Laserson KF, Bhushan G, Carter MD, et al. Association of acute toxic encephalopathy with litchi consumption in an outbreak in Muzaffarpur, India, 2014: A case-control study. Lancet Glob Health. 2017;5(4):e458-66.
11. Karthik G, Iyadurai R, Ralph R, Prakash V, Abhilash KP, Sathyendra S, et al. Acute oleander poisoning: A study of clinical profile from a tertiary care center in South India. J Family Med Prim Care. 2020;9(1):136.
12. de Silva HA, Fonseka MMD, Pathmeswaran A, Alahakone DGS, Ratnatilake GA, Gunatilake SB, et al. Multiple-dose activated charcoal for treatment of yellow oleander poisoning: A single-blind, randomised, placebo-controlled trial. Lancet. 2003;361(9373):1935-8.
13. Farooqui S, Tyagi T. Nerium oleander: It's application in basic and applied science: A review. Int J Pharm Pharm Sci. 2018;10(3):1.
14. Pillay VV, Sasidharan A. Oleander and datura poisoning: An update. Indian J Crit Care Med. 2019;23(S4):S250-5.
15. Thomas VV, Newbigging N, Johnson J, Kalimuthu M, Gunasekaran K, Iyadurai R. Review of current evidence in management of oleander poisoning. Current Medical Issues. 2022;20(2):82.
16. Eddleston M. Acute yellow oleander (Thevetia peruviana) poisoning: Cardiac arrhythmias, electrolyte disturbances, and serum cardiac glycoside concentrations on presentation to hospital. Heart. 2000;83(3):301-6.
17. Eddleston M, Juszczak E, Buckley NA, Senarathna L, Mohamed F, Dissanayake W, et al. Multiple-dose activated charcoal in acute self-poisoning: A randomised controlled trial. Lancet. 2008;371(9612):579-87.
18. Roberts DM, Southcott E, Potter JM, Roberts MS, Eddleston M, Buckley NA. Pharmacokinetics of digoxin cross-reacting substances in patients with acute yellow oleander (Thevetia peruviana) poisoning, including the effect of activated charcoal. Ther Drug Monit. 2006;28(6):784-92.
19. Antman EM, Wenger TL, Butler VP, Haber E, Smith TW. Treatment of 150 cases of life-threatening digitalis intoxication with digoxin-specific Fab antibody fragments. Final report of a multicenter study. Circulation. 1990;81(6):1744-52.

20. Eddleston M, Rajapakse S, Rajakanthan, Jayalath S, Sjöström L, Santharaj W, et al. Anti-digoxin Fab fragments in cardiotoxicity induced by ingestion of yellow oleander: A randomised controlled trial. Lancet. 2000;355(9208):967-72.
21. Jonasson M, Afshari R. Chronicle of datura toxicity in the 18th and 19th century. Asia Pac J Med Toxicol. 2016;5(4):101-6.
22. Khoshnam-Rad N, Heydari M, Mohammadi K, Mashayekhi M, Sahraei Z, Gholami K. Datura poisoning in a family: Case series and literature review. Clin Case Rep. 2022;10(7):e6091.
23. Choudhary M, Sharma I, Agrawal DC, Dhar MK, Kaul S. Neurotoxic potential of alkaloids from thorn apple (datura stramonium L.): A commonly used Indian folk medicinal herb. New York: SpringerLink; pp. 339-420.
24. Islam K, Khatun N, Seth S, Datta AK. Clinical features and adverse prognostic indicators in datura poisoning in children. Indian Pediatr. 2022;59(8):652-3.
25. Dawson AH, Buckley NA. Pharmacological management of anticholinergic delirium - theory, evidence and practice. Brit J Clin Pharma. 2016;81(3):516-24.
26. Ponraj L, Mishra A, Koshy M, Carey RB. A rare case report of Strychnos nux-vomica poisoning with bradycardia. J Family Med Prim Care. 2017;6(3):663-5.
27. Evans WC, Evans D. Chapter 26 - Alkaloids. In: Evans WC, Evans D, (Eds). Trease and Evans' Pharmacognosy, 16th edition. Philadelphia: W.B. Saunders; 2009 pp. 353-415.
28. Wood DM, Webster E, Martinez D, Dargan PI, Jones AL. Case report: Survival after deliberate strychnine self-poisoning, with toxicokinetic data. Crit Care. 2002;6(5):456.
29. Shadnia S, Moiensadat M, Abdollahi M. A case of acute strychnine poisoning. Vet Hum Toxicol. 2004;46(2):76-9.
30. Palatnick W, Meatherall R, Sitar D, Tenenbein M. Toxicokinetics of acute strychnine poisoning. J Toxicol Clin Toxicol. 1997;35(6):617-20.
31. Dasari S, Naha K. A rare case of strychnine poisoning by consumption of Strychnos nux-vomica leaves. Asian Pac J Trop Biomed. 2011;1(2):S303-4.
32. Chrispal A. Cleistanthus collinus poisoning. J Emerg Trauma Shock. 2012;5(2):160-6.
33. Parasuraman S, C M. GC–MS analysis of leaf extracts of Cleistanthus collinus Roxb. (Euphorbiaceae). Int J Pharm Sci. 2009;1:284-6.
34. Ramesh C, Ravindranath N, Ram TS, Das B. Arylnaphthalide lignans from Cleistanthus collinus. Chem Pharm Bull. 2003;51(11):1299-300.
35. Nampoothiri K, Chrispal A, Begum A, Jasmine S, Gopinath KG, Zachariah A. A clinical study of renal tubular dysfunction in *Cleistanthus collinus* (Oduvanthalai) poisoning. Clin Toxicol. 2010;48(3):193-7.
36. Kettimuthu KP, Lourthuraj AA, Manickam AS, Subramani S, Ramachandran A. Mechanisms of toxicity of *Cleistanthus collinus*: Vacuolar ATPases are a putative target. Clin Toxicol. 2011;49(6):457-563.
37. Kettimuthu KP, Kini A, Manickam AS, Lourthuraj AA, Venkatraman A, Subramani S, et al. Cleistanthus collinus poisoning affects mitochondrial respiration and induces oxidative stress in the rat kidney. Toxicol Mech Methods. 2019;1-8.
38. Subramani S, Maneksh D, Sidharthan A, Kettimuthu K, Kanthakumar P, Lourthuraj A, et al. Cleistanthus collinus induces type I distal renal tubular acidosis and type II respiratory failure in rats. Indian J Pharmacol. 2010;42(3):178.
39. Mohan A, Naik Gs, Harikrishna J, Kumar Dp, Rao M, Sarma K, et al. Cleistanthus collinus poisoning: Experience at a medical intensive care unit in a tertiary care hospital in south India. Indian J Med Res. 2016;143(6):793.
40. Monnet X, Shi R, Teboul JL. Prediction of fluid responsiveness. What's new? Ann Intensive Care. 2022;12(1):46.
41. Mohan A, Harikrishna J. Cleistanthus collinus poisoning. Indian J Crit Care Med. 2019;23(S4): S256-9.
42. Gaillard Y, Krishnamoorthy A, Bevalot F. Cerbera odollam: A "suicide tree" and cause of death in the state of Kerala, India. J Ethnopharmacol. 2004;95(2-3):123-6.
43. Menezes RG, Usman MS, Hussain SA, Madadin M, Siddiqi TJ, Fatima H, et al. Cerbera odollam toxicity: A review. J Forensic Legal Med. 2018;58:113-6.
44. Menon MS, Kumar P, Jayachandran CI. Clinical profile and management of poisoning with suicide tree: An observational study. Heart Views. 2016;17(4):136-9.
45. Renymol B, Palappallil D, Ambili N. Study on clinical profile and predictors of mortality in *Cerbera odollam* poisoning. Indian J Crit Care Med. 2018;22(6):431-4.
46. Bernshteyn M, Adams SH, Gada K. A case of attempted suicide by *Cerbera odollam* seed ingestion. Case Rep Crit Care. 2020;2020:1-5.
47. Abbes M, Montana M, Curti C, Vanelle P. Ricin poisoning: A review on contamination source, diagnosis, treatment, prevention and reporting of ricin poisoning. Toxicon. 2021;195:86-92.
48. Javadzadeh HR, Davoudi A, Davoudi F, Valizadegan G, Goodarzi H, Mahmoodi S, et al. Citrullus colocynthis as the cause of acute rectorrhagia. Case Rep Emerg Med. 2013;2013:652192.
49. Unnikrishnan R, Akhila C. Gloriosa superba poisoning—A case report. Indian J Respir Care. 2022;2(2):336-8.
50. Gupta P (Ed). Poisonous plants. In: Illustrated Toxicology. MA: Academic Press; 2018. pp. 309-29. (Chapter 11)
51. Karthikeyan A, Amalnath SD. Abrus precatorius poisoning: A retrospective study of 112 patients. Indian J Crit Care Med. 2017;21(4):224-5.

2.14 Poisonings and Envenomations by Marine Toxins

Ravikar Ralph, Ahmad Khaldun Ismail

INTRODUCTION

Marine poisonings and envenomations encompass a broad spectrum of injuries caused by exposure to various marine organisms. The clinical severity of these incidents can range from mild local pain to rapidly progressive organ failure. Envenomations typically occur when venomous animals inject a mixture of toxins, usually peptides and proteins, into the tissues of target organisms through stingers, spines, or fangs which cause mechanical injury to intact physical barriers.[1] In contrast, poisonings result from ingesting toxins present in certain marine species, often consumed as seafood.[1]

This chapter aims to outline the clinical aspects of major types of poisonings and envenomations from marine organisms that can lead to severe and life-threatening conditions requiring critical-care approaches for their management. The chapter is divided into two major sections: Marine food poisonings (Section 1) and marine envenomations (Section 2), respectively. Important principles of management have been discussed collectively at the end of each section in order to avoid repetition and maintain clarity.

SECTION 1: MARINE FOOD POISONING

Prompt identification and monitoring of seafood poisonings are crucial since patients can rapidly develop life-threatening neurological or cardiorespiratory disturbances. Detailed history-taking regarding exposure to seafood coupled with a comprehensive physical examination is vital in determining likely toxins and their effects on the body. While poisoning from marine biotoxins is classically associated with digestive symptoms, several types can cause acute and chronic neurological signs as seen in ciguatera, shellfish, and tetrodotoxin poisoning. The histaminergic effects of scombroid fish poisoning can lead to a wide range of symptoms, which may vary significantly based on the specific toxins present and their levels in the contaminated seafood.

Ciguatera

Ciguatera poisoning follows ingestion of large predatory fish, notably barracuda, grouper, snapper, and amberjack through accumulation of ciguatoxins in their flesh. Ciguatoxins are a potent nonprotein cyclic polyether neurotoxin with subtypes and related toxins. They are lipid soluble, colorless and tasteless, not destroyed by cooking or gastric acid, and can be transferred across the placenta and by breast milk. Their toxicological effects are attributed to their ability to cause persistent activation of voltage-gated sodium channels, increase neuronal excitability and neurotransmitter release, impair synaptic vesicle recycling, and induce cell swelling. Additionally, at high doses, they can block voltage-gated potassium channels.[2]

Ciguatoxins are produced by dinoflagellates like *Gambierdiscus* spp. and bioaccumulate in the marine food chain when toxic dinoflagellates are consumed by herbivorous fish that are then preyed upon by larger carnivorous fish. While the toxin is not overtly potent initially, ingestion by fish results in ciguatoxin biotransformation, creating much more potent analogs.

Epidemiology

With approximately 50,000 reported cases each year, ciguatera stands as the foremost preventable cause of fish-poisoning worldwide.[3] Endemic to tropical and subtropical coral reef waters, including the Pacific Basin, Indian Ocean, and Caribbean Sea, the prevalence is particularly pronounced in regions between 35° of northern and southern latitude.[3]

Clinical Features

Clinical manifestations exhibit considerable variability, demanding a heightened clinical suspicion for accurate diagnosis. Symptoms can be broadly categorized into gastrointestinal, cardiac, neurological, and pain. Gastrointestinal symptoms, such as nausea, vomiting, abdominal pain, and diarrhea, typically manifest within 1–6 hours. Neurological symptoms may take up to 48 hours to develop, encompassing paresthesia, especially perioral, a metallic taste, imbalance, dizziness, blurred vision, altered heat, and tactile perception, particularly a perception of burning pain on contact with cold objects and hallucinations. Cardiorespiratory complications, including bradycardia, respiratory depression, and cardiovascular collapse, while rare, are more likely to occur in the early stages of poisoning. Pain syndromes include odontalgia, myalgia, arthralgia, and painful micturition with regional variations in syndromes noted. The Pacific region predominantly experiences neurological effects, while the Caribbean sees greater gastrointestinal effects. Ingestion of affected fish in Indian waters presents with hallucinations, incoordination, depression, and nightmares.[2]

Neurological symptoms can recur even many years after the initial event, triggered by minor exposures to ciguatoxin or nonciguatoxin factors such as ethanol, stress, exercise, chicken, fish, and medications, including opiates and barbiturates. Fatalities are typically rare and associated with severe dehydration, cardiorespiratory failure, or cerebral edema.

Scombroid

Scombroid poisoning occurs following the consumption of spoiled fish that naturally contains high levels of histidine. Fish commonly implicated include tuna, mackerel, mahi mahi, walu walu, sardine, anchovy, bonito, herring, bluefish, amberjack, and marlin. The histidine is converted to histamine as a by-product of enzymatic decarboxylative action by histidine decarboxylase producing gram-negative enteric bacteria like *Morganella morganii, Proteus* spp., *Escherichia coli,* and *Klebsiella* spp. in fish muscle, during inadequate cold storage. When left at temperatures 20°C or higher, bacteria on the fish multiply rapidly, activating histidine decarboxylase and resulting in the accumulation of toxic levels of histamine within 2–3 hours.[4]

Epidemiology

Although initially associated with species from the *Scombridae* family, such as tuna and mackerel, scombroid poisoning has been observed in non-*Scombridae* fish like herrings, mahi-mahi, and sardines. Toxic histamine levels do not alter the taste or appearance of affected fish. Histamine is heat-stable and persists even after cooking, freezing, canning, or smoking. Many incidents occur during the summer months. However, the true global incidence of scombroid remains uncertain due to underreporting, often misdiagnosed as food allergy.[4] The USA, UK, and Japan report the highest frequency of scombroid poisoning cases, with only one recorded death worldwide.[4]

Clinical Features

Symptoms of scombroid poisoning typically manifest 10–90 minutes after ingestion, resembling classical histamine-related reactions.[5] These symptoms are frequently mistaken for food allergy. However, a negative history of previous food allergies and a history of similar symptoms in other individuals at the same location strongly suggest scombroid poisoning.[4] Symptoms encompass vomiting, diarrhea, abdominal pain, pruritus, urticaria, facial flushing, rhinorrhea, bronchospasm, and vasodilatory shock. Some patients report a metallic, bitter, or peppery taste while consuming the fish. Symptoms usually last for 6–8 hours; however, the sense of malaise can last for up to 24 hours.[4] Patients undergoing treatment with isoniazid or monoamine oxidase inhibitors tend to experience more severe and prolonged symptoms due to the inhibitory effects of these drugs on histamine catabolism.[4]

Tetrodotoxin Poisoning

Certain tetraodontiforme fish species, including pufferfish, porcupinefish, toadfish, and sunfish, can contain elevated levels of tetrodotoxin in their ovaries, viscera, and skin.[5] Tetrodotoxin, an amino perhydroquinazoline, is synthesized by various bacterial species, including *Pseudoalteromonas*, *Pseudomonas*, *Vibrio*, *Aeromonas*, and *Alteromonas* among other bacterial species.[6] This toxin exerts potent neurotoxic and cardiotoxic effects by blocking voltage-sensitive fast sodium channels, preventing neurotransmission centrally and in peripheral sensory and motor nerves.

Beyond tetraodontiforme fish, tetrodotoxin is also present in various marine organisms, including angelfish, blue-ringed octopi, moon snails (*Naticidae* spp.) and several species of starfish, xanthid crabs, horseshoe crabs, and marine worms.[6] Tetrodotoxin accumulates within these animals as bacteria move up the food chain and bioaccumulate in high-level tropic species. Being heat-stable, it remains undestroyed by cooking.[6] Most incidents of tetrodotoxin poisoning were from the consumption of improperly prepared pufferfish **(Fig. 1)**.

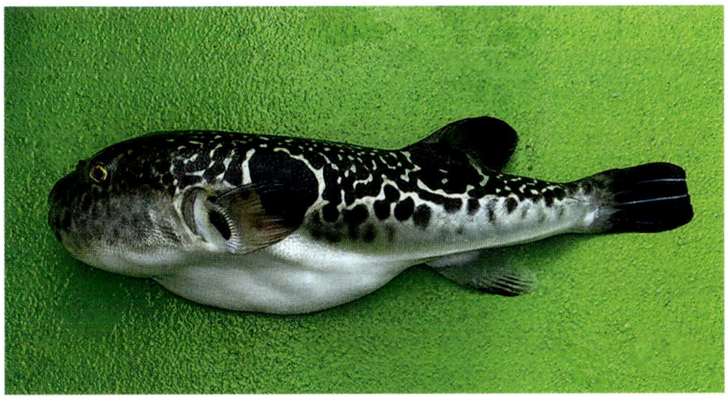

Fig. 1: Pufferfish.
Courtesy: Professor Dr Yoshito Kamijo.

Epidemiology

Accurate global data on the total number of pufferfish poisoning incidents and associated fatalities are currently unavailable. Most reported cases are from Japan, Taiwan, and other South-East Asian countries where the puffer fish (fugu) is a highly valued delicacy.[5,7] Pufferfish are also implicated in tetrodotoxin-related poisonings in Australia, Bangladesh, India, and the United States among other countries.[8-10]

Clinical Features

Clinical features of tetrodotoxin poisoning are closely related to the amount ingested. Significant poisoning primarily involves neurotoxic symptoms that manifest 10–45 minutes after ingestion. Symptoms of nausea and gastrointestinal distress closely follow. Perioral, buccal, and lingual paresthesia, altered taste, dizziness, headache, sweating, hypersalivation, and ataxia are associated with rapid ascending flaccid quadriparesis, which in severe cases can lead to respiratory failure and cardiorespiratory arrest.[5] Additional features include exfoliative dermatitis, hypotension, and arrhythmias. In instances of severe poisoning death occurs within 2–6 hours of consuming the fish.

Shellfish Poisoning

Various types of bivalve molluscs, such as mussels, clams, and oysters, filter-feed and accumulate a diverse array of toxins in microscopic algae containing these harmful substances. Most shellfish-related toxins poisoning manifest between 30 minutes and 24 hours post ingestion. It typically presents with nausea, vomiting, and diarrhea followed by additional toxin-specific clinical syndromes. These include:

- Neurotoxic shellfish poisoning (NSP)
- Paralytic shellfish poisoning (PSP)
- Amnesic shellfish poisoning (ASP)
- Diarrhetic shellfish poisoning (DSP)

Epidemiology

Accurate worldwide data on the total number of incidents and associated fatalities from shellfish poisoning are unavailable. Shellfish poisoning appears to be more prevalent in regions surrounded by temperate waters such as North America, Western Europe, and South Pacific. The frequency of certain types of shellfish poisonings like NSP and PSP increases during algal blooms, characterized by the rapid accumulation of toxin-containing dinoflagellates, sometimes resulting in a visible reddish coloration of the water known as red tide.[5,11,12]

Clinical Features

Individuals affected by NSP exhibit ciguatera-like paresthesias, involving sensations of tingling or numbness in the mouth, lips, and tongue. Additionally, distal paresthesias, including cold allodynia, are common and often accompanied by myalgias, imbalance, slurred speech, and a general loss of co-ordination.[5,13] In severe cases, symptoms can escalate to partial paralysis, and respiratory distress have been recorded.[13] Reports also frequently mention headaches, slurred speech, blurred vision due to pupillary dilatation, and general sense of fatigue. In some instances, victims may appear disoriented and exhibit signs akin to inebriation. The causative agent implicated in NSP are Brevetoxins, polycyclic ethers produced by *Karenia brevis* dinoflagellates.[13,14]

For PSP, tetrahydropurine neurotoxins like saxitoxin and gonyautoxins found in dinoflagellates such as *Alexandrium, Pyrodinium, and Gymnodinium* spp. cause predominant descending paralysis. This condition is associated with a case fatality of 8% in untreated cases.[5,13]

Amnesic shellfish poisoning is caused by domoic acid, derived from Pseudo-nitzschia diatoms consumed by bivalve molluscs and crustaceans. Symptoms include severe headache, seizures, short-term memory loss, agitation, or coma and evolve over 48 hours. Amnesia may persist permanently.

Diarrhetic shellfish poisoning caused by okadaic acid and related compounds primarily presents with gastrointestinal symptoms like nausea, vomiting, diarrhea, and abdominal pain. Symptoms commence 30 minutes to 4 hours post ingestion and can last up to 72 hours. A similar syndrome occurs in Europe after consuming mussels contaminated with Azaspiracids. These are polyether marine toxins produced by dinoflagellates of *Protoperidinium* spp. which bioaccumulate within the shellfish during filter-feeding. Symptoms begin within 6–18 hours of ingestion and can last for up to 5 days.[15]

Management of Marine Food Poisoning

Stabilization and Supportive Care

In the absence of specific treatments or antidotes, critical-care management strategies for patients with seafood poisoning prioritize effective supportive care. This encompasses airway and breathing support, hemodynamic stabilization, and close monitoring of vital parameters.

Decontamination

These measures involve the removal of gastrointestinal contents, but only if safely achievable within 1–2 hours of ingestion, and repeated dosing with activated charcoal to bind shellfish toxins and limit their enterohepatic circulation.

Specific Interventions

While the therapeutic effectiveness of early mannitol in ciguatera poisoning remains controversial, it is deemed safe in well-hydrated patients and often recommended.[5] Australian literature suggests that it is reasonable to consider early intravenous mannitol in the acute phase of the illness for maximal benefits.[16] Supporting evidence in favor of mannitol use for ciguatera poisoning includes four uncontrolled case series, one prospective, unblinded comparative trial, and several case reports.[16] Conversely, evidence against mannitol is based on a single randomized controlled trial (RCT) with a small sample size and potential limitations.[17]

Ethanol classically exacerbates ciguatera poisoning symptoms and must be avoided during the acute phase. Most cases resolve within 1 week, though severe cases may result in ongoing dysesthesias for several years.[5] While gabapentin and tricyclic antidepressants are commonly used as pain modulators in such instances, their efficacy remains unestablished.[16]

Mild to moderate scombroid poisoning symptoms respond well to antihistamines, while severe reactions may necessitate β_2-agonist bronchodilators, adrenaline, and fluid replacement.[5] Patients symptomatic of puffer fish poisoning should be admitted and monitored for peak clinical effects for at least 24 hours. The likelihood of life-threatening effects in those who have not developed them within the first 24 hours is minimal.[5]

SECTION 2: MARINE ENVENOMATIONS

Marine envenomations exhibit a wide range of severity, depending on the venomous species involved, the amount of venom injected, and the site of injury. Most injuries involve stings, bites, abrasions, and lacerations without a significant amount of venom injected into the tissue. However, envenomation from box jellyfish, cone snails, blue-ringed octopus, stonefish, or sea snakes can pose life-threatening risks. In such cases, prompt and effective treatment improves immediate outcomes but also reduces the likelihood of secondary complications.

Sea Snake Envenomations

Sea snakes are found in the warm, tropical waters of the Indian and Pacific oceans. They comprise of more than 57 species distributed across two major subfamilies (*Laticaudinae* and *Hydrophiinae*). Envenomation by sea snakes is particularly concerning due to the presence of potent neurotoxins in their venoms.[18,19]

Epidemiology

Most sea snake bites occur when fishermen attempt to remove inadvertently trapped sea snakes from fishing nets. It is an occupational hazard. Global estimates suggest that annually, 15,000–75,000 fishermen fall victims to sea snake bites. However, the accurate incidence of sea snake bites and envenomations remains uncertain, given that numerous cases occur at sea or in remote coastal fishing villages far from medical facilities. Over 90% of the victims are male and nearly 80% are fishermen bitten at their job.[20]

Sea snakes have small, fixed fangs that are easily dislodged during a bite. Most bites produce small puncture wounds or scratches without significant pain. It is estimated that only 20% of all sea snake bites result in envenoming.[19]

Clinical Features

Most sea snake species causing bites are unidentified. Typically, a sea snake bite induces minimal pain and exhibits no immediate local reaction or progressive swelling. However, in significant envenoming, patients may undergo a progression of symptoms within

30–60 minutes post bite incident. These include the onset of nausea, muscle stiffness, and pain, principally affecting muscles of the neck, trunk, and proximal limbs. Accompanying these are systemic neurotoxicity issues such as swallowing dysfunction, blurred or double vision, slurring of speech with associated difficulty in swallowing, limb paralysis, and potential for respiratory failure. These neurotoxic clinical manifestations are closely associated with systemic rhabdomyolysis, leading to dark-colored urine (myoglobinuria), myoglobin-induced acute kidney injury, and dyselectrolytemias. Notably, trismus, sustained tetanic spasms of the muscles of mastication, is a common clinical feature of myotoxic envenoming. It differs from tetanus in that it can be overcome by applying sustained pressure to the lower jaw.[21] Additional clinical features include painful extensor spasms (often triggered by touch stimulation), excessive sweating, drowsiness, and severe headache.

Cnidarian Stings

Cnidarians are members of phylum Cnidaria and encompass a diverse group of marine organisms such as jellyfishes, Portuguese Man O' War, sea anemones, and stinging corals. The hallmark of cnidarians is that they are armed with millions of specialized cells called cnidocytes. Each cnidocyte houses a specialized stinging organelle called a nematocyst. Each nematocyst consists of a cylindrical capsule loaded with venom attached to a long-coiled tube with a harpoon-like tip and hooks. Nematocyst deployment is triggered upon contact, with the spring-like tube being "explosively" expelled from within the capsule penetrating the skin accompanied by venom release into the subcutaneous tissue.[22] Cnidarian venoms are a complex mixture of peptides, vasoactive amines, prostaglandins, kinins, digestive enzymes, and ion-channel neurotoxins.[23]

Epidemiology

Jellyfish sting is the most common cause for cnidarian envenomation, with incidents more common in warm coastal waters. While most events are clinically mild, severe and potentially life-threatening envenomations are associated with stings from box jellyfish species such as *Chironex fleckeri*, *Carukia barnesi*, and *Malo kingi*, primarily reported in Australia and South-East Asia **(Fig. 2)**.[24-26] Cases largely involve younger individuals, aged between 10 and 29 years. The frequency of stinging incidents is nonuniform through the year with most cases clustering during certain months, usually between October and June.[24-26]

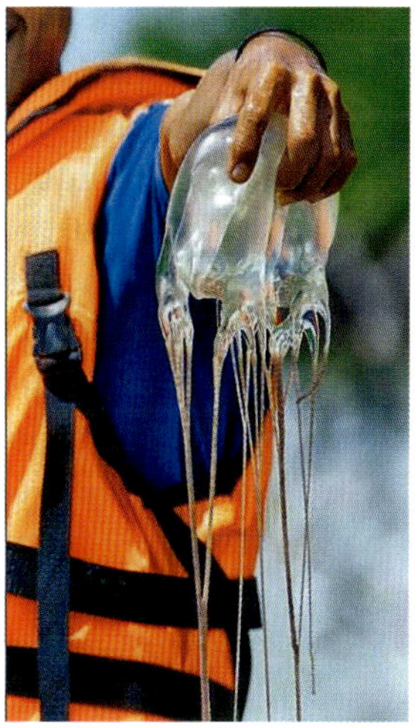

Fig. 2: Box jellyfish of *Chironex* species.
Courtesy: Professor Norhayati Ahmad.

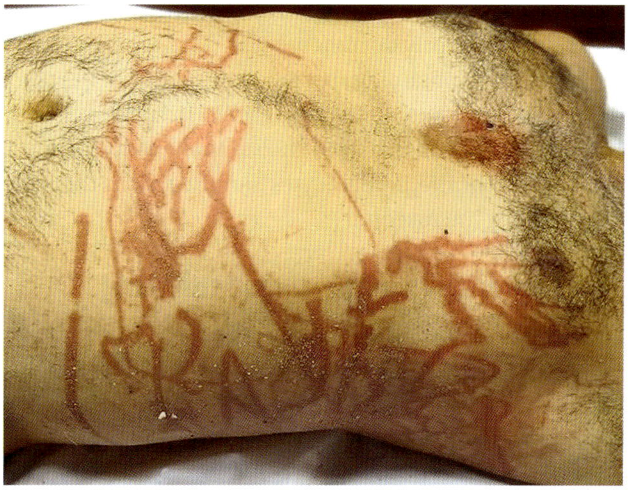

Fig. 3: Typical skin markings from a multitentacled box jellyfish sting.
Courtesy: Dr Ahmad Khaldun Ismail.

Clinical Features

Human contact with jellyfish results in the release of venom into the dermis, causing varying degrees of local discomfort, including immediate severe pain and strings of painful, irritant weal.[19] Nematocyst stings may leave a species-specific diagnostic pattern on the skin **(Fig. 3)**.[5] Systemic manifestations vary with species. Envenoming by multitentacled box jellyfish like *Chironex* spp. can lead to rapidly evolving series of cough, gastrointestinal symptoms, rigors, myalgia, and profuse sweating, progressing to pulmonary edema, seizures, and cardiorespiratory arrest.

Irukandji syndrome, most frequently associated with the smaller four tentacled box jellyfish (*Carukia barnesi, Malo kingi,* and others) is characterized by severe generalized musculoskeletal pain, delayed and persisting tremors, nausea, vomiting, anxiety, generalized sweating, headache, hypertension, raised troponin levels, and T-wave inversions on the ECG. These features manifest following a latent period of up to 60-minutes post sting.

Physalia spp. envenomation is associated with vasospasm, peripheral necrosis, nerve entrapment syndromes, intravascular hemolysis, and acute kidney injury. Individuals sensitized by prior stings may develop anaphylaxis upon subsequent exposure.[19]

There are many other jellyfish that are harmful to humans causing mixed envenomation features. However, these are still poorly documented.[27,28] This is partly due to the difficulty in obtaining species confirmation at the point of contact. Attempts at identifying jellyfish species causing the sting have been made via analyzing the morphological appearance of the nematocytes sampled from the sting sites under a microscope.

Scorpaenidae (Scorpionfish, Stonefish, and Lionfish) Stings

Numerous fish species within the *Scorpaenidae* family possesses venom glands embedded in the spines of their fins, shielded by integumentary sheaths. Venoms of these fish contain large proteinaceous toxins such as stonustoxin, verrucotoxin, and Sp-CTx. These toxins induce pores in cell membranes, resulting in cell death and triggering a cascade of pathological events that lead to many, though not all, symptoms following envenomation.[29] Additionally, fish venom contains peptides, enzymes, vasoactive kinins, 5-hydroxytryptamine, histamine, and catecholamines.[19] Among the *Scorpaenidae* family, lionfish (*Pterois* spp.) exhibit the lowest toxicity, followed by scorpionfish (*Scorpaena* spp.) with moderate toxicity, and stonefish (*Synanceia* spp.) with potent toxicity **(Figs. 4A and B)**.[19]

Epidemiology

Scorpaenidae fish predominantly inhabit the warm tropical waters of the Pacific and Indian Oceans while some species are also found in the Atlantic Ocean. Certain species like the lionfish, have become invasive nonnative species in regions such as the Caribbean and the eastern Mediterranean Sea. Though comprehensive data on the frequency of fish envenomation is lacking, case and case series reports suggest that it may be a relatively common issue among fishermen, aquarists, and fish handlers.[30,31] Most sting incidents occur when these fish are accidentally stepped on while wading near the shore and coral reefs, or handling with bare hands while cleaning the aquarium and preparing meals.

Clinical Features

Pain resulting from Scorpaenidae fish envenomation is immediate, reaching its peak at 60–90 minutes. It may

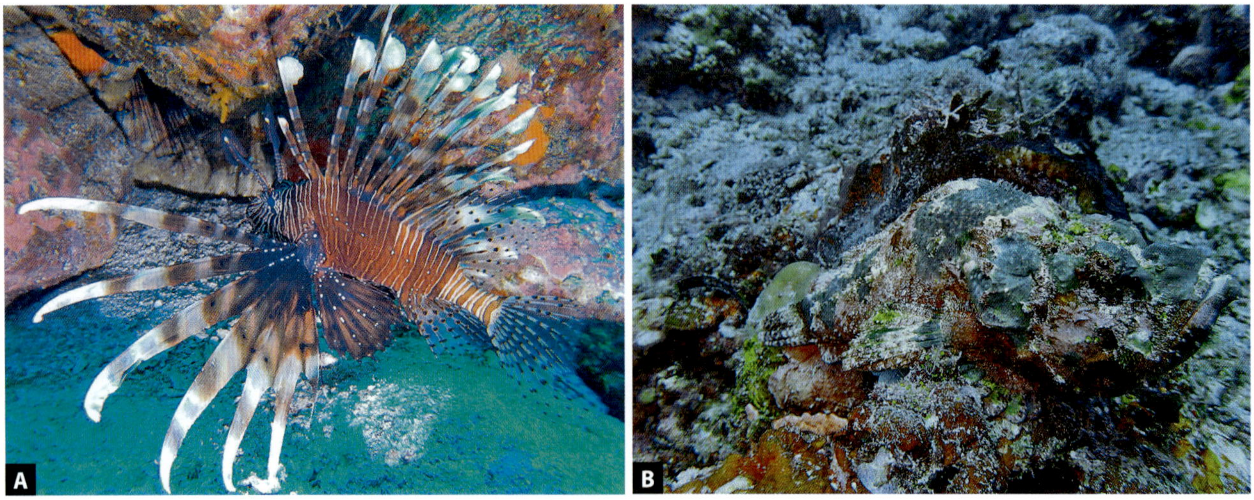

Figs. 4A and B: (A) Lionfish; (B) Stonefish.
Courtesy: (A) Professor Igor Iezhitsa; (B) Dr Muhammad Naim Ab Razak.

be intense enough to induce delirium and may persist from a few hours (scorpionfish) to days (stonefish). The puncture wound may appear ischemic and cyanotic and can progress to vesiculation, tissue sloughing, cellulitis, and necrotic ulceration. Systemic manifestations include headache, skin rash, fever, vomiting, diarrhea, abdominal pain, seizures, paralysis, pericarditis, atrioventricular blocks, and congestive cardiac failure. Death from severe stonefish envenomation is rarely reported and may occur within the first 6–8 hours post sting. Puncture wounds are often slow to heal in many instances, persisting for several months, especially when complicated with embedded foreign body and secondary marine bacterial infection.

Stingray Injuries

Stingrays are flat-bodied, cartilaginous fish that have whip-like tails with serrated, usually venomous spines made of a tough cartilaginous material called vasodentin **(Fig. 5)**. They are found around the world in both marine- and fresh-water aquatic environments. The entire structure is encased in an integumentary sheath that rips open during a sting. The barb can break off and be retained in the wound in up to 5% of cases. The serrations are directed proximally and can, therefore, cause further extensive tissue damage when the retained barb is pulled without caution out from a wound.

Envenomations can occur in up to 75% of stingray injuries. The venom is produced in secretory cells that line two ventral grooves in the spine and contains serotonin, 5′-nucleotidase, hyaluronidase, and phosphodiesterase among other toxins including cardiotoxins.

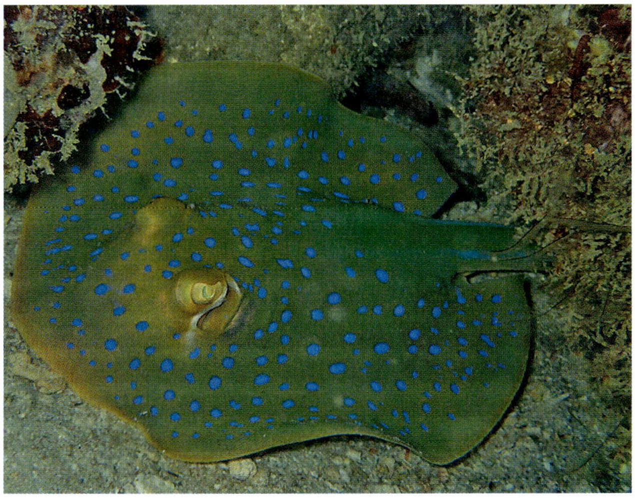

Fig. 5: Blue spotted stingray.
Courtesy: Dr Muhammad Naim Ab Razak.

Epidemiology

Stingray injuries are among the most common causes of fish-related envenomations/injuries in the world.[32] The most common site of injury is the lower limbs followed by the upper limbs.[33] The majority of marine incidents is associated with relatively low levels of morbidity.[32] However, stingray injuries can rarely result in death, either due to laceration of a major artery or organs such as heart or lungs or, less frequently, due to the envenomation itself.

Clinical Features

Patients usually present with a painful dusky laceration associated with local hemorrhage and necrosis at and around the sting site. Bleeding from the sting site can often be profuse. Local injury, especially with retained barbs, can be complicated by wound infections by *Vibrio* species and other bacteria including *Streptococcus, Staphylococcus, Aeromonas,* and *Clostridium* species. Wound infections can progress to ecthyma gangrenosum, necrotizing fasciitis, septic arthritis, septicemia, and osteomyelitis. Severe envenomations are associated with systemic symptoms including nausea, vomiting, diarrhea, salivation, muscle cramps, syncope, respiratory depression, seizures, myocardial necrosis, and arrhythmias.[33,34]

Mollusc Envenomations

Molluscs are a diverse group of invertebrates characterized by soft bodies with some being protected by an external shell. Notably, some molluscs, such as cone snails and octopus (*Hapalochlaena* spp.), produce potent neurotoxic venoms. Cone snails employ a modified harpoon-like radular tooth to inject venom into prey **(Fig. 6)**. The venom consists of neurotoxic peptides called conotoxins that target neuromuscular receptors, inducing paralysis.

Despite their small size, octopi in the genus *Hapalochlaena* are equipped with potent venom. They can be distinguished by iridescent blue rings and/or streaks on their bodies, which are vividly displayed when threatened **(Fig. 7)**. They deliver tetrodotoxin-containing venom through small bites from a retractable parrot-like beak situated ventrally in the buccal mass, surrounded by the muscular head appendages. The venom tetrodotoxins

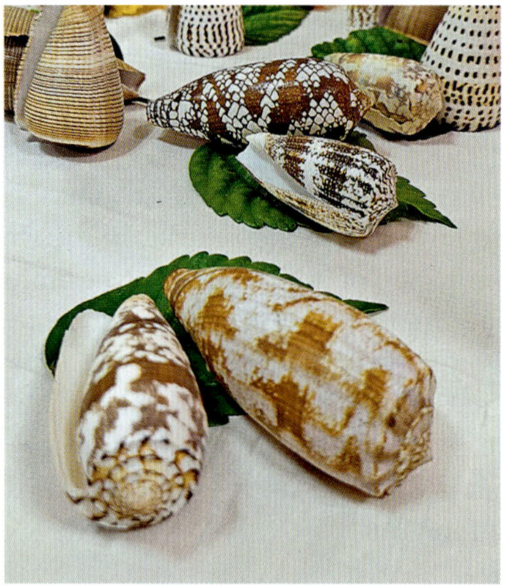

Fig. 6: Cone shells.
Courtesy: Dr Ahmad Khaldun Ismail.

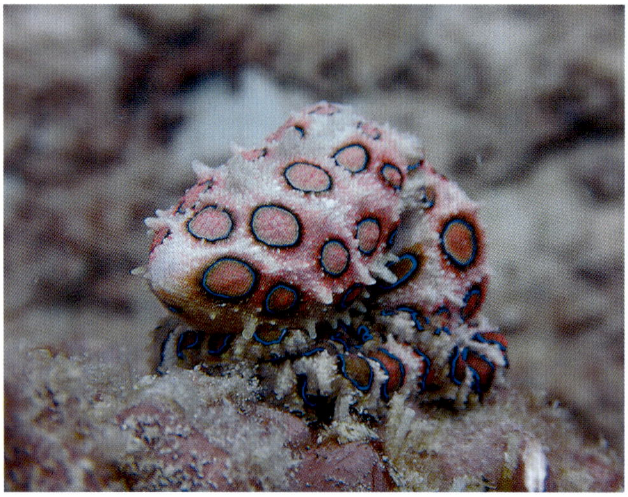

Fig. 7: Blue ring octopus.
Courtesy: Professor Igor Iezhitsa.

are produced by bacterial species residing in the posterior salivary glands of these octopi.

Epidemiology

Cone snails are predominantly found in warm waters of the Red Sea, the Caribbean and the Indian and Pacific Oceans. Due to the rarity of envenoming and limited global data, case-fatality estimates following envenomation range from 15 to 75%. The geographic cone, *Conus geometricus*, is the most toxic among known species and most human deaths were due to this species.

Venomous octopi of the genus *Hapalochlaena* are distributed in tropical to subtropical zones of the Indo-West Pacific and are particularly common in marine waters around Australia.[35] Bite envenoming incidents by venomous octopi are relatively rare, with most cases being recorded in Australia.[35]

Clinical Features

The puncture wound from cone snail stings resembles a bee sting and is associated with local cyanosis. Local paresthesia precedes progressive neuroparalysis lasting for 12–36 hours. Severe cases may result in respiratory failure, while milder envenoming presents with nausea, blurred vision, malaise, and weakness for a few hours.

Bites by venomous octopi typically result in one or two painless small-puncture wounds, often going unnoticed. Oral and facial numbness develop within 15 minutes and can rapidly progress to neuroparalysis and respiratory failure. Ingesting a poorly prepared blue-ring octopus may lead to tetrodotoxin poisoning.

Management of Marine Envenomations

Tailoring management strategies is essential for effective treatment of marine envenoming, considering the specific nature of the incident and the severity of the condition. Local protocols, medical facilities, and resources significantly influence the treatment plan. Successful management of marine envenomations typically encompasses the following key components.

Assessment and Stabilization

Given the dynamic nature of marine envenomations, rapid assessment of vital signs, airway, breathing, and circulation is imperative. Stabilization involves securing the airway, ensuring adequate oxygenation, and establishing intravenous access for fluid resuscitation.

Decontamination

Thorough removal of any remnants of marine organisms and toxins is crucial. For jellyfish stings, getting to safety and tentacle removal by carefully rinsing the affected area with seawater reduces the risk of more venom from entering the body. Vinegar application for jellyfish sting used to be a part of first-aid intervention; however, it remains controversial with recent studies suggesting that more venom is released by vinegar. The application of local anesthetic, lidocaine spray, appears to prevent nematocysts' activation and release of venom. Scorpaenidae stings may require wound irrigation and, if necessary, surgical exploration for spine extraction. Sting ray injuries require careful exploration, location, and surgical removal of the retained barb followed by serial debridement of necrotic tissue. Injuries due to a retained barb in the neck, thorax, abdomen, or groin must be treated as stab wounds.

Pain Management

Utilize analgesics, local anesthetics, or nerve blocks to effectively manage pain. Immersion of the affected limb in hot water (up to 45°C) can alleviate severe pain caused by Scorpaenidae envenomation and sting ray injuries. Regional anesthetic blocks are an effective alternative. However, to prevent scalding, hot water immersion is contraindicated in the anesthetized limb. This method may also provide pain relief for Cnidarian stings by *Chironex* and *Physalia* spp.[36]

Specific Antivenoms

Envenomations from sea snakes, multitentacled box jellyfish, and stonefish may require specific antivenom based on regional treatment guidelines. Timely administration of sea snake antivenom is crucial to prevent irreversible envenoming injury (rhabdomyolysis). Close serial observation of envenoming progression and regular blood and urine tests help to guide the decision for antivenom therapy. Box jellyfish antivenom is indicated for severe pain refractory to high-dose opioids or those with dysrhythmias or cardiorespiratory failure. Intravenous magnesium sulfate may be used for intractable pain, although evidence of its effectiveness is anecdotal. Stonefish antivenom is indicated for systemic envenoming or pain refractory to opioids, with the suggested dose being one ampoule (2000 units) per one or two puncture wounds via intramuscular (IM) injection or intravenously (IV). While this approach reliably alleviates pain, there is no evidence to suggest it reduces tissue damage.[19]

Cardiorespiratory Support

Severe neuroparalysis or cardiorespiratory arrest resulting from jellyfish or cone snail envenomations may require respiratory support. Invasive mechanical ventilation may be necessary in severe cases to maintain adequate oxygenation and support ventilation.

Adjunctive Treatment

Administer tetanus toxoid based on standard recommendations. Monitor serum electrolytes, creatine phosphokinase, and renal function closely in sea snake envenomations. Severe systemic rhabdomyolysis (CPK >10,000 U/L) may necessitate intravenous fluids, diuretics, and urinary alkalinization.[19] Acute kidney injury may require dialysis. Prophylactic cover with doxycycline 100 mg once daily or ciprofloxacin 500 mg twice daily must be considered for penetrating wounds following sting ray injuries and other fish stings, particularly when irrigation or debridement was delayed.[37]

CONCLUSION

Encounters with venomous marine organisms or ingestion of marine toxins can result in potentially life-threatening clinical consequences. The provision of critical care in marine poisonings and envenomations demands a thorough understanding of the diverse toxins, their effects, and appropriate management strategies. These strategies encompass timely recognition, prompt assessment, decontamination, continuous monitoring, supportive care, and the administration of targeted antidotes, such as antivenoms. To navigate these challenging scenarios in critical care settings, healthcare professionals and emergency response teams must stay informed and consistently trained, ensuring their readiness to address these complex and dynamic situations effectively.

REFERENCES

1. Nelsen DR, Nisani Z, Cooper AM, Fox GA, Gren ECK, Corbit AG, et al. Poisons, toxungens, and venoms: redefining and classifying toxic biological secretions and the organisms that employ them. Biol Rev Camb Philos Soc. 2014;89(2): 450-65.
2. Nicholson GM, Lewis RJ. Ciguatoxins: cyclic polyether modulators of voltage-gated Iion channel function. Mar Drugs. 2006;4(3):82-118.
3. Ting JY, Brown AF. Ciguatera poisoning: a global issue with common management problems. Eur J Emerg Med Off J Eur Soc Emerg Med. 2001;8(4):295-300.
4. Feng C, Teuber S, Gershwin ME. Histamine (Scombroid) fish poisoning: a comprehensive review. Clin Rev Allergy Immunol. 2016;50(1):64-9.
5. Warrell DA. Venomous bites, stings, and poisoning: an update. Infect Dis Clin North Am. 2019;33(1):17-38.
6. Lago J, Rodríguez LP, Blanco L, Vieites JM, Cabado AG. Tetrodotoxin, an extremely potent marine neurotoxin: distribution, toxicity, origin and therapeutical uses. Mar Drugs. 2015;13(10):6384-406.
7. Yang CC, Liao SC, Deng JF. Tetrodotoxin poisoning in Taiwan: an analysis of poison center data. Vet Hum Toxicol. 1996;38(4):282-6.

8. Islam QT, Razzak MA, Islam MA, Bari MI, Basher A, Chowdhury FR, et al. Puffer fish poisoning in Bangladesh: clinical and toxicological results from large outbreaks in 2008. Trans R Soc Trop Med Hyg. 2011;105(2):74-80.
9. Joseph TC, Goswami DB, Pradeep MA, Anupama TK, Parmar E, Renuka V, et al. Pufferfish poisoning from Arothron stellatus: the first confirmed case in India with exact DNA sequencing-based species identification. Toxicon Off J Int Soc Toxinol. 2021;200:180-2.
10. Isbister GK, Son J, Wang F, Maclean CJ, Lin CSY, Ujma J, et al. Puffer fish poisoning: a potentially life-threatening condition. Med J Aust. 2002;177(11-12):650-3.
11. Patel SS, Lovko VJ, Lockey RF. Red tide: overview and clinical manifestations. J Allergy Clin Immunol Pract. 2020;8(4):1219-23.
12. Hartigan-Go K, Bateman DN. Redtide in the Philippines. Hum Exp Toxicol. 1994;13(12):824-30.
13. Watkins SM, Reich A, Fleming LE, Hammond R. Neurotoxic shellfish poisoning. Mar Drugs. 2008;6(3):431-55.
14. Wang DZ. Neurotoxins from marine dinoflagellates: A brief review. Mar Drugs. 2008;6(2):349-71.
15. Twiner MJ, Rehmann N, Hess P, Doucette GJ. Azaspiracid shellfish poisoning: a review on the chemistry, ecology, and toxicology with an emphasis on human health impacts. Mar Drugs. 2008;6(2):39-72.
16. Mullins ME, Hoffman RS. Is mannitol the treatment of choice for patients with ciguatera fish poisoning? Clin Toxicol Phila Pa. 2017;55(9):947-55.
17. Schnorf H, Taurarii M, Cundy T. Ciguatera fish poisoning: a double-blind randomized trial of mannitol therapy. Neurology. 2002;58(6):873-80.
18. Walker MJ, Peng-Nam-Yeoh null. The in vitro neuromuscular blocking properties of sea snake (Enhydrina schistosa) venom. Eur J Pharmacol. 1974;28(1):199-208.
19. Hornbeak KB, Auerbach PS. Marine envenomation. Emerg Med Clin North Am. 2017;35(2):321-37.
20. Reid HA. Epidemiology of sea-snake bites. J Trop Med Hyg. 1975;78(5):106-13.
21. Reid HA. Sea-snake bite research. Trans R Soc Trop Med Hyg. 1956;50(6):517-38; discussion, 539-42.
22. Ozbek S. The cnidarian nematocyst: a miniature extracellular matrix within a secretory vesicle. Protoplasma. 2011;248(4):635-40.
23. Liao Q, Feng Y, Yang B, Lee SMY. Cnidarian peptide neurotoxins: a new source of various ion channel modulators or blockers against central nervous systems disease. Drug Discov Today. 2019;24(1):189-97.
24. Lippmann JM, Fenner PJ, Winkel K, Gershwin L. Fatal and severe box jellyfish stings, including irukandji stings, in Malaysia, 2000–2010. J Travel Med. 2011;18(4):275-81.
25. Nickson CP, Waugh EB, Jacups SP, Currie BJ. Irukandji syndrome case series from Australia's Tropical Northern Territory. Ann Emerg Med. 2009;54(3):395-403.
26. Mubarak AI, Wan Mohd Shukri WNA, Ismail AK. Estimation of local incidence of jellyfish envenomation in developed marine coastal areas and large populated island on the western coast of Peninsular Malaysia using case surveillance of government health facilities in Manjung, Perak and Langkawi Island. Int Marit Health. 2021;72(2):93-8.
27. Sivanasworn NK, Anantham G, Jamal SM, Hatta MM, Ismail AK. Managing an unidentified jellyfish sting with mixed envenomation syndrome at a noncoastal hospital: is this a new form of jellyfish envenomation? Wilderness Environ Med. 2023;34(2):225-30.
28. Loy JS, Khoo CC, Arumugam T, Ngian GH, Ismail AK. Rhabdomyolysis due to unidentified jellyfish envenomation in west Malaysian waters. Toxicon X. 2024;21:100170.
29. Ziegman R, Alewood P. Bioactive components in fish venoms. Toxins. 2015;7(5):1497-531.
30. Kizer KW, McKinney HE, Auerbach PS. Scorpaenidae envenomation. A five-year poison center experience. JAMA. 1985;253(6):807-10.
31. Lee JY, Teoh LC, Leo SP. Stonefish envenomations of the hand—a local marine hazard: a series of 8 cases and review of the literature. Ann Acad Med Singapore. 2004;33(4):515-20.
32. Diaz JH. The evaluation, management, and prevention of stingray injuries in travelers. J Travel Med. 2008;15(2):102-9.
33. Clark RF, Girard RH, Rao D, Ly BT, Davis DP. Stingray envenomation: a retrospective review of clinical presentation and treatment in 119 cases. J Emerg Med. 2007;33(1):33-7.
34. Meyer PK. Stingray injuries. Wilderness Environ Med. 1997;8(1):24-8.
35. Asakawa M, Matsumoto T, Umezaki K, Kaneko K, Yu X, Gomez-Delan G, et al. Toxicity and toxin composition of the greater blue-ringed octopus Hapalochlaena lunulata from Ishigaki Island, Okinawa Prefecture, Japan. Toxins. 2019;11(5):245.
36. Little M, Fitzpatrick R, Seymour J. Successful use of heat as first aid for tropical Australian jellyfish stings. Toxicon. 2016; 122:142-4.
37. Cevik J, Hunter-Smith DJ, Rozen WM. Infections following stingray attacks: a case series and literature review of antimicrobial resistance and treatment. Travel Med Infect Dis. 2022;47:102312.

2.15 Complementary and Alternative Medicines Toxicity

Ashish Bhalla, Mohan Kumar Hanumanthappa, Pooja Jangid

INTRODUCTION

Complementary and alternative medicine (CAM) refers to a diverse set of healthcare and medical practices, products, and systems that are not considered conventional or mainstream Western medicine. Complementary approaches are defined as those used together with conventional therapies, distinguishing them from alternative practices, those used as a substitute for standard care.

Complementary practices can roughly be divided into two major groups—mind and body practices and natural products. Mind and body practices and disciplines are usually administered by or taught to others by a clinician, trained practitioner, or teacher and include acupuncture, massage, meditation, and hypnosis. Natural products include a diverse group of orally or topically administered substances such as botanical products, unconventional diets, dietary supplements, herbal medicines, homeopathic remedies, probiotics, etc. The National Institutes of Health defined CAM as "healthcare approaches with a history of use or origins outside of mainstream medicine."[1]

Patients have become more interested and informed about CAM because of the increased availability of information on the Internet, increased contact with other cultures that traditionally use CAM, renewed interest in formerly countercultural ideologies, such as environmentalism, the perception that CAM is easier to understand, safer, and less expensive than conventional medications, distrust of and frustration with the healthcare system, and a growing recognition that many factors contribute to health and well-being.[1]

Indian systems of medicine recognize AYUSH (Ayurveda, Yoga, Naturopathy, Unani, Siddha, and Homeopathy) representing the tradition of codified, textual health knowledge systems other than the modern medicine.[2]

Traditional Chinese medicine (TCM) is another type of CAM formulations which is widely used in the world.[3] These medications are very easily available and are widely acceptable.

There are many other traditional medical systems practiced in the world. Some of them are being supported by the governments and being actively incorporated in the healthcare systems in those countries **(Table 1)**.

TABLE 1: Types of complementary and alternative medicine (CAM) available in the world.

Name	***Origin and developing nation***	***Characteristics of theory or application***	***Current role or status***	***Modern advances***
Traditional Chinese medicine (TCM)	China	• Based on Yin-yang and Wuxing concepts • A group of herbs that have a synergistic effect • Four elements: Monarch, Minister, Assistant, and Servant	• TCM and conventional medicine exist at every healthcare system in China • Covered under insurance in China • TCM services for both inpatients and outpatients	• Many TCM active compounds and compound-based therapeutics have been discovered • Efforts on to reveal underlying molecular mechanisms of TCM
Traditional Indian medicine (Ayurveda, Yoga)	India	• Natural elements to eradicate the cause of the illness • By balancing Vatt, Pitt, Kuff • To live a healthy • Ayurvedic formulations combine multiple herbs and metals	• >500,000 registered practitioners • AYUSH minister to control Ayurveda's educational quality, and practice integration with modern medicine	• Recognition of pharmacologically active compounds • Incorporation of Yoga as a preventive, health restoration practice

Contd...

Contd...

Name	Origin and developing nation	Characteristics of theory or application	Current role or status	Modern advances
Unani medicine	India Medicine system derived from *Greco-Arabic* medicine	• Treats body, mind, and soul • Body as a single unit consisting of four basic elements • Temperament reflects their physical characteristics and natural disposition	Unani is accepted by the World Health Organization (WHO) and India formally as a traditional healthcare system	Many bioactive ingredients have been separated from mangrove plants
Kampo (traditional Japanese medicine)	Kampo was introduced in Japan from China via the Korean peninsula	• Kampo treats every human being as one self-controlled whole in which body and mind impact mutually • Diseases result from disorders of psyche and soma. Herbs are supposed to affect the soul and the body equally	• Kampo is an approved modality in Japan • All Kampo herbal formulations are approved for use by the government	• All formulations are produced by certificated drug firms under strict quality management standards • The government and drug firms supervise all the processes to ensure the quality and safety
Traditional Korean medicine (TKM), Sasang constitutional medicine (SCM)	SCM is a division of Korean traditional medicine in vogue since last 100 years	• SCM classifies persons into four • *Sasang types:* Tae-Yang, So-Yang, Tae-Eum, and So-Eum • Based on the birth characteristics, • SCM believes in individualized, constitution-specific treatments	• 86% of Korean people use SCM • National medical insurance and private insurance cover Korean SCM services	Korean government initiated "The Lee Jema" project to generate scientific proof of SCM began in 2006
Traditional aboriginal medicine	Australia	Indigenous peoples believe that health problems have three types of causes: Natural bodily causes, harmful spirits, or witchcraft	Some government organizations support traditional medication	
Traditional medicine in Africa	Africa	Traditional medicine doctors treat patients holistically, mentally, and physically	80% of African people use traditional medicine either by itself or with conventional medicine. In some African countries, traditional medical system is incorporated in healthcare system	Research on some traditional products is being carried
Russian herbal medicine	In vogue in Russia since 10th century	The Russian Federation follows the State Pharmacopoeia, which has mention of many herbs	Herbal therapy is a formal and independent department. 14–40% Russians use these formulations	Researchers are focused on developing active ingredients from herbs and plants

(AYUSH: Ayurveda, Yoga, Naturopathy, Unani, Siddha, and Homeopathy; TCM: traditional Chinese medicine; TKM: traditional Korean medicine; SCM: Sasang constitutional medicine)

Source: Adapted from Yuan H, Ma Q, Ye L, Piao G. The traditional medicine and modern medicine from natural products. Molecules. 2016;21: 559-64.

CONCEPT OF TOXICITY IN COMPLEMENTARY AND ALTERNATIVE MEDICINES

Toxicity in CAM can arise from various sources, including herbal supplements, traditional remedies, and unconventional treatments. Individuals must be aware that just because a product or therapy is labeled as "natural" or falls under CAM does not necessarily mean that it is free of potential risks or side effects. Some common areas of concern related to toxicity in CAM are as follows:

- *Herbal supplements:* Some herbal remedies may contain active compounds that can be harmful in high doses or combined with certain medications. For example, herbal supplements may interact with prescription drugs, leading to adverse effects. Additionally, the purity and quality of herbal supplements can vary, and contamination with toxins or heavy metals is possible.
- *Heavy metal contamination:* Some traditional remedies, particularly those involving minerals or certain plants, may be contaminated with heavy metals such as lead, mercury, or arsenic. Prolonged exposure to these substances can lead to serious health problems.
- *Unregulated products:* The lack of regulation in the CAM industry can contribute to the availability of products with unknown or potentially harmful ingredients. Some products may be marketed without adequate testing or quality control.
- *Improper administration:* Certain CAM therapies, when administered incorrectly or without proper training, can lead to toxicity or adverse effects. Examples include acupuncture performed by untrained individuals or excessive use of specific essential oils.
- *Lack of scientific evidence:* Some CAM therapies need more scientific evidence regarding their safety and efficacy. Trying unproven treatments or therapies without proper oversight may expose individuals to unnecessary risks.
- *Allergic reactions:* Natural products used in CAM, such as herbs, can trigger allergic reactions in some individuals. It is essential to be aware of potential allergens and consult with healthcare providers before starting any new treatment.
- *Interactions with conventional medicine:* CAM therapies may interact with prescribed medications, reducing their effectiveness or causing harmful side effects. It is crucial to inform healthcare professionals about all CAM treatments being used to avoid potential interactions.[4]

TYPES OF COMPLEMENTARY AND ALTERNATIVE MEDICINES

Categorization of Various Complementary and Alternative Medicine Modalities

The National Centre for Complementary and Alternative Medicine (NCCAM) classified CAM into five categories, with many individual therapies crossing categories: Biologically based therapies, mind–body therapies, manipulative and body-based therapies, energy therapies, and systems of care.

Biologically Based Therapies

Biologically based therapies use substances typically found in nature, including herbs and essential oils, special diets (e.g., Ayurveda, hot–cold balance), nutritional and food supplements, and other products such as cartilage. According to NCCAM, these therapies are the most popular complementary therapies; nearly 18% of adults have reported using natural, nonvitamin, nonmineral products.

Biologicals in CAM could be in the form of herbs or a combination of naturally occurring metals and minerals with herbs. Ayurvedic formulations are a classic example of combination therapy with premixed herbs, minerals, and heavy metals in majority of the formulations.[5]

Another form which is a "drugless noninvasive rational and evidence-based system of medicine" is naturopathy. It revolves mainly around the principles of fasting and simple vegan diet supported by treatments with natural elements like water, pressure, and stretching. Hydrotherapy, chromotherapy, mud therapy, manipulative therapy, electrotherapy, acupuncture, magnetotherapy, and exercise are important components of naturopathy.[5]

Mind–body Therapies

Interventions that use various techniques to enhance the mind's ability to affect body functions and symptoms are known as mind–body therapies (or mind–body–spirit therapies, from a holistic perspective).

These therapies are among the most widely used categories of CAM and include guided imagery, visualization, progressive muscle relaxation, meditation, prayer, music therapy, light therapy, art therapy, journaling, storytelling, biofeedback, hypnosis, humor, animal-assisted therapy, and yoga. Manipulative and body-based therapies that apply pressure to, manipulate, or move one or more body parts are known as manipulative or body-based therapies. Chiropractic medicine, osteopathic manipulative medicine, movement therapy, massage, and other bodywork are some examples. Yoga aims to improve or develop one's inherent power (physical and mental) in a balanced manner and attain complete self-realization.[5]

Energy Therapies

These focus on the electromagnetic and biofield energies that are thought to originate in or near the body and on energy from other sources. These esoteric therapies may modify, manipulate, enhance, or support the energy fields.

Energy therapies may include healing touch, therapeutic touch, Reiki, acupuncture or acupressure, and reflexology. Concerns with some of the energy therapies include inaccurate diagnoses of conditions by practitioners and safety issues associated with the manipulative therapies.

Systems of Care Practices

These do not fit into the other categories and have evolved from cultural and spiritual traditions. These practices encompass whole systems of care built on theory and practices that evolved earlier than and apart from more conventional Western medicine. Some cultural healing systems, such as Hmong, Samoan, Somali, Latin American, and Native American, have persisted for centuries.[1]

Prevalence of Complementary and Alternative Medicines Use

In a systematic review, CAM usage estimates varied widely ranging from 9.8 to 76%.[6] The World Health Organization (WHO) estimates reveal that, in developing countries, up to 80% of the population rely on traditional medicines.[7] These are mainly in the form of herbs, either alone or in combination with other herbs and metals. Indian and Chinese diaspora are particularly at risk the world over[8] **(Table 1)**.

Trained physicians of modern medicine have difference in attitude and perception regarding the use of CAM. A recent study showed that a greater proportion of the trained modern medicine doctors utilized CAM in comparison to patients and preferred homeopathy over other therapies.[9] Similar results have been reported in earlier studies too.[8,10]

The patients prefer CAM as it was perceived it to be relatively safer due to fewer noted or documented side effects. Patients also perceive CAM to be economical, easily available, and well tolerated. CAM use was especially noted in patients suffering from chronic ailments like cancer, hypertension, and rheumatologic diseases.[9,11–13] At times, the end users are unaware that the CAM modality they are using to control or cure an illness may actually worsen the disease or may result in a complication, worse than the basic disease.[14]

IMPORTANCE OF UNDERSTANDING POTENTIAL RISKS

Complementary and alternative medicine includes diverse therapies, practices, and products that are not considered part of conventional medicine. While many individuals turn to CAM for various reasons, it is essential to recognize and understand the potential risks associated with these practices, which are listed in **Box 1**.

TOXIC COMPONENTS

Complementary and Alternative Medicines that Can Pose Toxicity Risks

The use of both Indian traditional formulations and TCM is associated with many clinically significant systematic toxicities. Chinese herbal nephrotoxicity is a condition directly linked to the toxicity of various compounds like aristolochic acid and various alkaloids, anthraquinones, flavonoids, and glycosides. Similar agents found in Indian traditional formulations may cause significant systematic toxicity. Some important toxins are as follows:

Aristolochic acids are nephrotoxic and carcinogenic phytochemicals found in many plant species, particularly the birthworts. Aristolochic acid nephropathy is characterized by rapidly progressive and hypocellular interstitial nephritis and fibrosis with end-stage renal disease as well as neuroepithelial malignancies.

Amygdalin is a naturally occurring plant glycoside produced from hydrolysis of amygdalin obtained from apricot kernels. Hydrogen cyanide production after oral ingestion of amygdaline (laetrile) can cause fatal cyanide poisoning, particularly in high oral doses or when ingested with fruit kernels, almonds, or high-dose vitamin C.

BOX 1: Potential risks associated with complementary and alternative medicine (CAM) practices.

Safety concerns
- CAM have adverse effects or interactions with conventional treatments

Toxicity concerns
- Risk of contamination of herbs with heavy metals in the soil or water
- Risk of contamination of herbs with pesticides
- Risk of contamination of stored herbs with organism (bacteria/fungi)

Lack of regulation
- Absence of standardized testing and quality control
- Risk of inconsistent product quality and potential harm to users

Delay in conventional treatment
- Relying solely on CAM may result in delayed diagnosis and treatment

Misinformation and lack of evidence
- CAM practices lack rigorous scientific studies
- There could be misinformation, false promises, and heightened expectations
- Lack of evidence: May result in ineffective or harmful interventions

Financial impact
- CAM treatments can be costly
- Lead to significant financial burden with lack of scientific efficacy
- Financial burden may divert resources from more effective treatments

Psychological impact
- The placebo effect is a significant factor in CAM
- Symptom relief is due to strong belief in the effectiveness of CAM

Cultural and ethical considerations
- Some CAM practices may be culturally rooted
- One must consider cultural and ethical aspects while evaluating these practices' potential risks and benefits

Interference with conventional therapies
- CAM users may stop or modify the conventional medications resulting in disease progression

(CAM: complementary and alternative medicine)

Vitamin D intoxication involves levels >375 ng/mL. Hypervitaminosis D presents with hypercalcemia (with findings including neuropsychiatric disturbances, hypovolemia from renal sodium and water losses, vomiting and abdominal pain, cardiac arrhythmias, or nephrocalcinosis and metastatic calcification of other) as well as suppressed parathyroid hormone level. This is frequently an iatrogenic condition resulting from excessive exogenous supplementation (typically at least 50,000 IU/day) due to either error in prescribing, manufacturing, or overenthusiastic self-administration.

In addition, soil contamination with *heavy metals* leads to bioaccumulation in herbal and medicinal plants and subsequent toxicity. Studies in plants have shown variable accumulation of various metals and metalloids with further differences among parts of the plant (roots, stems, or leaves) and the location of the samples.[4,15] Traditional formulations in addition may get contaminated with the pesticides in soil leading to possibility of acute high-dose or chronic low-dose exposures.[15]

Some of the traditional Indian formulations contain heavy metals as an essential component. During the preparation of the formulation for commercial purpose, the amount used may get altered, leading to unusually high levels of heavy metals in them.[15,16] Some authors have reported heavy metal levels in commonly used herbs in traditional Indian formulations to be within permissible limits.[17,18] This raises a possibility of some contamination being introduced during commercial manufacturing. It is recommended that strict monitoring and careful cultivation of medicinal herbs should be done to keep them safe from heavy metals and pesticide residue.[17,18] These practices are ideal but may be difficult to adhere to while cultivating medicinal plants commercially. Strict regulatory control during manufacturing and audit of practices followed should be adhered to.

Similar concerns have been raised regarding TCM. In a systematic review, it was noted that many factors govern toxicity, the important ones being misidentification, inappropriate combination of herbs, improper processing, and prolonged administration above the prescribed duration of administration.[19]

Traditional CAM formulations have been documented to be contaminated with many other toxic biologically active agents like alkaloids, glycosides, toxic proteins, polypeptide, amino acids, tannins, anthraquinones, phenols, aconitine, strychnine, and organic acids in addition to heavy metal elements.[20-22]

Another important factor is the inappropriate diagnosis. Nearly all the CAM prescribers depend solely on history and clinical examination, with very little importance to laboratory investigations.[19] This may mean lesser expenditure for the patient but may result in under- or overdiagnosis of certain diseases.

Most patients procure traditional CAM formulations over the counter, mostly without a valid prescription. Many times, the patients self-medicate and the dosage is guided by the package insert. These practices expose innocent patients to very high doses of various toxic compounds making them vulnerable to systemic toxicity of CAM formulations.

SCOPE OF THE PROBLEM

In a retrospective analysis of a Medicare population, it was noted that 15.1% of the population used CAM products and 5.8% were taking combinations considered to have a significant potential risk for adverse interaction. Most of the combinations with risk involved concurrent use of CAM products with a risk for bleeding (especially ginkgo and garlic) together with conventional drugs taken to reduce blood clotting (especially aspirin).[23]

Complementary and alternative medicine use has been noted to be associated with nearly 5% of emergency admissions.[24]

With increasing acceptance of CAM modalities by both physicians and patients,[9] the possibility of toxicity due to CAM intake is high. Since many practitioners of modern medicine do prescribe/use the CAM formulation with conventional therapies, the risk of associated drug–drug interactions increases significantly.

RISK FACTORS

While many CAM practices are generally considered safe, certain risk factors are associated with their use. Individuals must be aware of these factors to make informed decisions about their health care. Some common risk factors related to CAM are as follows:

Lack of scientific evidence: Many CAM therapies need robust scientific evidence to support their efficacy and safety. Proper research makes determining the benefits and potential risks associated with these treatments easier. Ineffective or unproven CAM treatments may delay or replace conventional medical interventions, potentially allowing conditions to worsen.

Interactions with conventional medications: Some CAM therapies, including herbal supplements, may interact with prescription medications, either reducing their effectiveness or causing adverse reactions. This can lead to unexpected health complications and compromise the efficacy of conventional medical treatments.

Contamination and quality control issues: Herbal supplements and other CAM products may be contaminated with heavy metals, pesticides, or other impurities due to inadequate quality control measures during cultivation, harvesting, or manufacturing. Exposure to contaminants can lead to health issues, including toxicity and allergic reactions.

Misdiagnosis or delay in diagnosis: Relying solely on CAM therapies may delay obtaining a proper medical diagnosis and treatment for severe health conditions. Delayed diagnosis and treatment may allow the progression of diseases that could have been effectively managed or treated with conventional medical approaches.

Unqualified practitioners: Some individuals offering CAM services may need more training, certification, or licensure. Inexperienced or unqualified practitioners may provide ineffective or harmful treatments, posing risks to the health and well-being of individuals seeking their services.

DETECTION AND DIAGNOSIS

A high index of clinical suspicion is a must for identifying CAM-related toxicity. Due to the lack of standardization of many agents used by patients, it is difficult to clearly establish a cause-and-effect relationship between CAM use and ill health. The most important cause for this is the fact that patients perceive these CAM modalities to be safe and healthy options, thereby hiding the fact from the physicians. The very fact that physicians practicing modern medicine are unsure about the CAM and pharmaceutical drugs interactions[9] further strengthens the belief that any unknown or unexplained clinical condition not explained by the toxicity of the prescribed modern medication should be evaluated for CAM toxicity.

Numerous case reports of clinical presentation of different kinds, related to heavy metal toxicity in CAM, are available and the number of reports is increasing. In one study, the levels of mercury and arsenic were found to be beyond permissible safe limits. These findings indicate that heavy metals should be looked for in case of renal, neurological, or hematological side effects related to CAM[16] **(Table 2)**.

Specialized laboratory tests looking at the blood/serum levels of heavy metals may be needed, but the results need to be interpreted in context of clinical presentation. These tests may or may not be available at many centers. In India,

TABLE 2: Toxicity of heavy metals, usually reported in traditional Indian formulations.

Lead	*Arsenic*	*Mercury*	*Nickel*	*Cadmium*	*Chromium*	*Zinc*
Memory impairment and neuropathy	Neuropathy and encephalopathy	Cognitive, memory, and motor dysfunction	Nausea and vomiting, diarrhea	Muscle and joint pain	Vomiting, diarrhea, acute liver failure	Nausea, vomiting, diarrhea
Difficulty in concentration	Muscle weakness	Headache, insomnia	Hair loss	Flu-like symptoms	Intravascular hemolysis	Lethargy
Hearing difficulty	Diarrhea and pain abdomen	Respiratory failure (inhalation)	Dermatitis	Renal failure	Occupational asthma, lung fibrosis	Metal fume fever (fumes)
Anemia	Cirrhosis and coagulopathy	Irritation of eyes (fumes)	Sinusitis, paranasal sinus cancer	Neuropathy	Sinusitis	Interstitial nephritis
Infertility	Renal failure	Renal failure	Occupational asthma and lung fibrosis	Infertility	Renal failure	Anemia
Abdominal pain	Skin mottling	Dermatitis	Heart failure	Atherosclerosis	Dermatitis	Neuropathy
Carcinogenic	Carcinogenic	Congenital malformation	Renal failure	Neurodegenerative disease	Lung cancer	Cancer

most of the National Accreditation Board for Hospitals & Healthcare Providers (NABH) accredited private laboratories now offer these investigations. The commonly used method is inductively coupled plasma mass spectrometry. This usually provides detailed information about the common heavy metals but can be customized to detect specific agents. The serum samples, blood samples, urine, the available CAM agents, hair, nails, etc., can be used as substrate, but specific techniques may be needed to evaluate different substrates.[16]

Most of the available laboratory tests do not go beyond the estimation of heavy metals, however at times; concerns regarding adulteration and substitution of components have been reported too.[19] Commercially grown medicinal herbs are likely to be more expensive and are replaced by similar-looking plants or cheaper options. This kind of adulteration may be very difficult to evaluate, but high-performance liquid/gas chromatography and polymerase chain reaction (PCR)-based tests to look for specific herbs are some of the tests that may be able to evaluate CAM agents.[25] These tests are usually not available in routine laboratories, but some research institutes or some specialized quality care laboratories may be able to provide these services. Many nationally accredited laboratories associated with quality control departments affiliated to the government should be able to standardize the formulations.[26]

PREVENTION

Preventing toxicity from CAM involves understanding the potential risks associated with these therapies and taking steps to ensure their safe use. The National Centre for Biotechnology Information (NCBI) provides valuable resources on this topic, and here are some general guidelines for preventing toxicity from CAM. In a recent review, it was noted that heavy metals in TIM are often the result of adulteration or improper manufacturing.

Making an integrative database of traditional medicines and its potential association/interaction with modern medicine is another way forward. This needs a dedicated team of experts to develop and disseminate. Such a database is available for some CAM agents.[19,27]

The government agencies and the researchers also recommend audit of the prescribing practices, and strict adherence to quality standards and protocols needs to be maintained to lower the risks associated with toxicity of the CAM.[26,28]

Some of the other potential mechanisms suggested are as follows **(Flowchart 1)**:

Flowchart 1: The way forward for standardizing herbal drugs for CAM.

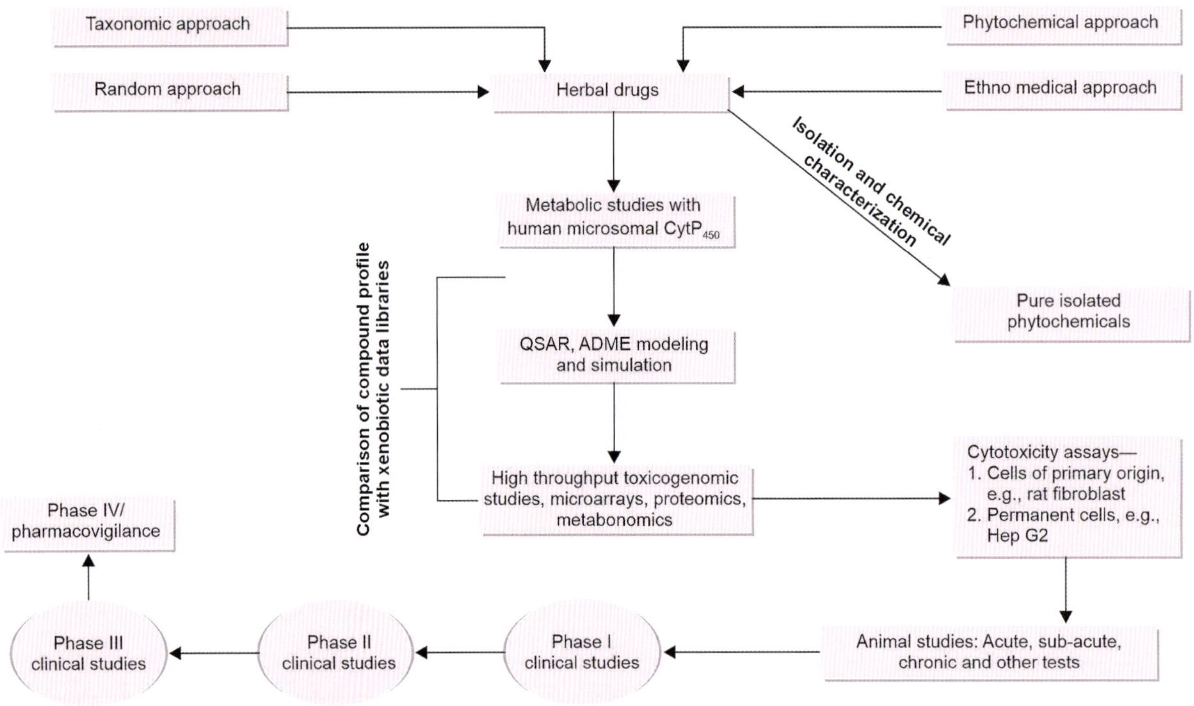

(CAM: complementary and alternative medicine; QSAR: quantitative structure–activity relationship)

Consultation with healthcare professionals: It is pertinent to note that many qualified practitioners of traditional medicine exist. A formal consultation and prescription must be mandatory before starting traditional medicine. As a user, one must always consult the primary healthcare professional before starting any new CAM therapy, especially if you are already taking prescribed medications or undergoing conventional medical treatments. If a traditional CAM has been started, one must inform the primary healthcare provider about all the CAM therapies you are consuming, as some may interact with medications or have contraindications.

Research and education: Thoroughly research the CAM therapy you want to understand its potential benefits and risks—utilize reputable sources such as scientific journals, health organizations, and government publications on the NCBI database. Trained clinical pharmacologists can play a vital role in developing such databases of traditional medicine. Some efforts have already been made in this regard, but more concentrated efforts are needed, especially for traditional Indian medicines.[27]

Quality and standardization: Choose CAM products and therapies that adhere to quality standards, such as good manufacturing practices (GMP) for supplements. Look for products that have been tested for safety and efficacy. The government guidelines and the efforts of researchers/experts of traditional CAM are needed for the same.[28]

Dosage and administration: Strictly adhering to the recommended dosages and administration guidelines for CAM products is the need of the hour. Unfortunately, many of the guidelines are not available. Avoiding self-prescription and not exceeding recommended doses are important components of CAM stewardship. One needs to be extra cautious with herbal remedies, as they may have many potential adverse effects or interactions.

Monitoring for adverse effects: Paying attention to the body's response to CAM therapies and being vigilant for any adverse effects may be needed. Reporting any unusual symptoms or side effects to the healthcare provider promptly should be advocated while prescribing/using CAM.

Avoiding risky practices: One must be cautious of therapies involving extreme or unproven practices, especially those with potential harm. Regular information about regulatory warnings and advisories related to specific CAM therapies should be issued by designated authorities.

Integration with conventional medicine: Use CAM as a complementary approach rather than a substitute for conventional medical treatments.

Patient education: Educating the patients about the principles and mechanisms of action behind the CAM therapy is an important consideration. Be aware of potential red flags, such as therapies that promise miraculous cures or those lacking scientific evidence.

REGULATORY ASPECTS

The Dietary Supplements Health and Education Act (DSHEA), passed in 1994, gives authority to the U.S. Food and Drug Administration (FDA) to regulate dietary supplements, but with expectations that differ in many respects from the regulation of drugs or food additives. Regulation of advertising and marketing claims is the purview of the Federal Trade Commission (FTC).[25] The FTC does take legal action against promoters or websites that advertise or sell dietary supplements with false or deceptive statements. There are appropriate laws available in India and many developing countries, but many producers or promoters of CAM exploit them. In the recent past, the judiciary in many countries have taken strict corrective measures and have cautioned the CAM producers to refrain from claiming cure for many chronic conditions.

For TCM and traditional Indian formulations, some regulations have been drafted but to make CAM safer and effective more such efforts at the international level are needed.[8]

THE WAY FORWARD (FLOWCHART 1)

An integral part of pharmacological/toxicological research in CAM is the need to develop the strategies of detoxification. One can use the age-old practices of checking the formulation and sticking to the timelines/methodology for processing medicinal herbs or use advanced strategies, such as chemical structural modification and molecular identification.[19,26]

Robust preclinical scientific studies and collating promising evidence from clinical/observational studies for classic CAM agents will surely provide us with evidence to successfully use CAM in the treatment of various fatal or previous untreatable diseases.[8]

CONCLUSION

Toxicity related to CAM refers to adverse effects or harmful reactions associated with nonconventional therapeutic approaches. CAM includes many practices, such as herbal remedies, dietary supplements, acupuncture, and other alternative therapies. While many people turn to CAM for its perceived natural and holistic qualities, it is essential to recognize that these interventions can carry risks, including potential toxicity.

ACKNOWLEDGMENT

The authors acknowledge Valliappan M for inspiring and helping in the chapter.

REFERENCES

1. Biro FM, Bloemer NL. “Complementary medicine”: complementary and alternative health approaches in pediatric and adolescent gynecology. J Pediatr Adolesc Gynecol. 2019;32(1):3-6.
2. Priya R, Shweta AS. Status and role of AYUSH and local health traditions under the National Rural Health Mission. New Delhi: National Health Systems Resource Centre; 2010.
3. Cheung F. TCM: Made in China. Nature. 2011;480:S82-3.
4. Charen E, Harbord N. Toxicity of herbs, vitamins, and supplements. Adv Chronic Kidney Dis. 2020;27(1):67-71.
5. Pengpid S, Peltzer K. Utilization of complementary and traditional medicine practitioners among middle-aged and older adults in India: Results of a national survey in 2017-2018. BMC Complement Med Ther. 2021:21:262-70.
6. Harris PE, Cooper KL, Relton C, Thomas KJ. Prevalence of complementary and alternative medicine (CAM) use by the general population: A systematic review and update. Int J Clin Pract. 2012;66:924-39.
7. Chan K. Some aspects of toxic contaminants in herbal medicines. Chemosphere. 2003;52:1361-71.
8. Liu R, Li X, Huang N, Fan M, Sun R. Toxicity of traditional Chinese medicine herbal and mineral products. Chapter 11. Du G (Ed). Adv Pharmacol. 2020;87:301-6.
9. Roy V, Gupta M, Ghosh RK. Perception, attitude and usage of complementary and alternative medicine among doctors and patients in a tertiary care hospital in India. Indian J Pharmacol. 2015;47(2):137-42.
10. Furlow ML, Patel DA, Sen A, Liu JR. Physician and patient attitudes towards complementary and alternative medicine in obstetrics and gynaecology. BMC Complement Altern Med. 2008;8:35.
11. Malhotra S, Bhatia GS, Pandhi P. Patterns of use of unconventional therapies in the medical outpatient department of a tertiary care hospital in India. J Ethnopharmacol. 2001;75(2-3):71-5.

12. Shafiq N, Gupta M, Kumari S, Pandhi P. Prevalence and pattern of use of complementary and alternative medicine (CAM) in hypertensive patients of a tertiary care center in India. Int J Clin Pharmacol Ther. 2003;41(7):294-8.
13. Wang ZX, Qi FH, Cui YG, Zhao L, Sun XG, Tang W, et al. An update on Chinese herbal medicines as adjuvant treatment of anticancer therapeutics. Biosci Trends. 2018;12:220-39.
14. Bara T Jr, Gurzu S, Sugimura H, Bara T, Beleaua MA, Jung I. A systematic review of the possible carcinogenic role of the aristolochic acid. Rom J Morphol Embryol. 2017;58:41-4.
15. Saper RB, Kales SN, Paquin J, Burns MJ, Eisenberg DM, Davis RB, et al. Heavy metal content of ayurvedic herbal medicine products. JAMA. 2004;292(23):2868-73.
16. Bhalla A, Pannu AK. Are ayurvedic medications store house of heavy metals? Toxicol Res (Camb). 2022;11(1): 179-83.
17. Sandhu A, Upadhya P, Singh PK, Aggarwal A, Karmakar D, Singh JPI, et al. Quantitative analysis of heavy metals in medicinal plants collected from environmentally diverse locations in India for use in a novel phytopharmaceutical product. Environ Monit Assess. 2015;187:542.
18. Deswal M, Deswal P, Laura JS, Study on heavy metals in some ayurvedic herbal products and risk assessment of their calculated average daily dose intake in humans. J Herb Med. 2022;34,100569.
19. Zhu H, Wang X, Wang X, Pan G, Zhu Y, Feng Y. The toxicity and safety of Chinese medicine from the bench to the bedside. J Herb Med. 2021;28:100450.
20. Efferth T, Kaina B. Toxicities by herbal medicines with emphasis to traditional Chinese medicine. Curr Drug Metab. 2011;12(10):989-96.
21. Kong X, Liu C, Zhang Z, Cheng M, Mei Z, Li X, et al. BATMAN-TCM 2.0: An enhanced integrative database for known and predicted interactions between traditional Chinese medicine ingredients and target proteins. Nucleic Acids Res. 2024;52(D1):D1110-20.
22. Lv W, Piao JH, Jiang JG. Typical toxic components in traditional Chinese medicine. Expert Opin Drug Saf. 2012;11(6):985-1002.
23. Elmer GW, Lafferty WE, Tyree PT, Lind BK. Potential interactions between complementary/alternative products and conventional medicines in a Medicare population. Ann Pharmacother. 2007;41(10):1617–24.
24. Kumar G, Sharma N, Bhalla A, Shafiq N, Harish CVN, Malhotra S. Evaluation of drug-related emergency department admissions in a tertiary care hospital. J Postgrad Med Edu Res. 2020;54(2):29-33.
25. Seethapathy GS, Raclariu-Manolica AC, Anmarkrud JA, Wangensteen H, de Boer HJ. DNA metabarcoding authentication of ayurvedic herbal products on the European market raises concerns of quality and fidelity. Front Plant Sci. 2019;10:68.
26. Yuan H, Ma Q, Ye L, Piao G. The traditional medicine and modern medicine from natural products. Molecules. 2016;21,559-64.
27. Xu H, Zhang Y, Wang P, Zhang J, Chen H, Zhang L, et al. Comprehensive review of integrative pharmacology-based investigation: a paradigm shift in traditional Chinese medicine. Acta Pharm Sin B. 2021;11(6): 1379-99.
28. Mukhopadhya S, Abraham SE, Holla B, Ramakrishna K, Gopalakrishna KL, Soman A, et al. Heavy metals in Indian traditional systems of medicine: a systematic scoping review and recommendations for integrative medicine practice. J Altern Complement Med. 2021;27(11): 915-29.

2.16 Hydrocarbon Poisoning

Rohit Bhowmick, Banani Poddar

INTRODUCTION

Hydrocarbons are a variety of chemical compounds consisting of hydrogen and carbons and are ubiquitous in nature. They are found in products used in the chemical industries and many household items like kerosene, solvents, natural gas, fuels, and petroleum derivatives. In developing countries like India, kerosene and similar low-cost hydrocarbon-containing fuels are used for lighting, heating, cooking, painting, or as a solvent of pesticides. Often, hydrocarbon derivatives are stored in bottles of drinking water or soft drinks, making them prone to accidental exposure to toddlers and young children.

Depending on their chemical properties, hydrocarbons are mainly classified into aliphatic (e.g., kerosene) and aromatic or cyclic hydrocarbons (e.g., benzene) **(Table 1)**. If the chemical structure contains a halogen compound (chloride, bromide, and fluoride), it is known as a halogenated hydrocarbon, which is the most toxic hydrocarbon.[1] The route, amount of exposure, and the type of hydrocarbon determine the

TABLE 1: Classification of common hydrocarbon compounds.

Type	Ingredients	Found in/example
Aliphatic	Kerosene, gasoline	Fuel
	Butane, naphtha	Lighter fuels and refills
	Mineral spirits, petroleum distillates	Paint thinner, machine lubricants
Aromatic	Xylene	Shoe glues, painter thinners
	Toluene	Glues
Halogenated	Trichloroethane	Paper correction fluid, spot remover
	Tetrachloroethylene	Brake cleaners
	Fluorinated products	Computer keyboard cleaners
Miscellaneous	Terpene	Thinner
	Pine oil	Wood and surface cleaning agents

severity of the illness. A spectrum of toxicity can vary from asymptomatic or mild disease to severe multiorgan dysfunction [multiple organ dysfunction syndrome (MODS)]. Though any organ can be affected by hydrocarbon poisoning, the respiratory system, central nervous system (CNS), and cardiovascular system (CVS) are the most significant ones.[2]

EPIDEMIOLOGY

Worldwide, hydrocarbon exposure remains one of the important poisonings, and annually, more than 25,000 cases are reported in the toxicological registry of the United States.[3] In adults and adolescents, the exposure can be intentional as a recreational agent by inhalation or unintentional, in most cases. In the Asian population, currently, pesticides are the most common poisoning, but hydrocarbons remain one of the critical poisons leading to hospital admission.[4,5] Due to their exploratory nature, children, especially under 5 years of age, are at a higher risk of hydrocarbon toxicity.[6] Though the incidence of pediatric hydrocarbon poisoning is decreasing globally, gasoline remains the most commonly ingested agent among children in developing countries.[7] The use of kerosene has significantly reduced in developed countries, but in India and other developing countries, kerosene poisoning still remains one of the important causes of emergency room admission.[8]

PATHOPHYSIOLOGY AND MECHANISM OF TOXICITY

The systemic effects of hydrocarbon depend on the chemical properties and route of exposure. Oral ingestion and inhalational routes are significant modes of toxicity, but other miscellaneous routes, like dermal exposure, may rarely affect humans.

Ingestion

Following ingestion, hydrocarbons act primarily as gastric irritants that cause spontaneous vomiting in about one-third of patients. The most important effect of oral hydrocarbon ingestion is the high risk of pulmonary aspiration and its subsequent complications.[9] Though aspiration and related lung injury most often occur in infants and toddlers who attempt to ingest liquid hydrocarbons, rarely similar damages result from patients playing a "fire-eating" game (spraying liquid hydrocarbons by mouth over a flame) or during diesel siphoning.[10,11]

Hydrocarbons induce lung injury by disrupting the surfactants, leading to alveolar instability and collapse, along with distal airway obstruction by the denatured and necrotic damaged epithelium. The final effect is due to ventilation-perfusion mismatch, bronchospasm, and shunt formation resulting in hypoxemia. Halogenated hydrocarbons, such as tetrachloroethylene, produce pulmonary mucosal irritation and can lead to chemical pneumonitis and acute lung injury.[12] Another unique form of pulmonary toxicity is the development of lipoid pneumonia (LP), a disease that results from the inhalation or aspiration of animal, vegetable, or mineral oils. LP results from prolonged foreign body reaction to fat or oil. After reaching the lungs by inhalation or aspiration, alveolar macrophages take the offending hydrocarbon.[13] These macrophages cannot metabolize the substance; therefore, repeated exposure to the offending agent leads to the death of the macrophage and subsequent granulomatous reactions.

Inhalation

In adolescents and adults, inhalational abuse of hydrocarbon occurs mainly as recreational agent exposure. Three main methods of inhalant use are sniffing (inhaling directly from the container), huffing (inhaling from a cloth soaked in the hydrocarbon), and bagging (breathing of vapors directly from a bag containing a hydrocarbon). Rarely, accidental inhalational injury occurs from volatile or gaseous hydrocarbons like propane or refrigerants.[14]

Following inhalation or ingestion, lipid-soluble hydrocarbons are systemically absorbed. They rapidly diffuse through systemic circulation to different body parts and into the CNS, leading to systemic effects. The CNS effects can be present as seizure or euphoria due to stimulation of excitatory neurons [like N-methyl-D-aspartate (NMDA) receptor], whereas CNS depression and altered sensorium can be seen due to the effects on inhibitory gamma-aminobutyric acid (GABA) receptor.[1,15] The cellular basis of hydrocarbon-induced myocardial damage is seen due to the inhibition of cardiac sodium, calcium, and potassium channels. The result is catecholamine-induced delayed after-depolarizations and ventricular dysrhythmias.[16]

CLINICAL FEATURES

Hydrocarbons can affect almost all body systems, but the lungs, brain, and heart are the most critical organs affected by acute poisoning. Aspiration may lead to acute-onset coughing or choking.[17,18] Due to low surface tension and low viscosity, hydrocarbon can penetrate the lungs, leading to severe necrotizing pneumonia. Damaged alveoli, airway epithelium, alveolar capillaries, and deranged surfactant may lead to atelectasis and ventilation-perfusion mismatch. These effects result in features of respiratory distress like tachypnea, dyspnea, retractions, grunting, and other elements of hypoxia. Secondary and tertiary bronchiolar epithelial damage leads to bronchospasm and wheezing. Chemical irritation of the alveoli results in an inflammatory response and causes temperature elevation, usually within hours of exposure.

The CNS manifestation of hydrocarbon poisoning may consist of two stages: The first stage involves excitation, impulsive behavior, and loss of inhibition; the second stage is characterized by CNS depression with confusion, hallucinations, tremors, ataxia, and weakness. Moreover, chemical pneumonitis leads to pulmonary injury, and severe hypoxia may cause secondary damage to the brain resulting in CNS depression or seizures.

The CVS effects are seen mainly following aromatic and halogenated hydrocarbon exposure. These agents sensitize the myocardium to catecholamines, leading to life-threatening arrhythmias [e.g., ventricular tachycardia (VT), ventricular fibrillation (VF), and sudden cardiac arrest]. Inhalation of volatile compounds, especially in children, can lead to sudden cardiovascular collapse or sudden sniffing death.[19]

Rarely, hydrocarbons can produce unique toxicities depending on their clinical properties. Some agents like toluene may cause a nonanion gap metabolic acidosis or renal tubular acidosis, hyperchloremia, and hypokalemia. Skin exposure may cause irritation, and with prolonged exposure, chemical burns can lead to superficial to full-thickness burns. Dermal lesions may also present as bullae or blisters. A particular type of skin irritation in the perioral area is known as a "glue sniffer's rash."

DIAGNOSIS

Focused History and Examination

Acute hydrocarbon exposure is a clinical diagnosis made based upon history and physical findings. A detailed history of the incident is essential to determine the nature of the exposure. In unconscious patients, it is necessary to enquire from the caregivers and bystanders to understand the complete picture of the event. Also, every effort should be made to obtain the container or bottle used to store the substance ingested or inhaled, to determine the exact chemicals the patient has been exposed to. A thorough past medical and psychological history is pertinent. A review of the patient's past medical records may give clues toward a history of abuse.

The patient may present with a cough or experience shortness of breath. An initial physical examination should focus on identifying inhalational or aspirational injuries. Evaluation of vital signs may show tachycardia, tachyarrhythmia, tachypnea, hypoxia, and fever. A thorough physical examination must include respiratory, cardiovascular, neurological, and dermatological examination. Respiratory system evaluation may reveal wheezes, rhonchi, or crepitations. Patients with CNS toxicity may present with euphoria, agitation, confusion, or may have seizures.

Investigations (Figs. 1 and 2)

Arterial or venous blood and pulse oximetry may identify hypoxemia and any associated acidosis if present. An initial chest radiograph may show normal findings, but following a significant aspirational insult, a chest X-ray may locate features suggestive of chemical pneumonitis. Asymptomatic patients who ingest hydrocarbons should

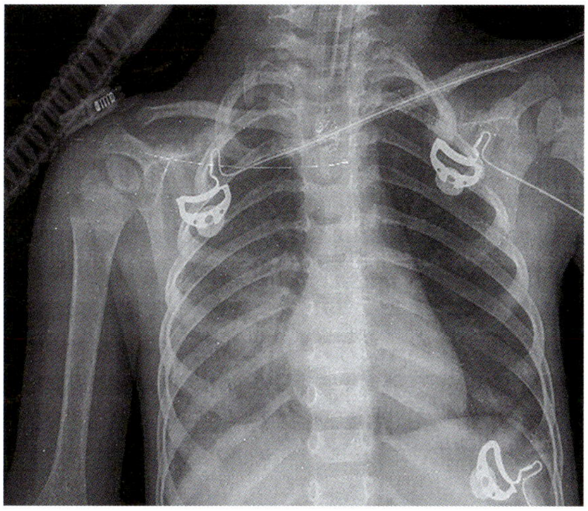

Fig. 1: Chest radiograph showing right lower lobe infiltrates in a patient following 6 hours of kerosene aspiration.

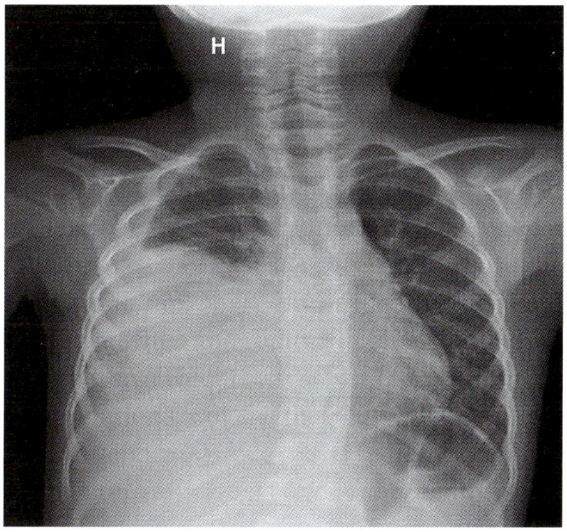

Fig. 2: Consolidation due to chemical pneumonitis following hydrocarbon ingestion.

receive a chest radiograph 4–6 hours after exposure to assess the subtle features of chemical pneumonitis. Continuous electrocardiogram (ECG) monitoring is necessary to detect arrhythmias (VT or VF) or associated prolonged QT intervals. A complete blood count (CBC) may show leukocytosis early in the clinical course of hydrocarbon aspiration, and leukocytosis may last as long as 1 week. Other rare hematological abnormalities like hemolysis, hemoglobinuria, and consumptive coagulopathy may occur following large ingestions and associated multiorgan dysfunction. Halogenated hydrocarbons may affect the kidneys and liver; hence, a liver function study may show transaminitis and renal function assessment may identify deranged urea and creatinine values.

MANAGEMENT

The management principles of hydrocarbon poisoning consist of decontamination, general care, timely recognition of pulmonary, cardiac, and/or neurologic toxicity, and rapid initiation of appropriate supportive care. Regional poison control centers should be contacted in all cases of intoxication.

Decontamination

Patients with skin exposure must have their clothes removed and be decontaminated with soap and warm water. Contact precautions should be used for the safety of staff and other healthcare providers. If exposed, eyes should be rinsed with copious saline or clean water. If the victims remain in a closed space, they should be moved to an open place and if needed, oxygen should be administered as soon as possible. Due to the risk of provoking vomiting and further aspiration, most patients with an isolated aliphatic or aromatic hydrocarbon ingestion should not receive activated charcoal or undergo gastric emptying. Although external decontamination is essential, it should not delay life-saving interventions like airway management for respiratory failure or coma, treatment of life-threatening arrhythmias, or initiation of anticonvulsant therapy.

Specific Treatment

Patients with mild-to-moderate respiratory symptoms on presentation are at risk for the development of chemical pneumonitis with progression to respiratory failure over the next 24–48 hours. Oxygen therapy should be initiated for all patients with respiratory distress. Any associated bronchospasm should be treated with inhaled beta-2 agonists. After initial oxygen therapy, a trial of high-flow nasal cannula oxygen delivery and/or noninvasive ventilation can be given in alert patients with progressive hypoxemia. Endotracheal intubation and mechanical ventilation are required for severe hypoxemic respiratory failure in patients with chemical pneumonitis. Lung-protective strategies should be initiated while ventilating patients with chemical pneumonitis, and other components of acute respiratory distress syndrome (ARDS) management protocol must be followed as indicated. Rarely high-frequency ventilation or extracorporeal membrane oxygenation therapy may be needed if the patient worsens despite maximum conventional ventilation support.

Unless there are any features of secondary infections, patients with chemical pneumonitis alone should not receive empirical antibiotics.[20] Corticosteroids have shown no beneficial effect on the course of hydrocarbon-related aspiration pneumonitis; moreover, they may have harmful effects. Some patients, predominantly children, may develop pneumatoceles that usually resolve spontaneously and do not require any treatment.

Prolonged QT, ST-segment elevation, bradycardia, atrioventricular (AV) blocks, atrial premature ventricular contractions, supraventricular tachycardia, and VF are all possible ECG findings with hydrocarbon toxicity. All patients should be placed on a cardiac monitor for prompt identification of life-threatening arrhythmias. Correction of electrolyte abnormalities is often required, as hypokalemia is common in hydrocarbon exposure. Age-appropriate algorithms, as per advanced cardiac life support or pediatric advanced life support, should be used for life-threatening arrhythmias (VF or VT or associated cardiac arrest). After hemodynamic stabilization, other types of arrhythmias can be managed with the advice of cardiologists. As the hydrocarbon sensitizes the myocardium to catecholamines, adrenaline should be avoided as much as possible.

Any patients with drowsiness or coma should be assessed carefully for airway protection; endotracheal intubation and mechanical ventilation may be required in some cases. Seizures should be treated with benzodiazepines apart from management of hypoxemia, and dyselectrolytemia should be corrected. For patients with status epilepticus, arrhythmogenic anticonvulsants like phenytoin should be avoided. Levetiracetam or phenobarbitone can be used for seizures refractory to benzodiazepines. If seizure remains refractory following appropriate management, associated co-ingestion of other agents, like organophosphates, must be considered, especially in the Indian setting.

No specific antidote is available for hydrocarbon-related chemical pneumonitis, cardiotoxicity, or neurotoxicity. N-acetylcysteine can be used for hepatotoxicity related to carbon tetrachloride and methylene blue may be used for methemoglobinemia seen with some specific hydrocarbon ingestion.

DISPOSITION

Patients can be discharged home with normal Glasgow Coma Scale (GCS), normal ECG, and no respiratory symptoms (cough, dyspnea, and wheezing). Asymptomatic patients should be observed for 6–8 hours, and normal pulse oximetry should be documented during the period of observation. If after an observation period of 4–6 hours, there are no signs of pulmonary or systemic toxicity, a chest radiograph with no infiltrates, the patient may be sent home with a follow-up advice mentioning the probable symptoms. If after observation, systemic or pulmonary symptoms appear, admission and prolonged observation may be necessary. For deliberate ingestion, a risk assessment should indicate that the patient is at low risk of further self-harm in the discharge setting.

PROGNOSIS

The typical clinical course of chemical pneumonitis ranges from 2 to 5 days and usually resolves completely without any long-term sequelae. CNS features like drowsiness or mild altered sensorium usually resolves in 24–48 hours. Rarely, chemical pneumonia may progress rapidly to hypoxemic respiratory failure and death.

CONCLUSION

Hydrocarbon exposure is an important cause of pediatric emergency admission, especially in rural India. Ingestion is the most common route of exposure among children and can result in aspiration pneumonia. Diagnosing chemical pneumonitis is essentially clinical, though chest X-ray and pulse oximetry may add valuable input to the management plan. Gastric emptying is contraindicated because aspiration is a risk. Treatment is mainly supportive, and meticulous monitoring until discharge is the key to improving the outcome.

REFERENCES

1. Ridenour TA, Bray BC, Cottler LB. Reliability of use, abuse, and dependence of four types of inhalants in adolescents and young adults. Drug Alcohol Depend. 2007;91(1):40-9.
2. Jolliff HA, Fletcher E, Roberts KJ, Baker SD, McKenzie LB. Pediatric hydrocarbon-related injuries in the United States: 2000–2009. Pediatrics. 2013;131(6):1139-47.
3. Gummin DD, Mowry JB, Beuhler MC, Spyker DA, Brooks DE, Dibert KW, et al. 2019 Annual Report of the American Association of Poison Control Centers' National Poison Data System (NPDS): 37th Annual Report. Clin Toxicol. 2020;58(12):1360-541.
4. Pannu AK, Bhalla A, Vamshi V, Upadhyay MK, Sharma N, Kumar S. Changing spectrum of acute poisoning in North India: A hospital-based descriptive study. Turk J Emerg Med. 2022;22(4):192-9.

5. Dayasiri MBKC, Jayamanne SF, Jayasinghe CY. Patterns and outcome of acute poisoning among children in rural Sri Lanka. BMC Pediatr. 2018;18(1):274.
6. Jayashree M, Singhi S. Changing trends and predictors of outcome in patients with acute poisoning admitted to the Intensive Care. J Trop Pediatr. 2011;57(5):340-6.
7. Palmer SB, Spiller HA, Kistamgari S, Casavant MJ, Rine NI, Yang J, et al. Hydrocarbon ingestions among individuals younger than 20 years old reported to United States Poison Centers, 2000–2021. Inj Epidemiol. 2023;10(1):48.
8. Mittal C, Singh S, Kumar MP, Varthya SB. Toxicoepidemiology of poisoning exhibited in Indian population from 2010 to 2020: A systematic review and meta-analysis. BMJ Open. 2021;11(5):e045182.
9. Ik K, Priyadarshini D, Nakka S, John J, Mahapatro S, Dwibedi B, et al. Profile and outcome of childhood hydrocarbon poisoning: An observational study. Cureus. 2021;13(12):e20144.
10. Butland BK, Field-Smith ME, Ramsey JD, Anderson HR. Twenty-five years of volatile substance abuse mortality: A national mortality surveillance programme. Addiction. 2013;108(2):385-93.
11. Jung CY, Chin HC, Tai CK. Hydrocarbon pneumonitis following fuel siphonage: A case report and literature review. World J Emerg Med. 2019;10(2):69.
12. Tenenbaum A, Rephaeli R, Cohen-Cymberknoh M, Aberbuch D, Rekhtman D. Hydrocarbon intoxication in children: Clinical and sociodemographic characteristics. Pediatr Emer Care. 2021;37(10):502-6.
13. Makrygianni EA, Palamidou F, Kaditis AG. Respiratory complications following hydrocarbon aspiration in children. Pediatr Pulmonol. 2016;51(6):560-9.
14. Forrester MB. Pediatric lamp oil injuries treated in US Emergency Departments. Pediatr Emer Care. 2022;38(1):e165-9.
15. Lubman DI, Yücel M, Lawrence AJ. Inhalant abuse among adolescents: Neurobiological considerations. Br J Pharmacol. 2008;154(2):316-26.
16. Sahin A, Ozer V, Akkaya F, Kaplan S. Successful resuscitation of prolonged cardiac arrest occurring in association with 'skunk' and toluene toxicity. Tur J Emerg Med. 2018;18(4):172-5.
17. Thompson KN, Oulhote Y, Weihe P, Wilkinson JE, Ma S, Zhong H, et al. Effects of lifetime exposures to environmental contaminants on the adult gut microbiome. Environ Sci Technol. 2022;56(23):16985-95.
18. Tsiaoussis J, Antoniou MN, Koliarakis I, Mesnage R, Vardavas CI, Izotov BN, et al. Effects of single and combined toxic exposures on the gut microbiome: Current knowledge and future directions. Toxicol Lett. 2019;312:72-97.
19. Alper AT, Akyol A, Hasdemir H, Nurkalem Z, Güler Ö, Güvenç TS, et al. Glue (toluene) abuse: Increased QT dispersion and relation with unexplained syncope. Inhal Toxicol. 2008;20(1):37-41.
20. Balme KH, Zar H, Swift DK, Mann MD. The efficacy of prophylactic antibiotics in the management of children with kerosene-associated pneumonitis: A double-blind randomised controlled trial. Clin Toxicol. 2015;53(8):789-96.

2.17 Alcohols

Yvonne Elisabeth Lao, Dag Jacobsen, Knut Erik Hovda

INTRODUCTION

Alcohols are organic compounds with a hydroxyl group attached to a carbon atom. The most common ones are ethanol, methanol, ethylene glycol, isopropanol, and diethylene glycol (DEG). Except for ethanol, the other alcohols are not for oral consumption due to their toxicity, hence the term toxic alcohols.

In India, the most common toxic alcohol poisoning is by methanol, a chemical easily available in everyday life, as it is used as an additive to consumer products as plastics, paint, and cosmetics. Methanol has also gained attention for use as an environmentally friendly fuel. Poisoning occurs mainly after oral consumption, but inhalation[1,2] and dermal exposure[3,4] can also lead to toxicity. Most poisonings occur as mass outbreak after unintentional ingestion of methanol added to ethanol,[5-8] whereas methanol from home distilled alcohol is less relevant.[9] Poisonings can also be individual cases of suicidal ingestion or unintentional exposure in children. Unintentional ingestion of hand sanitizers containing methanol during the coronavirus disease 2019 (COVID-19) pandemic resulted in single cases and outbreaks of poisoning.[10-12] If treatment is delayed or absent, the morbidity and mortality are high.[5-7,13-17]

Ethylene glycol is a liquid with a sweet taste, which can be found in consumer products such as antifreeze.

Most cases of poisonings are single cases of unintentional ingestion in children or self-harm/suicidal ingestion.[18] Recently, several deaths in children due to syrup medicines contaminated with ethylene glycol and/or DEG have been seen in Cameroon, Gambia, India, Indonesia, Iraq, and Uzbekistan.[19-21] Similar outbreaks with mass poisoning after exposure to pharmaceutical products contaminated with DEG have also occurred in Haiti, India, and Panama.[22-24] DEG can also be found in other products, such as automotive chemicals, that can lead to sporadic cases of poisoning after ingestion.[25]

Isopropanol is used in rubbing alcohol, in antiseptics, in concentrations of 60–70%, and in disinfectants for hand and surfaces. It can also be found in cosmetics, perfumes, and pharmaceutical preparations. Most cases of poisonings are accidental ingestion, dermal or inhalation exposure in children, as well as an ethanol substitute by alcoholics.[26]

METHANOL

Toxicity

After oral ingestion, the absorption is rapid[27] and the volume of distribution is approximately 0.7 L/kg.[27,28] Methanol elimination is mainly by liver metabolism. Elimination through kidneys and lungs is minimal.[29] It is slowly metabolized to formaldehyde by alcohol dehydrogenase (ADH) and then rapidly converted to the toxic metabolite formic acid by aldehyde dehydrogenase **(Fig. 1)**. Formic acid (pKa 3.74) dissociates almost completely to formate (and H^+) at physiological pH and is then metabolized to CO_2 and water, in a folate-dependent reaction. Primates are the only species with limited folate levels[30] and, therefore the only ones to be exposed by the toxic effects of methanol.[31] Formate is renally excreted, by a pH-dependent elimination. It is reabsorbed in the proximal tubule in a H^+/formate cotransport and by diffusion of formic acid that is indirectly connected to Na^+/H^+ exchange. The reabsorption of formate increases with decreasing pH; hence, renal formate excretion is reduced in acidosis.[32]

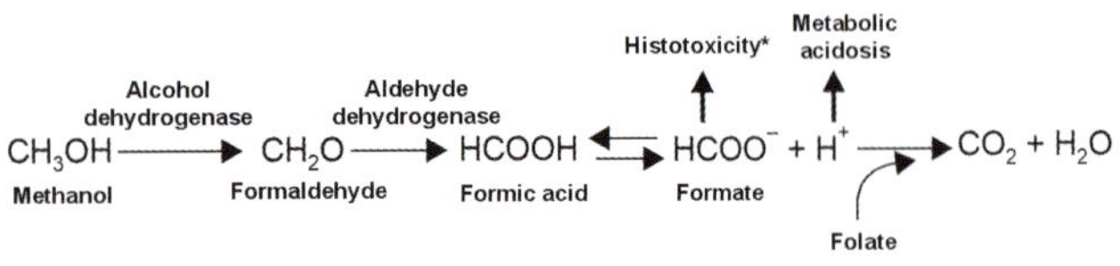

Fig. 1: Metabolism of methanol.
*Histotoxicity (see Fig. 2 for mechanisms).

In contrast to ethanol, methanol has little inebriating effect. The signs and symptoms of methanol poisoning will appear after a latency period of 12–24 hours or even longer if the ADH inhibitor ethanol is coingested.[15,16,33]

The toxic amount of methanol is reported between 30 and 240 mL. The estimated minimum lethal dose is 1 g/kg.[15,34] The mechanism for toxicity, in addition to the ensuing metabolic acidosis, is due to inhibition of cytochrome oxidase in the mitochondria by formate that binds to the ferric heme ion of cytochrome oxidase.[35] This is pH dependent, with increasing inhibition with decreasing pH. The result of the cytochrome oxidase inhibition produces oxidative stress.[35] Later, the effect on the mitochondrial respiration and anaerobic metabolism will increase lactate production and tissue hypoxia, which lowers the pH even more. This will also increase the diffusion of the toxic metabolite across the blood–brain barrier, cell membranes, and mitochondrial membranes, all due to an increased level of the undissociated formic acid. This is described as a vicious circle, named "circulus hypoxicus" **(Fig. 2)**.[36]

The brain and the eyes are the organs mostly affected by methanol poisoning. Formate has a direct toxic effect on the eye which causes retinal and optic nerve damage.[37] In addition, it also reduces the levels of glutathione in the retina and thereby reduces protection against oxidative stress. The neurotoxicity occurs in the late phase of the poisoning. The lenticular nucleus (putamen and globus pallidus) is particularly vulnerable to this toxicity. Why so and the exact mechanism are unknown, but it is assumed that this is due to the histotoxic effect of formate in the late stages, and areas with higher energy consumption are likely to be more vulnerable **(Fig. 2)**.

Clinical Presentation

After the latency phase of 12–24 hours (later if ethanol is coingested), the patient will present features of toxicity, due to metabolic acidosis and formate accumulation. Initially, the patient may have a feeling of severe "hangover" despite methanol not giving an inebriating effect. In addition to this, the patient often suffers from nonspecific gastrointestinal features (nausea, vomiting, and abdominal pain), hyperventilation (due to the metabolic acidosis), and visual disturbances (typically blurred vision, altered visual fields, or even complete blindness). Late presenters may have coma and respiratory and circulatory failure.[16,33] The few reported cases of methemoglobinemia may

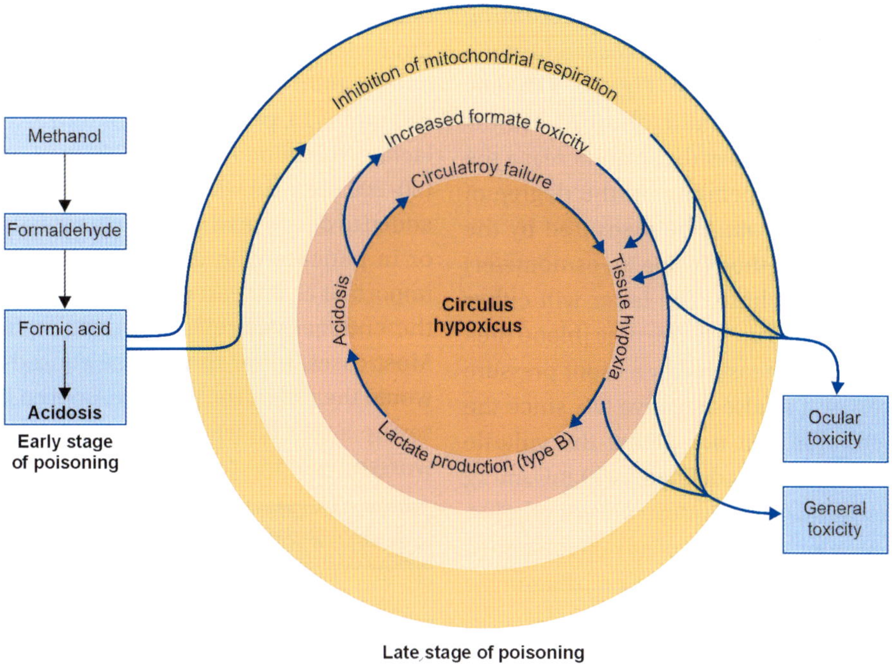

Fig. 2: Circulus hypoxicus, the vicious circle of methanol poisoning.
Source: Adapted with permission from Drangsholt et al. (2018).[36]

possibly be explained by binding of formate to the ferric part of hemoglobin.[15]

Diagnosis

The diagnosis is challenging due to the nonspecific signs and symptoms and limited access to analytical options for methanol or formate detection. It is based on medical history, clinical presentation, and analytical options, depending on what is available.

A detailed medical history is particularly important in case of limited access to analytical options. Recent ingestion of illegal/bootleg alcohol and the source, as well as knowledge of whether there have been other cases of confirmed methanol poisoning in the surroundings, provides important information. The time of ingestion and (delayed) onset of symptoms may also give an indication of possible methanol poisoning. In comatose patients, information from friends and family should be obtained.

Hyperventilation due to the metabolic acidosis is the most important and consistent clinical feature. A respiration rate of 20–25 breaths or more/min will gradually appear as the acidosis develops, often perceived as dyspnea or breathing difficulties. The respiration rate increases as the metabolic acidosis progresses. In the late phase, it may be absent due to decompensation and lack of ability to hyperventilate. The presence of visual disturbances may indicate methanol poisoning but is not always present. Visual disturbances can occasionally also be seen in metabolic acidosis of other causes. It is also not possible to evaluate in comatose patients. Pseudopapillitis is a specific diagnostic sign, again not always present.[15,34]

The detection of methanol by gas chromatography is often considered the gold standard,[33] but it is rarely available. Less known, formate detection by an enzymatic assay is an alternative,[38,39] although still requiring trained laboratory personnel. A point-of care test is under development,[40,41] but there is no commercial product on the market as of 2024. A negative methanol detection does not exclude poisoning since late presenters can have metabolized all methanol to formate, whereas the formate test may be negative in early presenters, especially if ethanol is coingested. However, in the latter group, no symptoms from methanol will be present as long as the patient has ethanol in the blood to stop metabolism.

Measurement of osmolal gap (OG) and anion gap (AG) is an indirect method that can be used if available. Increased OG and normal AG are seen in the early phase due to the presence of methanol. The OG then decreases with increasing methanol metabolism (= decreasing methanol level) with correspondingly increased formate concentration and AG in the late phase **(Fig. 3)**.[42] Diabetic and alcoholic ketoacidosis[43,44] and chronic kidney disease[45] are differential diagnoses that can increase the OG (moderately) and AG (depending on the degree of the acidosis). The osmolality *must* be measured by the freezing-point depression method (using an osmometer) and *not* by a blood gas machine. The latter will either calculate the osmolality based on a fictive urea [blood urea nitrogen (BUN)] or it will be measured by a vapor pressure technique.[46] This can give a false-negative OG since the vapor pressure technique will not detect the volatile alcohols. An upper normal OG is defined as 19 mOsm/kg H_2O (5 ± 2 SD), whereas an OG below can never exclude a toxic alcohol being present.[5] Presence of any ethanol must be subtracted for the calculation to be of any diagnostic value **(Table 1)**.

Commonly, an arterial blood gas or detection of metabolic acidosis is the only available analytical option, if at all present. In patients with metabolic acidosis of unknown origin, methanol poisoning should be considered. Diabetic and alcoholic ketoacidosis are both common differential diagnoses. A high blood sugar (>20 mmol/L) may indicate the former (but is not a requirement, especially in patients with SGLT2-inhibitors), while the latter is more difficult to diagnose in the absence of analytical options. The so-called fluid trial may be of valuable help in these settings.[47] In case of mild-moderate metabolic acidosis (base deficit <20 mmol/L), provide 1–2 L of Ringer's acetate or Ringer's lactate, thiamine (e.g., 100–250 mg), and dextrose 5–20% (50–200 mg/mL) within 30–60 minutes. Insulin should be added to dextrose where the blood sugar seems to increase or in patients with a low relative insulin level. This is important as increased α-adrenergic stimulus will inhibit the endogenous release of insulin from the pancreas. Most cases, other than those caused by toxic alcohols, would then stabilize, improve, or even be corrected (if less severe acidosis) within 1–2 hours. Absence of effect or worsening of the patient's condition may indicate a toxic

TABLE 1: Osmolal contribution from acetone and common alcohols per 100 mg/dL.

	Molecular weight (g/mol)	***Osmolal contribution per 100 mg/dL (mOsm/kg H_2O)***
Acetone	58	18
Diethylene glycol	106	10
Ethanol	46	24
Ethylene glycol	62	17
Isopropanol	60	17
Methanol	32	34

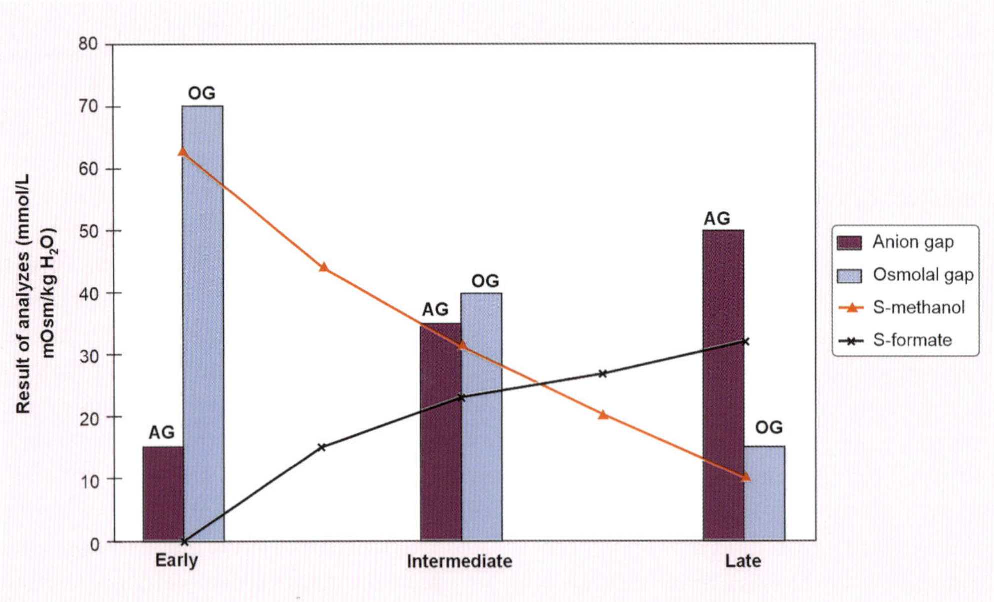

Fig. 3: Changes in osmolal gap (OG) and anion gap (AG) in methanol poisoning. Note that the AG may be normal/low in the early stage and the OG normal/low in the late stage of poisoning.
Source: Adapted with permission from Hovda et al. (2004).[42]

alcohol poisoning.[47] In lack of any specific analytical equipment, a flowchart has been suggested to support the clinical evaluation using mentioned fluid trial **(Flowcharts 1 and 2)**.[48]

Treatment

The goal of the targeted treatment is to correct the acidosis with sodium bicarbonate, block the metabolism of methanol with antidote, and remove methanol and/or formate with dialysis.[15–17] Treatment with dialysis will also help correcting the metabolic acidosis. Folinic acid will theoretically reduce formate levels by increasing the endogenous metabolism of formate.[16] Gastrointestinal decontamination is not recommended due to rapid absorption of methanol.

Flowchart 1: Diagnosis algorithm for methanol poisoning when no blood gas (arterial or venous) is available.

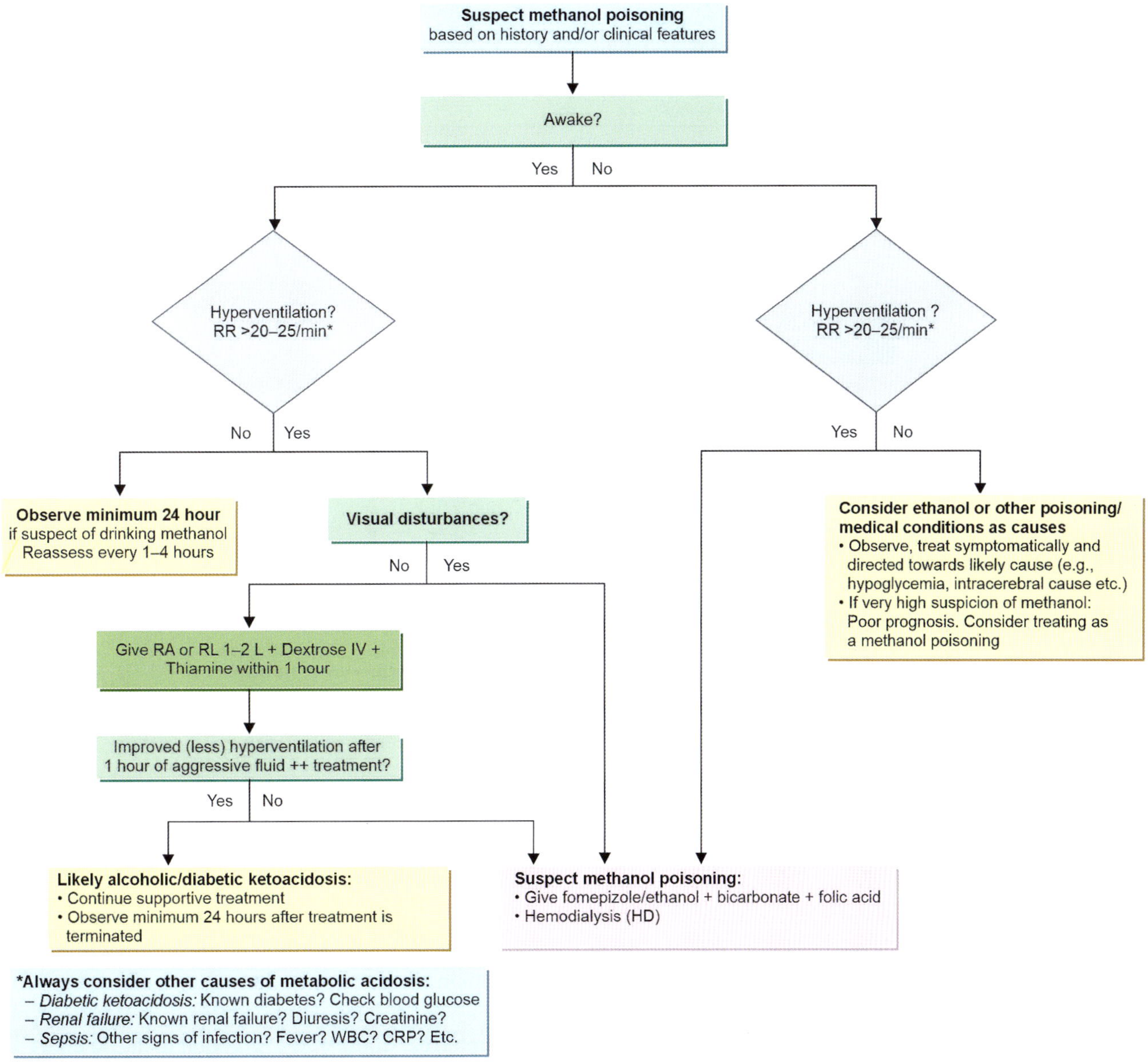

(CRP: C-reactive protein; RA: Ringer acetate; RL: Ringer lactate)

Source: Adapted from Medicines sans Frontieres (2023).[48]

Flowchart 2: Diagnosis algorithm for methanol poisoning when blood gas (arterial or venous) is the only analytic available.

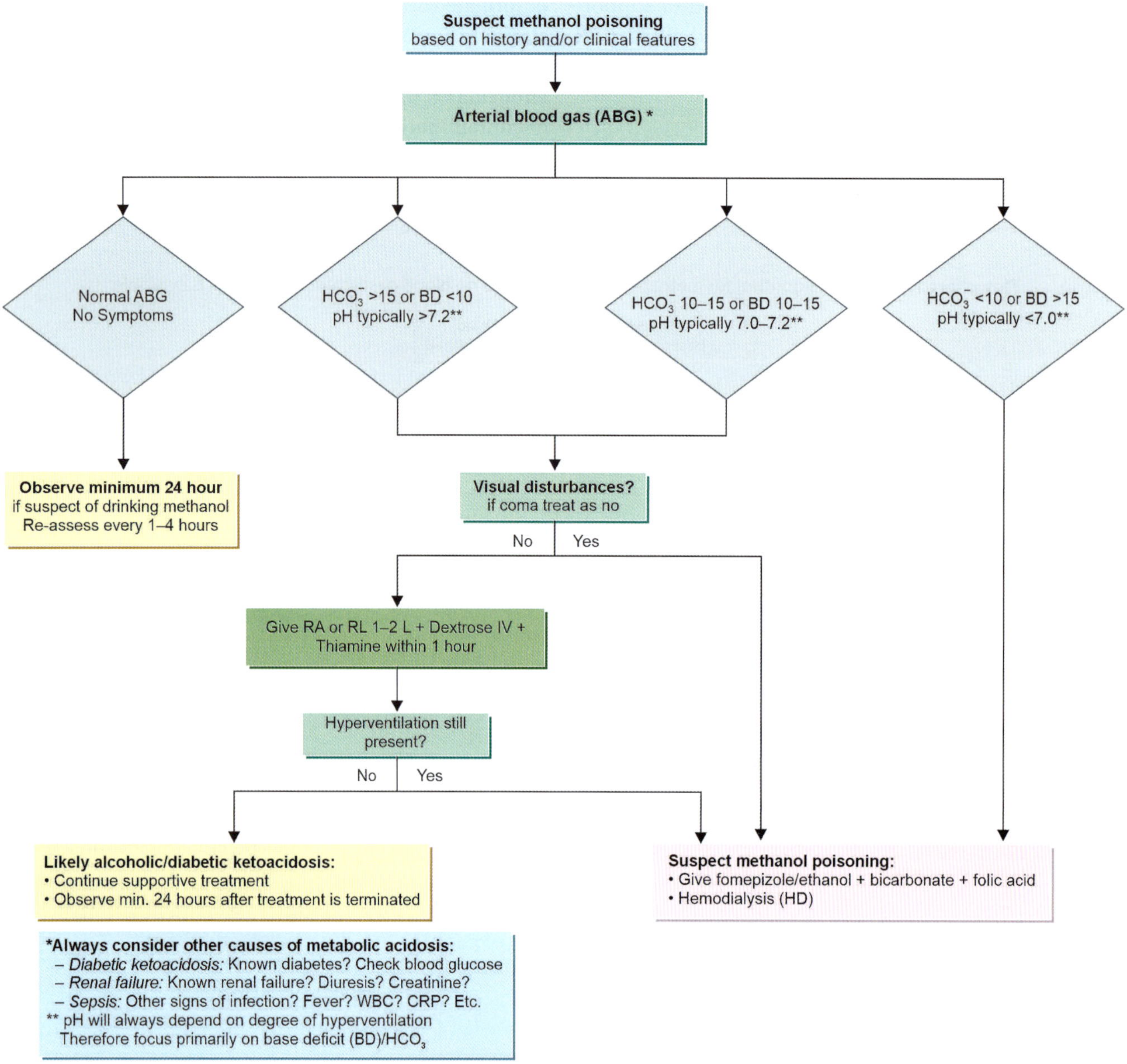

(BD: base deficit; RA: Ringer acetate; RL: Ringer lactate)
Source: Medecins sans Frontieres (2023).[48]

BICARBONATE

Sodium bicarbonate will correct the metabolic acidosis and thus reduce the toxicity by decreasing the fraction of undissociated formic acid. Correction of acidosis will also increase the renal excretion of formate. Full correction of the acidosis is recommended **(Table 2)**. Monotherapy with bicarbonate is not sufficient, as the toxic effect of formate on the mitochondria will continue **(Fig. 2)**.

Antidote

Fomepizole inhibits the enzyme ADH, while ethanol occupies the enzyme resulting in no/minimal methanol metabolism. A difference in outcome between the antidotes has not been demonstrated,[7,49] but fomepizole is still preferred. Compared to ethanol, it has no effect on the central nervous system (CNS), there is no need for monitoring of the serum concentration, and it is easier

TABLE 2: Dosing of sodium bicarbonate in metabolic acidosis from toxic alcohol poisoning.

Dosing of bicarbonate		
Blood gas available	***Blood gas not available***	***Oral treatment***
Dose bicarbonate (mmol) = 0.3 × patient weight (kg) × base deficit (mmol/L or mEq/L)	150–200 mmol bicarbonate *or more* over 1–2 hours until respiratory rate is below 20/minute. Repeat if necessary	Only preferred if IV treatment is not available. Give 3–10 g bicarbonate tablets every hour until hyperventilation is corrected

TABLE 3: Dosing of fomepizole.

	Fomepizole dose without dialysis	***Fomepizole dose with intermittent hemodialysis***	***Fomepizole dose with continuous renal replacement therapy***
Loading dose	15 mg/kg	15 mg/kg	15 mg/kg
Maintenance dose 1–3	10 mg/kg × 2	10 mg/kg × 6 (= every 4 hours)	10 mg/kg × 3 (= every 8 hours)
Maintenance dose 4 (= 5th dose incl. loading dose) and further dosing	15 mg/kg × 2	15 mg/kg × 6	15 mg/kg × 3

TABLE 4: Dose suggestion for oral or intravenous ethanol.

	5% ethanol	***10% ethanol***	***20% ethanol***	***40% ethanol***
Loading dose	15 mL/kg	7.5 mL/kg	4 mL/kg	2 mL/kg
Maintenance dose—normal	2 mL/kg/h	1 mL/kg/h	0.5 mL/kg/h	0.25 mL/kg/h
Maintenance dose—regular drinker	4 mL/kg/h	2 mL/kg/h	1 mL/kg/h	0.5 mL/kg/h
Maintenance dose—normal during intermittent hemodialysis	4 mL/kg/h	2 mL/kg/h	1 mL/kg/h	0.5 mL/kg/h
Maintenance dose—regular drinker during intermittent hemodialysis	6 mL/kg/h	3 mL/kg/h	1.5 mL/kg/h	0.8 mL/kg/h

to administer. However, it is more expensive. For dose recommendations, see **Table 3**.

Ethanol has a greater affinity for ADH as compared to methanol, and serum concentration of ethanol should be at least a quarter of methanol concentration. For simplicity, a serum concentration of >22 mmol/L is recommended, and if available, this should be monitored every 1–2 hours due to extensive inter- and intraindividual variations in ethanol metabolism.[15-17,50] Ethanol is removed by dialysis,[28] and a doubling of the dose has been suggested during intermittent hemodialysis (IHD).[50] Ethanol administration can be oral, by a nasogastric tube, or intravenous. To avoid gastrointestinal irritation with oral administration or venous irritation for intravenous administration, concentrated ethanol should be diluted. For dose recommendations, see **Table 4**.

Recommended indications for antidote treatment when documented/suspected methanol ingestion are[50]:

- Serum methanol ≥10 mmol/L
- Osmolal gap ≥25 mOsm/kg H_2O with ethanol subtracted
- Two or more of the following criteria:
  - Arterial pH <7.3
  - Serum bicarbonate <20 mmol/L
  - Osmolal gap >25 mOsm/kg H_2O with ethanol subtracted

The duration of treatment depends on whether it is used in a combination with dialysis or not. Combined with dialysis, continue antidote for 12–24 hours after the dialysis has ended. Without dialysis, give an antidote for 5–7 days. If recurrent metabolic (acidosis evaluate 24 hours after stopping antidote treatment), restart antidote, stop after another 2 days, and look for recurrent acidosis.[47] In these situations, a medical toxicologist or a poisons information center should preferably be consulted.

FOLIC ACID/FOLINIC ACID

The effect of folic/folinic acid is a theoretical assumption, and case reports/series are the only human data.[51] This vitamin B has a good safety profile, giving a low risk with treatment. It is, therefore, commonly recommended as a part of the treatment.[16,33] The suggested dose is 1 mg/kg (maximum 50 mg) IV every 4–6 hours.[16]

Dialysis

Dialysis removes methanol and the toxic metabolite formate, and it contributes to the correction of the metabolic acidosis. IHD is the preferred modality due to faster elimination of methanol and formate,[52] as well as a faster correction of the acidosis.[53] Continuous renal replacement therapy (CRRT) can be used in the absence of IHD[54] or in hemodynamic unstable patients. No difference in outcome has been shown as regards mortality or morbidity.[55] Peritoneal dialysis is not recommended, due to a lower efficiency compared to hemodialysis.[56] However, it can be used if the other modalities are not available.

There are no strict indications for dialysis in methanol poisoning. An absolute indication is a new visual impairment in a patient with a verified methanol poisoning or a metabolic acidosis with suspect methanol poisoning. Relative indications include severe metabolic acidosis (BD > 20 mmol/L) (particularly if unresponsive to buffer and antidote treatment), a blood methanol level >16 mmol/L (50 mg/dL), or ingestion of more than 1g/kg of methanol. While there are possibilities to postpone or even ameliorate hemodialysis in patients with little or no metabolic acidosis who are given fomepizole (not ethanol), most patients should still be provided dialysis to shorten the treatment with fomepizole (T½ of methanol while on fomepizole treatment is 50–80 hours).[33] The duration of treatment is controlled by serum methanol and is recommended terminated when methanol concentration is <10 mmol/L and acidosis corrected.[33] In the absence of methanol concentration, the suggested duration is 8 hours for IHD[33,54] and 18 hours for CRRT.[54] Restart treatment in case of recurrent metabolic acidosis.

Prognosis

The patient's clinical features on admission can give an indication of the prognosis. Coma, pH, and the ability to hyperventilate in patients with metabolic acidosis are prognostic markers for outcome.[5-7,49] Low pH (<7.00) is the strongest risk factor for poor outcome, followed by coma and a reduced ability to hyperventilate.[49]

In an event of an outbreak of methanol poisoning, there may be limited access to equipment for diagnosis and treatment. A consensus statement on how to handle this has been published,[57] emphasizing the importance of making emergency plans ahead of any events. The use of a triage system with level of consciousness, pH, and pCO_2 is recommended. If possible, prehospital antidote treatment should be started as early as possible.[58] Where fomepizole is available in limited quantities, it should be reserved for those with severe poisoning, pregnant women, and children <14 years. The rest should be given ethanol. IHD is the preferred dialysis modality, but use what is available and prioritize patients with visual disturbances and severe acidosis with a fair prognosis.

ETHYLENE GLYCOL

Ethylene glycol is metabolized to glycolaldehyde by ADH, further to glycolic acid, which will dissociate to glycolate and H^+, and be responsible for the metabolic acidosis.[15,17,18] A small part of the glycolic acid will be further metabolized to oxalic acid, where the corresponding anion forms insoluble calcium oxalate crystals, leading to cellular toxicity[59] **(Fig. 4)**.

Ethylene glycol has an inebriating effect similar to that of ethanol, and the patient will often initially present with a CNS depression. Compared to methanol, the latency phase is shorter (typically 6–12 hours); upon when the patient will present with signs and symptoms of metabolic acidosis with hyperventilation and multiorgan failure, of which renal failure is the most common.[15,17,18] Without treatment, seizures, coma, and death may occur.

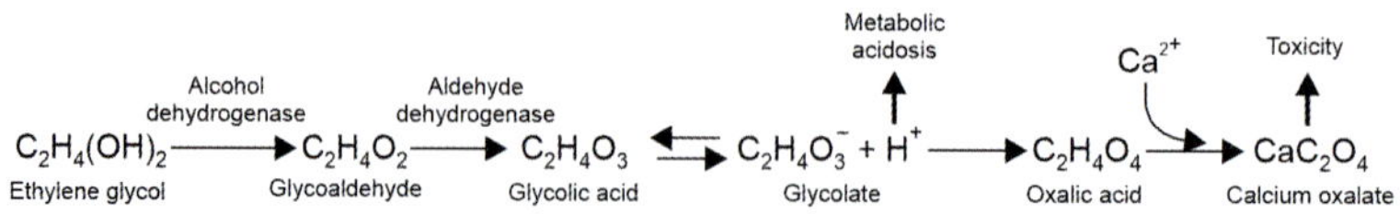

Fig. 4: Metabolism of ethylene glycol.

Similar to methanol poisoning, ethylene glycol poisoning can be challenging to diagnose, unless known ingestion of ethylene glycol or access to analysis of ethylene glycol with an enzymatic[60] or chromatographic method.[61] OG and AG can also be used as nonspecific diagnostic methods.[15,18] The presence of calcium oxalate crystals in the urine can support the diagnosis but is not always present.[15,18] These crystals are usually enveloped-shaped in the early phase (depending on the relative oxalate concentration) and gradually change to needle-shaped in the later stage (>36–48 hours' post ingestion).[62]

Treatment consists of blocking the metabolism of ethylene glycol to glycolate with an ADH inhibitor (ethanol or fomepizole), correction of the metabolic acidosis with bicarbonate, and removal of ethylene glycol and its toxic metabolites with dialysis.[15,18] Approximately 20% of the ethylene glycol is excreted by the kidneys,[18] and the half-life is approximately 15 hours if its metabolism is blocked by fomepizole and renal function is normal.[63] Therefore, with little or no acute kidney injury and/or only moderate metabolic acidosis, monotherapy with fomepizole without dialysis may also be considered.[64]

DIETHYLENE GLYCOL

The toxic metabolite of DEG is 2-hydroxyethoxyacetic acid, which causes a metabolic acidosis.[65] This is further metabolized to the nephrotoxic diglycolic acid.[66] The enzymes involved in the formation of 2-hydroxyethoxyacetic acid are ADH and aldehyde dehydrogenase.[67] Initially, the clinical presentation is metabolic acidosis and gastrointestinal features, followed by acute kidney injury after 1–3 days. Thereafter, neurological features such as bilateral facial nerve palsy, peripheral neuropathy, coma, and death may follow after 5–7 days.[67] Treatment is similar to the ethylene glycol poisoning, although the documentation for this recommendation is scarce.[63]

ISOPROPANOL

Isopropanol is metabolized by ADH to acetone in rats.[68] This metabolite is also detected in human cases and most probably explains why there is no metabolic acidosis.[69] The patient will present with nausea, vomiting, and abdominal pain, due to the gastrointestinal irritation of isopropanol. In addition, CNS depression and ketosis may occur, but usually without ketoacidosis.[26] Treatment is mainly supportive care, and there is no specific antidote.[26] An ADH inhibitor will block isopropanol metabolism,[70] but the toxicity is mainly due to isopropanol and ADH inhibitors are, therefore, contraindicated.[26] Isopropanol and acetone are removed by hemodialysis[71] and may be considered in addition to supportive care in very severe poisonings.[26] These patients are often circulatory unstable and continuous hemodialysis may, therefore, be preferred.

CONCLUSION

Methanol and ethylene glycol share many of the same properties: None are toxic themselves, but they both have toxic metabolites that can give a severe metabolic acidosis. They are often difficult to diagnose, but effective treatment exists in the form of buffer (to correct acidosis), antidote and dialysis (removing the alcohols and its toxic metabolites). Treatment is also similar for the much more rarely seen diethylene glycol, whereas isopropanol metabolizes to acetone and therefore does not lead to a metabolic acidosis.

REFERENCES

1. Frenia ML, Schauben JL. Methanol inhalation toxicity. Ann Emerg Med. 1993;22(12):1919-23.
2. Wallace EA, Green AS. Methanol toxicity secondary to inhalant abuse in adult men. Clin Toxicol (Phila). 2009;47(3):239-42.
3. Downie A, Khattab TM, Malik MIA, Samara IN. A case of percutaneous industrial methanol toxicity. Occup Med (Lond). 1992;42(1):47-9.
4. Sahbudak Bal Z, Can FK, Anil AB, Bal A, Anil M, Gokalp G, et al. A rare cause of metabolic acidosis: Fatal transdermal methanol intoxication in an infant. Pediatr Emerg Care. 2016;32(8):532-3.
5. Hovda KE, Hunderi OH, Tafjord AB, Dunlop O, Rudberg N, Jacobsen D. Methanol outbreak in Norway 2002–2004: Epidemiology, clinical features and prognostic signs. J Intern Med. 2005;258(2):181-90.
6. Paasma R, Hovda KE, Tikkerberi A, Jacobsen D. Methanol mass poisoning in Estonia: Outbreak in 154 patients. Clin Toxicol (Phila). 2007;45(2):152-7.
7. Zakharov S, Pelclova D, Urban P, Navratil T, Diblik P, Kuthan P, et al. Czech mass methanol outbreak 2012: Epidemiology, challenges and clinical features. Clin Toxicol (Phila). 2014;52(10):1013-24.
8. Rostrup M, Edwards JK, Abukalish M, Ezzabi M, Some D, Ritter H, et al. The methanol poisoning outbreaks in Libya 2013 and Kenya 2014. PLoS One. 2016;11(3):e0152676.
9. Lao Y, Pham BD, Le HT, Van HN, Hovda KE. Methanol content in homemade alcohol from a province in North Vietnam. Drug Alcohol Rev. 2019;38(5):537-42.

10. Holzman SD, Larsen J, Kaur R, Smelski G, Dudley S, Shirazi FM. Death by hand sanitizer: Syndemic methanol poisoning in the age of COVID-19. Clin Toxicol (Phila). 2021;59(11):1009-14.
11. Hassanian-Moghaddam H, Zamani N, Kolahi A-A, McDonald R, Hovda KE. Double trouble: Methanol outbreak in the wake of the COVID-19 pandemic in Iran-a cross-sectional assessment. Crit Care. 2020;24(1):402-3.
12. Mahdavi SA, Zamani N, McDonald R, Akhgari M, Kolahi A-A, Gheshlaghi F, et al. A cross-sectional multicenter linkage study of hospital admissions and mortality due to methanol poisoning in Iranian adults during the COVID-19 pandemic. Sci Rep. 2022;12(1):9741.
13. Hassanian-Moghaddam H, Pajoumand A, Dadgar SM, Shadnia S. Prognostic factors in methanol poisoning. Hum Exp Toxicol. 2007;26(7):583-6.
14. Paasma R, Hovda KE, Jacobsen D. Methanol poisoning and long term sequelae - A six years follow-up after a large methanol outbreak. BMC Clin Pharmacol. 2009;9:5.
15. Jacobsen D, McMartin KE. Methanol and ethylene glycol poisonings. Mechanism of toxicity, clinical course, diagnosis and treatment. Med Toxicol. 1986;1(5):309-34.
16. Barceloux DG, Bond GR, Krenzelok EP, Cooper H, Vale JA. American Academy of Clinical Toxicology practice guidelines on the treatment of methanol poisoning. J Toxicol Clin Toxicol. 2002;40(4):415-46.
17. Kraut JA, Mullins ME. Toxic alcohols. N Engl J Med. 2018;378(3):270-80.
18. Barceloux DG, Krenzelok EP, Olson K, Watson W. American Academy of Clinical Toxicology practice guidelines on the treatment of ethylene glycol poisoning. J Toxicol Clin Toxicol. 1999;37(5):537-60.
19. WHO. (2023). Medical Product Alert N°6/2023: Substandard (contaminated) syrup medicines. [online] Available from https://www.who.int/news/item/07-08-2023-medical-product-alert-n-6-2023--substandard-(contaminated)-syrup-medicines. [Last accessed October, 2024].
20. Das KN, Khanna S. (2023). India finds two more toxic syrups months after poisoning deaths. Reuters. [online] Available from https://www.reuters.com/world/india/india-regulator-finds-more-syrups-toxic-government-report-2023-10-04/. [Last accessed October, 2024].
21. The Indian EXPRESS. (2022). After Gambia, an Indian syrup linked to deaths of 18 kids in Uzbekistan. [online] Available from https://indianexpress.com/article/india/uzbekistan-children-died-consumption-of-india-made-syrup-8349555/. [Last accessed October, 2024].
22. Singh J, Dutta AK, Bhatia R, Sokhey J, Khare S, Dubey NK, et al. Diethylene glycol poisoning in Gurgaon, India, 1998. Bull World Health Organ. 2001;79(2):88-95.
23. O'Brien KL, Selanikio JD, Hecdivert C, Placide MF, Louis M, Barr DB, et al. Epidemic of pediatric deaths from acute renal failure caused by diethylene glycol poisoning. Acute Renal Failure Investigation Team. JAMA. 1998;279(15):1175-80.
24. Rentz ED, Lewis L, Mujica OJ, Barr DB, Schier JG, Weerasekera G, et al. Outbreak of acute renal failure in Panama in 2006: A case-control study. Bull World Health Organ. 2008;86(10):749-56.
25. Marraffa JM, Holland MG, Stork CM, Hoy CD, Hodgman MJ. Diethylene glycol: Widely used solvent presents serious poisoning potential. J Emerg Med. 2008;35(4):401-6.
26. Slaughter RJ, Mason RW, Beasley DMG, Vale JA, Schep LJ. Isopropanol poisoning. Clin Toxicol (Phila). 2014;52(5):470-8.
27. Graw M, Haffner HT, Althaus L, Besserer K, Voges S. Invasion and distribution of methanol. Arch Toxicol. 2000;74(6):313-21.
28. Jacobsen D, Jansen H, Wiik-Larsen E, Bredesen JE, Halvorsen S. Studies on methanol poisoning. Acta Med Scand. 1982;212(1-2):5-10.
29. Jacobsen D, Ovrebø S, Arnesen E, Paus PN. Pulmonary excretion of methanol in man. Scand J Clin Lab Invest. 1983;43(5):377-9.
30. Noker PE, Tephly TR. The role of folates in methanol toxicity. Adv Exp Med Biol. 1980;132:305-15.
31. Makar AB, Tephly TR, Mannering GJ. Methanol metabolism in the monkey. Mol Pharmacol. 1968;4(5):471-83.
32. Hovda KE, Andersson KS, Urdal P, Jacobsen D. Methanol and formate kinetics during treatment with fomepizole. Clin Toxicol (Phila). 2005;43(4):221-7.
33. Hovda KE, McMartin K, Jacobsen D. Methanol and formaldehyde. In: Brent J, Burkhart K, Dargan P, Hatten B, Megarbane B, Palmer R, et al. (Eds). Critical Care Toxicology: Diagnosis and Management of the Critically Poisoned Patient. Cham: Springer International Publishing; 2017. pp. 1769-86.
34. Röe O. Species differences in methanol poisoning. Crit Rev Toxicol. 1982;10(4):275-86.
35. Nicholls P. The effect of formate on cytochrome aa3 and on electron transport in the intact respiratory chain. Biochim Biophys Acta. 1976;430(1):13-29.
36. Drangsholt E, Vangstad M, Zakharov S, Hovda KE, Jacobsen D. The hypothesis of circulus hypoxicus and its clinical relevance in patients with methanol poisoning—An observational study of 35 patients. Basic Clin Pharmacol Toxicol. 2018;123(6):749-55.
37. Martin-Amat G, McMartin KE, Hayreh SS, Hayreh MS, Tephly TR. Methanol poisoning: Ocular toxicity produced by formate. Toxicol Appl Pharmacol. 1978;45(1):201-8.
38. Hovda KE, Urdal P, Jacobsen D. Increased serum formate in the diagnosis of methanol poisoning. J Anal Toxicol. 2005;29(6):586-8.
39. Zakharov S, Kurcova I, Navratil T, Salek T, Komarc M, Pelclova D. Is the measurement of serum formate concentration useful in the diagnostics of acute methanol poisoning? A prospective study of 38 patients. Basic Clin Pharmacol Toxicol. 2015;116(5):445-51.

40. Hovda KE, Gadeholt G, Evtodienko V, Jacobsen D. A novel bedside diagnostic test for methanol poisoning using dry chemistry for formate. Scand J Clin Lab Invest. 2015;75(7):610-4.
41. Lao YE, Heyerdahl F, Jacobsen D, Hovda KE. An enzymatic assay with formate oxidase for point-of-care diagnosis of methanol poisoning. Basic Clin Pharmacol Toxicol. 2022;131(6):547-54.
42. Hovda KE, Hunderi OH, Rudberg N, Froyshov S, Jacobsen D. Anion and osmolal gaps in the diagnosis of methanol poisoning: Clinical study in 28 patients. Intensive Care Med. 2004;30(9):1842-6.
43. Schelling JR, Howard RL, Winter SD, Linas SL. Increased osmolal gap in alcoholic ketoacidosis and lactic acidosis. Ann Intern Med. 1990;113(8):580-2.
44. Sulway MJ, Malins JM. Acetone in diabetic ketoacidosis. Lancet. 1970;2(7676):736-40.
45. Sklar AH, Linas SL. The osmolal gap in renal failure. Ann Intern Med. 1983;98(4):481-2.
46. Walker JA, Schwartzbard A, Krauss EA, Sherman RA, Eisinger RP. The missing gap. A pitfall in the diagnosis of alcohol intoxication by osmometry. Arch Intern Med. 1986;146(9):1843-4.
47. Hovda KE, Jacobsen D. Comment on "Elevated osmol gap in patients with alcoholic ketoacidosis". Clin Toxicol (Phila). 2025;63(1):68-70.
48. Medicines sans frontieres. MSF methanol poisoning protocol 2023. [online] Available from https://methanolpoisoning.msf.org/en/resource-centre/. [Last accessed October, 2024].
49. Paasma R, Hovda KE, Hassanian-Moghaddam H, Brahmi N, Afshari R, Sandvik L, et al. Risk factors related to poor outcome after methanol poisoning and the relation between outcome and antidotes – A multicenter study. Clin Toxicol (Phila). 2012;50(9):823-31.
50. McMartin K, Jacobsen D, Hovda KE. Antidotes for poisoning by alcohols that form toxic metabolites. Br J Clin Pharmacol. 2016;81(3):505-15.
51. Theobald J, Lim C. Folate as an adjuvant therapy in methanol poisoning. Nutr Clin Pract. 2019;34(4):521-7.
52. Zakharov S, Pelclova D, Navratil T, Belacek J, Kurcova I, Komzak O, et al. Intermittent hemodialysis is superior to continuous veno-venous hemodialysis/hemodiafiltration to eliminate methanol and formate during treatment for methanol poisoning. Kidney Int. 2014;86(1):199-207.
53. Zakharov S, Pelclova D, Navratil T, Belacek J, Latta J, Pisar M, et al. Efficiency of acidemia correction on intermittent versus continuous hemodialysis in acute methanol poisoning. Clin Toxicol (Phila). 2017;55(2):123-32.
54. Roberts DM, Yates C, Megarbane B, Winchester JF, Maclaren R, Gosselin S, et al. Recommendations for the role of extracorporeal treatments in the management of acute methanol poisoning: A systematic review and consensus statement. Crit Care Med. 2015;43(2):461-72.
55. Zakharov S, Rulisek J, Nurieva O, Kotikova K, Navratil T, Komarc M, et al. Intermittent versus continuous renal replacement therapy in acute methanol poisoning: Comparison of clinical effectiveness in mass poisoning outbreaks. Ann Intensive Care. 2017;7(1):77-11.
56. Keyvan-Larijarni H, Tannenberg AM. Methanol intoxication: Comparison of peritoneal dialysis and hemodialysis treatment. Arch Intern Med. 1974;134(2):293-6.
57. Hassanian-Moghaddam H, Zamani N, Roberts DM, Brent J, McMartin K, Aaron C, et al. Consensus statements on the approach to patients in a methanol poisoning outbreak. Clin Toxicol (Phila). 2019;57(12):1129-36.
58. Zakharov S, Pelclova D, Urban P, Navratil T, Nurieva O, Kotikova K, et al. Use of out-of-hospital ethanol administration to improve outcome in mass methanol outbreaks. Ann Emerg Med. 2016;68(1):52-61.
59. Hovda KE, Guo C, Austin R, McMartin KE. Renal toxicity of ethylene glycol results from internalization of calcium oxalate crystals by proximal tubule cells. Toxicol Lett. 2010;192(3):365-72.
60. Standefer J, Blackwell W. Enzymatic method for measuring ethylene glycol with a centrifugal analyzer. Clin Chem. 1991;37(10 Pt 1):1734-6.
61. Aarstad K, Dale O, Aakervik O, Ovrebø S, Zahlsen K. A rapid gas chromatographic method for determination of ethylene glycol in serum and urine. J Anal Toxicol. 1993;17(4):218-21.
62. Jacobsen D, Hewlett TP, Webb R, Brown ST, Ordinario AT, McMartin KE. Ethylene glycol intoxication: Evaluation of kinetics and crystalluria. Am J Med. 1988;84(1):145-52.
63. Hovda KE, McMartin K, Jacobsen D. Ethylene glycol and other glycols. In: Brent J, Burkhart K, Dargan P, Hatten B, Megarbane B, Palmer R, et al. (Eds). Critical Care Toxicology: Diagnosis and Management of the Critically Poisoned Patient. Cham: Springer International Publishing; 2017. pp. 1743-60.
64. Beaulieu J, Roberts DM, Gosselin S, Hoffman RS, Lavergne V, Hovda KE, et al. Treating ethylene glycol poisoning with alcohol dehydrogenase inhibition, but without extracorporeal treatments: A systematic review. Clin Toxicol (Phila). 2022;60(7):784-97.
65. Besenhofer LM, McLaren MC, Latimer B, Bartels M, Filary MJ, Perala AW, et al. Role of tissue metabolite accumulation in the renal toxicity of diethylene glycol. Toxicol Sci. 2011;123(2):374-83.
66. Landry GM, Martin S, McMartin KE. Diglycolic acid is the nephrotoxic metabolite in diethylene glycol poisoning inducing necrosis in human proximal tubule cells in vitro. Toxicol Sci. 2011;124(1):35-44.
67. Schep LJ, Slaughter RJ, Temple WA, Beasley DMG. Diethylene glycol poisoning. Clin Toxicol (Phila). 2009;47(6):525-35.

68. Nordmann R, Ribiere C, Rouach H, Beauge F, Giudicelli Y, Nordmann J. Metabolic pathways involved in the oxidation of isopropanol into acetone by the intact rat. Life Sci. 1973;13(7):919-32.
69. Pappas AA, Ackerman BH, Olsen KM, Taylor EH. Isopropanol ingestion: A report of six episodes with isopropanol and acetone serum concentration time data. J Toxicol Clin Toxicol. 1991;29(1):11-21.
70. Bekka R, Borron SW, Astier A, Sandouk P, Bismuth C, Baud FJ. Treatment of methanol and isopropanol poisoning with intravenous fomepizole. J Toxicol Clin Toxicol. 2001;39(1):59-67.
71. Rosansky SJ. Isopropyl alcohol poisoning treated with hemodialysis: Kinetics of isopropyl alcohol and acetone removal. J Toxicol Clin Toxicol. 1982;19(3):265-71.

2.18 Common Household Poisons

Vikas Suri, Ashish Bhalla

INTRODUCTION

Poisoning is a serious public health concern, defined as the exposure to substances that can harm the body and endanger an individual's life. This exposure can occur through ingestion, inhalation, or contact with the skin or mucous membranes. According to the World Health Organization (WHO), approximately 0.3 million people die each year due to various poisoning agents.[1] The modern lifestyle, characterized by increasing complexity and stress, has contributed to a rise in the incidence of suicidal poisoning. India is ranked 49th in the world as far as the rates of self-harm are concerned.[2] Every year, 14.04 people/lakh population commit suicide.[2]

HOUSEHOLD POISONS

Household poisoning, often attributed to accidental ingestion of substances, is a prevalent issue, particularly among children under the age of 5 years. This demographic is more susceptible due to their curious and adventurous nature rather than any negligence on the part of parents or caregivers. Moreover, the confined spaces of small houses make household objects easily accessible to young children, further increasing the risk of accidental ingestion.[3]

Burden of the problem in India

The data about exposure to poisonous compounds and resultant morbidity and mortality is variable. The National Crime Bureau of India reports a gradual and sustained rise in the rate of completed suicides in India.[4] In the year 2022, a total of 1,70,924 suicides were reported in India, with an absolute increase of 4.2% in comparison to 2021.[4] Out of the total completed suicides, 25.8% were due to poisoning. Nearly 15% (14.9%) had consumed pesticides.[4] Recent studies indicate that in the cities, pesticides remain the major killers but household compounds (corrosives, pharmaceutical drugs, and other chemical agents) are fast becoming the preferred methods for attempting self-harm.[5] It has been observed that the percentage of victims consuming pharmaceutical agents and available household compounds has been steadily rising.[6] In the southern part of India, accidental poisoning accounted for a significant portion (68.40%) of reported poisoning cases with toxic compounds available at home (household poisons) being responsible for 25% of these incidents.[7]

In an important 10-year data review from a poison center in north India, household agents were implicated in poisoning in nearly 30% cases.[8] These included compounds such as household cleaners (21.8%), naphthalene balls (5%), antiseptics (3%), kerosene (2%), and paint thinner (2%).[8] The other household compounds commonly implicated are camphor, hair dye, nail polish remover, cosmetics, and adhesives.[8] These substances, often found in everyday household items, pose a significant risk, especially in individuals who may inadvertently come into contact with them.

Household poisons **(Table 1)** can be hazardous acutely or even after a prolonged exposure.

Corrosives

These include alkaline and acidic agents found in household products like disinfectants, detergents, and cleaners. Exposure can lead to intense local symptoms

TABLE 1: Household poisons.

Common	*Uncommon*
Windshield washer solutions	Detergents/dishwashers
Drain cleaners	Furniture polish
Toilet bowl cleaners	Perfumes/aftershave
Artificial nail removers	Mouthwash
Rat poisons	Mothballs
Drugs	• Alcoholic beverages • Miniature batteries

such as pain, redness, and burning, as well as systemic manifestations like hypovolemia and hypoxia. Corrosives (acid and alkali) have been separately discussed in the book. Here, we are discussing household agents which can have corrosive actions.

Household Detergents

A typical household detergent contains builders (50% by weight, approximately), surfactants (15%), bleach (7%), enzymes (2%), soil antideposition agents, foam regulators, corrosion inhibitors, optical brighteners, dye transfer inhibitors, fragrances, dyes, fillers, and formulation aids.[9] Of these, anionic surfactants and builders can cause corrosive injuries upon ingestion.[9] Some detergents may contain unusual chemicals; one such example is 1.2 g of potassium permanganate ($KMNO_4$) and 12.5 g of oxalic acid containing detergent for washing clothes. Nonionic and anionic detergents are of low toxicity, but cationic detergents can produce corrosive effects, especially in concentrated solutions.

Specific types of detergent products also pose unique risks:

- *Toilet rim blocks:* These disinfectants are made from anionic surfactants and have low systemic toxicity but can cause local corrosive action if ingested.
- *Bleaches:* Household bleaches containing sodium hypochlorite or hydrogen peroxide are unpalatable and unlikely to cause serious damage. However, mixing bleach with ammonia or toilet cleaners can produce toxic gases. Some of these gases can be irritant and may cause respiratory distress or precipitate acute attacks of asthma in predisposed individuals.

Clinical manifestations of cationic detergent poisoning: These include acute-onset vomiting, cough, nausea, drowsiness, and rash.[10] Serious life-threatening manifestations, especially in children, could be

- Corrosive injury to the gastrointestinal (GI) (hematemesis/melena), respiratory, and corneal mucosa depending on the route of exposure
- Acute kidney injury (AKI) with rhabdomyolysis
- Myocardial dysfunction with or without tachyarrhythmias
- Acute respiratory distress syndrome (ARDS), both early and late onset

Treatment: It usually involves removing the patient from the source and irrigation of the exposed skin/eyes/mucous membrane with water. The mainstay of treatment is good supportive care.[9,10] In patients reporting oral ingestion, early endoscopy (within the first 12–24 hours) helps assess the extent of injury. All patients reporting ingestion should be observed for at least 6–8 hours. The ones remaining asymptomatic after 6–8 hours may be discharged.[10]

Patients with superficial injuries (Grades I and IIA) typically do not require admission and specific therapy. All patients with serious GI lesions (Grade II and above) should be admitted. Nasojejunal tube insertion or feeding jejunostomy may be needed for injuries that are grade II and above.[9] Antibiotics must be considered in all admitted patients. The patients should be closely observed for at least 48 hours for any evidence of perforation before considering discharge. Long-term sequelae of corrosive ingestion may include the development of esophageal strictures or squamous cell carcinoma.[10]

Button Batteries

Button batteries are commonly used in various electronic devices such as cameras, watches, calculators, hearing aids, and electronic games and pose a unique and serious risk of toxicity if ingested. These small, round batteries, typically <15 mm in size, contain chemicals such as potassium hydroxide and heavy metals, some of which are poisonous.

Foreign body ingestion like button batteries is a common occurrence in young children and infants and can cause injury through several different mechanisms.[11] The most common mechanism of injury, from most foreign bodies, is simply the result of prolonged pressure effects of the foreign body. Some foreign bodies like button batteries have specific toxicity.[11]

Impaction, local pressure effect and local effect of the direct current are factors responsible for gastrointestinal (GI) injury. The narrowest parts of the esophagus are the common sites of impaction. The most common sites

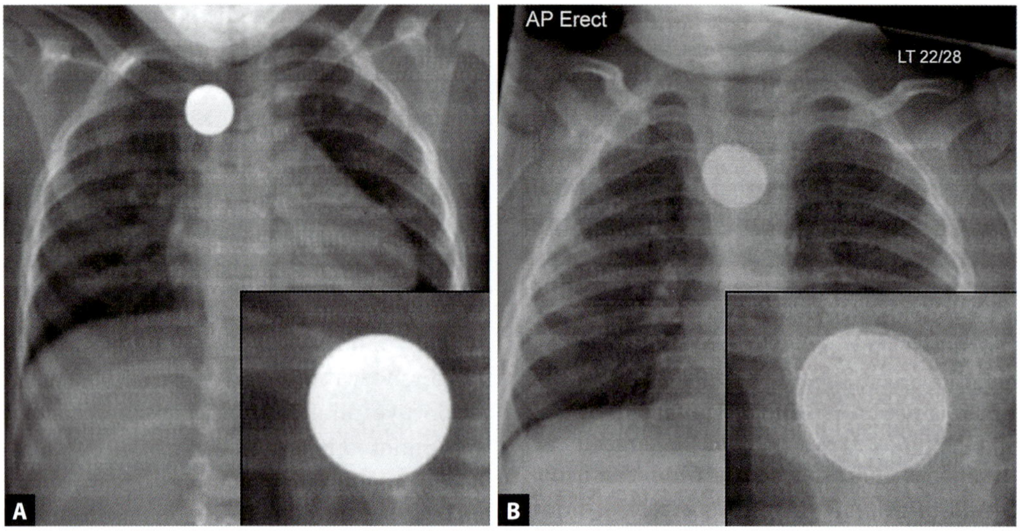

Figs. 1A and B: Frontal chest X-ray (AP view)

involved are the thoracic inlet, the region of the aortic arch, and the gastroesophageal junction.[12]

The corrosive action of button batteries occurs due to leakage of the battery contents at the site of contact with tissue. Children are specifically vulnerable, and the history of ingestion may be lacking in many. Subtle symptoms should be looked for and a high index of clinical suspicion is needed. Button batteries are known to cause serious complications like tracheoesophageal fistula and aortoesophageal fistula.[12]

When button battery ingestion is suspected, a comprehensive radiographic examination from the nasopharynx to the anus should be conducted to localize the site of the battery. Routine frontal chest X-ray will commonly demonstrate "double rim" or "halo" sign **(Figs. 1A and B)** which distinguishes a button battery from a coin (the latter appearing solid).[11]

Different button batteries may contain specific agents **(Table 2)**. These agents are responsible for some local or systemic symptoms.

Endoscopic examination will act as a diagnostic as well as a therapeutic procedure; endoscopic removal is the preferred method if the battery is lodged in the esophagus. If the button battery has crossed the gastroesophageal (GE) junction and the patient is asymptomatic, most of the times it will be expelled from the body without causing significant harm. In this situation, expectant management may be appropriate.[11] However, if the battery fails to pass through the lower bowel after 1 week of ingestion, enemas may be given to facilitate its passage. Surgical intervention is warranted only if the patient is initially symptomatic or if physical examination and diagnosis suggest gut perforation.[12]

TABLE 2: Types of button batteries.[11]

Code battery	*Chemistry*
L	Alkaline
LR	Alkaline
AG	Alkaline
BR/CR	Lithium
SR	Silver oxide
SG	Silver oxide
AG	Alkaline

Overall, prompt identification and management of button battery ingestion are crucial to prevent serious complications such as tissue damage, perforation, and systemic toxicity. Vigilance, timely intervention, and appropriate medical care are essential to ensure the best possible outcomes for affected individuals.

Alcohols/Perfumes/Mouthwash

Commonly found in alcoholic beverages and household products, can be ingested by young children accidentally or given intentionally by caretakers. It acts as a central nervous system (CNS) sedative in overdose, mediated by its interaction with the gamma-aminobutyric acid-A (GABA-A) receptor, leading to increased CNS inhibition. Additionally, ethanol suppresses excitatory

BAC	Clinical symptoms
0.02–0.05%	Decreased inhibition, diminished fine motor coordination
0.05–0.10%	Impaired judgment, impaired coordination
0.10–0.15%	Difficulty with gait and balance
0.15–0.25%	Lethargy, difficulty sitting upright without assistance
0.30%	Coma in nonhabituated drinker
0.40%	Respiratory depression

TABLE 3: Dose-related ethanol toxicity: Blood alcohol concentration (BAC) and central nervous system (CNS) effects.[14]

neurotransmission by activating the N-methyl-D-aspartate (NMDA) type glutamate receptor **(Table 3)**.[13]

Children under 6 years of age, particularly toddlers, are at risk of ethanol ingestion due to their exploratory behaviors. Household products such as aftershave lotion, glass cleaners, mouthwashes, and perfumes contain varying concentrations of ethanol, ranging from 10 to 95%.[13]

One must be careful as some cosmetic agents may contain acetone (nail polish removers) or acetonitrile (false nail removers). The clinical manifestations may overlap.

Ethanol intoxication can result in nausea and vomiting if a large amount is consumed by the uninitiated. It is not uncommon to find a young child walking unsteadily, confused or stupor, after inadvertent/accidental consumption of nonbeverage ethanol.[14]

Massive ingestion may cause coma and hypoglycemia. Hypoglycemia is due to inhibition of gluconeogenesis in the liver and may add to confusion or coma.[13]

Initial symptoms of acetone, nitroethane, and acetonitrile poisoning may be similar to ethanol ingestion.[15] These include vomiting, lethargy, slurred speech, ataxia, stupor, coma, and respiratory depression. Delayed vomiting may be important in alerting healthcare providers to acetonitrile/nitroethane toxicity in exposed children.[15]

Conventional methods of GI decontamination, such as gastric lavage and activated charcoal administration, are not recommended for ethanol ingestion because ethanol does not bind to activated charcoal, and these methods pose a risk of pulmonary aspiration.

Supportive care is the mainstay of managing ethanol intoxication.[13] This includes treatment of hypoglycemia (IV infusion of dextrose), hypovolemia (IV fluids), respiratory depression (ventilation), seizures (benzodiazepines), and hypothermia (external rewarming).[14]

Acetonitrile poisoning may result in severe cyanosis which is not associated with respiratory distress.[15] In such clinical situations, methemoglobinemia should always be suspected. In such cases, after the diagnosis is established, therapy with methylene blue results in prompt relief.[16] Timely intervention and appropriate medical care are essential to ensure good outcomes in cases of ethanol intoxication in children.

Insect Repellent

Insect repellents applied to exposed skin serve as an essential measure for protecting against mosquito bites. Effective repellents include synthetic preparations such as DEET (N,N-diethyl-m-toluamide), Picaridin (KBR3023), IR 3535, and PMD (P-menthane-3,8-diol) derived from lemon eucalyptus. Among these, DEET is considered preferable for maximal protection against mosquitoes.[17]

The toxicity of insect repellents largely depends on the route and extent of exposure. Common unintentional routes of exposure include skin contact, eye contact, inhalation, and unknowing ingestion. Ocular and nasal exposure are frequently encountered due to the formulation of repellents, often in liquid or spray form.[18] Picaridin, for instance, may be inhaled when sprays are used around the body, especially in indoor spaces where vapors can linger.[18] Accidental ingestion can occur if users fail to wash their hands after applying repellent and then handle food or smoke.

DEET, another commonly used repellent, can cause local irritation and discomfort when introduced into the eyes or oral cavity.

A majority of these accidental ingestions are reported during summer months. Ingestion of DEET has been associated with a range of symptoms, including nausea, vomiting, hypotension, encephalopathy, seizure, coma, and ataxia.[17] Excessive dermal application of DEET, particularly in children, can lead to seizures, bradycardia, nausea, vomiting, bullous eruptions, lethargy, ataxia, encephalopathy, and anaphylaxis. In some studies, mild-to-moderate ARDS has been reported as a presenting symptom. This usually responds to supplemental oxygen with or without positive airway pressure. Most of the intoxications are nonfatal.[17]

Clinical manifestations of accidental ingestion of liquid mosquito repellent vaporizer include vomiting, convulsions, cough, and respiratory distress.[18] Which component of the vaporizer causes toxicity is debatable.[19] It could be the parent compound or solvent which results in toxicity.

Treatment is largely symptomatic and supportive in the form of intravenous fluids, oxygen supplementations, and benzodiazepines to control the seizures and oxygenation/ventilation for hypoxia.[17,18]

Insect repellents are effective in preventing mosquito bites; accidental exposures, particularly in children, can lead to serious health consequences. Proper education on the safe use and storage of repellents, along with prompt medical attention in case of ingestion or exposure, is essential in mitigating risks and ensuring the well-being of individuals.

Rodenticides

Rodenticides are substances used to kill rodents, and they often contain hydroxycoumarin anticoagulants. When resistance to warfarin, a first-generation anticoagulant, began to emerge in rodents, second-generation *superwarfarins* and *indandione* derivatives were introduced. Other rodenticides may include *bromethalin*, *cholecalciferol*, *alphachloralose*, *strychnine*, yellow phosphorus, and zinc phosphide.[20]

Alphachloralose, for example, induces CNS depression.[20] While most one-time warfarin ingestions are insignificant accidental poisonings and do not typically lead to bleeding problems, toxicity may occur with large amounts in a single exposure or repetitive exposures over several days. The *superwarfarins*, having a longer biological half-life, can lead to marked anticoagulation effects for weeks to months with a single ingestion. Acute intentional or repeated ingestions of *superwarfarins* can result in severe bleeding.[21]

Patients with symptomatic *superwarfarin* exposure present with bleeding-related manifestations such as gross hematuria, mucosal bleeding, GI bleeding, soft-tissue bleeding, menorrhagia, and hemoptysis, and nonbleeding-related symptoms and signs such as abdominal pain, flank pain, and headache.[22] Prothrombin time (PT) and international normalized ratio (INR) are the investigations of choice in *superwarfarins'* poisoning. Serum levels can be measured but are not routinely used. In patients with acute ingestion, activated charcoal can be administered although there is no robust proof of its efficacy.[20] Management in a bleeding patient is guided by PT and INR. It includes vitamin K1 therapy, and early and rapid correction of coagulopathy can be achieved by administration of fresh frozen plasma and four-factor prothrombin complex concentrate.[23]

Yellow phosphorus ingestion leads to acute nausea and vomiting, followed by jaundice and acute liver failure. GI hemorrhage and perforation are some other reported complications.[24] Untreated exposures can be fatal. All patients with *yellow phosphorus* ingestion should be admitted and observed. Most of the mildly poisoned patients will respond to supportive therapy. Administration of N-acetylcysteine is commonly practiced but has not been substantiated as standard of care for acute *yellow phosphorus* poisoning.[25] Therapeutic plasma exchange (TPE) has sown mortality benefit in patients with fulminant hepatic failure secondary to *yellow phosphorus* exposure.[25] TPE may act as a bridge to liver transplant in severe acute liver failure.

Zinc phosphide poisoning clinically presents as aluminum phosphide toxicity. In both the ingestions, it is the cytotoxic phosphine which acts like mitochondrial poison to cause symptoms. Unresponsive hypotension and severe metabolic acidosis are classic clinical manifestations.[26] This needs to be treated like aluminum phosphide poisoning with inotropes, sodium bicarbonate, glucose–insulin–potassium (GIK) infusion, and extracorporeal membrane oxygenation (ECMO) if indicated and available.[26]

Hair Dyes

Hair dyes are categorized into oxidative dyes (permanent), direct dyes (semipermanent or temporary), metal salts, and natural salts. Modern oxidative dyes, commonly used in permanent hair coloring, typically consist of two components that react chemically upon mixing to generate the dye within the hair through an oxidative process.[27]

These dyes contain various ingredients, including primary intermediates such as *para*-phenylenediamine (PPD), para-toluenediamine (PTD), substituted *para*-diamines, and *ortho*- or *para*-aminophenols, as well as couplers or modifiers like *m*-phenylene-diamines, m-aminophenols, and resorcinol, along with oxidants and alkalinizing agents.[28]

Para-phenylenediamine, an aromatic amine, undergoes a chemical reaction with hydrogen peroxide during the dyeing process, forming Bandrowski's base, which is highly allergenic and toxic.

The principal adverse effects of high oral doses of PPD in humans are angioedema leading to acute respiratory distress. This can be sudden and may be fatal. Patients having history of allergies should be cautioned regarding this complication and should not be using hair dyes. A milder degree of allergic reactions is seen in nearly every adult using hair dye. The more severe complication is seen in the form of rhabdomyolysis, which can lead to acute renal failure. Rhabdomyolysis is seen mainly in patients following ingestion and is rarely seen after local application.[29] Other mechanisms of acute renal failure associated with PPD poisoning may involve hypovolemia, intravascular hemolysis, and direct toxic effects of PPD or its metabolites on the kidneys. Some other commonly reported features of PPD poisoning include liver failure, drowsiness, altered sensorium, convulsions, GI symptoms, exophthalmos, and chronic renal failure.[28] Acute-onset motor paralysis with PPD toxicity is extremely rare, with only isolated case reports being documented.

Treatment of systemic PPD poisoning primarily involves supportive care as there is no specific antidote. Early clinical suspicion, prompt diagnosis, and therapeutic interventions, such as tracheostomy, intravenous fluid administration, and hemodialysis, can lead to full recovery.[27–29]

Miscellaneous Household Poisons

Miscellaneous household poisons encompass a variety of substances found in common household products, each with its own toxic effects and management considerations:

- *Imidazoline decongestants*: Active components of over-the-counter nasal sprays and nasal decongestant drops can cause toxicity in children on ingestion. Naphazoline, oxymetazoline, and tetrahydrozoline are the common active ingredients.[30] Most common symptoms are somnolence, sweating, hypothermia, bradycardia, and hypotension. Sometimes, it may cause respiratory distress.[30] Treatment primarily involves symptomatic and supportive care. Most patients recover completely within 24 hours.[30]
- *Paint thinners/turpentine substitutes*: Paint thinners and organic solvents may be available in certain households. Thinner is an organic solvent that contains aromatic hydrocarbons such as toluene and xylene and is easily accessible in products such as gasoline, paint, varnish, and plastic production industries.[31] While relatively low in toxicity when ingested in small quantities, these substances can cause severe oral symptoms and GI irritation. Toluene and xylene once absorbed from the GI tract can cause rhabdomyolysis, metabolic acidosis, and hepatic and renal dysfunction.[31] CNS depression occurs if consumed in large amounts.

  The main concern is aspiration, which can lead to chemical pneumonitis. Lung injury may occur due to aspiration of the compound or secondary to aspiration of the vomitus.[31] Even a few milliliters of hydrocarbon ingestion/aspiration may cause severe chemical pneumonitis.[31] Mortality is generally attributed to secondary infections.[32] Symptoms may develop up to 24 hours post ingestion, emphasizing the need for respiratory assessment in all patients. Treatment with surfactant in pediatric patients with ARDS has been of some benefit. Budesonide and nitric oxide for bronchospasm may help.[33] Severe cases of chemical pneumonitis may require ECMO support.
- *Camphor:* It is a colorless to white substance commonly available at homes. It has a characteristic strong odor and very pungent taste. Camphor is usually available in solid form, but liquid form is also available.[34] It is a common ingredient in vaporized or topical cold preparations, like Vicks VapoRub, Tiger Balm, topical musculoskeletal anesthetics, and moth repellents, as an important component in religious ritual ceremonies and in antimicrobial preparations.[35] The easy availability of these products at home puts people, especially children, at high risk of camphor poisoning. Camphor can cause severe toxicity even when ingested in small amounts.[36]

  The onset of action is very rapid (5–15 minutes); after ingestion, the first symptoms are burning sensation in the mouth and pharynx. A strong camphor smell in the breath can be an important clue. Pain in epigastrium and vomiting follow local oral symptoms.[34] CNS manifestations are in the form of confusion, restlessness, delirium, and hallucinations. Muscle twitching and myoclonus are common. Hyperreflexia and fasciculations are important signs. Gait is usually ataxic. Seizure may be the first sign of systemic toxicity and may occur soon after ingestion without any preceding symptoms. Seizures denote severe toxicity. Camphor can also lead to hepatic and renal injury. Mortality usually occurs due to seizures or respiratory failure.[34,35]

  All symptomatic patients should be admitted to the intensive care unit. Asymptomatic patients should be observed for a minimum period of 6 hours. If they remain asymptomatic after 6 hours, they may be discharged.[37] The treatment is supportive with a focus on airway management and seizure control. Dermal and ocular decontamination, in patients with local exposure, is done by flushing the affected site with a large amount of water. Gastric lavage and activated charcoal have a limited role in management; therefore, these are not advocated.[34] Seizures can be aborted with benzodiazepines. Intravenous midazolam or lorazepam may be used. IV patients with difficult-to-control seizures, repeated doses of benzodiazepines, or an IV infusion may be needed. For difficult-to-control seizures, phenobarbitone or phenytoin can be added.[38]

- *Naphthalene:* Mothballs are common in nearly every household, and naphthalene is a major ingredient in them. It is commonly used as a household pesticide for preventing damage to clothes from moths.[39] The size and the amount of naphthalene in mothballs are variable. Usually, mothballs may contain naphthalene varying from 0.5 to 5 g.[40] The fatal dose of naphthalene is unknown, but accidental ingestion of even a single mothball can result in clinically significant toxicity. In most of the developed countries, naphthalene has been replaced with 1,4-dichlorobenzene, which is harmless. In many countries, naphthalene mothballs are widely available.[39]

Naphthalene ingestion is uncommon due to its pungent smell and taste. It is insoluble in water but is rapidly absorbed when inhaled. Both dermal and GI absorption is erratic.[40]

The clinical manifestations of toxicity are related to acute hemolysis. This is common in children with glucose-6-phosphate dehydrogenase (G6PD) deficiency.[39] The usual symptoms are headache, vomiting, abdominal pain, and altered mental status. Acute, severe intravascular hemolysis leads to anemia.[40]

Intracellular hemoglobin further dissociates into heme and globin. Presence of free heme in the cells leads to cytotoxicity. Free hemoglobin in renal tubules manifests pathologically as pigment cast nephropathy. The end result of this is AKI.[40]

Complete blood count is mandatory in all patients. Peripheral blood film should be carefully evaluated for evidence of hemolysis. Presence of free hemoglobin in urine and elevated level of plasma hemoglobin, lactate dehydrogenase (LDH), renal and liver function tests, acid–base status, urine routine examination, methemoglobin levels, and G6PD levels need to be monitored serially.[34,39]

The treatment is generally supporting. Anemia is managed by transfusion of compatible packed red blood cells. AKI requires monitoring of fluid and electrolyte balance. Administration of alkali (sodium bicarbonate) to reduce the precipitation of free hemoglobin in tubules may be tried. Significant renal dysfunction will warrant renal replacement therapy.[40]

PREVENTION OF HOUSEHOLD POISONING

Legislative strategies aimed at preventing household poisoning are crucial in safeguarding public health. Enacting stringent laws to regulate the procurement of lethal drugs and potentially harmful products can significantly reduce the risk of accidental exposures. This may involve imposing restrictions on the sale of certain chemicals or substances, requiring proper labeling and packaging of hazardous products, and implementing penalties for noncompliance.[3]

Promoting product engineering to develop safer alternatives for household items is another important legislative approach. Encouraging manufacturers to innovate and create products with lower toxicity or reduced risk of harm can contribute to preventing accidental poisonings.

Education plays a vital role in preventing household poisoning. Educating individuals, especially parents and caregivers, on safe handling and storage of chemicals and household products is essential. This includes raising awareness about common household items that may pose a poisoning risk, even if they are not typically considered poisonous. Providing information on proper storage practices, such as keeping toxic products locked away and out of reach of children, can help mitigate the risk of accidental ingestion or exposure.[1]

Protecting young children, who are most vulnerable to household poisons, should be a priority. Parents should be encouraged to regularly clean their homes to identify and remove potential hazards. Additionally, storing toxic products in small quantities and disposing them properly when no longer needed can help prevent unintentional exposures.[1]

Segregating consumables from potentially harmful products and storing them separately can further reduce the risk of accidental ingestion. This includes keeping medicines, insecticides, rat poison, and household cleaners locked away in cupboards or cabinets, away from areas accessible to children.[1,3]

CONCLUSION

Legislative efforts to prevent household poisoning should focus on enacting laws to regulate the procurement of harmful substances, promoting product engineering for safer alternatives, and educating the public on safe handling and storage practices. By implementing these strategies, policymakers can help protect individuals, particularly young children, from the dangers of household poisons.

REFERENCES

1. World Health Organization. Poison control and unintentional poisoning. (2021). [online] Available from: https://www.who.int/data/gho/data/themes/topics/indicator-groups/poison-control-and-unintentional-poisoning. [Last accessed October, 2024].
2. Yadav S, Aathavan KK, Cunningham SA, Bhandari P, Mishra US, Aditi A, et al. Changing pattern of suicide deaths in India. Lancet Reg Health Southeast Asia. 2023;16:100265.
3. Suri V, Bhalla A, Varma S. Household poisoning – a review. Household Personal Care Today. 2010;2:16-20.
4. National Crime Records Bureau. (2022). Accidental deaths and suicides in India: Published by National Crime Records Bureau; 2022 [online] Available from https://data.opencity.in/dataset/6af5e9d7-9de5-4689-9fe3-3418790bb0d5/resource/493c904b-d83b-48bc-bf55-678594ffffff/download/1701611156012adsi2022publication2022.pdf. [Last accessed October, 2024].
5. Pagdhune A, Kunal K, Patel KA, Patel AB, Mishra S, Palkhade R, et al. Poisoning cases reported to poison information centre: a three year observation study. Cent Asian J Glob Health. 2020;9(1):2166-7403.
6. Pannu AK, Bhalla A, Vamshi V, Upadhyay MK, Sharma N, Kumar S. Changing spectrum of acute poisoning in North India: a hospital-based descriptive study. Turk J Emerg Med. 2022;22:192-9.
7. Jesslin J, Adepu R, Churi S. Assessment of prevalence and mortality incidences due to poisoning in a South Indian tertiary care teaching hospital. Indian J Pharm Sci. 2010;72(5):587-91.
8. Peshin SS, Gupta YK. Poisoning due to household products: A ten years retrospective analysis of telephone calls to the National Poisons Information Centre, All India Institute of Medical Sciences, New Delhi, India. J Forensic Leg Med. 2018;58:205-11.
9. Suri V, Mahi S, Bhalla A, Varma S. Detergents: uncommon household poisons. Indian J Med Sci. 2009;63(7):311-2.
10. Bonney AG, Mazor S, Goldman RD. Laundry detergent capsules and pediatric poisoning. Can Fam Physician. 2013;59(12):1295-6.
11. Semple T, Calder AD, Ramaswamy M, McHugh K. Button battery ingestion in children—a potentially catastrophic event of which all radiologists must be aware. Br J Radiol. 2018;91:20160781.
12. Mirshemirani A, Khaleghnejad-Tabari A, Kouranloo J, Sadeghian N, Rouzrokh M, Roshanzamir F, et al. Clinical evaluation of disc battery ingestion in children. Middle East J Dig Dis. 2012;4:107–10.
13. LaHood AJ, Kok SJ. Ethanol toxicity. 2023. Treasure Island (FL): StatPearls Publishing; 2024.
14. Vonghia L, Leggio L, Ferrulli A, Bertini M, Gasbarrini G, Addolorato G, et al. Acute alcohol intoxication. Eur J Intern Med. 2008;19:561.
15. Losek JD, Rock AL, Boldt RR. Cyanide poisoning from a cosmetic nail remover. Pediatrics. 1991;88:337-40.
16. Patra S, Sikka G, Khaowas AK, Kumar V. Successful intervention in a child with toxic methemoglobinemia due to nail polish remover poisoning. Indian J Occup Environ Med. 2011;15(3):137-8.
17. Reddy MV, Ganesan SL, Narayanan K, Jayashree M, Singhi SC, Nallasamy K, et al. Liquid mosquito repellent ingestion in children. Indian J Pediatr. 2020;87(1):12-6.
18. Naeem B, Saleem J, Haider Naqvi ASA, Kausar S, Arshad A, Kumar K, et al. Systematic review of clinical manifestations, management and outcome following accidental ingestion of liquid mosquito repellent vaporiser in children. BMJ Paediatr Open. 2024;8(1):e002476.
19. Chandelia S, Dubey NK. Mosquito repellent vaporizer poisoning – Is the culprit transfluthrin or Kerosene? Indian Paediatr. 2014;51:319.
20. Isackson B, Irizarry L. Rodenticide toxicity. In: StatPearls [Internet]. Treasure Island (FL): StatPearls Publishing; 2024.
21. Deaton JG, Nappe TM. Warfarin toxicity. StatPearls [Internet]. Treasure Island (FL): StatPearls Publishing; 2023.
22. Chong YK, Mak TWL. Superwarfarin (long-acting anticoagulant rodenticides) poisoning: from pathophysiology to laboratory-guided clinical management. Clin Biochem Rev. 2019;40(4):175-85.
23. Rubinstein I, Weinberg G, van Breemen R, Hershow RC, Feinstein DL. Treatment for long acting anticoagulant rodenticide poisoning – beyond INR monitoring? Toxicol Commun. 2018;2:59-61.
24. Ravikanth R, Sandeep S, Philip B. Acute yellow phosphorus poisoning causing fulminant hepatic failure with parenchymal hemorrhages and contained duodenal perforation. Indian J Crit Care Med. 2017;21(4):238-42.
25. Marin GA, Montoya CA, Sierra JL, Senior JR. Evaluation of corticosteroid and exchange-transfusion treatment

of acute yellow-phosphorus intoxication. N Engl J Med. 1971;284:125-8.
26. Anbalagan LC, Pannu AK, Bhalla A, Dhibar DP, Sharma N. Prognostic significance of poison-related factors and consumption patterns in acute aluminum phosphide poisoning. Turk J Emerg Med. 2023;23(2):88-95.
27. Kumar PAS, Talari K, Dutta TK. Super vasomol hair dye poisoning. Toxicol Int. 2012;19(1):77-8.
28. Asghar S, Mahbub S, Asghar S, Shahid S. Paraphenylenediamine (hair dye) poisoning: a prospective study on the clinical outcome and side effects profile. Cureus. 2022;14(9):e29133.
29. Hamdouk M. Paraphenylenediamine (Hair Dye) Acute Systemic toxicity. PPD Nephrotoxicity. Sheffield: Sheffield Kidney Institute; 2001. pp. 34-47.
30. Bucaretchi F, Dragosavac S, Vieira RJ. Exposição aguda a derivados imidazolínicos em crianças [Acute exposure to imidazoline derivatives in children]. J Pediatr (Rio J). 2003;79(6):519-24.
31. Koçak M, Açıksarı K. Chemical pneumonia due to paint thinner ingestion: A case report and literature review. Eurasian J Emerg Med. 2019;18(1):55-7.
32. Jayashree M, Singhi S, Gupta A. Predictors of outcome in children with hydrocarbon poisoning receiving intensive care. Indian Pediatr. 2006;43:715-9.
33. Horoz OO, Yildizdas D, Yilmaz HL. Surfactant therapy in acute respiratory distress syndrome due to hydrocarbon aspiration. Singapore Med J. 2009;50:e130-2.
34. Kumar S, Kavitha TK, Angurana SK. Kerosene, camphor, and naphthalene poisoning in children. Indian J Crit Care Med. 2019;23(Suppl 4):S27881.
35. Sahana KS, Rajiv D. Camphor poisoning. Indian Pediatr. 2012;49(10):841-2.
36. Matteucci J. One pill can kill: assessing the potential for fatal poisonings in children. Pediatr Ann. 2005;34(12):964-8.
37. Mathen PG, Sreekrishnan TP, Kumar KPG, Mohan N. Camphor poisoning: a rare cause of acute symptomatic seizures in children. J Emerg Trauma Shock. 2018;11(3):2289.
38. Manoguerra AS, Erdman AR, Wax PM, Nelson LS, Caravati EM, Cobaugh DJ, et al. Camphor poisoning: an evidence-based practice guideline for out-of-hospital management. Clin Toxicol. 2006;44(4):357-70.
39. Ekambaram S, Chandan Kumar KM, Mahalingam V. Acute kidney injury: a rare complication of mothball (Naphthalene) poisoning. Saudi J Kidney Dis Transpl. 2017;28(6):1412-5.
40. Uthuman AAA, Jayasinghe CS, Fernando AHN. Acute intravascular hemolysis due to naphthalene toxicity: a case report. J Med Case Rep. 2019;13(1):91.

2.19 Reducing Agents that Cause Methemoglobinemia

Ranajit Chatterjee, Lalit Gupta

INTRODUCTION

Methemoglobinemia is a condition where levels of methemoglobin, an altered form of hemoglobin, are elevated. This can happen when hemoglobin undergoes oxidation, changing from ferrous (Fe^{2+}) to ferric (Fe^{3+}) iron. Normal methemoglobin levels are under 3%.[1] Higher levels can lead to symptoms related to decreased oxygen delivery to tissues. Certain drugs and chemicals act as reducing agents, and they can trigger methemoglobinemia by causing oxidation of hemoglobin to methemoglobin.[2] Methemoglobin cannot bind and transport oxygen effectively, resulting in functional anemia and tissue hypoxia. Methemoglobinemia is a serious condition that requires prompt treatment. Management involves removing the inciting agent and providing supportive care. In severe cases, methylene blue or ascorbic acid may be given to accelerate the reduction of methemoglobin back to hemoglobin.[3] An interprofessional team approach is key for the effective diagnosis and management of methemoglobinemia. This chapter will provide an overview of methemoglobinemia induced by reducing agents, including the mechanisms, clinical manifestations, diagnosis, treatment, and prevention.

ETIOLOGY

Methemoglobinemia arises from genetic or acquired causes. Inherited forms result from deficiencies in cytochrome b5 reductase (CYB5R), which impairs enzymatic reduction of methemoglobin, or mutations in hemoglobin subunits that destabilize ferrous iron binding.[4] These rare congenital types include methemoglobinemia types I and II based on cell specificity of the CYB5R defect, along with multiple hemoglobin M variants from alpha or beta chain mutations near the heme group.[5] Acquired methemoglobinemia is more common and induced by exogenous agents that overwhelm natural reductase systems through direct oxidization or metabolic activation.

Well-known triggers are drugs like benzocaine from procedures and nitrites' ingestion from contaminated water. Benzocaine is a particular concern, implicated in most cases from topical anesthetic use, prompting Food and Drug Administration (FDA) warnings about benzocaine oral product risks.[6] While congenital forms are uncommon, acquired methemoglobinemia has a higher incidence, typically from inadvertent or occupational exposures that generates methemoglobin more rapidly than the body can physiologically reduce iron back to its oxygen-binding ferrous state.[7] Overall, this dangerous hemoglobin disorder can arise from inherited enzyme or hemoglobin abnormalities but more often results from exposure to potent exogenous oxidizing substances.

What are reducing agents?

Reducing agents are substances that oxidize ferrous iron in hemoglobin to ferric state, leading to the formation of methemoglobin. Methemoglobin forms when hemoglobin is oxidized, changing the iron atoms from ferrous (Fe^{2+}) to ferric (Fe^{3+}) state. Ferric iron cannot bind oxygen. This oxidation also causes allosteric changes in hemoglobin that increase its affinity for oxygen. As a result, oxygen binds more tightly to the remaining ferrous iron atoms in methemoglobin. However, this increased binding affinity impairs the release of oxygen to tissues. The end result is less oxygen delivery to tissues, leading to hypoxia.[8]

Many aromatic amines and compounds containing nitroso or nitro groups act as reducing agents in vivo.[9-13] Examples include nitrites, aniline dyes, antimalarial drugs like primaquine, and others. Nitrites are commonly ingested from processed and cured meats or through contamination of water sources. Aniline dyes are found in textiles, leather, and cosmetics. Many pharmaceutical agents such as dapsone and primaquine are also potent reducing agents. These compounds gain enzymatic access to erythrocytes where they induce electron deficiency and oxidize ferrous hemoglobin to ferric methemoglobin, ultimately disrupting its oxygen-binding capacity **(Table 1)**.

TABLE 1: Drugs that induce methemoglobinemia.

Reducing agent	*Examples*
Nitrites	Various medications (amyl nitrite, bismuth subnitrate, sodium nitroprusside, nitric oxide)
Nitrates	Nitroglycerin, isosorbide dinitrate, silver nitrate
Local anesthetics	Benzocaine, prilocaine, lignocaine
Antimalarials	Primaquine
Analgesics	Acetanilide, fentanyl, celecoxib
UTI drug	Phenazopyridine
Antibiotics	Dapsone, sulfonamides
Hormones	Flutamide
Anticonvulsants	Phenobarbital, phenytoin, sodium valproate
Chemicals/dyes	Aniline dyes, naphthalene, etc.

(UTI: urinary tract infection)

MECHANISM OF METHEMOGLOBINEMIA

Methemoglobinemia represents an interplay between oxidizing agents, intrinsic enzyme function, and individual susceptibility that allows abnormal methemoglobin to accumulate to pathologic levels. Under normal circumstances, inherent nicotinamide-adenine dinucleotide hydrogen (NADH)–methemoglobin reductase (NADH—cytochrome b5 reductase) enzyme systems continually convert methemoglobin back to functional, oxygen-binding hemoglobin.[4] However, upon exposure to high concentrations of potent oxidizing reducing agents, these endogenous protective enzymes can become overwhelmed and saturated. This prevents efficient reduction of methemoglobin back to functional hemoglobin, allowing build-up of the abnormal form.

Some individuals also have inherent deficiencies in the enzymes that normally reduce methemoglobin or they have other conditions like glucose-6-phosphate dehydrogenase (G6PD) deficiency that impair this process. These individuals are more susceptible to methemoglobin accumulation and hypoxia when exposed to oxidizing substances.[14]

Several other factors also influence a drug's potential to induce methemoglobinemia[15-17] **(Table 2)**.

CLINICAL MANIFESTATIONS

Clinical manifestations of methemoglobinemia vary based on the circulating level of methemoglobin in the

TABLE 2: Factors affecting drug's potential to induce methemoglobinemia.

Factors	*Influence on methemoglobinemia*
Potency of the oxidizing agent	Strong oxidizers are more likely to cause methemoglobinemia than weak oxidizers
Presence of aniline, nitroso, or hydroxylamine groups	Drugs metabolized into these compounds tend to be more methemoglobinemic. For example, phenacetin metabolizes into a nitroso compound that can induce methemoglobinemia after overdose
Route of administration	Local anesthetics are more likely to cause methemoglobinemia when injected or used topically, as opposed to orally. Prilocaine has a higher risk than other local anesthetics
Dose	Methemoglobinemia is more likely with overdoses or higher than recommended therapeutic doses (high dose of trimethoprim/sulfamethoxazole for long duration)
Duration	Prolonged or chronic use of oxidizing medications can increase the risk of methemoglobinemia over time (repetitive doses of metoclopramide over long duration)
Concomitant administration of more than one oxidant drugs	Using multiple oxidizing medications together, especially potent combinations in vulnerable populations like infants, increases the risk of clinically significant methemoglobinemia • Combining primaquine and dapsone in patients with human immunodeficiency virus (HIV) can cause clinically significant methemoglobinemia if given within 24 hours • Combining isosorbide dinitrate and nitroglycerin ointments increased methemoglobin levels
Individual susceptibility	Factors like anaerobic gut bacteria, malnutrition, pediatric age group, and genetic deficiencies can increase risk in certain people

bloodstream. The severity of symptoms increases with higher concentrations of methemoglobin. The spectrum of clinical manifestations ranges from subtle symptoms in mild cases to severe neurological and cardiovascular complications in critical instances[3,8,18] **(Table 3)**.

TABLE 3: Clinical manifestations at different methemoglobin levels.

Methemoglobin level	*Symptoms*	*Clinical presentation*
10%	Headache, fatigue, dizziness, shortness	Generally mild with early signs of oxygen delivery impairment
20–50% "chocolate-brown" cyanosis	Rapid heart rate, increased respiratory rate, metabolic acidosis	Pronounced signs of oxygen deficiency, central cyanosis unresponsive to oxygen
50–70%	Disorientation, lethargy, seizures, arrhythmias	Critical impairment of oxygen delivery, potential life-threatening complications
>70%	Frequently fatal	Profound inability to deliver oxygen to tissues, often leading to death

DIAGNOSIS

Methemoglobinemia is diagnosed based on blood co-oximetry, which can rapidly measure functional oxygen-carrying hemoglobin versus nonfunctional methemoglobin through spectrophotometry. Provisional diagnosis is made on suspicious history, symptoms like refractory hypoxemia, and chocolate-colored blood. Pulse oximetry (SpO_2) is inaccurate due to interference from methemoglobin's light absorbance. It tends to falsely elevate readings. Arterial blood gas (SaO_2) is falsely normal because it assumes that all hemoglobin is oxy/deoxyhemoglobin.[19]

The gap between the low SpO_2 and normal SaO_2 is a clue pointing toward methemoglobinemia or other hemoglobinopathies. An elevated methemoglobin level on co-oximetry in a patient with consistent symptoms is diagnostic. Testing for the presence of a causative reducing agent can support the diagnosis. Other laboratory findings of metabolic acidosis and elevated lactate may be present due to hypoxia. A comprehensive approach that integrates clinical, laboratory, and historical aspects is crucial for accurate diagnosis and appropriate management **(Box 1)**.[6,20]

TREATMENT

Methemoglobinemia is effectively treated with methylene blue, serving as the primary antidote intervention.[9] The treatment involves addressing the impaired

BOX 1: Diagnosis of methemoglobinemia.

Blood co-oximetry:
- *Methodology:* Co-oximetry enables the precise measurement of different hemoglobin species, including methemoglobin, in the blood
- *Diagnostic significance:* An elevated methemoglobin level detected by co-oximetry, especially in the presence of consistent clinical symptoms, serves as a key diagnostic criterion for methemoglobinemia

Causative reducing agents:
- *Supporting the diagnosis:* Identifying and testing for the presence of specific reducing agents known to induce methemoglobinemia can further support the diagnosis
- *Common reducing agents:* Nitrites, local anesthetics, antimalarials, analgesics, and certain antibiotics are among the substances that may act as causative reducing agents

Laboratory findings:
- *Metabolic acidosis:* Laboratory tests may reveal metabolic acidosis, reflecting the overall physiological impact of impaired oxygen delivery to tissues
- *Elevated lactate:* Hypoxia resulting from methemoglobinemia can lead to elevated lactate levels, contributing to the characterization of the metabolic disturbance associated with this condition

Clinical correlation:
- *Symptom consistency:* A thorough correlation with the patient's symptoms is essential for a comprehensive diagnosis
- Elevated methemoglobin levels, coupled with clinical manifestations such as central cyanosis, neurological symptoms, and cardiovascular complications, contribute to a more robust diagnostic picture

Additional considerations:
- *Patient history:* Understanding the patient's medical history, including exposure to potential reducing agents, assists in identifying the underlying cause of methemoglobinemia
- *Timing of testing:* Co-oximetry should be performed promptly when methemoglobinemia is suspected to facilitate timely diagnosis and intervention

oxygen-carrying capacity of hemoglobin due to elevated methemoglobin levels **(Table 4)**.[7,17,21,22]

PREVENTION

Preventing exposure to causative reducing agents is a crucial strategy to avert acquired methemoglobinemia. This involves careful consideration of patient susceptibility, screening for specific enzyme deficiencies, and implementing public health measures to minimize community-wide risks.[22-27]

TABLE 4: Treatment and interventions for methemoglobinemia.

Treatment and interventions	***Details***
Methylene blue as antidote treatment	• *Mechanism:* Methylene blue acts as an exogenous reducing agent, providing an alternative pathway for the conversion of methemoglobin to functional hemoglobin • *Dosing:* Administered intravenously (IV) at a dose of 1–2 mg/kg (0.1–0.2 mL/kg of 1% solution) over 5 minutes. The dose can be repeated in 30–60 minutes if symptoms persist or methemoglobin levels remain elevated
Additional interventions	• *Discontinuing causative agent:* Cease exposure to the causative reducing agent to prevent further methemoglobin formation • *Supportive oxygen therapy:* Administer supplemental oxygen to address tissue hypoxia and alleviate symptoms associated with impaired oxygen delivery. Consider hyperbaric oxygen if available • *High-dose vitamin C:* Up to 10 g/dose, IV. Caution in renal insufficiency due to potential oxalate kidney stones/renal failure • *Red blood cell transfusions:* Severe cases may require transfusions to replace dysfunctional hemoglobin
Exchange transfusion for severe cases	• *Indication:* In life-threatening methemoglobinemia cases unresponsive to methylene blue • *Purpose*: Exchange transfusion involves replacing the patient's blood with donor blood to rapidly decrease methemoglobin levels and improve oxygen delivery

- *Avoiding exposure to reducing agents*:
  - *Causative agents*: Identification and avoidance of substances known to act as reducing agents and induce methemoglobinemia are essential preventive measures.
  - *Common agents*: Nitrites, local anesthetics, antimalarials, analgesics, and certain antibiotics are among the substances that can contribute to methemoglobinemia.
- *Screening for G6PD deficiency*:
  - *Oxidant drug prescription*: Prior to prescribing drugs with oxidant properties, such as primaquine and dapsone, screening for G6PD deficiency is recommended.

- *Avoidance in susceptible patients*: Identifying G6PD deficiency allows healthcare providers to avoid prescribing drugs that may trigger methemoglobinemia in susceptible individuals.

- *Risk mitigation for oxidant drugs*:
  - *Lower doses and close monitoring*: For patients requiring drugs with oxidant properties, such as primaquine and dapsone, prescribing lower doses and closely monitoring their response can help mitigate the risk of methemoglobinemia.
  - Co-administering antioxidants like ascorbic acid may prevent hemoglobin oxidation by drugs undergoing enterohepatic recycling. However, vitamin C is not recommended for acute acquired methemoglobinemia.
  - N-acetylcysteine can act as a glutathione precursor and directly reduce toxic metabolites, potentially preventing oxidation. It can be given orally on a weekly basis in susceptible cases.
  - Cytochrome P450 inhibitors may prevent formation of toxic metabolites when given concurrently with oxidizing drugs.
- *Public health measures*:
  - *Limiting industrial chemical exposures*: Implementing public health measures to restrict exposure to industrial chemicals that act as reducing agents can effectively lower the community-wide risk of methemoglobinemia.
  - *Occupational safety practices*: Ensuring proper occupational safety practices in industries dealing with potentially harmful chemicals contributes to a safer working environment.

CONCLUSION

Methemoglobinemia is an abnormal condition where hemoglobin's oxygen-carrying capacity is reduced. Diagnostically, elevated methemoglobin levels on co-oximetry confirm the diagnosis. Therapeutically, methylene blue administration and removal of inciting agents comprise mainstays of treatment. Preventatively, avoidance of known hemoglobin-oxidizing agents, screening for G6PD deficiency, and implementation of public health measures to curtail exposure risks are imperative. Early recognition and intervention remain crucial, with dose reductions and close monitoring attenuating methemoglobinemia risk in susceptible patients. This comprehensive approach, utilizing diagnosis, treatment, and prevention strategies, enables thorough understanding and effective management of methemoglobinemia as a disease process. Such an approach optimizes positive health outcomes in individual patients and promotes broader public health through risk reduction in affected communities.

REFERENCES

1. Rehman HU. Methemoglobinemia. West J Med. 2001;175(3):193-6.
2. Keohane EM, Otto CN, Walenga JM. Rodak's hematology: Clinical Principles and Applications, 6th edition. Philadelphia: Saunders; 2019.
3. Iolascon A, Bianchi P, Andolfo I, Russo R, Barcellini W, Fermo E, et al. Recommendations for diagnosis and treatment of methemoglobinemia. Am J Hematol. 2021;96(12):1666-78.
4. Curry S. Methemoglobinemia. Ann Emerg Med. 1982;11(4):214-21.
5. Kedar PS, Gupta V, Warang P, Chiddarwar A, Madkaikar M. Novel mutation (R192C) in CYB5R3 gene causing NADH-cytochrome b5 reductase deficiency in eight Indian patients associated with autosomal recessive congenital methemoglobinemia type-I. Hematology. 2018;23(8):567-73.
6. Nappe TM, Pacelli AM, Katz K. An atypical case of methemoglobinemia due to self-administered benzocaine. Case Rep Emerg Med. 2015;2015:670979.
7. Bradberry SM. Occupational methaemoglobinaemia. Mechanisms of production, features, diagnosis and management including the use of methylene blue. Toxicol Rev. 2003;22(1):13-27.
8. Wright RO, Lewander WJ, Woolf AD. Methemoglobinemia: etiology, pharmacology, and clinical management. Ann Emerg Med. 1999;34(5):646-56.
9. Skold A, Cosco DL, Klein R. Methemoglobinemia: pathogenesis, diagnosis, and management. South Med J. 2011;104(11):757-61.
10. Jay U. Methemoglobin--It's not just blue: a concise review Am J Hematol. 2007;82:134-44.
11. Burke P, Jahangir K, Kolber MR. Dapsone-induced methemoglobinemia: case of the blue lady. Can Fam Physician. 2013;59(9):958-61.
12. Ramsay RR, Dunford C, Gillman PK. Methylene blue and serotonin toxicity: Inhibition of monoamine oxidase A (MAO A) confirms a theoretical prediction. Br J Pharmacol. 2007;152(6):946-51.
13. Guay J. Methemoglobinemia related to local anesthetics: a summary of 242 episodes. Anesth Analg. 2009;108(3):837-45.
14. Palmer K, Dick J, French W, Floro L, Ford M. Methemoglobinemia in patient with G6PD deficiency and SARS-CoV-2 infection. Emerg Infect Dis. 2020;26(9):2279-81.
15. Ashurst J, Wasson M. Methemoglobinemia: a systematic review of the pathophysiology, detection, and treatment. Del Med J. 2011;83(7):203-8.

16. Ng JS, Edwards EM, Egelund TA. Methemoglobinemia induced by rasburicase in a pediatric patient: a case report and literature review. J Oncol Pharm Pract. 2012;18(4):425-31.
17. Bradberry SM, Aw TC, Williams NR, Vale JA. Occupational methaemoglobinaemia. Occup Environ Med. 2001; 58(9):611-5.
18. Wilkerson RG. Getting the blues at a rock concert: a case of severe methaemoglobinaemia. Emerg Med Australas. 2010;22(5):466-9.
19. Akhtar J, Johnston BD, Krenzelok EP. Mind the gap. J Emerg Med. 2007;33(2):131-2.
20. Chan ED, Chan MM, Chan MM. Pulse oximetry: Understanding its basic principles facilitates appreciation of its limitations. Respir Med. 2013;107(6):789-99.
21. Cho Y, Park SW, Han SK, Kim HB, Yeom SR. A case of methemoglobinemia successfully treated with hyperbaric oxygenation monotherapy. J Emerg Med. 2017;53(5):685-7.
22. Lee KW, Park SY. High-dose vitamin C as treatment of methemoglobinemia. Am J Emerg Med. 2014;32(8):936.
23. Claro LM, Leonart MSS, Comar SR, Nascimento NJD. Effect of vitamins C and E on oxidative processes in human erythrocytes. Cell Biochem Func. 2006;24: 531-5.
24. Tenório MCDS, Graciliano NG, Moura FA, Oliveira ACM, Goulart MOF. *N*-acetylcysteine (NAC): Impacts on human health. Antioxidants (Basel). 2021;10(6):967.
25. Benrahmoune M, Therond P, Abedinzadeh Z. The reaction of superoxide radical with N-acetylcysteine. Free Radic Biol Med. 2000;29:775-82.
26. Guengerich FP. A history of the roles of cytochrome P450 enzymes in the toxicity of drugs. Toxicol Res. 2021; 37:1-23.
27. Zhao M, Ma J, Li M, Zhang Y, Jiang B, Zhao X, et al. Cytochrome P450 enzymes and drug metabolism in humans. Int J Mol Sci. 2021;22(23):12808.

2.20 Snakebite Envenoming

SP Kalantri

INTRODUCTION

Snakebites take a heavy toll globally, with an estimated 5.4 million incidents each year. This causes 1.8–2.7 million cases of envenomation and between 81,410 and 137,880 deaths.[1-3] Moreover, nearly 400,000 individuals are left with lasting disabilities, including musculoskeletal deformities, amputations, visual impairment, chronic kidney disease, and neurological deficits.[4] Worldwide, the estimated number of annual deaths due to snake envenomation is similar to the estimate for drug-resistant tuberculosis and for multiple myeloma.[5]

EPIDEMIOLOGY

Snakebite primarily affects people in rural areas of low-income countries with limited resources and inadequate public health systems. South Asia, including Bangladesh, India, Nepal, Pakistan, and Sri Lanka, bears the brunt of this burden, contributing to nearly 70% of global snakebite mortality.[6] India, in particular, experiences substantial burdens of mortality and disability from snakebite envenoming.[2,7]

Unfortunately, these regions often lack the necessary infrastructure and capacity for comprehensive data collection and reporting, making it challenging to obtain accurate and reliable data on the true incidence and mortality of snakebite.[8] The healthcare-seeking behavior of patients in resource-limited settings further compounds the lack of data.[9] Delays in accessing medical care, particularly in rural areas where traditional healers may initially manage cases, are common due to factors such as cost, sociocultural beliefs, and geographical remoteness.[10]

The lack of reliable national data underscores the inadequacies of current global mortality estimates. A lower global snakebite mortality rate, such as the claim of 63,400 deaths in 2019, is misleading due to their lack of data from regions where snakebite fatalities are common.[11]

Each year, an estimated 5.4 million people get bitten by snakes, with 1.8–2.7 million developing clinical illness. Sadly, between 81,410 and 137,880 people die. Additionally, snakebites result in approximately three times as many cases of amputations and other permanent disabilities each year.[12,13]

Community-based epidemiological studies challenge these figures, revealing a much higher mortality toll, particularly in Asia. For instance, in India alone, snakebite-related deaths exceed 58,000 annually,[2] with significant mortality being also recorded in Bangladesh, Sri Lanka,

Nepal, and China. These findings emphasize the critical need for improved data collection methods to accurately assess the true burden of snakebite and inform effective public health interventions.

In 2009, the World Health Organization (WHO) recognized snakebite as a neglected tropical disease (NTD), expanding access to funding for research and antivenoms. In 2017, snakebite was added back onto the WHO list of NTDs, after being struck off the list in 2013.[14] In 2019, the WHO set a target to halve the number of deaths and cases of snakebite envenoming by 2030, underscoring the importance of these measures in reducing mortality and morbidity associated with snakebite.[4]

DEMOGRAPHICS AND SNAKEBITE RISK

Rural populations in tropical areas are at a higher risk.[7,10,15] Those at risk include farmers and agricultural workers, hunter-gatherers, herders, fishermen, and villagers, who often work barefoot, engage in activities such as crop deweeding or harvesting cotton or sugarcane, and live in basic houses with outside toilets.[6,9,11,16] These situations make it more likely that they will meet venomous snakes. Both men and women aged between 10 and 40 years are more affected.[10]

UNDERSTANDING VENOMOUS SNAKES AND THEIR VENOM

Venomous snakes encompass around 4,000 species, with the main families being Elapidae (like cobras, mambas, coral snakes, and kraits) and Viperidae (including vipers, adders, and rattlesnakes). These families are responsible for most snakebite envenomings globally.[11]

Snake venoms generally comprise a blend of 20 to more than 100 elements, with peptides and proteins constituting the majority (>90%). These venoms exhibit prominent bioactivities like neurotoxicity, hemotoxicity, and cytotoxicity, which vary depending on the snake species. Composition can differ significantly not only between species but also within the same species.[17]

Venom composition varies within a species due to factors like age, gender, prey availability, diet, geographic location (hot and dry or wet and humid), age of the snake, gender, and time of the year.[17] These differences affect how people get sick from snakebites and how well they respond to treatment. Antivenom that works for one group of snakes or people might not work as well for others.

Elapid venoms primarily consist of peptides and proteins, with secreted phospholipases A2 (PLA2s) and three-finger toxins (3FTxs) being major components that play a crucial role in venom action. In contrast, Viperid venoms typically contain PLA2, snake venom metalloproteinase (SVMP), and snake venom serine protease (SVSP). Most viperid PLA2s are myotoxic, despite sharing significant sequence similarity with elapid PLA2s, many of which are neurotoxic.[17]

Viperidae venom is typically hemotoxic and necrotoxic, while Elapidae venom tends to be neurotoxic. The severity of envenomation severity ranges from "dry" bites with no intoxication to mild (local edema and pain), moderate (pain, edema spreading beyond the bite area, and systemic signs), and severe (shock, severe coagulopathy, and massive edema).[18]

The primary paralytic toxins comprise nonenzymatic α-neurotoxins, categorized as 3FTxs, exclusive to elapid venoms, and enzymatic β-neurotoxins, notably type I and type II secretory PLA2s (sPLA2s), present in both elapid and viperid venoms. Many elapids use both α- and β-neurotoxins for prey capture, but viper venom paralytic neurotoxins are exclusively from the β class. Krait venom contains β-bungarotoxins, which are presynaptic neurotoxins with PLA2 activity.[19] The presynaptic action is irreversible and is the reason that once paralysis develops it is not usually reversed with antivenom administration,[20] however, antivenom can mop up the circulating venom, reducing the duration of neuroparalysis.

CLINICAL PRESENTATION

Snakebite envenoming primarily affects young, particularly agricultural workers, making it both an occupational and environmental health concern.

Patients suffering from snakebite envenomation exhibit both local and systemic symptoms. They may also appear anxious. Many receive traditional first-aid treatments such as tourniquets, local incisions, or application of ice, fire, or electric shocks, which can cause harm, resulting in painful, swollen, or even gangrenous limbs, bleeding, or infections.[21]

In many snakebite incidents, the victim may receive only a dry bite; however, distinguishing between a dry and wet bite can be challenging as both typically result in inflammation and swelling, making initial envenoming diagnosis difficult.[18,22]

Local envenoming presents with increasing pain at the bite site (krait bites are typically painless), accompanied by swelling that spreads proximally and tender, painful swelling of regional lymph nodes draining the bite site. Other signs include fang marks, persistent local bleeding, bruising, lymphangitis, inflammation (swelling, redness, and heat), blistering (blebs, bullae, and vesicles), infection, abscess formation, and necrosis.[23]

Krait bites are distinctly painless. Kraits leave no fang marks, and there is absence of local swelling, or bleeding. Most of the krait bites go unnoticed as the snake escapes. Victims are usually asleep on the ground at night discovered to be unresponsive by others. Initial tests for envenomation, such as the 20-minute whole blood clotting test (20WBCT) and kidney function tests, typically yield normal results. Early symptoms include droopy eyes, difficulty swallowing and speaking, and protrusion of the tongue, followed by respiratory distress.

In contrast, most victims are bitten by vipers while actively working in the field, engaging in activities like deweeding, harvesting cotton or sugarcane, or walking barefoot. Bites most commonly involve the extremities. A viper bite commonly results in intense pain and local envenoming, marked by swift swelling and bleeding at the wound site. Fang marks are evident as vipers deliver venom intramuscularly with their lengthy fangs. Moreover, local lymph nodes quickly swell and become tender. Patients frequently present with bleeding and clotting disturbances, shock, or acute kidney injury (AKI). The victim of a viper bite may also experience symptoms such as nausea, vomiting, visual disturbances, abdominal or loin pain, and profound weakness.

A cobra bite elicits local envenoming along with neurological symptoms such as ptosis, ophthalmoplegia, and respiratory paralysis, accompanied by systemic effects like vomiting and shock upon presentation.

Doctors must be trained to distinguish between venomous and nonvenomous. They should be aware of key features of envenoming and should anticipate complications such as respiratory, circulatory, or renal failure. Antivenom treatment should be initiated by a trained doctor and should be avoided in field setting.

Hemostatic Disturbances

Signs of hemostatic disturbances encompass ongoing bleeding from the fang punctures and from newly formed or recently healed wounds. Systemic bleeding may also manifest at distant sites from the bite, including the gingival sulci, nose, conjunctivae, floor of the mouth, or vagina. Additionally, symptoms may include hematuria, hematemesis, melaena, bleeding gums, and ecchymoses.

Several snake venoms impact platelets. SVMPs cause microvascular damage, while C-type lectin-like proteins also reduce platelet counts. Additionally, disintegrins, C-type lectin-like proteins, snake venom serine proteinases, and certain SVMPs hinder platelet aggregation by either blocking platelet receptors or interacting with von Willebrand factor. Thrombocytopenia has been linked to a higher risk of systemic bleeding in envenomations caused by hemorrhagic venoms.[21]

Neurotoxicity

Neurotoxic envenoming typically begins with a "descending paralysis," starting from smaller muscle groups and progressing to larger ones. Ocular muscles, akin to myasthenia gravis, are notably vulnerable. Initially, weakness may cause ptosis, followed by ophthalmoplegia and diplopia. Facial nerve weakness, speech slurring, and weakened masseter muscles often follow. Subsequently, neck and bulbar muscles are affected, leading to dysphagia, dysarthria, drooling, and compromised airway. Eventually, paralysis extends to limb muscles. Reduced tidal volume due to intrinsic breathing muscle failure may necessitate ventilatory support.[24]

The patient may appear sleepy, but the levator palpebrae superioris muscle function is normal. Drooping or closed eyelids might erroneously suggest bilateral ptosis, often the initial sign of neurotoxicity.

Pooling of saliva and mucus, along with paralysis of the tongue and oropharynx, can lead to aspiration and airway obstruction, potentially resulting in cardiopulmonary arrest. Simple tests like single-breath count and breath-holding time, performed serially, can give us a trend of worsening respiratory paralysis. Tests such as the three-ball incentive spirometer, peak expiratory flow, and maximum expiratory pressure with a sphygmomanometer can also be performed.

Glasgow Coma Score to evaluate consciousness in the setting of neuroparalytic snake envenomation may be misleading. Even though these patients may be fully conscious, they may fail to respond to vocal commands and open their eyes or move, resulting in lower scores. Patients with severe neuroparalysis may meet the criteria for brain death (dilated fixed pupils and absent Doll's eye reflex) misleading the clinicians.[11]

Neurotoxicity is attributed to two main types of neurotoxins: α-neurotoxins and β-neurotoxins. α-Neurotoxins, a part of the 3FTx family, target postsynaptic sites at neuromuscular junctions. In contrast, such as PLA2 enzymes act at presynaptic nerve terminals. α-Neurotoxins from *Naja naja* act postsynaptically, binding reversibly to acetylcholine receptors at neuromuscular junctions. Neuroparalysis may improve within 30–60 minutes after the initial dose of antivenom. In these patients, anticholinesterase drugs like neostigmine act rapidly. In contrast, krait venoms contain presynaptic toxins (β-neurotoxins) that bind irreversibly to presynaptic nerve endings, leading to their destruction. Early antivenom treatment may prevent paralysis by neutralizing β-bungarotoxins, but once paralysis develops, it cannot be reversed, and anticholinesterases (neostigmine) are ineffective in krait envenomation. Prolonged/repeated administration of antivenom to paralyzed and mechanically ventilated victims is not recommended.

Antivenoms have been shown to reverse α-toxin-induced early signs of neurotoxicity, a feature of cobra envenomation.[24] Antivenom fails to reverse or improve established neurotoxicity in patients envenomed with β-neurotoxins, commonly found in kraits. In a recent review, the authors found no randomized placebo-controlled trials demonstrating the efficacy of antivenom in reversing established neuroparalysis.[25] Similar results have been reported in confirmed Russell's viper envenomation with antivenom failing to improve neurotoxicity.[26]

Acute Kidney Injury

Following bites from snakes such as Russell's viper, saw-scaled viper, and hump-nosed pit viper, AKI is a common complication. A comprehensive review covering five decades and 28 studies analyzed 534 renal biopsies, with Russell's viper bite,[27] and revealed acute tubular necrosis as the predominant finding. This was followed by acute interstitial nephritis, acute cortical necrosis (ACN), and thrombotic microangiopathy (TMA). The presence of ACN and TMA was associated with poor outcomes.[27]

Prolonged AKI with oliguria may suggest ACN or acute tubular necrosis in association with interstitial nephritis or extracapillary glomerulonephritis. Venom-induced direct injury, hemodynamic changes (shock and hemorrhage), and release of vasoactive mediators may contribute to AKI. Kidney injury may also be exacerbated by venom-induced consumption coagulopathy (VICC), intravascular hemolysis, and rhabdomyolysis.[27] The incidence of AKI varies from 5% to 29% depending on snake species and envenomation severity. The onset usually occurs within a few hours to 96 hours post bite and usually lasts for 2–3 weeks.[28,29]

Acute kidney injury usually responds to fluid management but if it persists despite conservative management, renal replacement therapy may become necessary.

Shock

Hypotension or shock is usually due to hypovolemia, hemorrhage, myocardial dysfunction, or venom-induced vasodilation. These patients should receive fluid resuscitation followed by vasopressors, should fluid resuscitation fail to restore tissue perfusion. Excess volume resuscitation may cause pulmonary edema in a setting of oliguric AKI. Point-of-care ultrasonography may guide resuscitation.

Venom-induced Consumption Coagulopathy

Venom-induced consumption coagulopathy, commonly caused by *Daboia russelii* and *Echis carinatus*, is the most clinically important coagulopathy, because it can be complicated by serious and life-threatening hemorrhage.[30] These toxins activate clotting factors, leading to decreased fibrinogen levels, which can result in bleeding from the bite or IV cannula site.[30] Most of the times, bleeding is localized, but some may develop bleeding from the gums, gastrointestinal tract (melena or hematemesis), or hematuria.[31]

Diagnosis and monitoring are particularly challenging in resource-poor settings. Antivenom is the primary treatment for VICC, although high-quality evidence supporting its effectiveness is lacking. Neither heparin nor fresh frozen plasma (FFP) after antivenom administration in patients with Russell's viper bites have been shown to hasten recovery of coagulopathy.[32] Persistent/unresponsive coagulopathy or bleeding may suggest a bite with hump nosed or pit vipers, not neutralized by available antivenom.

POINT-OF-CARE TESTS FOR COAGULOPATHY

Bedside clotting assessments like the 20WBCT continue to be the most suitable and feasible approach for identifying coagulopathy in resource-limited settings.

The 20WBCT was introduced in 1977 by Warrell and colleagues to assess patients bitten by saw-scaled or carpet vipers in Nigeria.[33] This test involves placing a small amount of freshly collected blood into a clean, dry glass test tube and leaving it undisturbed for 20 minutes and then tipping it to check for clotting. If the blood fails to clot within 20 minutes, it indicates coagulopathy and systemic envenoming. Conversely, if clotting occurs, it suggests the absence of coagulopathy. Guidelines have adopted the 20WBCT as a method to detect systemic hemotoxic envenoming.[34]

A recent meta-analysis of 12 studies from six countries, encompassing a total of 2,270 patients, was conducted.[35] Using an international normalized ratio (INR) >1.4 as the reference standard, the 20WBCT showed a sensitivity of 0.84 [confidence interval (CI) 0.61–0.94] and a specificity of 0.91 (0.76–0.97), with an area under the curve (AUC) of 0.94 (*CI* 0.91–0.96). When using fibrinogen <100 mg/dL, the sensitivity was 0.72 (CI 0.58–0.83), specificity was 0.94 (CI 0.88–0.98), and the summary receiver operating characteristic (SROC) AUC was 0.93 (0.91–0.95). The meta-analysis concluded that in the absence of laboratory clotting assays, the 20WBCT remains a highly specific and moderately sensitive bedside test for detecting coagulopathy following snakebite. The healthcare workers need to be adequately trained; use new, clean, and dry test tubes; and read the test results precisely at the 20-minute mark.

In resource-limited settings, standard laboratory tests like INR, activated partial thromboplastin time, fibrinogen, and D-dimer may not be an option due to cost or availability.[36] To address this, researchers are exploring simpler alternatives. Options, like using synthetic fibrinogen for INR tests, are affordable but lack reliability. D-dimer measurement shows promise for early clotting detection after snakebites; its cost limits its use in poorer areas.[37] Advanced tests like thromboelastography and rotational thromboelastometry are expensive and require skilled operators, making them challenging to implement.[38]

MANAGEMENT

Management of snake envenomation involves first aid, judicious use of antivenom, management of local and systemic effects followed by management of complications, and follow-up for addressing any sequalae or disability.[21]

Physicians must rely on evidence-based treatment. They should quickly establish clinically a venomous or nonvenomous bite. The treating clinician should be trained in knowing the dose of antivenom and the methodology to administer it.

Our current knowledge of snake envenomation management, including the effectiveness and safety of first aid, antivenoms, and other treatments, lacks solid evidence.[39] Critical aspects such as late adverse reactions, wound outcomes, quality of life, hospitalization duration, cost, and disability are insufficiently studied. This emphasizes the pressing need for further research to enhance snakebite management protocols and enhance patient outcomes.

Management of venomous snakebites in an intensive care unit (ICU) demands a blend of clinical expertise, intuition, and experience to administer evidence-based interventions effectively at the patient's bedside. This often entails extended ICU stays, necessitating prolonged mechanical ventilation or hemodialysis, which can significantly increase healthcare costs. Additionally, patients may require blood transfusions, plasma or platelet infusions, and costly antibiotics to manage worsening wound infections. Extended stays in the ICU often result in high costs, which are frequently unaffordable for patients.

Treatment of the Bitten Part

- *Wound management*: Large and tense blisters, bullae, or blebs should not be deroofed and aspirated only if they threaten to rupture. Abscesses should be aspirated with a needle. Amputation may be required if toes or the limb develop gangrene.
- *Bacterial infections*: Evidence does not support the use of empiric antibiotics to prevent secondary infection after the snakebite. Cellulitis or abscess after a snakebite needs antibiotic therapy. Necrosis on the bitten limb may require surgery and skin grafts, particularly in the case of cobra bites. One should wait for surgery till a clear demarcation of the necrosis has developed.
- *Compartment syndrome*: Victims of snakebite occasionally present with an immobile, tense swollen, hypoesthesia, cold, and apparently pulseless snake-bitten limb, a condition called compartment syndrome. This is the result of an increased intracompartmental pressure in the affected limb. The syndrome is uncommon, but the clinician must be aware of this complication and must always look for. It is difficult to

diagnose clinically. Serial evaluation of the temperature and peripheral pulses can help in early detection. Ultrasonic evaluation of the affected limb along with doppler for flow can help. Most such patients with tense swelling can be managed conservatively and do not need fasciotomy. Compartmental syndromes are often overdiagnosed, and patients have to endure distressing effects of unnecessarily performed fasciotomies.

- *Tetanus prophylaxis*: Snakebites are considered tetanus-prone wounds and require tetanus prophylaxis. In patients with coagulopathy, tetanus prophylaxis should be postponed until after antivenom therapy and normalization of abnormalities.
- Snakebite victims deserve effective pain relief. Krait bites are usually painless, unless the bitten limb gets infected. Pain management should involve the use of paracetamol or morphine, although morphine is often underutilized in hospital settings. Aspirin or nonsteroidal anti-inflammatory drugs (NSAIDs) should be avoided due to the risk of exacerbating bleeding issues.

Antivenom

Currently, the only clinically proven specific treatment for snakebite envenoming is polyclonal antivenoms. Despite antivenom's initial development in the 1890s, manufacturing technology has remained largely unchanged over the past 135 years[40] **(Table 1)**.

The antivenoms are still developed by immunizing animals, typically horses, with specific snake venoms to stimulate the production of polyclonal neutralizing immunoglobulin G (IgG) antibodies. Once a sufficient antibody level is reached, plasma is collected and processed to isolate and concentrate the antibodies, creating the final product for human use. Before being released to the market, antivenoms undergo rigorous testing in both laboratory settings and clinical studies, following internationally accepted guidelines such as those established by the WHO.

While cutting-edge human monoclonal antibodies pave the way for cancer treatment, outdated and inadequately purified equine polyclonal antibodies continue to be used for snake envenoming, leading to a stark disparity in efficacy and safety.[41]

In India, most venomous snakebites are caused by four main species: Spectacled cobra, common krait, Russell's viper, and saw-scaled viper. There are geographic areas reporting envenomation with pit vipers and other krait species, which are not currently covered by the available polyvalent antivenom. The antivenom currently available in India only targets these four species, leaving out other important snakes. The effectiveness of antivenom depends on the composition of the snake's venom, which can vary both within and between species. All of India's snake venom for making antivenom comes from snakes in Tamil Nadu. Studies indicate that none of the commercially available brands of antivenom displayed strong binding to common krait venom from North India, despite being specifically designed to counter it.[42] This antigenic variability is the prime reason for the current antivenom being not effective against bites from some neglected snakes.[42] These findings highlight the urgent need for better antivenom for snakebite therapy in India. New antivenoms that are highly effective against a wider range of snake species are essential to improve outcomes for snakebite victims.

TABLE 1: Differentiating between the snake envenomation clinically.

Clinical parameters	*Cobra*	*Krait*	*Russell's viper*	*Saw scaled viper*	*Himalayan Pit viper*	*Hump nosed pit viper*
Swelling at bite site	+	–	++	+	+	+
Bleeding at bite site	–	–	+++	+	+	±
Systemic bleeding	–	–	++	++	++	–
Paresthesia/pain at bite site	+	++	+	±	–	+
Pain abdomen	–	++	–	–	–	+
Ptosis	++	++	±	–	–	–
Neuroparalysis	++	+++	±	–	–	–
Oliguria	–	–	++	+	+	+
Compartment syndrome	–	–	+	–	±	±

Clotting factors in the blood can start to return to normal within about 6 hours after receiving enough antivenom.[43] This forms the basis of repeat testing at 6 hours and repeat dosing of antisnake venom (ASV) if 20WBCT is still prolonged. However, there is not enough evidence available to dictate the right initial dose of antivenom for most snakes.[44]

It is important for treating doctors to follow national guidelines for the correct dosage and mode of administration of antivenom. Antivenom is typically administered intravenously over a period of 30–60 minutes. If bleeding continues, weakness worsens, or signs of cardiovascular problems persist after 2 hours, or if clotting tests remain abnormal after 6 hours, additional doses of antivenom may be necessary.[23] Since antivenoms may not be effective for treating certain complications like nerve damage, tissue damage, and kidney injury, so additional treatments may be needed for these conditions.[23,25,45]

A systematic review comparing low-dose (20–220 mL) versus high-dose (40–550 mL) antivenom, encompassing five randomized controlled trials with a total of 473 participants, revealed varied dosages in both groups. Surprisingly, no significant differences were observed between the two groups across all outcomes assessed. The overall evidence quality was deemed "very low," primarily due to the majority of trials being open-label.[46]

In another study for treating neurotoxic snakebites, there was no difference in mortality, need for respiratory support, or additional antivenom between the low- and the high-dose groups.[47]

In a clinical trial involving patients with severe krait envenomation conducted in 2024, a low-dose antivenom regimen was found to be comparable to the standard dose in terms of the median duration of mechanical ventilation, median length of stay, and in-hospital mortality.[48]

Antivenom is often in short supply, expensive, and can cause serious adverse effects, so it should be used judiciously only when indicated and in the prescribed dose. The dose of antivenom may or may not make a major difference but the type of snake responsible for envenomation does. It has been noted that neuroparalytic patients bitten by kraits fare worse than those bitten by cobras.[47]

Risk of Adverse Reactions with Antivenom

Acute reactions to antivenom are common, with up to 40% progressing to severe anaphylaxis. The practice of administering hydrocortisone and antihistamines prior to antivenom infusion is not supported by evidence and should be discouraged. Performing a skin test to predict antivenom reactions is unsupported by evidence, so it is not advocated. In a large clinical trial involving 1,007 patients, with a 75% acute reaction rate, a small dose of subcutaneous adrenaline (250 µg) notably reduced severe reactions by 43% within the first hour. This trial affirmed the safety of a small subcutaneous adrenaline dose post snake bite in preventing severe adverse reactions, even in patients having vasculotoxic snakebite.[49]

Other Treatments

Neostigmine combined with atropine can be helpful for patients bitten by certain snakes like cobras, which produce postsynaptic neurotoxins in their venom. However, this treatment does not work for patients with neurotoxicity from krait bites. Additionally, while antivenom may be effective for patients with cobra-induced neurotoxicity, it may not work for those with krait-induced neuromuscular envenomation once they reach the hospital and have full-blown neurotoxicity. These differences in antivenom efficacy for established neurotoxicity between kraits and cobras are crucial to ensure that antivenom is used effectively and not wasted.

Neostigmine Challenge

Neostigmine, an anticholinesterase drug, can partially overcome blockade by postsynaptic neurotoxins and has shown efficacy in cobra bite envenoming. It is, however, not effective in krait bites due to presynaptic toxins causing nerve-ending destruction. Baseline assessment before neostigmine administration is essential for comparison. In the absence of local symptoms/signs at bite site with neuroparalysis, there is very little one may gain by administering neostigmine; hence, it should be avoided. In suspected cobra bites, it is fair to give neostigmine challenge.

After pretreatment with 0.6 mg of atropine, neostigmine at a dose of 0.02 mg/kg should be administered intramuscularly. If ptosis resolves and ventilatory capacity improves, neostigmine at a dose of 0.5 mg can be repeated hourly, alongside an 0.6 mg atropine infusion over 8 hours, with a maximum of two such injections. Neostigmine may obviate the need for advanced airway management and mechanical ventilation or facilitate early liberation from mechanical ventilation.

Neuroparalytic patients experiencing loss of gag reflex, inability to cough, or respiratory distress require endotracheal intubation and mechanical ventilation. Victims may require prolonged ventilator support depending on the severity of envenomation and delay in administration of antivenom.

Local soft-tissue damage is a common occurrence with both cobra and viper bites. It is important to address large, tense bullae by aspirating them to achieve three goals: Better care for the affected limb, prevent spontaneous rupture, and reduce the risk of secondary infection. While broad-spectrum antibiotics are commonly used in centers managing snakebites, they should only be administered if the wound has been incised or if there are signs of necrosis, infection, or abscess formation. Surgical interventions may be opted for in severe cases. Fasciotomies are generally not recommended since compartment pressures typically remain within normal limits despite apparent muscle swelling and tension.[21]

PROGNOSIS

Because many victims of venomous snakebites die before reaching medical facilities, mortality estimates derived solely from hospital records may underestimate the actual mortality rate of snakebite incidents.

Mortality in snake envenomation varies from 7.5% to 18%.[50,51] Factors associated with a higher risk of death include vomiting, neurotoxicity, requirement of ventilation, and AKI.[50,51] Another important factor is prehospital delay. Patients with a prehospital delay exceeding 24 hours experienced an 18% mortality rate, compared to 5% among those admitted within the specified period.[51]

Persistent sequelae following snakebites are frequent and encompass a range of conditions such as tissue loss, amputations, contractures, septic arthritis, hypertrophic and keloid scars, tendon damage, chronic skin ulcers, and osteomyelitis. At times, inappropriate fasciotomies and arthrodeses cause more harm than good, leading to significant morbidity.[21]

PREVENTION

Effective snakebite prevention relies on understanding snake epidemiology and habitats. Measures like covering feet and hands, using light at night, and sleeping under mosquito nets are proven against krait and cobra bites, backed by studies across India, Nepal, and Sri Lanka. Cultural barriers hinder proposals like protective footwear in rural areas. Limited awareness, financial constraints, and high illiteracy rates hinder preventive measures like maintaining domestic areas free of rubbish, rubble, and firewood; controlling rodent populations; and constructing snake-proof houses in villages.[52] Targeted prevention and first-aid training, including what not to do, are crucial.

CONCLUSION

Collaboration between health workers and communities is essential for education and early hospital care. However, deterring victims from relying on traditional healers, deeply ingrained in rural Indian communities, remains a formidable challenge.

REFERENCES

1. Kasturiratne A, Wickremasinghe AR, de Silva N, Gunawardena NK, Pathmeswaran A, Premaratna R, et al. The global burden of snakebite: a literature analysis and modelling based on regional estimates of envenoming and deaths. PLoS Med. 2008;5(11):e218.
2. Mohapatra B, Warrell DA, Suraweera W, Bhatia P, Dhingra N, Jotkar RM, et al. Snakebite mortality in India: a nationally representative mortality survey. PLoS Negl Trop Dis. 2011;5(4):e1018.
3. Suraweera W, Warrell D, Whitaker R, Menon G, Rodrigues R, Fu SH, et al. Trends in snakebite deaths in India from 2000 to 2019 in a nationally representative mortality study. eLife. 2020;9:e54076.
4. GBD 2019 Snakebite Envenomation Collaborators. Global mortality of snakebite envenoming between 1990 and 2019. Nat Commun. 2022;13(1):6160.
5. Seifert SA, Armitage JO, Sanchez EE. Snake envenomation. N Engl J Med. 2022;386(1):68-78.
6. Afroz A, Siddiquea BN, Chowdhury HA, Jackson TN, Watt AD. Snakebite envenoming: a systematic review and meta-analysis of global morbidity and mortality. PLoS Negl Trop Dis. 2024;18(4):e0012080.
7. Dandona R, Kumar GA, Kharyal A, George S, Akbar M, Dandona L. Mortality due to snakebite and other venomous animals in the Indian state of Bihar: findings from a representative mortality study. PLoS One. 2018;13(6):e0198900.
8. Warrell DA. Snake bite. Lancet. 2010;375(9708):77-88.
9. Chaaithanya IK, Abnave D, Bawaskar H, Pachalkar U, Tarukar S, Salvi N, et al. Perceptions, awareness on snakebite envenoming among the tribal community and health care providers of Dahanu block, Palghar District in Maharashtra, India. PLoS One. 2021;16(8):e0255657.
10. Menon JC, Bharti OK, Dhaliwal RS, John D, Menon GR, Grover A, et al. ICMR task force project-survey of the incidence, mortality, morbidity and socio-economic burden of snakebite in India: a study protocol. PLoS One. 2022;17(8):e0270735.

11. Warrell DA, Williams DJ. Clinical aspects of snakebite envenoming and its treatment in low-resource settings. Lancet. 2023;401(10385):1382-98.
12. World Health Organization. (2023). Snakebite envenoming. [online] Available from https://www.who.int/news-room/fact-sheets/detail/snakebite-envenoming#:~:text=Key%20facts,are%20caused%20by%20snakebites%20annually [Last accessed October, 2024].
13. Minghui R, Malecela MN, Cooke E, Abela-Ridder B. WHO's snakebite envenoming strategy for prevention and control. Lancet Glob Health. 2019;7(7):e837-e8.
14. The Lancet. Snake-bite envenoming: a priority neglected tropical disease. Lancet. 2017;390(10089):2.
15. Bawaskar HS, Bawaskar PH, Punde DP, Inamdar MK, Dongare RB, Bhoite RR. Profile of snakebite envenoming in rural Maharashtra, India. J Assoc Phys India. 2008;56:88-95.
16. Longbottom J, Shearer FM, Devine M, Alcoba G, Chappuis F, Weiss DJ, et al. Vulnerability to snakebite envenoming: a global mapping of hotspots. Lancet. 2018;392(10148):673-84.
17. Oliveira AL, Viegas MF, da Silva SL, Soares AM, Ramos MJ, Fernandes PA. The chemistry of snake venom and its medicinal potential. Nat Rev Chem. 2022;6(7):451-69.
18. Adukauskienė D, Varanauskienė E, Adukauskaitė A. Venomous snakebites. Medicina (Kaunas). 2011;47(8):461-7.
19. Harris JB, Scott-Davey T. Secreted phospholipases A2 of snake venoms: effects on the peripheral neuromuscular system with comments on the role of phospholipases A2 in disorders of the CNS and their uses in industry. Toxins. 2013;5(12):2533-71.
20. Dixon RW, Harris JB. Nerve terminal damage by beta-bungarotoxin: its clinical significance. Am J Pathol. 1999;154(2):447-55.
21. Gutiérrez JM, Calvete JJ, Habib AG, Harrison RA, Williams DJ, Warrell DA. Snakebite envenoming. Nat Rev Dis Primers. 2017;3:17063.
22. Pucca MB, Knudsen C, Oliveira IS, Rimbault C, Cerni FA, Wen FH, et al. Current knowledge on snake dry bites. Toxins. 2020;12(11).
23. World Health Organization. (2016). Guidelines for the management of snakebites, 2nd edition. [online] Available from https://apps.who.int/iris/handle/10665/249547 [Last accessed October, 2024].
24. Ranawaka UK, Lalloo DG, de Silva HJ. Neurotoxicity in snakebite—the limits of our knowledge. PLoS Negl Trop Dis. 2013;7(10):e2302.
25. Silva A, Hodgson WC, Isbister GK. Antivenom for neuromuscular paralysis resulting from snake envenoming. Toxins. 2017;9(4):143.
26. Silva A, Maduwage K, Sedgwick M, Pilapitiya S, Weerawansa P, Dahanayaka NJ, et al. Neurotoxicity in Russell's viper (Daboia russelii) envenoming in Sri Lanka: a clinical and neurophysiological study. Clin Toxicol (Phila). 2016;54(5):411-9.
27. Meena P, Bhargava V, Gupta P, Panda S, Bhaumik S. The kidney histopathological spectrum of patients with kidney injury following snakebite envenomation in India: scoping review of five decades. BMC Nephrol. 2024;25(1):112.
28. Chugh KS. Snake-bite-induced acute renal failure in India. Kidney Int. 1989;35(3):891-907.
29. Dharod MV, Patil TB, Deshpande AS, Gulhane RV, Patil MB, Bansod YV. Clinical predictors of acute kidney injury following snake bite envenomation. N Am J Med Sci. 2013;5(10):594-9.
30. Isbister GK. Snakebite doesn't cause disseminated intravascular coagulation: coagulopathy and thrombotic microangiopathy in snake envenoming. Semin Thromb Hemost. 2010;36(4):444-51.
31. Phillips RE, Theakston RD, Warrell DA, Galigedara Y, Abeysekera DT, Dissanayaka P, et al. Paralysis, rhabdomyolysis and haemolysis caused by bites of Russell's viper (Vipera russelli pulchella) in Sri Lanka: Failure of Indian (Haffkine) antivenom. Q J Med. 1988;68(257):691-715.
32. Isbister GK, Jayamanne S, Mohamed F, Dawson AH, Maduwage K, Gawarammana I, et al. A randomized controlled trial of fresh frozen plasma for coagulopathy in Russell's viper (Daboia russelii) envenoming. J Thromb Haemost. 2017;15(4):645-54.
33. Warrell DA, Davidson N, Greenwood BM, Ormerod LD, Pope HM, Watkins BJ, et al. Poisoning by bites of the saw-scaled or carpet viper (Echis carinatus) in Nigeria. Q J Med. 1977;46(181):33-62.
34. White J, Mahmood MA, Alfred S, Thwin KT, Kyaw KM, Zaw A, et al. A comprehensive approach to managing a neglected, neglected tropical disease; The Myanmar Snakebite Project (MSP). Toxicon: X. 2018;1:100001.
35. Lamb T, Abouyannis M, de Oliveira SS, Shenoy K R, Geevar T, Zachariah A, et al. The 20-minute whole blood clotting test (20WBCT) for snakebite coagulopathy: a systematic review and meta-analysis of diagnostic test accuracy. PLoS Negl Trop Dis. 2021;15(8):e0009657.
36. O'Rourke KM, Correlje E, Martin CL, Robertson JD, Isbister GK. Point-of-care derived INR does not reliably detect significant coagulopathy following Australian snakebite. Thromb Res. 2013;132(5):610-3.
37. Isbister GK, Noutsos T, Jenkins S, Isoardi KZ, Soderstrom J, Buckley NA. D-dimer testing for early detection of venom-induced consumption coagulopathy after snakebite in Australia (ASP-29). Med J Aust. 2022;217(4):203-7.
38. Mullins ME, Freeman WE. Thromboelastometry (ROTEM) and thromboelastography (TEG) in copperhead snakebites: a case series. Clin Toxicol (Phila). 2020;58(9):931-4.
39. Bhaumik S, Beri D, Tyagi J, Clarke M, Sharma SK, Williamson PR, et al. Outcomes in intervention research on snakebite envenomation: a systematic review. F1000Res. 2022;11:628.
40. Pucca MB, Cerni FA, Janke R, Bermúdez-Méndez E, Ledsgaard L, Barbosa JE, et al. History of envenoming

therapy and current perspectives. Front Immunol. 2019;10:1598.
41. Stone SF, Isbister GK, Shahmy S, Mohamed F, Abeysinghe C, Karunathilake H, et al. Immune response to snake envenoming and treatment with antivenom; complement activation, cytokine production and mast cell degranulation. PLoS Negl Trop Dis. 2013;7(7):e2326.
42. Senji Laxme RR, Khochare S, de Souza HF, Ahuja B, Suranse V, Martin G, et al. Beyond the 'big four': venom profiling of the medically important yet neglected Indian snakes reveals disturbing antivenom deficiencies. PLoS Negl Trop Dis. 2019;13(12):e0007899.
43. Gulati A, Isbister GK, Duffull SB. Effect of Australian elapid venoms on blood coagulation: Australian Snakebite Project (ASP-17). Toxicon. 2013;61:94-104.
44. Watson JA, Lamb T, Holmes J, Warrell DA, Thwin KT, Aung ZL, et al. A Bayesian phase 2 model based adaptive design to optimise antivenom dosing: application to a dose-finding trial for a novel Russell's viper antivenom in Myanmar. PLoS Negl Trop Dis. 2020;14(11):e0008109.
45. Alfred S, Bates D, White J, Mahmood MA, Warrell DA, Thwin KT, et al. Acute kidney injury following Eastern Russell's Viper (Daboia siamensis) snakebite in Myanmar. Kidney Int Rep. 2019;4(9):1337-41.
46. Das RR, Sankar J, Dev N. High-dose versus low-dose antivenom in the treatment of poisonous snake bites: a systematic review. Indian J Crit Care Med. 2015;19(6): 340-9.
47. Alirol E, Sharma SK, Ghimire A, Poncet A, Combescure C, Thapa C, et al. Dose of antivenom for the treatment of snakebite with neurotoxic envenoming: evidence from a randomised controlled trial in Nepal. PLoS Negl Trop Dis. 2017;11(5):e0005612.
48. Pannu AK, Chand D, Bhalla A, Dhibar DP. Efficacy of a low dose of antivenom for severe neuroparalysis in Bungarus caeruleus (common krait) envenomation: a pilot study. Toxicol Res. 2024;13(2):tfae023.
49. de Silva HA, Ryan NM, de Silva HJ. Adverse reactions to snake antivenom, and their prevention and treatment. Br J Clin Pharmacol. 2016;81(3):446-52.
50. Kalantri S, Singh A, Joshi R, Malamba S, Ho C, Ezoua J, et al. Clinical predictors of in-hospital mortality in patients with snake bite: a retrospective study from a rural hospital in central India. Trop Med Int Health. 2006;11(1): 22-30.
51. David S, Matathia S, Christopher S. Mortality predictors of snake bite envenomation in southern India—a ten-year retrospective audit of 533 patients. J Med Toxicol. 2012;8(2):118-23.
52. Ralph R, Sharma SK, Faiz MA, Ribeiro I, Rijal S, Chappuis F, et al. The timing is right to end snakebite deaths in South Asia. BMJ. 2019;364:k5317.

2.21 Scorpion and Spider Bites

Badria Ali Alhatali

SCORPION STINGS

INTRODUCTION

The exact prevalence of scorpion sting envenomation is unknown as many victims do not seek medical evaluation. It is considered one of the neglected health issues in many parts of the world including Africa, Middle East, southern states of USA, Mexico and parts of South America, and the Indian sub-continent.[1] Despite that, most of the patients experience minor envenomation with localized pain and minimal systemic manifestations.[2] There are around 650 species known around the world, of which the Buthidae family is the most lethal one, but only few are considered dangerous.[3,4]

MECHANISM OF ENVENOMATION

Scorpion venoms contain several protein fractions, peptides, enzymes, nucleotides, lipids, mucoproteins, and other substances.[5] These protein fractions and peptides modulate specific ion channels, such as sodium (Na^+), potassium (K^+), calcium (Ca^{2+}), and chloride (Cl^-) ion channels, and hence toxins are classified into four groups according to their effects on these ions or based on the length of peptides.[6] The venom composition varied with different species, age, and nutritional state of the scorpion, which explain the differences in signs and symptoms after the sting.[4] The long-chain toxins affecting sodium channels are subdivided into two major subtypes, α- and β-toxins, based on their pharmacological effects on sodium channels.[7,8] The toxins that carry a major medical consequence are the α-toxins which bind to a specific site on the mammalian voltage-gated sodium channel in a membrane-dependent manner, leading to prolonged depolarization of the nerves and muscles and hence neurological excitation.[2,7]

Scorpion stings produce tissue injury that may induce a systemic inflammatory along with the concomitant release of different cytokines. It also stimulates the release of catecholamines, bradykinin, and prostaglandins resulting in the release of interleukin-1 (IL-1) and IL-6.[9]

CLINICAL MANIFESTATIONS

Scorpion stings are associated with a wide range of clinical manifestations due to activation of the autonomic nervous system (sympathetic and parasympathetic) and neuromuscular excitation.[2] Mostly, the venom causes a local intense pain, erythema, itching and burning sensation, and occasionally discoloration due to the local reaction of the venom, which last for few hours.[3] When the critical threshold of scorpion toxin plasma concentration is reached, a massive release of neurohormonal mediators occurs in association with systemic vasoconstriction, manifesting as a sudden and severe increase in systemic arterial pressure, left ventricle (LV) filling pressure, impaired LV emptying, increase in capillary critical pressure, and decreased cardiac output leading to pulmonary edema and cardiogenic shock.[10,11] Lung edema and cardiac dysfunction are the main causes of death after systemic envenomation or scorpionism.[12] Excitation of the parasympathetic and sympathetic autonomic nervous systems results in a cholinergic toxidrome and adrenergic excitations. Patients expressing cholinergic manifestations present with profuse diaphoresis, hypersalivation, lacrimation, miosis, diarrhea, vomiting, bradycardia, hypotension, increased respiratory secretions, and priapism. With the excitation of the sympathetic nervous system, patients usually present with different degrees of tachycardia, hypertension, mydriasis, hyperthermia, hyperglycemia, agitation, restlessness, and convulsions.[2]

Increased release of neurohormonal mediators including catecholamines, increases oxygen consumption the myocardium as well as alters the membrane permeability at a cellular level resulting in abnormalities in the electrolyte fluxes and shifts across the cellular membranes. This is also associated with coronary microvascular spasm leading to reduction in the myocardial perfusion. There is also a risk of direct effect of the venom on cardiac muscles called scorpion myocarditis.[13]

Stimulation of the peripheral nervous system leads to uncoordinated neuromotor hyperactivity, oculomotor movements, visual abnormalities, and muscle fasciculation and spasm of the face, tongue, and limbs.[2,14] Some scorpion species like *Tityrus serrulatus* are associated with development of acute pancreatitis due to exocrine secretion.[15]

There are three categories of envenomation that have been accepted worldwide. The first category is "mild" envenomation which includes mainly local manifestations. The second category or "moderate envenomation" involves abdominal pain, vomiting, sweating, hypertension, tachycardia or bradycardia, agitation, excessive salivation, dysphagia, and hyperglycemia. The last category is considered "severe" envenomation where victims suffer from severe cardiovascular complications including congestive heart failure, dilated cardiomyopathy, cardiogenic shock, dysrhythmias, malignant hypertension, pulmonary edema, acute pancreatitis, hypertensive encephalopathy, coma, and seizures.[3]

DIAGNOSTIC INVESTIGATIONS

Diagnosing scorpion envenomation can be challenging, as symptoms may mimic other medical conditions making the history of exposure as well as clinical presentation crucial for accurate diagnosis. There are no specific diagnostic investigations for scorpion envenomation; however, laboratory investigations can be used to assess systems' involvement and hence complications as well as to categorize the severity of envenomation. A renal function test and pancreatic enzymes can be used to assess renal injury and pancreatitis.[2] Scorpion envenomation may cause hyperglycemia, hypokalemia, neutrophil leukocytosis, coagulation disorders, and metabolic acidosis.[16] Echocardiographic abnormalities include sinus tachycardia, T-wave changes, ST elevation or depression in a pattern like acute myocardial infarction, Q waves, QTc prolongation, QRS changes, atrial or ventricular ectopics, variable atrioventricular (AV) blocks, and incomplete right bundle branch block (RBBB).[17,18] Echocardiographic abnormalities may include decrease in LV contractility [left ventricular ejection fraction (LVEF) <55%] and right ventricle (RV) end-systolic pressure which return toward the normal range in few days after recovery.[11]

CURRENT TREATMENT APPROACHES

The management of scorpion envenomation involves supportive care and, in systemic envenomation, the administration of antivenom. The approach may vary depending on the severity of the envenomation. Aggressive supportive care including pain management, hydration, and monitoring for respiratory and cardiovascular complications is the mainstay of treatment in severe envenomation. In most cases, the treatment involves local wound care, including tetanus prophylaxis and pain management only.[3] Scorpion antivenom is derived from the plasma of animals immunized with scorpion venom, and it binds to the toxins to prevent them from reaching target sites and increase rate of elimination.[2] It is usually recommended for moderate-to-severe envenomation as the literature approved its effectiveness in rapid resolution of symptoms and reduction in hospital stay and associated morbidity and mortality.[3,19] Due to the extensive variation in the venom composition and immunogenicity, antivenoms are usually manufactured using venoms relevant to a specific geographical region.[1] In patients with acute pulmonary edema and cardiogenic shock, postenvenomation aggressive intensive care is required including inotropic agents, prazocin, atropine, vasodilators, benzodiazepines, and ventilator support.[2,11] Dobutamine was considered the drug of choice in cases with cardiogenic shock due to severe envenomation and was proven to decrease mortality.[11,20] It is a selective β-2 agonist that improves the function of LV and RV leading to a sustained increase in cardiac output and systemic arterial pressure.[21] It was indirectly evident from observation and uncontrolled trials that prazosin, a postsynaptic α-adrenergic blocker, reduced the preload and afterload and treated malignant hypertension associated with the catecholamine surge, and hence decreased the mortality.[22,23] Extracorporeal membrane oxygenation (ECMO) and intraaortic balloon pump (IABP) have been used in patients with refractory cardiogenic shock.[24]

SPIDER BITES

INTRODUCTION

There are more than 41,000 recorded species of spider; however, very few are medically important.[25] Most of the bites are caused by female spiders as the male spiders have fangs that are too short and fragile to cause envenomation in human. Children are more likely to develop severe envenomation with higher morbidity and mortality.[26] A small number of research focused on the clinical effects of bites of spiders worldwide. Majority of the cases with spider bites develop minor symptoms that resolve spontaneously and only few cases require specific therapy including antivenoms.[27] The most common types of medical importance are Widow spiders (genus *Latrodectus*), Recluse spiders (genus *Loxosceles*), Funnel web and mouse spiders (limited to Australia), armed or banana spiders (genus *Phoneutria*), and other spider species that can cause variable effects, mainly local pain with limited duration.[28]

DIFFERENT SPECIES

Widow Spiders (Genus *Latrodectus*)

Venom and Pathophysiology of Envenomation

Alpha-latrotoxin is the main component in the venom of *Latrodectus* spp. and is a potent neurotoxin that binds to specific presynaptic receptors, neurotoxin I-α and Ca^{2+} independent receptor for α-latrotoxin causing massive release of certain neurotransmitters like norepinephrine, dopamine, acetylcholine, glutamate, and γ-aminobutyric acid, leading to a toxidrome called latrodectism.[3,29,30]

Clinical Manifestations

Latrodectism usually starts few minutes after the bite and persists over 48 hours and then declines. The bite itself is painless or produces a minimal prick pain followed by, few minutes later, generalized signs and symptoms including vomiting, abdominal pain due to muscle rigidity, lymphadenitis, sweating, hypertension, lacrimation, salivation, increased bronchial secretions, and respiratory failure due to muscle paralysis.[30,31] Latrodectism myopathy begins 15–60 minutes after the bite with muscle cramps that may extend beyond the bite's site involving mainly chest, abdomen, and face muscles.[3] Occasionally, these symptoms may last for several days whereas weakness and muscle pain may last for weeks.[30]

Latrodectism myopathic syndrome begins 15–60 minutes after the bite with muscle cramps that may extend beyond the bite's site involving mainly chest, abdomen, and face muscles.[3,31] Myocardial infarction, myocarditis, cardiovascular failure, and gangrene have been reported.[3,30–33] Priapism has been reported as an unusual, rare clinical finding from most of *Latrodectus* species.[34]

Diagnostic Investigations

Laboratory findings may include oliguria, albuminuria, high levels of creatinine kinase (CK), hyperglycemia, leukocytosis, and decrease in eosinophils count.[30]

Current Treatment Approach

The treatment consists of supportive care, wound care, pain management, muscle relaxants, narcotics, intravenous calcium, and antivenom.[35] There are different types of antivenom produced against specific *Latrodectus* spp. in different regions worldwide. Although it is recognized treatment in severe latrodectism, caution in administration should be exercised as it is associated with hypersensitivity manifestations and serum sickness. Prophylactic administration of antihistamines and steroids prior to antivenom administration has been practiced.[36,37]

Recluse Spiders (Genus *Loxosceles*)

Venom and Pathophysiology of Envenomation

Recluse spiders, of the genus *Loxosceles*, are known for their venomous bites that cause a condition called loxoscelism. The mechanism of action for recluse spider's venom at the site of the bite and systemic effects is still not clearly understood. The venom contains a mixture of toxic components including sphingomyelinase D and hyaluronidase enzymes which play a crucial role in the toxic effects by inhibiting neutrophil chemotaxis as well as depleting total hemolytic complement, leading to disruption of the cell integrity.[3,38] Endothelial damage of the skin can occur as soon as 3 hours after the bite, accompanied by thrombocytopenia, altered prothrombin and partial thromboplastin times, and decreased fibrinogen levels. Small capillaries become occluded with thrombi leading to tissue hypoxia and death.[39]

Clinical Manifestations

The main concern with brown recluse spider bites is the potential for tissue necrosis. The clinical manifestation ranges from a mild local reaction to death due to loxoscelism depending on the amount of the venom injected. At the bite site, the patient may get little or no pain, followed by itching, swelling, mild-to-severe tenderness and redness, 2–8 hours after the bite followed by blistering, bleeding, and ulceration.[3,40] In 1 week, central necrosis starts to appear with eschar formation followed by wound induration and ulceration that heal with secondary intention in 14 days.[3] Progression and the lesion's size are the main factors to determine the time required for the lesion to heal.

Systemic loxoscelism occurs 24–48 hours after the bite and is shown to be more severe in children. This syndrome consists of fever, chills, malaise, weakness, nausea and vomiting, joint pain, and petechiae eruption. This can progress to severe rhabdomyolysis, disseminated intravascular coagulation, hemolysis, acute kidney injury, and convulsions.[3,40,41] Transverse myelitis, facial nerve palsy, and myopericarditis have been reported after brown recluse spider bite.[41-44]

Diagnostic Investigations

Laboratory investigations should evaluate associated hemolysis and leukocytosis. Blood film may show toxin-induced spherocytosis and stomatocytosis. Coagulopathy is often present and manifests with elevated fibrin split products, decrease fibrinogen concentration, and positive D-dimer assay.[3] Evidence of acute renal failure, hypokalemia, hematuria, and hemoglobinuria should be monitored. Rhabdomyolysis is evident with elevated CK. Transaminitis has been reported in such cases.[41]

Current Treatment Approach

Constant monitoring of the renal function is utterly important. Protective measures should be in place in treating loxoscelism, e.g., fluid replacement, urinary alkalinization, and hemodynamic support. Cases with signs and symptoms of severe hemolysis should be treated with blood transfusion.[41] Wound care of dermatonecrosis at the bite's site should include immobilization, tetanus prophylaxis, and analgesics. Corrective surgery of the necrotic area should be delayed until adequate tissue demarcation occurred.[3] Early treatment with dapsone, 100 mg twice daily for 2 weeks, in the first 6–8 hours after the bite, has reduced the need for surgical intervention.[3,45] It inhibits polymorphonuclear leukocyte function and hence theoretically plays a dominant role in reducing toxin-induced skin necrosis.[46] Dapsone is associated with significant side effects including hemolysis, agranulocytosis, aplastic anemia, methemoglobinemia, hypersensitivity, and toxic epidermal necrolysis syndrome and cannot be used in patients with glucose-6-phosphate dehydrogenase (G6PD) deficiency.[47] There is a wide use of antivenom in South America due to the considerable morbidity and mortality associated with the bite; however, the evidence to support its benefits is little.[27] Hyperbaric oxygen therapy has been proposed to treat the necrotic lesions as this therapy promotes angiogenesis and hence decreases the wound's severity and increases the healing rate. It also produces elevated oxygen tension required for fibroblast activation and collagen matrix production to enhance capillary endothelial cell growth.[48,49]

Armed or Banana Spiders (Genus *Phoneutria*)

Venom and Pathophysiology of Envenomation

These spiders are located mainly in Central America, South America, East of Andes, and North of Argentina. The venom of different species in this genus has different components, but mainly a complex mixture of neurotoxins, short-chain peptides, and enzymes including hyaluronidase and peptidases.[50]

Clinical Manifestations

Most of the bites are associated with mild effects, e.g., pain at the site of the bite, localized diaphoresis, and piloerection. Rarely, systemic envenomation occurs due to parasympathetic nervous system stimulation that manifests with bradycardia, hypotension, and priapism and can be severe in children and elderlies.[29]

Current Treatment Approach

Majority of the cases do not require more than supportive treatment, wound care, and pain management. There is a specific antivenom in Brazil that is administered intravenously in <5% of the cases. It is associated with early allergic reactions but there is little data on frequency.[29-50]

Funnel-web Spiders (*Atrax* and *Hadronyche* spp.)

Venom and Pathophysiology of Envenomation

Funnel-web spider (FWS), located in Australia, is considered the deadliest spider envenomation in the world. The main neurotoxin in FWS venom is δ-atracotoxins which affect voltage-gated Na^+ channels causing delay in their activation leading to repeated stimulation and hence release of a massive number of neurotransmitters in nerve endings.[25,35]

Clinical Manifestations

The severe envenomation of FWS consists of neuromuscular excitation (paresthesia and fasciculation); massive autonomic simulation in the form of bradycardia or tachycardia, hypertension, hypersalivation, lacrimation and miosis or mydriasis; noncardiogenic pulmonary edema; and generalized systemic effects. This will be complicated with refractory hypotension, neuromuscular paralysis, coma coagulopathy, and multiorgan failure.[27]

Current Treatment Approach

The mainstay of treatment is aggressive supportive measures, limb immobilization, wound care, and pain management.[35] Hemodynamic and ventilatory support is required in severe envenomation. There is a specific antivenom that should be administered urgently in severe envenomation. It is highly effective and can reverse neurotoxic effects, particularly with early administration.[25]

CONCLUSION

Scorpion stings and spider bites are commonly encountered in clinical practice. The symptoms are likely to differ with different species. Aggressive supportive therapy and pain relief are the main stays of management and should be initiated as soon as possible. Scorpion antivenom, if available, should be administered in patients with severe systemic envenomation. Antivenom administration helps ameliorate systemic symptoms rapidly, but non availability is a bottle neck. In areas with a high prevalence of scorpion envenomation, every effort should be made to stockpile antivenom. Management of autonomic dysfunction and diligent watch for systemic complications are important priorities in the management of these cases.

REFERENCES

1. World Health Organization. Rabies and envenomings: a neglected public health issue. Report of a consultative meeting, World Health Organization, Geneva, January 10, 2007.
2. Isbister GK, Bawaskar HS. Scorpion envenomation. N Engl J Med. 2014;371(5):457-63.
3. Repplinger DJ, Hahn IH. Arthropods. In: Nelson LS, Howland M, Lewin NA, Smith SW, Goldfrank LR, Hoffman RS (Eds). Goldfrank's Toxicologic Emergencies, 11th edition. New York: McGraw-Hill Education; 2019. pp. 1540-58.
4. Yarom R. Scorpion venom: A tutorial review of its effects in men and experimental animals. Clin Toxicol. 1970;3(4):561-9.
5. Bosmans F, Tytgat J. Voltage-gated sodium channel modulation by scorpion α-toxins. Toxicon. 2007;49(2):142-58.

6. Srinivasan KN, Gopalakrishnakone P, Tan PT, Chew KC, Cheng B, Kini RM, et al. SCORPION, a molecular database of scorpion toxins. Toxicon. 2002;40(1):23-31.
7. Petricevich VL. Scorpion venom and the inflammatory response. Mediators Inflamm. 2010;2010:903295.
8. Possani LD, Becerril B, Delepierre M, Tytgat J. Scorpion toxins specific for Na^+-channels. Eur J Biochem. 1999;264(2):287-300.
9. D'suze G, Moncada S, González C, Sevcik C, Aguilar V, Alagón A. Relationship between plasmatic levels of various cytokines, tumour necrosis factor, enzymes, glucose and venom concentration following Tityus scorpion sting. Toxicon. 2003;41(3):367-75.
10. Abroug F, Ouanes-Besbes L, Tilouche N, Elatrous S. Scorpion envenomation: State of the art. Intensive Care Med. 2020;46(3):401-10.
11. Abroug F, Souheil E, Ouanes I, Dachraoui F, Fekih-Hassen M, Ouanes Besbes L. Scorpion-related cardiomyopathy: clinical characteristics, pathophysiology, and treatment. Clin Toxicol. 2015;53(6):511-8.
12. Reis MB, Zoccal KF, Gardinassi LG, Faccioli LH. Scorpion envenomation and inflammation: beyond neurotoxic effects. Toxicon. 2019;167:174-9.
13. Gokdemir M, Sezer T. Evaluation of myocardial function using tissue Doppler imaging in children with moderate scorpion envenomation. Clin Toxicol. 2013;51(3):156-61.
14. Boyer LV, Theodorou AA, Berg RA, Mallie J; Arizona Envenomation Investigators; Chávez-Méndez A, García-Ubbelohde W, et al. Antivenom for Critically Ill Children with Neurotoxicity from Scorpion Stings. N Engl J Med. 2009;360(20):2090-8.
15. Chen JW, Shi CX, Teng MJ, Schloithe AC, Toouli J, Saccone GT. Scorpion venom stimulates biliary/duodenal motility and pancreatic exocrine secretion. Neurogastroenterol Motil. 2004;16(4):447-54.
16. Warrell DA. Venomous and poisonous animals. In: Manson's Tropical Infectious Diseases. London: Routledge. 2014. pp. 235-50.
17. Kamalakar MV. A study of electrocardiographic abnormalities in patients with scorpion string. Int J Contemp Med. 2015;32.
18. Rao CL, Murthy KV. Analysis of electrocardiographic changes in patients with scorpion sting. Ind J Forensic Med Toxicol. 2017;11:17-21.
19. Bond GR. Antivenin administration for Centruroides scorpion sting: risks and benefits. Ann Emerg Med. 1992;21(7):788-91.
20. Bouaziz M, Hamida CB, Chelly H, Bahloul M, Kallel H. Dobutamine in the treatment of severe scorpion envenoming. Toxicon. 2020;182:54-8.
21. Khalaf MA, El-Zaher MA, Paulis MG, Ahmed MB. Can the addition of prazosin or dobutamine to the antivenom improve scorpion envenomation-induced cardiotoxicity in children. J Forensic Toxicol Medicol Anal. 2016;1:29-33.
22. Rodrigo C, Gnanathasan A. Management of scorpion envenoming: a systematic review and meta-analysis of controlled clinical trials. Systematic Rev. 2017;6(1):1-2.
23. Gupta V. Prazosin: A pharmacological antidote for scorpion envenomation. J Trop Pediatr. 2006;52(2):150-1.
24. D'sa SR, Peter JV, Chacko B, Pichamuthu K, Sathyendra S. Intraaortic balloon pump (IABP) rescue therapy for refractory cardiogenic shock due to scorpion sting envenomation. Clin Toxicol. 2016;54(2):155-7.
25. Isbister GK, Fan HW. Spider bite. Lancet. 2011;378(9808): 2039-47.
26. Blackman JR. Spider bites. J Am Board Family Practice. 1995;8(4):288-94.
27. Isbister GK, White J. Clinical consequences of spider bites: recent advances in our understanding. Toxicon. 2004;43(5):477-92.
28. Seifert SA, Dart RC, White J. Envenomation, Bites, and Stings. In: Goldman-Cecil Medicine. 24th ed. 2025. p. 705-713.e1.
29. Vetter RS, Isbister GK. Medical aspects of spider bites. Ann Rev Entomol. 2008;53:409-29.
30. Rauber A. Black widow spider bites. J Toxicol. 1983;21(4-5):473-85.
31. Maretić Z. Latrodectism: variations in clinical manifestations provoked by Latrodectus species of spiders. Toxicon. 1983;21(4):457-66.
32. Emara AG, Aboshady AA, Aboshady OA, Shawqi MM. Reversible myocarditis following black widow spider (Latrodectus spp.) bite in Egypt: a case report. Sultan Qaboos Univ Med J. 2023;23(2):251-5.
33. Müller GJ. Black and brown widow spider bites in South Africa: A series of 45 cases. South Afr Med J. 1993;83(6):399-405.
34. Hoover NG, Fortenberry JD. Use of antivenin to treat priapism after a black widow spider bite. Pediatrics. 2004;114(1):e128-9.
35. Rahmani F, Khojasteh SM, Bakhtavar HE, Rahmani F, Nia KS, Faridaalaee G. Poisonous spiders: bites, symptoms, and treatment; an educational review. Emergency. 2014; 2(2):54.
36. Timms PK, Gibbons RB. Latrodectism—effects of the black widow spider bite. Western J Med. 1986;144(3): 315-7.
37. Clark RF. The safety and efficacy of antivenin Latrodectus mactans. J Toxicol. 2001;39(2):125-7.
38. Babcock JL, Marmer DJ, Steele RW. Immunotoxicology of brown recluse spider (Loxosceles reclusa) venom. Toxicon. 1986;24(8):783-90.
39. Forks TP. Brown recluse spider bites. J Am Board Family Practice. 2000;13(6):415-23.
40. Wasserman GS, Siegel C. Loxoscelism (brown recluse spider bites): A review of the literature. Clin Toxicol. 1979;14(3):353-8.

41. Loden JK, Seger DL, Spiller HA, Wang L, Byrne DW. Cutaneous-hemolytic loxoscelism following brown recluse spider envenomation: new understandings. Clin Toxicol. 2020;58(12):1297-305.
42. Sauer GC. Transverse myelitis and paralysis from a brown recluse spider bite. Mo Med. 1975;72(10):603-4.
43. Stolzenberg L, Koch A, Huang A, Usman M, Subhedar S, Decker T, et al. Spider bite-induced facial nerve palsy. Cureus. 2022;14(12):e32162.
44. Carroll MM, Palmen R, Grodzinsky A. The girl with a big heart: a case of myopericarditis following a brown-recluse spider bite. J Am Coll Cardiol. 2023;81(8 Supplement): 2806.
45. Rees RS, Altenbern DP, Lynch JB, King Jr LE. Brown recluse spider bites. A comparison of early surgical excision versus dapsone and delayed surgical excision. Ann Surg. 1985;202(5):659.
46. Wolf R, Matz H, Orion E, Tuzun B, Tuzun Y. Dapsone. Dermatol Online J. 2002;8(1):2.
47. Wright SW, Wrenn KD, Murray L, Seger D. Clinical presentation and outcome of brown recluse spider bite. Ann Emerg Med. 1997;30(1):28-32.
48. Strain GM, Snider TG, Tedford BL, Cohn GH. Hyperbaric oxygen effects on brown recluse spider (Loxosceles reclusa) envenomation in rabbits. Toxicon. 1991;29(8): 989-96.
49. Andersen RJ, Campoli J, Johar SK, Schumacher KA, Allison Jr EJ. Suspected brown recluse envenomation: a case report and review of different treatment modalities. J Emerg Med. 2011;41(2):e31-7.
50. Fernandes FF, Moraes JR, Santos JL, Soares TG, Gouveia VJ, Matavel A, et al. Comparative venomic profiles of three spiders of the genus Phoneutria. J Venom Anim Toxins Incl Trop Dis. 2022;28:e20210042.

2.22 Bee, Wasp, and Hornet Stings

YP Singh, Gaurav Pratap Singh, Saurabh Jain

INTRODUCTION

Bee, wasp, and hornet stinging is a neglected clinical entity, especially in tropical regions. These stings might appear in a variety of ways. On one end of the spectrum are modest localized skin reactions, while on the other end, toxin-induced multiorgan involvement and death can occur.

As per literature, hornet, wasp, and bee stings lead the tally for the highest number of fatalities among venomous bites in USA over a 10-year period (2011–2021) accounting for 788 deaths, i.e., 72 deaths/year.[1] Fatality rate due to wasp sting has been found to be 0.02 and 0.2 per million population per year in an Australian study and Swedish registry, respectively.[2,3]

The comprehensive national data for this entity is not available in India but its significance has been identified in some states, leading to the inclusion of deaths caused due to honeybee, hornet, and wasp sting in their respective Disaster and Relief Norms.

These stinging insects belong to the order Hymenoptera and class *Insecta*. Hymenoptera include *Apidae* (bees) and *Vespidae* (wasps and hornets).

VENOM

Venom of these insects is a highly concentrated and complex mixture of various bioactive enzymes, amines, peptides, and kinins.[4] A brief review of various components and their action is provided in **Table 1**.

CLINICAL MANIFESTATIONS

Wasp and bee stings can cause a variety of clinical disorders, ranging from modest local reactions to catastrophic systemic reactions accompanied by multiorgan failure. Organ dysfunction can be caused by anaphylactic shock or by direct effect of poisons themselves.

Toxin-mediated organ injury may result in acute renal failure (ARF), acute liver injury (ALI) with or without fulminant hepatic failure, disseminated intravascular coagulation (DIC), hemolysis, rhabdomyolysis, myocarditis and acute respiratory distress syndrome (ARDS) or pulmonary hemorrhage. This multiorgan involvement can be attributed to a systemic hyperinflammatory state caused by cytokine storm.

In the later stages, immune system activation may cause hypersensitivity or autoimmunity manifesting as interstitial nephritis, encephalopathy, or vasculitis.

Anaphylaxis

The first reported human fatality from anaphylaxis was Egyptian Pharaoh Menes, who was stung by a wasp.[11]

TABLE 1: Composition of venom.

Venom components	Actions
• Phospholipases (PLA-1 and PLA-2) • Hyaluronidase	• Both act on the cell membranes, leading to cell lysis, including hemolysis[5] • Cytotoxic and immunostimulatory effects, causing immune activation[5] • They act as antigen, binds to IgE, causing allergic and anaphylactic reactions[5,6] • Hyaluronidase aids in local spread of the venom by lysing the extracellular matrix and entering blood vessels, resulting in systemic envenomation[5,6]
Amines (histamine, serotonin, catecholamines)	• Histamine increases vascular permeability and enhances cytolysis[7] • Serotonin causes vasoconstriction and along with histamine induces pain[7] • Catecholamines cause tachycardia and helps in venom spread as it enters circulation[5]
Wasp kinins	• Increase vascular permeability and edema • Pain • Weak mast cell degranulation
Mastoparans	• Cell lysis • Mast cell degranulation • Triggers cell apoptosis • Inhibits Na^+/K^+ ATPase of the renal • Tubular cells causing ATN[8]
• Melittin • Apamin	• Weak allergens[9] • Pain • Cell lysis • Activation of inflammatory response[9]
Antigen-5[10]	Strong allergen
Others (mast cell degranulating peptide, Adolapin, Tertiapins, Scapins, Acetylcholine)[5]	• First three have anti-inflammatory action • Scapins cause leukotriene-induced hyperalgesia and edema • Acetylcholine causes pain by intense depolarization of nociceptors in dermis

(ATN: acute tubular necrosis; IgE: immunoglobulin E)

Anaphylaxis is the leading cause of death and organ damage after bee and wasp stings, caused by immunoglobulin E (IgE) mediated type 1 hypersensitivity reactions.[12]

Hyperinflammatory Response and Multisystem Involvement

Hymenoptera envenomation causes elevated cytokine levels, mainly interleukin-6 (IL-6), IL-8, IL-10, IL-2, IL-17, tumor necrosis factor-α (TNF-α), and interferon-γ (IFN-γ). These cause activation of leukocytes, neutrophilic degranulation, and humoral immunity, resulting in a systemic hyperinflammatory response leading to multiorgan dysfunction.[13,14]

The effects of Hymenoptera envenomation on major organs are as follows:

- *Renal effects*: Acute kidney injury (AKI) from wasp envenomation can happen in 10–58% of patients.[4,15,16] A case series with 1,091 patients from China showed an incidence of AKI as 21.0%.[13] In this case series, >80% who had AKI had a severe course and required dialysis.[17-19]

  The AKI is characteristically oliguric with gross hematuria in a minor percentage of patients.[13,15] Multiple factors coexist to cause AKI including acute tubular necrosis (ATN), pigment nephropathy, hypoperfusion, and acute tubulointerstitial nephritis (AIN).[20]

  The ATN is caused by direct nephrotoxic chemicals in wasp venom, hypotension-induced renal ischemia, and microvascular circulatory dysfunction. Phospholipases (PLA) and Mastoparan also contribute to ATN by disrupting renal cell membranes and inducing cell necrosis.[21] Rarely, renal cortical necrosis and thrombotic microangiopathy can induce AKI.

  The incidence and severity of AKI are proportional to the number of wasp stings and levels of IL-6, IL-2, IL-10, and IL-17.[14] Elderly and patients with macroscopic hematuria are more prone to a severe course of illness.[15,22] Most patients recover completely with a minority (around 10%) progressing to *end-stage renal disease* (ESRD).[23,24]
- *Hepatic effects*: Hepatotoxicity can be found in 30% of patients following wasp stinging.[13,16] *Hepatitis is the most common pattern among patients with ALI, with a disproportionate rise in transaminases relative to an elevation of alkaline phosphatase (ALP) and gamma-glutamyl transferase (GGT).*[13] Identifying hepatic injury can be a dilemma, as transaminases can also be raised by concurrent rhabdomyolysis, hemolysis, and cardiac injury. Presence of direct, mixed hyperbilirubinemia along with decreased synthetic functions points toward a hepatic injury. A significant proportion of these may progress to acute fulminant hepatic failure.[25]

  Liver biopsy characteristically shows centrilobular hepatic necrosis along with some fat infiltration.

- *Cardiovascular effects*: *Circulatory collapse* following bee or wasp envenomation can be multifactorial due to anaphylaxis or due to direct vasodilatory effects of the toxins or both.

  Myocardial injury is frequently seen following wasp stings. *Myocardial infarction (MI), hypersensitivity myocarditis, and Takotsubo cardiomyopathy* are the three mechanisms of myocardial injury in these patients.[26] MI occurs secondary to shock or coronary vasoconstriction,[27,28] induced by chemical mediators [histamine, cathepsin D, leukotrienes, thromboxane A2 (TXA2), and platelet activating factor (PAF)] and treatment with epinephrine.[11]

  Kounis syndrome, i.e., anaphylaxis-associated acute coronary syndrome (ACS), can be seen after wasp stings.[29]

Takotsubo cardiomyopathy or stress cardiomyopathy, myocarditis secondary to direct toxin effect, and various arrhythmias [atrial fibrillation, flutter, and paroxysmal supraventricular tachycardia (PSVT)] have been described following Hymenoptera stings.[30-33]

- *Effects on hematological system*: Hemolysis may be seen in 17–22% of patients[13,15] due to disruption of the RBC cell membrane by PLA and other toxins[5] and can be present even after a single wasp sting.[34,35] The other pathological effects are thrombocytopenia, coagulopathy, and DIC.

  Endogenous hyper-heparinization: Prolonged activated partial thromboplastin time (APTT) and reduced factor Xa activity (secondary to heparin release from mast cells) and hypofibrinogenemia (effect of tryptase on fibrinogen and its ability to activate plasminogen) may be seen.[36,37]

  The coagulopathy usually correlates with the venom dose.[16] Wasp venom itself has anticoagulant properties. The venom affects multiple steps in intrinsic, extrinsic, and common pathways and has fibrinogen-degrading properties.[38]

  Magnvesin, a serine protease derived from the venom of Vespa magnifica, acts as an anticoagulant by hydrolyzing tissue factor and clotting factors VII, VIII, IX, and X.[39]

- *Effects on skeletal muscles*: PLA and melittin in wasp venom lead to disruption of skeletal muscle cell membrane causing elevated creatine phosphokinase (CPK) levels (53.7%) which may proceed further to rhabdomyolysis (24.1%).[13,40]

  Other molecules, e.g., Mastoparan, which promote myonecrosis, apoptosis, and cytokine activation in muscles, are also important in the pathogenesis of skeletal muscle injury.[41]

  Patients typically report weakness, myalgia, and muscular edema following sting. Skin necrosis may be seen and is typically a bad prognostic sign.[42] As expected, the incidence of AKI is much higher in patients suffering rhabdomyolysis.

- *Neurological effects*: Wasps' venom contains neurotoxins; however, neurological consequences are rare.

  Early signs include hypotension, anaphylaxis, and direct neurotoxicity from venom, whereas delayed manifestations are immune-mediated hypersensitivity reactions.

  Ischemic strokes have been reported following bee and wasp stings with pathophysiology being similar to that of Kounis syndrome.[43]

  Rarely, neuromyotonia and Myasthenia Gravis have also been reported following bee stings and *molecular mimicry* has been postulated as the mechanism in these. Other neurological manifestations have been summarized in the **Table 2**.

TABLE 2: Clinical manifestations.

Organ system	*Manifestations*
Respiratory system	• Diffuse alveolar hemorrhage[44] • Pleural effusions[44] • Acute pulmonary edema[44] • ARDS[45]
Gastrointestinal	• Fatal GI bleeding[46] • Nonocclusive mesenteric ischemia[47] • Pancreatitis[48] • Spontaneous splenic rupture[49]
Rheumatological	Henoch–Schonlein purpura[50]
Skin	Skin necrosis and hemorrhage[51]
Ocular	Corneal decompensation and cataracts[52]
Central nervous system	• Acute encephalopathy, coma • Extrapyramidal symptoms • Acute disseminated encephalomyelitis • Posterior reversible encephalopathy syndrome[53]
Peripheral nervous system	• Guillain-Barré syndrome[54] • Miller Fisher syndrome • Trigeminal neuralgia[55] • Autoimmune neuromyotonia • Myasthenia gravis[56]

(ARDS: acute respiratory distress syndrome; GI: gastrointestinal)

- *Other organ system effects*: Various other organ systems may get involved and are elaborated in **Table 2**.

MANAGEMENT OF A PATIENT WITH HYMENOPTERA ENVENOMATION

Evaluation

- *Airway, breathing, and circulation (ABCs)*: Evaluation and urgent management of ABC first
- *Uncomplicated local reactions*: Comprised of a small area of local edema, warmth, and tenderness
- *Large local reactions (LLRs)*: Comprised of >10 cm area of erythema, edema, and warmth. It is larger and last longer than uncomplicated local reactions.
- *Systemic reactions (including anaphylaxis)*: Include histaminic manifestations such as generalized urticaria, angioedema/facial swelling, stridor, respiratory distress/wheezing secondary to bronchospasm, abdominal pain, nausea, vomiting, and flushing.

Treatment

There are no established guidelines on the management of systemic Hymenoptera envenomation.

Management should primarily focus upon:
- Managing anaphylaxis
- Preventing organ injury
- Providing organ support

Anaphylaxis, occurring in up to 3% of patients post Hymenoptera sting, can be particularly severe and is a leading cause of anaphylactic deaths. Treatment of anaphylaxis due to Hymenoptera venom is similar to anaphylaxis due to any other cause.

Organ injury can be largely prevented by maintaining tissue perfusion. Shock should be treated on an urgent basis as it can hasten the development of AKI, which is a poor prognostic factor. Fluids and vasopressors should be used to maintain adequate organ perfusion pressure. Electrolyte imbalances, if any, should be treated at the earliest.

The elimination of venom poisons and toxic by-products of organ damage, such as myoglobin and hemoglobin, is the next critical step in preventing organ destruction. Forced alkaline diuresis has been used to remove hemoproteins,[47] but it requires a high urine production, which may not be available in cases of shock and accompanying oliguria.

Ordinary renal replacement therapy cannot effectively remove venom and endogenous toxins as they have high molecular weights; therefore, incorporating adsorbent therapies like *hemoperfusion* is an effective way to remove them. *Continuous renal replacement therapy* (CRRT) and more specifically *high-volume hemofiltration* (HVHF) have been shown to be more efficacious in removing these compounds than intermittent hemodialysis alone.[57] Hemoperfusion uses an *adsorbent charcoal cartridge or an ion exchange resin* in series with CRRT. So, toxins, superantigens, and other endogenous compounds that are not removed by dialysis or hemofiltration get adsorbed to the material in the cartridge.

Plasma exchange (PE) has also been utilized to treat multiorgan dysfunction caused by wasp envenomation. PE combined with hemoperfusion has been shown to be more effective than PE alone.[58] There is no evidence supporting the routine use of steroids and pooled human immunoglobulins (IVIG) in Hymenoptera envenomation.

Extracorporeal membrane oxygenation (ECMO) has also been used in patients with pulmonary hemorrhage following Hymenoptera stings.[59]

PROGNOSIS FOLLOWING HYMENOPTERA STING

The mortality is in the range of 4–10% after Hymenoptera envenomation.[15,23] Although immediate mortality post sting is almost always due to anaphylaxis, organ dysfunction post envenomation has much higher overall mortality than anaphylaxis. The more the number of stings, the more the mortality.[13] The presence of an organ injury, especially AKI, significantly increases the mortality rate. High creatinine levels, presence of shock, oliguria, hematuria, and anemia are the strong predictors of bad prognosis.[24]

CONCLUSION

Hymenoptera venom is a complicated collection of proteins that affects several organ systems in the body. This envenomation may result in acute hypersensitivity reactions (anaphylaxis), direct toxin-mediated cell injury, and related systemic inflammation, leading to diverse organ dysfunction and, finally, delayed immunological responses.

The kidneys, liver, hematological system, skeletal muscles, and cardiovascular system are the most commonly impacted organ systems. Although rare, neurological signs may appear caused by type II or III hypersensitivity reactions. Hymenoptera envenomation is primarily treated with supportive care, while therapies such as hemoperfusion, PE, and ECMO have been used effectively on occasion.

REFERENCES

1. Morbidity and Mortality Weekly Report. Number of Deaths from Hornet, Wasp and Bee Stings Among Males and Females - National Vital Statistics system, United States, 2011-2021. MMWR Morb Mortal Wkly Rep. 2023;72:756.
2. McGain F, Harrison J, Winkel KD. Wasp sting mortality in Australia. Med J Aust. 2000;173:198-200.
3. Johansson B, Eriksson A, Ornehult L. Human fatalities caused by wasp and bee stings in Sweden. Int J Legal Med. 1991;104:99-103.
4. Gong J, Yuan H, Gao Z, Hu F. Wasp venom and acute kidney injury: the mechanisms and therapeutic role of renal replacement therapy. Toxicon. 2019;163:1-7.
5. Moreno M, Giralt E. Three valuable peptides from bee and wasp venoms for therapeutic and biotechnological use: Melittin, apamin and mastoparan. Toxins (Basel). 2015;7:1126-50.
6. Gräler MH, Goetzl EJ. Lysophospholipids and their G protein-coupled receptors in inflammation and immunity. Biochem Biophys Acta. 2002;1582:168-74.
7. Mortari MR, do Couto LL, dos Anjos LC, Mourão CBF, Camargos TS, Vargas JAG, et al. Pharmacological characterization of Synoeca cyanea venom: an aggressive social wasp widely distributed in the neotropical region. J Toxicon. 2012;59:163-70.
8. Choi MB, Lee YH. The structure and antimicrobial potential of wasp and hornet (Vespidae) mastoparans: a review. Entomol Res. 2020;50:369-76.
9. Pucca MB, Cerni FA, Oliveira IS, Jenkins TP, Argemí L, Sørensen CV, et al. Bee updated: current knowledge on bee venom and envenoming therapy. Front Immunol. 2019;10:2090.
10. Bazon ML, Perez-Riverol A, Dos Santos-Pinto JRA, Fernandes LGR, Lasa AM, Justo-Jacomini DL, et al. Heterologous expression, purification and immuno-reactivity of the antigen 5 from Polybia paulista wasp venom. Toxins (Basel). 2017;9:259.
11. Kounis NG, Cervellin G, Koniari I, Bonfanti L, Dousdampanis P, Charokopos N, et al. Anaphylactic cardiovascular collapse and Kounis syndrome: systemic vasodilation or coronary vasoconstriction? Ann Transl Med. 2018;6:332.
12. Schmidt JO. Clinical consequences of toxic envenomations by Hymenoptera. Toxicon. 2018;150:96-104.
13. Xie C, Xu S, Ding F, Xie M, Lv J, Yao J, et al. Clinical features of severe wasp sting patients with dominantly toxic reaction: analysis of 1091 cases. PLoS One. 2013;8: e83164.
14. Li F, Liu L, Guo X, Luo Z, Zhang Y, Lu F, et al. Elevated cytokine levels associated with acute kidney injury due to wasp sting. Eur Cytokine Netw. 2019;30:34-8.
15. Wang M, Prince S, Tang Y, Zhong X, Chen S, Li G, et al. Macroscopic hematuria in wasp sting patients: a retrospective study. Ren Fail. 2021;43:500-9.
16. Xuan BHN, Le MH, Thi TXN, Thi MTH, Nguyen HN, Rabenou RA. Swarming hornet attacks: shock and acute kidney injury–a large case series from Vietnam. Nephrol Dial Transplant. 2010;25:1146-50.
17. Paudel B, Paudel K. A study of wasp bites in a tertiary hospital of western Nepal—PubMed. Nepal Med College J. 2009;52-6.
18. Vikrant S, Jaryal A, Parashar A. Mortality due to mass Hymenoptera attacks: a serious but underrecognized public health problem in a mountainous state of India. Indian J Public Health. 2019;63:154-6.
19. Sigdel MR, Raut KB. Wasp bite in a referral hospital in Nepal—PubMed. J Nepal Heal Res Counc. 2013;11: 244-50.
20. Dhanapriya J, Dineshkumar T, Sakthirajan R, Shankar P, Gopalakrishnan N, Balasubramaniyan T. Wasp sting-induced acute kidney injury. Clin Kidney J. 2016;9:201.
21. Agarwal A, Dong Z, Harris R, Murray P, Parikh SM, Rosner MH, et al. Cellular and molecular mechanisms of AKI. J Am Soc Nephrol. 2016;27:1288-99.
22. Deng YY, Shen JM, Mao YN, Gou R, Li WW, Ye TT. Sustained low-efficiency diafiltration is superior to hemodialysis in promoting renal function recovery in elderly wasp sting victims with stage III acute kidney injury: a retrospective study. Ren Fail. 2019;41:814-20.
23. Zhang L, Yang Y, Tang Y, Zhao Y, Cao Y, Su B, et al. Recovery from AKI following multiple wasp stings: a case series. Clin J Am Soc Nephrol. 2013;8:1850-6.
24. Yuan H, Lu L, Gao Z, Hu F. Risk factors of acute kidney injury induced by multiple wasp stings. Toxicon. 2020; 182:1-6.
25. Chen TH, Liao WT, Chen CS, Lin PC, Wu MY. An envenoming syndrome from massive vespa stings induces multiple organ failure. Insects. 2020;11:219.
26. Sirur FM, Wilson W, Gopinathan V, Chethana AS, Lekha N. Hymenoptera heartaches—cardiac manifestation with hymenoptera stings, a retrospective study from a tertiary care hospital in South India. Am J Emerg Med. 2021;50:294-300.
27. Levine HD. Acute myocardial infarction following wasp sting. Report of two cases and critical survey of the literature. Am Heart J. 1976;91:365-74.
28. Scherbak D, Lazkani M, Sparacino N, Loli A. Kounis syndrome: a stinging case of ST-elevation myocardial infarction. Heart Lung Circ. 2015;24:e48-50.
29. Ralapanawa DMPUK, Kularatne SAM. A case of Kounis syndrome after a hornet sting and literature review. BMC Res Notes. 2014;7:867.

30. Diaz JH. A wasp sting and a broken heart. Wilderness Environ Med. 2016;27:326-9.
31. Ferreira DB, Costa RS, De Oliveira JAM, Muccillo G. An infarct-like myocardial lesion experimentally induced in Wistar rats with Africanized bee venom. J Pathol. 1995;177:95-102.
32. Fisher BAC, Antonios TFT. Atrial flutter following a wasp sting. J Postgrad Med. 2003;49:254-5.
33. Patel SC, Detjen PF. Atrial fibrillation associated with anaphylaxis during venom and pollen immunotherapy. Ann Allergy Asthma Immunol. 2002;89:209-11.
34. Monzon C, Miles J. Hemolytic anemia following a wasp sting. J Pediatr. 1980;96:103940.
35. Schulte KL, Kochen MM. Haemolytic anaemia in an adult after a wasp sting. Lancet. 1981;2:478.
36. Wang J-L, Shen E-Y, Ho M-Y. Isolated prolongation of activated partial thromboplastin time following wasp sting. Acta Paediatr Taiwan. 2005;46:164-5.
37. Lai D, Tian Y, Zhang J, Weng CF. Hyperendogenous heparinization suggests a guideline for the management of massive wasp stings in two victims. Wilderness Environ Med. 2021;32:344-50.
38. Czaikoski PG, Menaldo DL, Marcussi S, Baseggio ALC, Fuly AL, Paula RC, et al. Anticoagulant and fibrinogenolytic properties of the venom of Polybia occidentalis social wasp. Blood Coagul Fibrinolysis. 2010;21:653-9.
39. Han J, You D, Xu X, Han W, Lu Y, Lai R, et al. An anticoagulant serine protease from the wasp venom of Vespa magnifica. Toxicon. 2008;51:914-22.
40. Constantino K, Pawlukiewicz AJ, Spear L. A case report on rhabdomyolysis after multiple bee stings. Cureus. 2020;12:e9501.
41. Rocha T, Soares de Barros LL, Fontana K, Monson de Souza B, Palma MS, Alice da Cruz-Höfing M. Inflammation and apoptosis induced by mastoparan Polybia-MPII on skeletal muscle. Toxicon. 2010;55:1213-21.
42. Ito K, Imafuku S, Nakayama J. Rhabdomyolysis due to multiple wasp stings. Case Rep Dermatol Med. 2012;2012:1-2.
43. Mirijello A, Pepe G, Zampiello P, Manfrini A. Ischemic stroke after wasp sting: another manifestation of Kounis syndrome? J Emerg Med. 2017;52:e215.
44. In S-H, Shin Y-C, Hwang E-K, You H-W, Kim J-I, Park J-H, et al. Unusual reaction to Hymenoptera stings. Allergy Asthma Respir Dis. 2016;4:305–7.
45. Ou WF, Huang WH, Chiu HF, Mao YC, Wen MC, Chen CH, et al. Clinical manifestation of multiple wasp stings with details of whole transcriptome analysis: two case reports. Medicine (Baltimore). 2021;100:e24492.
46. Vikrant S, Pandey D, Machhan P, Gupta D, Kaushal SS, Grover N. Wasp envenomation-induced acute renal failure: a report of three cases. Nephrology (Carlton). 2005;10:548-52.
47. Yamazaki H, Yasumura R, Miyashita K, Ishii Y, Kobayashi Y. Nonocclusive mesenteric ischemia following multiple wasp stings. Am J Emerg Med. 2014;32:689.e3-4.
48. Shilpakar O, Rajbhandari B, Karki B, Bogati U. Multiple organ dysfunction and acute pancreatitis following wasp stings. J Nepal Health Res Counc. 2020; 18:566-8.
49. Kang W, Zhang J, Xie Y, Zhang Y, Lian J. Spontaneous splenic rupture: an unusual complication following wasp stings. ANZ J Surg. 2017;87:315-6.
50. Burke DM, Jellinek HL. Nearly fatal case of Schoenlein–Henoch syndrome following insect bite. AMA Am J Dis Child. 1954;88:772-4.
51. Yanagawa Y, Morita K, Sugiura T, Okada Y. Cutaneous hemorrhage or necrosis findings after Vespa mandarinia (wasp) stings may predict the occurrence of multiple organ injury: a case report and review of literature. Clin Toxicol (Phila). 2007;45:803-7.
52. Arcieri ES, França ET, De Oliveria HB, De Abreu FL, Ferreira MA, Rocha FJ. Ocular lesions arising after stings by hymenopteran insects. Cornea. 2002;21:328-30.
53. Loh HH, Tan CHH. Acute renal failure and posterior reversible encephalopathy syndrome following multiple wasp stings: a case report. Med J Malaysia. 2012;67: 133-5.
54. Bachman DS, Paulson GW, Mendell JR. Acute inflammatory polyradiculoneuropathy following hymenoptera stings. JAMA. 1982;247:1443-5.
55. Kahilogullari G, Ugur HC, Tatli M, Kanpolat Y. Trigeminal neuropathic pain following honeybee sting: a case report. Turk Neurosurg. 2010;20(2):261-4.
56. Brumlik J. Myasthenia gravis associated with wasp sting. JAMA. 1976;235:2120-1.
57. Si X, Li J, Bi X, Wu L, Wu X. Clinical evaluation of high-volume hemofiltration with hemoperfusion followed by intermittent hemodialysis in the treatment of acute wasp stings complicated by multiple organ dysfunction syndrome. PLoS One. 2015;10:e0132708.
58. Yuan H, Chen S, Hu F, Zhang Q. Efficacy of two combinations of blood purification techniques for the treatment of multiple organ failure induced by wasp stings. Blood Purif. 2016;42:49-55.
59. Wang YC, Hsu CY, Chen YL, Lin PC, Wu MY. Massive Vespa basalis stings induce an envenoming syndrome. Am J Emerg Med. 2021;46:625-7.

2.23 Chemical Warfare Agents

Rawan Eskandarani

INTRODUCTION

Over centuries, naturally occurring substances from plants and animals that were maliciously used were the earliest forms of chemical warfare agents. The utilization of incapacitating chemical substances in warfare dates back to the First World War, where a large number of fatalities were caused by exposure to chlorine and phosgene gas, similarly, exposure to organophosphates and nerve agents as incapacitating substances in the Persian Gulf War, as they were produced and stocked during the periods of the Cold war by extremists as chemical weapons for mass destruction.

Toxic chemicals have also been used incapacitating agents by governments and leaders against rebels and to disperse and control crowds in certain situations; these were named as riot control agents (RCAs). However, these have also been justified to be used for opposing civilians, such as in the Moscow theater hostage crisis where fentanyl was used in 2002 and the use of carbon monoxide and Zyklon B during the Holocaust.

Terrorist cults have used chemical substances such as sarin, which was used by the Cult leader Aum Shinrikyo for religious reasons in the Tokyo subway in Japan in 1994.

The unintentional release of such devastating chemicals has occurred in history, such as the accidental release of methyl isocyanate in Bhopal, India, in 1984, which caused deaths in several thousands and injuries in more than one million.

Over the years, with the global rising concern of the misuse of certain chemical substances for law enforcement purposes, the negotiating of Chemical Weapon Convention (CWC) was developed in Geneva in 1992, where the agreement was concluded to completely ban the use of an entire class of weapons and firmly limit and strictly monitor activities that may contribute to malicious production of other weapons.[1]

The different types of chemical agents from the military point of view were generalized into three main categories based on their tactical functions:

1. *Lethal agents:* Used to kill or severely injure the enemy
2. *Incapacitating agents:* Used to put the enemy completely out of function for several hours or even days, but disablement is for a short term, where full recovery can be expected without medical aid.
3. *Short-term incapacitating (harassing agents):* Temporary disablement during the period of exposure.

The general agreement is to merge all definitions under (chemical weapon) to include any chemical substance used for purposes prohibited by the CWC. There is a continuous rise in psychochemical incapacitants that are increasingly harmful and have the potential to be weaponized, such as RCAs and other central nervous system (CNS)-acting chemicals that have been used by governments.[2]

WHAT IS AN INCAPACITATING CHEMICAL AGENT?

An incapacitating chemical agent is an ideal biochemical agent that would incapacitate personnel without causing a fatality.

The balance between lethality and acceptable safety margin is highly variable and interpretable, where the ratio of risks to benefits depends highly on morals, type of military operation, and political, ethical, and societal considerations.

To be an ideal incapacitating agent, it should fulfill the following:[2,3]

- Rapid onset
- Short duration of action
- Potent in low concentrations
- Reversible effects
- Easy to store and deliver
- Have predictable effects
- Controlled and predictable dissemination and distribution
- High safety margin
- Low fatality rate with high concentrations

CHEMICAL WARFARE AGENTS

Traditionally, chemical warfare agents have been categorized into the following categories based on their toxicological behaviors:[4]

- Nerve agents
- Psychomimetic and incapacitating chemical agents
- RCAs
- Choking agents
- Blood agents
- Vesicants
- Biological toxins

Organophosphate and Nerve Agents

Anticholinesterase agents such as Tabun, Sarin, Soman, VX, and Novichok are organophosphate and nerve agents. They are organophosphate substances that are deliberately formulated for significant debilitation or death and have been used by multiple nations for military purposes during times of war **(Table 1)**.

Nerve agents are divided mainly into two groups, G and V (from Germany and Victory, the British who first synthesized it). The oldest and most common agent is the VX.

The G-series agents (Tabin, Sarin, and Soman) are all viscous liquids with variable volatility.

The high vapor pressure of the G-series agents allows them to be rapidly disseminated.

Agent VX is deliberately formulated to be less volatile and more persistent on contacted surfaces. It spreads slowly and can remain on exposed surfaces for weeks before it dissipates.[5]

It is a major threat from cutaneous exposure but still compromises vapor inhalational risk at higher temperatures.[6]

Nerve agents are known to work by blocking the breakdown of acetylcholine by binding to the acetylcholinesterase (AChE) enzyme. This will cause acetylcholine to stimulate the muscle and cause uncontrolled continuous contractions, eventually resulting in muscular paralysis.

The irreversible phosphorylation of the serine-containing active site of AChE (aging) gives the nerve agent its characteristic toxic manifestation and lethality.

TABLE 1: Organophosphate and nerve agents.

Agent	*LD50 (mg)*	*Aging t½*	*Volatility*
VX	10	2.1–5.4 days	Neglectant
Soman	100	40 seconds to 10 minutes	Moderate
Tabun	1,000	46 hours	Low
Sarin	1,700	5.2–12 hours	High

Note: Estimates are based on the chemical and physical properties of each agent, which can be variable depending on other variables and environmental factors.

Red blood cell (RBC) AChE is usually used as the specific enzyme for diagnosing organophosphate-related compound toxicity. Measurement of butyrylcholinesterase (pseudocholinesterase) is less specific but can be used as a more sensitive test for organophosphate toxicity.[7]

Clinical signs and symptoms related to nerve agent exposure are more dose-dependent but usually follow the expected classic description of headache, mitosis, rhinorrhea, vomiting, shortness of breath, muscular weakness, and fasciculations. These have been described consistently on multiple nerve agent exposure events on variable occasions.[8-10]

In cases of a high number of casualties in a nerve agent attack, efforts in management are highly aimed at effectively and adequately removing casualties from the affected scene and providing adequate ventilation means to both individual patients and exposed areas to allow for the dissemination of the substance. Decontamination, airway, breathing, and circulation supportive care can effectively decrease toxicity and fatalities associated with nerve agent exposure. Particular emphasis on using atropine, oxime agents, and seizure control needs to be considered in critical care settings as controlling excessive airway secretions and bronchoconstriction plays a crucial role in toxicity optimization, and full recovery can be expected when aggressive supportive measures are ensued.[7]

Incapacitating Chemical Agents

Central Nervous System-acting Chemicals

Central nervous system-acting chemicals are chemicals that selectively modify the CNS functions. Fentanyl, from the opioid class, can be considered safe to use in a supervised medical setting but needs to be safely controlled and administered under experienced medical supervision as it is deemed to have low safety margins and can have variable human responses. CNS-acting chemicals from the fentanyl class opioids do not have a sufficient safety margin to be considered for the so-called nonlethal operations as they have very low safety margin when aerosolized as all forms chemical toxicity is a matter of dosage, and many factors can affect this dispersion such as environment, dissemination, temperature, variable human responses, and presence of risk factors.[1]

Fentanyl and its analogs, such as carfentanil, remifentanil, and sufentanil, are synthetic opioids that were found to be of beneficial use as analgesic agents in medical use for pain management or for veterinarian uses. It is listed as a Schedule II controlled substance in the United States but has been clandestinely produced as powder or counterfeit tablets and widely abused.[11] Illicit fentanyl analogs have no legitimate uses and are listed under Schedule I controlled substances.

Fentanyls act by binding to and stimulating the activity of opioid receptors in the brain and spinal column. In high doses and susceptible patients, they cause CNS depression and coma.

The use of fentanyl as an "incapacitating chemical agent" in the unfortunate event in the Dubrovka Theatre as a means to end the Moscow theater siege, where it was used by the Russian special forces when storming the theater, emphasizes the importance of the international role of the CWC in monitoring and controlling the use of incapacitating agents in military operations and clearly differentiating incapacitating agents that can pose a life-threatening risk from RCAs which are sometimes used for crowd control and dispersion and are meant to disable or cause discomfort without causing significant harm or lethality.

Psychotomimetic Agents

The psychotomimetic effects are attributed to the anticholinergic effects noted since the ancient times of using Atropa belladonna.

BZ (also known as 3-quinuclidinyl benzilate), a glycolated anticholinergic substance, was among early chemicals researched as a psychomimetic incapacitating agent. Its less-than-ideal properties made it less favorable to be used in military, mainly because of its prolonged onset of action and unpredictable variable effects when deployed to the target which can even lead to stimulation and overactivity rather than incapacitating the person.

Of the major known anticholinergic symptoms, dry mouth, pupillary dilatation, and tachycardia are common. Higher doses are expected to cause central excitation leading to irritability, disorientation, and hallucinations or delirium.

Central nervous system effects increase considerably in the following order: Atropine, scopolamine, benactyzine, ditran, and, finally, BZ. BZ has been noted to cause confusion and hallucinations even in smaller doses and thus was not suitable for most medical usage.[12]

Riot Control Agents

Riot control agents are chemical substances that primarily work on the peripheral sensory nervous system, mainly as an irritant to the eyes, nose, and respiratory system. They can cause immediate discomfort and disable a person as long as he is exposed to the substance. Effects quickly dissipate once the person is removed from exposure.

Riot control agents do not affect the CNS system and are not considered to be of the CNS-acting chemicals class. RCAs are mostly known for their use by law enforcement personnel to disperse crowds and clear large gatherings. They are often considered as either tear gas or pulmonary irritants, depending on their predominant toxicity. But modern RCAs comprise diverse chemical compounds and can affect a wide variety of systems.

Examples of such compounds are chloroacetophenone (CN), ortho-chlorobenzylidene malononitrile (CS), Dibenz(b,f)-1:4-Oxazepine (CR), oleoresin capsicum, and other capsaicinoids.

Riot control agents are mostly expected to cause irritation and burns on the skin; however, depending on the class, they can cause a wide array of symptoms varying from nasal (rhinorrhea, sneezing, burning pain), ophthalmic (lacrimation, conjunctivitis, blepharospasms), oral (excessive salivation, stomatitis), respiratory (wheezing, cough, chest tightness, bronchorrhea), dermal (pruritus, dermatitis, vesication, pigmentation), gastrointestinal (gagging, gastritis, emesis), and neuronal (paresthesia, neuropathic pain).[13-16]

Choking Agents

Choking or pulmonary irritants are substances that characteristically cause severe irritation of the respiratory tract. They can affect the upper or lower airway depending on their water solubility.

Chemicals such as chlorine, phosgene, and ammonia are common examples of irritant gases that have been known and used as chemical warfare agents in early World War I.

Chlorine gas produces acids that react with the respiratory tract mucosa and cause respiratory symptoms. Its medium water solubility allows it to reach further in the lower airway with its high reactivity and oxidizing potential, causing further alveolar damage in contrast to the higher water-soluble agents such as ammonia. Phosgene is characterized by more alveolar damage and further reactivity owing to its low water solubility.[17] Its damage is further pronounced due to its mild upper respiratory, eye, and skin irritation and being colorless with a mildly pleasant odor leaving victims liable for significant exposure and inhalation before escaping the affected areas.

Treatment of all pulmonary irritants involves removing the victim from the suspected areas, providing adequate ventilation and respiratory support, using humidified oxygen and inhaled beta-adrenergic agents, endotracheal intubation, and mechanical ventilation in extreme cases.

Blood Agents

Blood agents are blood or systemic agents or the cyanide group of chemicals that are absorbed systemically and prevent normal utilization of oxygen from the blood. Their function does not directly affect blood components, but they exert their toxic effects by affecting cellular functions and the electron transport chain in the inner membranes of mitochondria. Hydrogen cyanide (HCN), cyanogen chloride (CNCl), and hydrogen sulfide (HS) are the main chemical warfare agents in this category. They are also known as knockdown agents because they can cause a sudden loss of consciousness, disruption of mental status, seizure, and cardiac arrest in a rapid manner.

The most prominent use of HCN was during World War II by the Nazis in what was known at the time as Zyklon B, which comprised of calcium sulfate and HCN used to exterminate millions of civilians and opposing enemy soldiers in death camps.[18]

Exposure to low levels of cyanide can lead to various nonspecific symptoms such as headache, dizziness, nausea, vomiting, confusion, coma, and urinary incontinence. Higher concentrations can quickly result in seizures, coma, and cardiac and/or respiratory failure. Death is not an uncommon outcome seen with cyanide exposures.[19]

In situations where exposure to cyanide is possible, care should be taken to limit further exposure in the environment by removing the victim from the contaminated atmosphere. Proper decontamination by removing any liquid on skin or clothing as soon as possible, removing all contaminated clothing, copious rinsing of skin with soap and water are suggested.

Supportive therapy can be sufficient in certain situations where ventilatory support and mechanical ventilation are provided. Specific antidotal therapy may be needed. Definitive antidote treatment differs worldwide, and there is no international consensus on the most effective definitive antidote therapy to be used. Three categories of agents that are agreed upon are methemoglobin inducers (amyl nitrite and sodium nitrite), sulfur donors (sodium thiosulfate), and cobalt compounds (hydroxocobalamin in the Cyanokit).[20]

Vesicants or Blistering Agents

Vesicants are toxic compounds that cause painful skin injuries resembling those caused by burns. They can also cause severe respiratory symptoms as they burn respiratory mucosa causing pulmonary inflammation, alveolar damage, and pulmonary edema.

The most known categories of vesicant agents are mustards and arsenicals. With Sulfur Mustard being known as the king of this class of chemical warfare. Other substances like nitrogen mustard and lewisites have been used as well.

Mustards are lipophilic and extremely toxic to dividing cells as they readily penetrate the skin, rubber gloves, and most textiles.[21]

Symptoms of mustard exposure depend on the route and length of exposure, concentration of the agent, and the surrounding environment. Dermal exposure can cause pain that has a delayed onset of a few hours after exposure and is caused by coagulation necrosis of the dermis. Presentation can range from erythema to vesicles and large skin blisters. Eye exposure can lead to corneal opacification, ulceration, and rupture. Respiratory tract swelling and erythema up to laryngeal edema and necrosis that can lead to deadly respiratory failure can be seen.[22,23]

PRINCIPLES OF PERSONAL PROTECTION

Recognition and identification of hazardous materials, assessment, and providing proper protection for healthcare staff play a vital role in any contingency plan. Efforts to understand, anticipate, and apply emergency decontamination and appropriate treatment principles have a higher chance of better outcomes in keeping staff and patient protection as an essential priority.

Personal protection clothing has four levels for handling any hazardous substances, known as A, B, C, and D, aimed at different chemical protection levels and respiratory protection, with level A providing the highest level of respiratory, skin, eye, and mucous membrane protection.[24]

Protection should provide proper, fully encapsulated, vapor-tight, chemical-resistant suit, boots, and gloves along with self-contained breathing apparatus.

CHEMICAL WEAPONS CONVENTION

Chemical Weapons Convention is an international treaty that was founded in 1997 and aims to regulate the use of chemical weapons and their development. Its main objectives are to prohibit the development, production, acquisition, retention, stockpiling, transfer, and the use of chemical weapons worldwide.

It is a scientifically grounded global agreement that incorporates a verification system for overseeing adherence and necessitates scientific and technical proficiency for efficient execution.

As of date, it is comprised of 193 member states where all member states are required to destroy existing stockpiles of chemical weapons and related facilities. The treaty maintains a strict verification regimen to ensure global compliance.[25]

It has been approximated that around 100,000 substances are regulated within the framework of the CWC.

The Organization for the Prohibition of Chemical Weapons (OPCW) ensures continuous efforts to identify and monitor analytical data of the chemicals that fall under the CWC under the Central Analytical Database, which is a compilation maintained by the OPCW laboratory.

CONCLUSION

The risk of mass hazmat exposure and the use of chemical weapons in warfare have been steadily increasing in the past years. It is of paramount significance to increase knowledge and awareness among medical practitioners and facilities by learning and planning a preparedness plan ahead of any emergency situation to be able to provide maximum safety and protection for staff and patients. Recognition and identification of hazmat, assessment of the conditions, protection of staff and facilities, and decontamination principles are essential elements of any hazmat contingency plan.

REFERENCES

1. Mathews RJ. Central nervous system-acting chemicals and the Chemical Weapons Convention: a former scientific adviser's perspective. Pure Appl Chem. 2018;90(10):1559-75.
2. Pearson A. Incapacitating Biochemical Weapons. Nonproliferation Rev. 2006;13(2):151-88.
3. Klotz L, Furmanski M, Wheelis M. Beware the Siren's Song: Why "non lethal" incapacitating chemical agents are lethal. 2003. [online] Available from https://programs.fas.org/bio/chemweapons/documents/sirens_song.pdf. [Last accessed October, 2024].
4. Kosal ME. Romano JA Jr, Lukey BJ, Salem H, (Eds). Chemical Warfare Agents: Chemistry, Pharmacology, Toxicology, and Therapeutics, 2nd edition. Boca Raton, FL: CRC Taylor & Francis; 2007.
5. Dunn MA, Sidell FR. Progress in medical defense against nerve agents. JAMA. 1989;262(5):649-52.
6. National Academies of Sciences, Engineering, and Medicine, Division on Earth and Life Studies, Board on Environmental Studies and Toxicology, Committee on Acute Exposure Guideline Levels Committee on Toxicology. Acute Exposure Guideline Levels for Selected Airborne Chemicals: Volume 20. Washington (DC): National Academies Press; 2016. p. 195.
7. Sidell FR, Borak J. Chemical warfare agents: II. Nerve agents. Ann Emerg Med. 1992;21(7):865-71.
8. Okumura T, Takasu N, Ishimatsu S, Miyanoki S, Mitsuhashi A, Kumada K, et al. Report on 640 victims of the Tokyo subway sarin attack. Ann Emerg Med. 1996;28(2):129-35.
9. Yanagisawa N, Morita H, Nakajima T. Sarin experiences in Japan: a cute toxicity and long-term effects. J Neurol Sci. 2006;249(1):76-85.
10. Leikin JB, Thomas RG, Walter FG, Klein R, Meislin HW. A review of nerve agent exposure for the critical care physician. Crit Care Med. 2002;30(10):2346-54.
11. DEA. Drug Enforcement Administration. 2016. [online] Available from: https://www.dea.gov/index.shtml [Last accessed October, 2024].
12. National Research Council (US) Panel on Anticholinesterase Chemicals, National Research Council (US) Panel on Anticholinergic Chemicals. Possible Long-Term Health Effects of Short-Term Exposure to Chemical Agents: Volume 1 Anticholinesterases and Anticholinergics. 1982. Washington (DC): National Academies Press (US). [online] Available from http://www.ncbi.nlm.nih.gov/books/NBK217774/. [Last accessed October, 2024].
13. Quiroga-Garza ME, Ruiz-Lozano RE, Azar NS, Mousa HM, Komai S, Sevilla-Llorca JL, et al. Noxious effects of riot control agents on the ocular surface: pathogenic mechanisms and management. Front Toxicol. 2023;5:1118731.
14. Beswick FW. Chemical agents used in riot control and warfare. Hum Toxicol. 1983;2(2):247-56.
15. Debarre S, Karinthi L, Delamanche S, Fuché C, Desforges P, Calvet JH. Comparative acute toxicity of o-chlorobenzylidene malononitrile (CS) and oleoresin capsicum (OC) in awake rats. Hum Exp Toxicol. 1999;18(12):724-30.
16. Menke BA, Ryu C, Justin GA, Chundury RV, Hayek BR, Debiec MR, et al. Ophthalmic manifestations and management considerations for emerging chemical threats. Front Toxicol. 2023;5:1281041.

17. Zellner T, Eyer F. Choking agents and chlorine gas—History, pathophysiology, clinical effects and treatment. Toxicol Lett. 2020;320:73-9.
18. Satu MS, Lukey BJ, Jr JAR, Romano JA, Salem H (Eds). Chemical Warfare Agents: Toxicity at Low Levels. Boca Raton, FL: CRC Press; 2000. p. 464.
19. Baskin SI, Rockwood GA. Neurotoxicological and behavioral effects of cyanide and its potential therapies. Mil Psychol. 2002;14(2):159-77.
20. Cummings TF. The treatment of cyanide poisoning. Occup Med Oxf Engl. 2004;54(2):82-5.
21. Ganesan K, Raza SK, Vijayaraghavan R. Chemical warfare agents. J Pharm Bioallied Sci. 2010;2(3):166-78.
22. Davis KG, Aspera G. Exposure to liquid sulfur mustard. Ann Emerg Med. 2001;37(6):653-6.
23. Kehe K, Szinicz L. Medical aspects of sulphur mustard poisoning. Toxicology. 2005;214(3):198-209.
24. Chan J, Yeung R, Tang S. Hospital preparedness for chemical and biological incidents in Hong Kong. Hong Kong Med J. 2002;8(6):440-6.
25. Pitschmann V. Overall view of chemical and biochemical weapons. Toxins (Basel). 2014;6(6):1761-84.

2.24 Biological Warfare Agents

Jonathan Looms, Muhammad EMO Elamin

INTRODUCTION

Biological warfare agents consist of either microorganisms or toxic substances produced by living organisms that are produced and deliberately released to cause injury to humans, animals, or plants. They form part of a wider class of unconventional weapons, which includes chemical, nuclear, and radioactive agents.

Biological warfare agents can pose major threats to public safety and national security. They also have the potential to mimic natural epidemics, and it can be difficult to differentiate between attacks and naturally occurring outbreaks. Many diseases caused by biological weapons no longer occur naturally or are encountered rarely in clinical practice, adding to diagnostic challenges and the need for specific training for managing outbreaks.

The US Centers for Disease Control and Prevention (CDC) categorizes bioterrorism agents into three categories in terms of risk to national security, ease of dissemination, and potential to cause disruption and panic, in addition to emerging pathogens which can constitute a future risk[1] **(Table 1)**.

GENERAL APPROACH AND INTENSIVE CARE CONSIDERATIONS

Suspicion of Exposure

Disease caused by a microorganism or its toxins can present indistinguishably between natural infective processes and biological warfare. A series of differentiation criteria have been proposed that should promote suspicion of bioterrorism.[2] For example, an epidemic curve with a high number of cases presenting initially, rather than an insidious onset, would be highly unusual for a natural epidemic. Other suggestive features include a change to expected seasonal variation (such as spikes of Q fever outside of spring during lambing season), occurrence of a zoonotic disease in an area without the natural animal reservoir, or unexplainable changes to geographic distributions without any travel or contact history. Altered pathogenic variants, unexpected antimicrobial resistance, or changes to expected mortality rates could suggest intentional human manipulation of the pathogen. For biological weapons, the expected delivery method would be via aerosol; for many organisms (such as anthrax), this is different to their typical route of infectivity and produces different clinical presentations and incubation periods. There are also important wider factors, including environmental conditions such as wind direction which can determine pathogenic spread or claims of bioterrorist activity by organizations.

Decontamination

Most biological weapons are delivered by aerosol. If a release is known, removal of clothing and cleaning the patient with soap and water are likely to minimize organism deposits on the skin. Clothing should be securely disposed of to prevent retransmission of these deposits. Decontamination in ambulance areas is ideal to minimize the risk of further contamination in hospitals.[3]

TABLE 1: Centers for Disease Control and Prevention (CDC) class of bioterrorism agents.[1]

Category A	*Category B*	*Category C*
Anthrax (*Bacillus anthracis*)	Brucellosis (*Brucella* species)	Emerging infectious diseases such as Nipah virus and hantavirus
Botulism (*Clostridium botulinum* toxin)	Epsilon toxin of *Clostridium perfringens*	
Plague (*Yersinia pestis*)	Food safety threats (*Salmonella* species, *Escherichia coli* O157:H7, *Shigella*)	
Smallpox (*Variola* major)	Glanders (*Burkholderia mallei*)	
Tularemia (*Francisella tularensis*)	Melioidosis (*Burkholderia pseudomallei*)	
Viral hemorrhagic fevers, including Filoviruses (Ebola, Marburg), Arenaviruses (Lassa, Machupo)	Psittacosis (*Chlamydia psittaci*)	
	Q fever (*Coxiella burnetii*)	
	Ricin toxin from Ricinus communis (castor beans)	
	Staphylococcal enterotoxin B	
	Typhus fever (*Rickettsia prowazekii*)	
	Viral encephalitis (alphaviruses, such as eastern equine encephalitis, Venezuelan equine encephalitis, and western equine encephalitis)	
	Water safety threats (*Vibrio cholerae, Cryptosporidium parvum*)	

Deceased patients present risks of transmission for certain biological weapons, such as smallpox and plague. Mortuary precautions would be necessary, with postmortem examination avoided if possible and cremation a preferred option.[4]

Triage

In the event of a mass casualty scenario with the potential to overwhelm healthcare, triage will be needed to determine the best use of limited resources. Intensive care can play a role in both immediate treatment and assessment of needs and survivability. Patients are placed into one of four categories: (1) Expectant (death inevitable), (2) immediate (immediate life-saving treatment required), (3) delayed (treatment can be delayed), and (4) minor (or walking wounded).[3]

Respiratory Isolation

Several agents can be spread by human-to-human transmission through respiratory droplets. If these agents are suspected or confirmed, strict adherence to inflection guidelines must be carried out to minimize the risk of further transmission. This includes isolation of patients and ensuring that staff are wearing appropriate personal protective equipment. Enhanced measures such as negative pressure isolation and high-efficiency particulate air (HEPA) filtration are needed in the case of highly transmissible pathogens such as smallpox and viral hemorrhagic fevers. Rapid spread of disease through trained hospital staff can cripple a healthcare response to an attack. In the 2003 severe acute respiratory syndrome (SARS) outbreak, 94% of cases in Taiwan resulted from in-hospital exposure.[4] With higher numbers of cases, patient cohorting by infection may be pragmatically necessary. In the event of delayed identification of a bioterrorism attack, postexposure prophylaxis may need to be considered for affected staff.

Specialist Involvement

It is important to involve infectious disease specialists early in the time course of disease, particularly when dealing with rare or exotic organisms that may be outside of local experience. An awareness of national and international guidelines on healthcare reporting for these diseases is also important.

Supportive Intensive Care

In the event of a small number of casualties, intensive treatments such as invasive ventilation and advanced hemodynamic monitoring are likely to be essential in the management of biological warfare agents. However, as case numbers rise, the capacity of supportive intensive care unit

(ICU) management will quickly be exhausted.[4] Intensivists should, therefore, be mindful of these limitations and understand the pathways to rapidly increasing capacity through acquisition of space, ventilators, and trained staff, such as was required globally during the coronavirus disease 2019 (COVID-19) pandemic.

Education

Staff should be adequately trained on the features and risks of potential biowarfare agents, because of the possibility for misdiagnosis with many of these pathogens and the need for timely intervention, to both prevent secondary spread through populations and in cases where early treatment significantly reduces mortality, such as in plague and smallpox. Simulations and tabletop exercises are important opportunities for aiding preparedness, especially in situations where these systems are unlikely to be stress tested before the event.[5]

SPECIFIC AGENTS

Category A

Anthrax

Bacillus anthracis is a gram-positive spore-forming bacterium. It is distributed worldwide in affected soil. It exists in the environment with infective potential as a spore and is commonly contracted by animals while grazing. Humans can become exposed due to contact with infected animals' wool or hides, from ingesting infected meat, or from inhaling spores during the processing of wool for textiles. The spores can remain viable in the environment for decades, but human-to-human transfer does not occur.[6] Anthrax is widely recognized for its potential as a biological weapon and would most likely be distributed as an aerosol leading to the inhalational form. The United States military weaponized it in the 1950s and 1960s, and Iraq has admitted to researching how to weaponize it in the Persian Gulf War.[6] An accidental release in the former Soviet Union led to the attributable deaths of at least 66 people.[7] In 2001, 23 cases of anthrax, including 11 cases of inhalational anthrax, with 5 fatalities, were reported in the United States associated with suspected bioterrorist activity via suspicious letters mailed to recipients.[8]

There are three distinct phenotypes in humans: (1) Cutaneous, (2) gastrointestinal, and (3) inhalational (also known as wool-sorter's disease, due to the almost exclusive occupational link). Cutaneous anthrax presents as an ulcerating, painless red lesion following inoculation of minor skin lesions with spores. Most cases heal spontaneously, although a minority progress to sepsis and death if not treated with antibiotics. Gastrointestinal anthrax occurs as a result of ingesting infected meat and consists of gastrointestinal symptoms including vomiting and abdominal pain. Ascites is common and develops within 2–4 days. Mucosal ulceration can arise as a complication and often leads to hemorrhage and death despite treatment.[9] Inhalational anthrax presents following exposure to aerosolized spores and presents similar to a bacterial pneumonia with cough, fever, and malaise. This mild initial presentation usually persists for several days, before rapidly deteriorating into severe respiratory distress and mediastinitis. Complications include septic shock and meningitis, which often has a hemorrhagic component and is seen in up to 50% of inhalational cases.[10] This condition was thought to be universally fatal once complications are seen; however, this has been revised following the 2001 outbreak.[11]

Bacillus anthracis can be diagnosed with Gram staining of blood and isolated from cultures but is often not seen until relatively late in disease. Enzyme-linked immunosorbent assays (ELISA) exist to allow for rapid diagnosis of circulating toxin, which appears 2–3 days following exposure. Chest radiographs demonstrate a widened mediastinum with pleural effusions but do not usually show infiltrates.[6]

Antibiotic therapy is with ciprofloxacin or doxycycline, with IV preparations used for inhalational cases and oral preparations used for prophylaxis or cutaneous cases. Additional antibiotics are also used for inhalational cases alongside this, with previous strategies involving agents used to inhibit protein synthesis and halt toxin production or with demonstrated in vitro activity against anthrax.[11] Prolonged courses of antibiotics are needed due to presentations being described 6 weeks following exposure, and a 60-day course of antibiotics is recommended.[7] Intensive care management includes supportive management of septic shock and the need for intubation and ventilation in respiratory distress.

Botulism

The anaerobic bacterium *Clostridium botulinum* produces seven distinct neurotoxins, which if inhaled or ingested lead to the disease of botulism. This occurs most commonly in the ingestion of improperly prepared or canned food. They are the most toxic compounds known and are 100,000 times more toxic than sarin.[12] Iraq has performed research on botulinum toxins before the Persian Gulf War, and there is evidence that munitions containing the toxin were deployed. The agent could be used to sabotage the food supply, although an aerosol attack is more likely.[6]

Botulinum toxins produce a dose-dependent response in humans and act as neurotransmitter blockers by preventing the presynaptic release of acetylcholine at neuromuscular junctions. This manifests initially with bulbar palsies causing diplopia, ptosis, dysarthria, and dysphagia. This is then followed by a symmetrical descending progressive weakness, leading to respiratory failure and death if untreated. Cases can progress rapidly.

The diagnosis is made clinically, and the presence of multiple cases of similar progressive paralysis should lead to clinical suspicion. Laboratory tests are of limited value, with studies demonstrating that aerosolized toxin is not usually identified and survivors rarely producing a sufficient antibody response. The tensilon test can be falsely positive in botulism and therefore cannot differentiate it from myasthenia.[13]

Supportive management of respiratory failure is key to reducing mortality, with severe cases requiring intubation and ventilation. Weaning and recovery can be prolonged, lasting months. Botulism antitoxin is available and has been demonstrated to shorten the course of illness and reduce mortality. It is more effective when given earlier. Botulism antitoxin neutralizes unbound toxin; therefore, it is ineffective in already paralyzed muscles. It is, therefore, important to administer early when the diagnosis is suspected.[14]

Plague

Yersinia pestis is a gram-negative enterobacterium. It has an animal reservoir in rats and can be transmitted to humans via flea bites from infected hosts. Human-to-human transmission can occur via respiratory droplets. Historically, it has been implicated in multiple worldwide pandemics. Japan investigated the use of plague as a biological weapon during World War II, and it was later studied by the United States military in the 1950s. Other countries have also been suspected of weaponizing plague.[6]

Plague can present in humans as bubonic, septicemic, or pneumonic disease. Bubonic diseases manifest up to 10 days following exposure with fever and painful enlarged lymph nodes known as buboes. Complications include pustular skin lesions and microvascular arterial thrombosis, leading to necrosis, as well as conversion to the other forms of the disease. Bubonic disease is by far the most common initial presentation and has a mortality of up to 60% without treatment.[15] Septicemia can be primary or secondary and presents primarily as septic shock with vasoplegia and hypotension. Pneumonia can arise following droplet inhalation or following disseminated spread through a host. It presents with fever and hemorrhagic cough, before rapidly progressing to respiratory distress and cardiovascular collapse. While treatable, if antibiotics are not started within 24 hours of symptoms, it is invariably fatal.[6]

Gram staining of blood or lymph node aspirate reveals gram-negative coccobacilli and has a typical safety-pin appearance.[16] The organism can be cultured, although it grows slowly and there is a narrow time window to treat.

Pneumonic cases should be treated with IV gentamicin or streptomycin; the use of chloramphenicol and doxycycline has also been described. Postexposure prophylaxis regimens consist of ciprofloxacin or doxycycline.[6] Strict adherence to infection-control guidelines is needed given the potential for disease spread across patients, with isolation and personal protective equipment for respiratory droplets and special consideration applied to aerosol-generating procedures such as intubation.

Smallpox

The DNA orthopoxvirus variola causes smallpox disease. It can infect monkeys, although humans were the natural host for the disease before its eradication in 1980.[17] There are two known World Health Organization (WHO)—approved stockpiles of the variola virus, but further stockpiles are suspected in various countries.[18] In 1970, the WHO stated that smallpox "can be easily produced in large quantities in the laboratory and freeze-dried, and its virulence thus preserved for months and years."[19] That, combined with the high mortality and a civilian population that is no longer routinely vaccinated, gives grave potential for its use as a biological weapon. The US military began vaccinating their personnel against smallpox again in 2002.[20] Given its eradicated status, even a single case of smallpox would be highly significant and would need immediate disclosure to public health authorities.

Smallpox is transmitted via respiratory droplets and aerosols. The incubation period lasts 2 weeks, following which patients present with fever, malaise, and headaches. They then classically develop oropharyngeal lesions (which shed infectious secretions and are a major form of transmission) and a papular rash across the face and upper limbs followed by the lower limbs and abdomen. The rash progresses to a vesicular followed by pustular form, before scabbing and leaving hypopigmented scars. Patients remain febrile throughout. Neurological symptoms including delirium are a common complication. Superadded bacterial infection leading to pneumonia is common and is a major contributor to mortality, which in the unvaccinated population is 30%.[17]

Clinically, it is difficult to differentiate smallpox from chickenpox, with the key difference being the time course; lesions appear at the same time on body parts, whereas they vary in chickenpox.

Respiratory isolation is of paramount importance and is recommended for 17 days to all people in direct contact with the index case.[6] Cidofovir and ribavirin are two antivirals that have been proven to have in vitro effectiveness against smallpox but are unlikely to be effective after the development of symptoms.[21] Vaccination within 1–2 days of exposure confers good protection as postexposure prophylaxis, especially if the individual has been previously vaccinated.

Tularemia

Francisella tularensis is a small nonmotile aerobic facultative gram-negative coccobacillus, found in rodents and rabbits. It is spread to humans by contact with infected animal material or from the bites of arthropods (usually ticks or deer flies). The organism can remain viable for weeks in the environment or for years in frozen rabbit meat.[22] Human-to-human spread is unusual. *F. tularensis* was weaponized by the United States Military program in the 1950s and 1960s. Aerosolized bacteria would be more likely to cause the typhoidal variety of the disease.[6]

Tularemia can present in either the ulceroglandular or the typhoidal form. The ulceroglandular form predominates and presents as local ulceration with lymphadenopathy, fever, and malaise. The typhoidal form presents similarly, but without dermal features or lymphadenopathy. A nonproductive cough is common, and pneumonia with associated pleural effusion is possible with both manifestations but is more likely with the typhoidal form. If untreated, the mortality rate for typhoidal tularemia is 35%.[22]

Diagnosis can be challenging given the nonspecific features. Organism isolation is difficult in the laboratory, although it can be established retrospectively by serological testing. Gentamicin IV or streptomycin IM are the standard antibiotics of choice, with other antimicrobials such as chloramphenicol shown to be effective but having higher relapse rates.[23] As human-to-human spread is rare, respiratory isolation is not routinely recommended.

Viral Hemorrhagic Fevers

Several different RNA viruses are capable of producing a syndrome categorized as viral hemorrhagic fever. These include Arenaviridae (Lassa fever, Brazilian hemorrhagic fever), Bunyaviridae (Rift Valley fever, Congo-Crimean hemorrhagic fever, hantaviruses), *Filoviridae* (Ebola, Marburg disease), and *Flaviviridae* (yellow fever, Dengue fever). Transmission is usually via contact with an infected animal or via arthropod vector. Each has a particular geographic distribution where it is endemic, with cases outside of these areas without recent travel being highly unusual. If aerosolized, these viruses are highly infectious. They can cause high morbidity and mortality and are easy to produce, making them potential targets for biological weapons.

Patients usually present with high fevers and myalgia, before subsequently developing distributive shock with microvascular damage and changes to vascular permeability. This can present as petechial hemorrhages through to disseminated intravascular coagulation and varies from virus to virus.[24]

Diagnosis can be made by ELISA or reverse transcription polymerase chain reaction (RT-PCR) testing for viremia.

Management is supportive. Special consideration should be given to the need for invasive devices on ICU given the high potential for damage to the capillary bed and high risk of secondary infection in these patients.[6] Hemorrhage and DIC require conventional hematological management. These patients can be challenging to manage from a fluid balance perspective, given the altered vascular permeability and hypotension; pulmonary edema is a frequent complication following resuscitation. Ribavirin has been proven to reduce mortality in high-risk patients suffering from Lassa fever[25] and shows promise with some other viral hemorrhagic fevers, although preclinical studies have predicted ineffectiveness against filoviruses and flaviviruses.

Selected Category B

Brucellosis

Brucellae (*Brucella melitensis*, abortus, suis, and canis) are gram-negative aerobic nontoxicogenic, nonspore-forming coccobacilli, generally disease-producing in grazing livestock. Each species has a preference for a specific animal vector. Most human exposure is via eating contaminated meat or dairy, or aerosol contact from infected animals. Human-to-human transfer does not typically occur, but aerosol droplets are highly infectious and can survive for up to 10 weeks in soil or water. Brucella suis was weaponized by the United States Military in the 1940s and 1950s, and other countries are also suspected to have weaponized brucellae. Delivery of the organism has been proposed via either a dry aerosol or slurry in a bomb.[6]

Brucellosis presents nonspecifically with fever, chills, and a general malaise. Brucellae are facultative macrophage parasites, and disease complications are reflected in organs with high numbers of macrophages. There is respiratory involvement in up to 20% of patients, with rarer complications including osteoarticular, genitourinary, and hematological.[26] Endocarditis and nervous system involvement is rare, occurring in <2% of untreated individuals, but when it does occur mortality is 25% (accounting for the overwhelming majority of mortality in brucellosis).[27]

Diagnosis can be made by culture, serological testing, and nucleic acid amplification assays (NAAT). Culture can require substantial incubation periods. Serological testing is useful in low-income countries but lacks specificity. NAAT allows for rapid diagnosis and is sensitive and specific but is limited by persistent positivity following recovery.[28]

Combination antibiotic therapy is required, given the potential for relapse with single agents. The standard recommended treatment is oral doxycycline and rifampicin for a 6-week course.[21]

Q Fever

Q fever is caused by *Coxiella burnetii*, an obligate rickettsia-like bacterium. It has high infectivity but low virulence and typically affects domesticated livestock. It causes infection in humans following indirect exposure to infected animals (or their by-products), and its spore-like form can survive heat and drying and persist in the environment for weeks and months post exposure.[29] The Q in Q fever originally represented "Query," as the pathogen was unknown when the condition was first described. Q fever is recognized as a potential biological warfare agent and was studied by the United States military before their research program ended. It has an infectivity and casualty production comparable to anthrax.[19]

Up to 50% of infections are asymptomatic, and following a prolonged incubation period of up to 40 days it presents as a febrile illness associated nonspecifically with myalgias and malaise. The pyrexia often fluctuates, with peaks up to 40°C. Patchy pleural infiltrates, pleural effusions, and consolidation are reported radiologically in up to 50% of patients, although far fewer patients complain of cough or chest pain. Other complications include hepatitis, endocarditis, and meningoencephalitis. Mortality is low from untreated disease, but postinfective malaise lasting several months has been reported in up to a third of patients.[29]

It is most commonly diagnosed by serological antibody detection, which is not diagnostic in the first 2 weeks of illness.

Treatment shortens disease duration and can prevent disease occurrence when given during the incubation period. The first-line treatment is with doxycycline, although macrolides are also effective. The standard acute duration of antibiotics is 2 weeks, although chronic forms of the disease can require treatment for up to 24 months.[30]

Staphylococcal Enterotoxin B

Staphylococcal enterotoxin B is one of several exotoxins produced by the bacteria *Staphylococcus aureus*. They are heat stable and are a common cause of food poisoning in humans if improperly prepared. They lead to T-cell activation, causing the production and release of cytokines leading to widespread immune system activation. There have been reports of military laboratory researchers being exposed to staphylococcal enterotoxin B.[31]

Clinical symptoms occur 3–12 hours following ingestion, and patients present with nausea, vomiting, diarrhea, fever, headache, nonproductive cough, and myalgia. Most cases are self-limiting, although there are often pronounced fluid losses, and patients can be incapacitated for up to 2 weeks. Rarely, a widespread cytokine storm reaction can be observed leading to toxic septic shock and death.[32]

The diagnosis is made clinically, and due to the nonspecific symptoms it can be delayed. However, if used as a biological weapon there would be expected high numbers of patients presenting over a very short time course given the short incubation period.[6]

Management is supportive, with particular attention to managing fluid losses. Pulmonary edema can occur as a complication, necessitating noninvasive or invasive ventilation.

Viral Encephalitis

Venezuelan equine encephalitis (VEE), eastern equine encephalitis (EEE), and western equine encephalitis (WEE) viruses are antigenically related members of the alphavirus of the Togaviridae family. They are transmitted by mosquitoes, and horses provide a natural reservoir of these viruses. These viruses have high potential for use in biological warfare; if aerosolized, they are highly infective. They can be produced at high volume cheaply and easily and are relatively stable. The presence of these viruses should be regarded with suspicion when seen outside of known endemic areas.

All three viruses are known for their potential for neurological involvement in humans. EEE and WEE classically present with a febrile prodrome for up to 11 days, before neurological progression with delirium deteriorating into coma. EEE causes high morbidity and mortality, with mortality rates up to 75% and a third of survivors left with seizures and neuropathies.[33] WEE has a reported mortality rate of 10%, with infants and elderly patients being more susceptible. VEE is generally milder and causes a debilitating febrile illness with prolonged recovery, although neurological involvement is rare (up to 4%) and survivors usually have complete neurological recovery.[34]

Viremia can often be detected and isolated during the febrile prodrome, although is absent by the onset of neurological symptoms. The virus has been isolated from cerebrospinal fluid (CSF) in encephalitis cases. Serologic antibody testing is usually positive by the second week of illness. Biochemical findings include an early leucopenia followed by a leukocytosis, and common lumbar puncture findings include an elevated opening pressure and lymphocytic pleocytosis on CSF examination.[35]

Management is symptomatic, with the major considerations being airway protection as coma develops and seizure management with anticonvulsants. WEE can provoke a significant fever above 40°C and may need active cooling measures to control.[6]

CONCLUSION

The intentional use of a pathogen or biological product to cause harm to a human, animal, plant, or other living organisms is a real threat in the war stricken word. Biological agents can be easily developed, tend to be more lethal, are cheaper to procure/manufacture and very difficult to detect. An appropriate response to bioterrorism needs prioritization in recent times. Preparedness, planning, timely surveillance, adequate availability/stockpiling of drugs/vaccines, and protection of key functionaries remain priorities to deal with possible biological warfare.

REFERENCES

1. Center for Disease Control and Prevention. (2018). Bioterrorism agents/diseases. [online] Available from https://emergency.cdc.gov/agent/agentlist-category.asp. [Last accessed October, 2024].
2. Noah DL, Sobel AL, Ostroff SM, Kildew JA. Biological warfare training: infectious disease outbreak differentiation criteria. Mil Med. 1998;163(4):198-201.
3. White SM. Chemical and biological weapons. Implications for anaesthesia and intensive care. Br J Anaesth. 2002;89(2):306-24.
4. Stephens RS, Wiener CM, Rubinson L. Bioterrorism and the intensive care unit. Clin Crit Care Med. 2006:685-95.
5. Richards CF, Burstein JL, Waeckerle JF, Hutson HR. Emergency physicians and biological terrorism. Ann Emerg Med. 1999;34(2):183-90.
6. Franz DR, Jahrling PB, Friedlander AM, McClain DJ, Hoover DL, Bryne WR, et al. Clinical recognition and management of patients exposed to biological warfare agents. JAMA. 1997;278(5):399-411.
7. Meselson M, Guillemin J, Hugh-Jones M, Langmuir A, Popova I, Shelokov A, et al. The Sverdlovsk anthrax outbreak of 1979. Science. 1994;266(5188):1202-8.
8. Centers for Disease Control and Prevention (CDC). Suspected cutaneous anthrax in a laboratory worker—Texas, 2002. MMWR Morb Mortal Wkly Rep. 2002;51(13): 279-81.
9. Dixon TC, Meselason M, Guillemin J, Hanna PC. Medical progress. Anthrax N Engl J Med. 1999;341:815-26.
10. Abramova FA, Grinberg LM, Yampolskaya OV, Walker DH. Pathology of inhalational anthrax in 42 cases from the Sverdlovsk outbreak of 1979. Proc Natl Acad Sci. 1993;90(6):2291-4.
11. Inglesby TV, O'Toole T, Henderson DA, Bartlett JG, Ascher MS, Eitzen E, et al. Anthrax as a biological weapon, 2002: Updated recommendations for management. JAMA. 2002;287(17):2236-52.
12. Gill DM. Bacterial toxins: a table of lethal amounts. Microbiol Rev. 1982;46(1):86-94.

13. Edell T, Sullivan Jr C, Osborn K, Gambin J, Brenman R. Wound botulism associated with a positive tensilon test. West J Med. 1983;139(2):218.
14. Franz DR, Pitt LM, Clayton MA, Hanes MA, Rose KJ. Efficacy of prophylactic and therapeutic administration of antitoxin for inhalation botulism. Botulinum and tetanus neurotoxins: neurotransmission and biomedical aspects. NY, USA: Springer; 1993. pp. 473-6.
15. McGovern TW, Christopher GW, Eitzen EM. Cutaneous manifestations of biological warfare and related threat agents. Arch Dermatol. 1999;135(3):311-22.
16. Prentice MB, Rahalison L. Plague. Lancet. 2007;369(9568): 1196-207.
17. Fenner F, Henderson DA, Arita I, Ježek Z, Ladnyi ID. Smallpox and its eradication / F. Fenner, et al. World Health Organization; 1988. pp. 1371-1409. [online] Available from https://iris.who.int/handle/10665/39485 [Last accessed October, 2024].
18. Breman JG, Henderson D. Poxvirus dilemmas—monkeypox, smallpox, and biologic terrorism. N Engl J Med. 1998;339(8):556-9.
19. World Health Organization. (1970). Health aspects of chemical and biological weapons: Report of a WHO group of consultants. [online] Available from https://iris.who.int/handle/10665/39444 [Last accessed October, 2024].
20. Barkdoll T, Cabiad R, Tankersley M, Adkins J. Secondary and tertiary transfer of vaccinia virus among US military personnel-United States and worldwide, 2002-2004. MMWR Morb Mortal Wkly Rep. 2004;53(5):103.
21. Drugs and vaccines against biological weapons. Conn Med. 2001;65(12):719-20.
22. Evans ME, Gregory DW, Schaffner W, McGee ZA. Tularemia: a 30-year experience with 88 cases. Medicine. 1985;64(4):251-69.
23. Sawyer WD, Dangerfield HG, Hogge AL, Crozier D. Antibiotic prophylaxis and therapy of airborne tularemia. Bacteriol Rev. 1966;30(3):542-50.
24. Borio L, Inglesby T, Peters C, Schmaljohn AL, Hughes JM, Jahrling PB, et al. Hemorrhagic fever viruses as biological weapons: medical and public health management. JAMA. 2002;287(18):2391-405.
25. McCormick JB, King IJ, Webb PA, Scribner CL, Craven RB, Johnson KM, et al. Lassa fever. N Engl J Med. 1986;314(1):20-6.
26. Young EJ. An overview of human brucellosis. Clin infect Dis. 1995;21(2):283-9.
27. Narimisa N, Razavi S, Khoshbayan A, Masjedian Jazi F. Prevalence of Brucella endocarditis: a systematic review and meta-analysis. Health Sci Rep. 2023;6(5):e1301.
28. Yagupsky P, Morata P, Colmenero JD. Laboratory diagnosis of human brucellosis. Clin Microbiol Rev. 2019;33(1):10.1128/cmr. 00073-19.
29. Smith D, Ayres J, Blair I, Burge P, Carpenter M, Caul E, et al. A large Q fever outbreak in the West Midlands: Clinical aspects. Respir Med. 1993;87(7):509-16.
30. Kersh GJ. Antimicrobial therapies for Q fever. Expert Rev Anti-infective Ther. 2013;11(11):1207-14.
31. Rusnak JM, Kortepeter M, Ulrich R, Poli M, Boudreau E. Laboratory exposures to staphylococcal enterotoxin B. Emerg Infect Dis. 2004;10(9):1544.
32. Fries BC, Varshney AK. Bacterial Toxins-Staphylococcal Enterotoxin B. Microbiol Spectr. 2013;1(2):10.1128/microbiolspec.AID-0002-2012.
33. Armstrong PM, Andreadis TG. Eastern equine encephalitis virus-old enemy, new threat. 2013; N Engl J Med. 2013;368(18):1670-3.
34. Martin DH, Eddy GA, Sudia WD, Reeves WC, Newhouse VF, Johnson KM. An epidemiologic study of Venezuelan equine encephalomyelitis in Costa Rica, 1970. Am J Epidemiol. 1972;95(6):565-78.
35. Deresiewicz RL, Thaler SJ, Hsu L, Zamani AA. Clinical and neuroradiographic manifestations of eastern equine encephalitis. N Engl J Med. 1997;336(26):1867-74.

3

SECTION

Supportive Therapy in Poisoning

Section Editors: *Vivek Gupta, Sandeep Dewan, Ranajit Chaterjee*

3.1 Cardiovascular Support in Poisoned Patients

Rajesh Vijayvergiya

INTRODUCTION

Poisoning can be defined as cellular injury or death due to exposure to exogenous substances.[1] Various poisons related to cardiotoxicity lead to significant morbidity and mortality. They can affect blood pressure, cardiac output, cardiac rhythm, and myocardial perfusion. All physicians should know the cardiovascular effects of commonly encountered poisons and their management.

CARDIAC INVOLVEMENT IN POISONING

A poison can adversely affect the cardiovascular system directly or indirectly. Direct effects include vasoconstriction, leading to hypertension, and vasodilatation, leading to hypotension. Effects on the myocardial tissue include decreased cardiac output, while impact on the conduction system can cause tachy- or bradyarrhythmias. Indirect effects on the cardiovascular system can occur due to the neurohormonal impacts of toxins, preexisting comorbidities, and drug interactions. Prompt identification of these effects is necessary to initiate appropriate treatment. The clinical presentation of commonly encountered cardiovascular poisons and their management is enlisted in **Table 1**.

Toxicology screening, as well as routine biochemistry, should be performed in all patients. Specific investigations like blood levels of drugs/toxic agents are helpful in prompt and effective management. A basic assessment of any poisoned patient for cardiovascular toxicity includes measurement of the blood pressure, heart rate, jugular venous pressure, oxygen saturation, and auscultation of the precordium and lung fields. An electrocardiogram (ECG) should be done in each patient for electrolyte imbalance, myocardial ischemia/injury, and cardiac arrhythmias. Based on preliminary tests and type of poisoning, certain specific tests such as echocardiogram, Holter monitoring, and coronary angiography may be required in some patients. Echocardiography can provide useful information about cardiac functions and fluid resuscitation as per the inferior vena cava (IVC) dimensions. A list of known cardiac poisons is mentioned in **Table 2**.

Treatment of a poisoned patient should include supportive care, prevention of additional exposure, administration of medications that reverse or bypass the effect of the poison on its molecular target (antidotes), and prompt elimination of the poison from the body whenever possible. **Table 3** describes the antidotes of specific poisons.

Supportive care entails patient stabilization and ensuring airway, breathing, and circulation (ABC). In most instances, fluid resuscitation and vasopressor support are adequate for hypotension; however, in some cases, temporary extracorporeal cardiovascular support may be required for survival and recovery.[2]

The management of individual cardiovascular side effects of poisoning is described in the following sections.

Hypertension

The most common causes of elevated blood pressure in poisoned patients are withdrawal of benzodiazepine or ethanol and discontinuation of a therapeutically prescribed antihypertensive medication such as clonidine or minoxidil, resulting in rebound hypertension. Cardiac stimulant like cocaine is known to cause life-threatening hypertension and pulmonary edema. Poison-induced hypertensive emergency is often of short duration and does not require aggressive and prolonged antihypertensive therapy. Benzodiazepine, a sedative and tranquilizer, is quite effective in controlling high blood pressure and tachycardia **(Table 1)**. It is preferred for hypertension caused by drugs with indirect adrenergic activity and drug-of-abuse withdrawal. Intravenous vasodilator drugs like nitroglycerine and nitroprusside are effective for hypertension due to overdose of sympathomimetic drugs like amphetamines **(Table 1)**. Labetalol, a selective α-blocker, is also effective for sympathomimetic poisoning. Propranolol, a nonselective β-blocker, should be avoided as it may lead to unopposed α-adrenergic stimulation and worsening hypertension.

Myocardial Ischemia

Cocaine can cause myocardial ischemia by an adrenoceptor-mediated coronary artery vasospasm

TABLE 1: Cardiovascular manifestations of commonly encountered poisons and their management.

Drug class	*Example*	*Cardiac effects*	*Other effects*	*Antidote*	*Other treatment*
Sympathomimetic	Cocaine, amphetamine, theophylline, caffeine, ephedrine, salbutamol	Hypertension, tachycardia, hyperthermia	Hyperalert, agitation, hallucination, paranoia, seizures, diaphoresis, tremors, hyperreflexia, mydriasis	Benzodiazepine	• No treatment may be needed • Benzodiazepines for agitation • Intravenous nitro-glycerine/sodium nitroprusside for hypertension
Anticholinergic	Antihistaminics, TCA, antiparkinsonism drugs, atropine, antispasmodics, Datura plant	Hypertension, tachycardia, hyperthermia, tachypnea	Agitation, hallucinations, delirium, coma, dry skin and mucosa, urinary retention, decreased bowel sounds, myoclonus, mydriasis	Physostigmine	• Symptomatic treatment for hypertension and hyperthermia • Intravenous sodium bicarbonate and magnesium sulfate for ventricular arrhythmias
Hallucinogenic	Phencyclidine, MDMA	Hypertension, tachycardia, hyperthermia, tachypnea	Hallucinations, agitation, depersonalization, perceptual distortions, nystagmus, mydriasis	Dantrolene	• No treatment if mild • Intravenous nitroglycerine/ sodium nitroprusside
Opioid	Heroin, morphine	Bradypnea, apnea	CNS depression, coma hyporeflexia, pulmonary edema, miosis	Naloxone	Mechanical ventilation
Sedative-hypnotic	Benzodiazepines, barbiturates, alcohol	Hypotension, bradycardia, hypothermia, bradypnea, apnea	CNS depression, confusion, stupor, coma, hyporeflexia	Flumazenil	• Atropine, isoproterenol, electrical pacing for bradycardia • Crystalloids, vasopressors, inotropes, mechanical support for hypotension
Cholinergic	Organophosphate and carbamate insecticide, nerve agents, nicotine, physostigmine	Bradycardia, hypotension/ hypertension, tachypnea/ bradypnea	Confusion, coma, Salivation, lacrimation, diarrhea, emesis, diaphoresis, urinary incontinence, bronchoconstriction, fasciculations, seizures, miosis	Atropine, Pralidoxime	Mechanical ventilation, symptomatic management
Serotonin syndrome	SSRIs, TCA, dextromethorphan	Hypertension, tachycardia, tachypnea, hyperthermia	Confusion, agitation, coma, tremors, hyperreflexia, myoclonus, flushing, diaphoresis, rigidity, diarrhea	Cyproheptadine	Supportive treatment, sedation

(CNS: central nervous system; MDMA: methylenedioxymethamphetamine; TCA: tricyclic antidepressants; SSRI: selective serotonin reuptake inhibitor)

TABLE 2: Known myocardial toxins.

Examples	*Toxic myocarditis agents*
Drugs	Amphetamines, anthracyclines, cocaine, cyclophosphamide, ethanol, fluorouracil, lithium, catecholamines, hemetine, interleukin-2, trastuzumab, clozapine, immune checkpoint inhibitors (anti-PD-I and/or anti-CTLA4) for cancer treatment
Heavy metals	Copper, iron, lead
Miscellaneous	Scorpion sting, snake and spider bites, bee and wasp stings, carbon monoxide, inhalants, phosphorus, arsenic, sodium azide
Hormones	Phaeochromocytoma, vitamin-B1 deficiency: Beriberi
Physical agents	Radiation, electric shock

(anti-CTLA4: cytotoxic T-lymphocyte–associated antigen 4; anti-PD-1: programmed cell death protein 1)

TABLE 3: Antidotes for cardiac toxins.

Toxin	*Antidote*
Anticholinergics	Physostigmine
β-blockers	Glucagon, high dose of insulin with glucose
Calcium channel blockers	Calcium, glucagon, high insulin, and glucose
Cyanide	Hydroxocobalamin, sodium thiosulphate
Digoxin	Digoxin-specific Fab fragments
Oxidants	Methylene blue
Stimulants (theophylline/cocaine)	Benzodiazepine
Organophosphates and carbamates	Atropine, pralidoxime
Paracetamol	N-acetylcysteine
Carbon monoxide/hydrogen sulfide	Oxygen, hyperbaric oxygen therapy
Phosphine (zinc/aluminum phosphide)	High-dose insulin with glucose, LV support devices, extracorporeal membrane oxygenators

(LV: left ventricular)

and also by increasing myocardial oxygen demand. It also increases platelet aggregation, which can result in thrombus formation and fulminant myocardial infarction.[3] Nitroglycerine and phentolamine (α-blocker) do reverse cocaine-induced vasoconstriction.[4] In acute coronary syndrome resistant to these treatments, intracoronary administration of coronary vasodilators should be considered.

Toxic Myocarditis

Toxic gases like phosphine, carbon monoxide, hydrogen cyanide, and hydrogen sulfide exposure can result in significant cardiovascular toxicity **(Table 2)**. These agents can result in coronary vasospasm and direct myocardial depression, resulting in toxic myocarditis. Vasopressors may help in mild cases, but those with severe cardiovascular collapse may require mechanical circulatory support (MCS) devices and extracorporeal membrane oxygenation (ECMO) to support the failing heart.

Vasoplegic Syndrome

Vasoplegic syndrome is defined as low systemic vascular resistance, normal or high cardiac output, and resistant hypotension unresponsive to vasopressor agents and fluid resuscitation. It is determined when systemic vascular resistance is <700 dyn/sec/cm^{-5}, systolic blood pressure is <90 mm Hg, mean arterial pressure is <60 mm Hg, and cardiac output is >5 L/min or cardiac index >2.2 L/min/m^2.

Overdose of many drugs, such as angiotensin-converting enzyme inhibitors/angiotensin receptor blockers, metformin, protamine, amiodarone, nitrates, calcium channel blockers, phosphodiesterase inhibitors, and β-blockers, can cause paraplegic syndrome. Since these drugs are routinely prescribed, there is always a risk of drug overdose and self-harm in susceptible patients.[5] The current treatment strategies include volume replacement and vasopressor support **(Table 1)**. Epinephrine and vasopressin are the preferred vasopressors for it. In catecholamine-resistant vasoplegic syndrome, methylene blue, high-dose hydroxocobalamin, vitamin C, thiamine, and corticosteroids can be considered **(Table 3)**.

MANAGEMENT OF SHOCK IN POISONED PATIENTS

Shock in a poisoned patient can be cardiogenic due to decreased cardiac output or distributive due to decreased systemic vascular resistance. Poisons can cause myocardial depression directly as well as indirectly due to hypoxia and metabolic acidosis, leading to impaired cardiac contractility. Dysrhythmias also exacerbate myocardial dysfunction. Measurement of central venous pressure and IVC dimensions helps to assess the patient's volume status.[6]

In hypovolemic shock, initial treatment includes a fluid challenge to optimize preload. If shock persists after adequate fluid challenge, a vasopressor must be started. Evidence supports dopamine as the most effective agent in mild-to-moderate poisoning.[7] Dopamine-resistant shock indicates a low systemic vascular resistance and needs more potent and high-dose vasopressors, like norepinephrine and phenylephrine. Vasopressin must be added if ventricular arrhythmias develop following vasopressor infusion or secondary to direct cardiac toxicity. Dobutamine and isoproterenol decrease systemic vascular resistance and should be avoided in distributive shock. In drug-induced cardiogenic shock, inotropic agents like dobutamine, isoproterenol, calcium, glucagon, insulin, and amrinone may be required. These agents increase cardiac contractility and cardiac output, but concomitant vasopressor may be necessary due to decreased systemic vascular resistance.

Nonadrenergic vasoactive drugs are effective for treating overdose of β-adrenergic blockers and calcium channel blockers-induced shock. Glucagon, a peptide hormone, stimulates adenyl cyclase and increases intracellular cyclic adenosine monophosphate (cAMP) through a nonadrenergic mechanism **(Table 3)**. This increase in cAMP causes an increase in intracellular calcium, which leads to positive chronotropic and inotropic action in such patients. A high-dose insulin euglycemia therapy is also used to treat β-adrenergic blockers, calcium channel blockers, and aluminum phosphide toxicity **(Table 3)**. It also improves myocardial utilization of carbohydrates for energy, thus increasing cardiac contractility and perfusion.[8]

Lipid emulsion therapy in critically ill poisoned patients reverses the toxicity of local anesthetics, calcium channel blockers, tricyclic antidepressants, benzodiazepines, anticonvulsants, and β-adrenergic blockers.[9] An intravenous bolus of lipid emulsion therapy is effective in restoring rhythm in cardiac arrest patients due to overdose poisoning due to these drugs.

MANAGEMENT OF ARRHYTHMIAS IN POISONED PATIENTS

Some drugs slow heart rate and can inhibit atrioventricular conduction by increasing the refractory time of the atrioventricular node, resulting in various degrees of heart block. In patients with symptomatic, hemodynamically unstable bradycardia, atropine and temporary pacing support are required. Atropine is effective and lifesaving in acute organophosphate or carbamate poisoning[3] **(Table 1)**.

High-dose isoproterenol can be effective, though it can worsen hypotension and precipitate ventricular arrhythmias in patients with β-blocker poisoning.[3] Digoxin-specific Fab antibody fragments are highly effective in treating ventricular arrhythmias and heart block due to digoxin/cardiac glycoside poisoning **(Table 3)**. Temporary cardiac pacing may be required for symptomatic, persistent bradycardia when a definitive antidote is not available. Percutaneous transvenous pacing is needed if external pacing is not tolerated or fails.

Drug-induced hemodynamically significant atrial or ventricular tachyarrhythmias may induce myocardial ischemia, myocardial infarction, ventricular tachycardia/fibrillation, high-output heart failure, and shock. Pharmacological measures are preferred when rate control is necessary. Calcium channel blockers are relatively contraindicated in those with hypotension and depressed cardiac functions. Adenosine and synchronized cardioversion may not be effective, as tachycardia is likely to recur or may be refractory. Benzodiazepines such as diazepam or lorazepam are generally safe and effective in drug-induced tachycardia **(Table 1)** but should be used cautiously to avoid respiratory depression. Physostigmine is a specific antidote for drug-induced tachycardia due to central anticholinergic poisoning[3] **(Table 3)**. Nonselective β-blockers such as propranolol may be effective in patients with tachycardia due to sympathomimetic poisoning.[3]

Ventricular tachycardias (VT) are life-threatening complications of poisoning and can result from cardiac hyperexcitability secondary to sodium or potassium channel blockers. Sodium channel blockade reduces conduction velocity in the ventricle and bundle of His, prolonging the QRS complex duration and increasing the risk of re-entrant ventricular tachycardia. Sodium bicarbonate injection and correction of electrolytes and hypoxemia improve the conduction in such toxicity.[10] Prolonged repolarization (increased QT interval in ECG) predisposes the myocardium to early after-depolarizations and the multifocal ventricular tachycardia termed "torsades de pointes." This often occurs in bursts, causing transient syncope, but can degenerate into ventricular fibrillation (VF), leading to cardiac arrest. A corrected QT interval (QTc) of >500 ms or a drug-induced increase of >60 ms confers a high risk of torsades de pointes.[3] The use of antiarrhythmic drugs to treat poisoning-induced arrhythmias is challenging as many of these drugs can increase the QT interval or further block the sodium channels.[11] Procainamide is contraindicated in tricyclic antidepressant poisonings. Magnesium has beneficial effects in some instances of drug-induced VT, specifically torsades de pointes, but it can aggravate hypotension. In most cases of drug-induced monomorphic VT, lidocaine is the antiarrhythmic of choice.[12,13] Electrical overdrive pacing at 100–120 beats/min or pharmacological overdrive pacing with isoproterenol can terminate torsades de pointes.[13] Hypertonic saline and systemic alkalinization can reverse adverse electrophysiological effects of sodium channel blockers and tricyclic antidepressant poisoning.[14] Repetitive boluses of 1–2 mEq/kg sodium bicarbonate can establish systemic alkalinization by achieving a pH of 7.50–7.55.

EXTERNAL SUPPORT DEVICES FOR MYOCARDIAL DYSFUNCTION

Mechanical cardiovascular support, including an intra-aortic balloon pump (IABP), left ventricular (LV) assist device, and/or extracorporeal membrane oxygenation, may be required in severe refractory hemodynamic compromise not responding to standard resuscitative measures as a bridge to recovery.

Intra-aortic Balloon Pump

Percutaneous IABP placement at the descending thoracic aorta is beneficial for ECG-gated synchronized counterpulsation, which increases mean arterial blood pressure, coronary perfusion pressure, and cardiac output (by approximately 1 L/min) and decreases the LV end-diastolic pressure, LV wall stress, and myocardial oxygen demand.[13] The quality of support an IABP provides depends on heart rate, rhythm, and systemic vascular resistance. Contraindications to IABP use include severe peripheral vascular disease and aortic dissection, tortuosity, aneurysm, and significant aortic regurgitation. This has been tried in patients having toxic myocarditis, mainly due to aluminum or zinc phosphide, with variable success.[15-17]

Percutaneous Left Ventricular Devices

The two major percutaneous LV support devices are microaxial flow pumps (such as Impella from Abiomed, MA, USA) and extracorporeal centrifugal devices. Both devices allow increases in cardiac output and mean arterial blood pressure, with corresponding increases in coronary and systemic perfusion pressures. Microaxial flow devices traverse the aortic valve and continuously remove blood from the LV cavity to achieve unloading. Effective LV "unloading" reduces LV end-diastolic pressure, decreasing wall tension and myocardial oxygen demand.[18] The left-sided Impella comes in various sizes and can deliver 2.5–5.5 L/min of flow. These devices are inserted percutaneously through the femoral artery across the aortic valve. Impella device is contraindicated in patients with severe aortic valve stenosis, severe aortic regurgitation, LV thrombus, mechanical aortic valve, and peripheral arterial disease of the aorta and iliofemoral arteries.[19]

TandemHeart (LivaNova) percutaneous assist device is a continuous flow, centrifugal pump, left atrium to femoral artery system. A 21F trans-septal inflow cannula is inserted via the femoral vein into the left atrium, while an outflow cannula (15F–19F) is placed into the descending aorta, bypassing the left ventricle. The device is powered by an extracorporeal electromagnetic motor that drives a plastic impeller at 3,000–7,500 rpm and can deliver flows up to 5 L/min.[20] Despite the hemodynamic benefits observed with TandemHeart, its widespread use is limited due to technical challenges in device insertion and monitoring. It has not been used in patients with toxic myocarditis.[21,22]

Percutaneous Right Ventricular Devices

Like the temporary LV support options as discussed above, options for percutaneous right ventricular (RV) support include microaxial and extracorporeal centrifugal devices. These devices directly reduce right atrial and RV pressures and increase blood flow across the pulmonary artery, increasing mean pulmonary arterial pressure, LV preload, and cardiac output in the setting of preserved or assisted LV function.[23] The Impella RP system is a percutaneous microaxial RV assist device that operates on the same principles as the left-side device. A 22F catheter is placed in IVC, which delivers blood from the inlet area to the outlet opening in the pulmonary artery. Contraindications to right-sided device placement include mechanical tricuspid or pulmonary valves, severe tricuspid or pulmonary stenosis or regurgitation, disorders of the pulmonary artery wall that prohibit device placement, and mural thrombus of the right atrium, RV, or IVC.[21]

Extracorporeal membrane oxygenation is indicated in poisoned patients in refractory shock who do not show improvement with conventional treatment. ECMO serves as a bridge until the toxins are metabolized or eliminated. Its role in poisoning is discussed in another chapter in the textbook.

Mechanical Circulatory Support Device-related Complications

Temporary MCS devices are associated with cardiovascular, hematological, immune, and neurological complications. These complications should be weighed against the potential clinical benefit for individual patients.

Cardiovascular complications are related to cardiac or local vascular access injuries. These include valvular injury, chamber perforation, pericardial effusion, and tamponade. Vascular complications include acute limb ischemia and dissection of cannulated vessels.

Hematological complications include hemorrhage, anemia, platelet dysfunction, thrombocytopenia, and thrombosis. Despite routine anticoagulation, the risk of pump thrombosis persists. MCS-related bleeding is multifactorial due to coagulation defects, hemolysis from high shear forces, thrombocytopenia, access-related issues, and requisite anticoagulation.

Infectious complications are commonly encountered in the setting of MCS, given the multiple sites of external cannulation access combined with critical illness and prolonged hospital stays. Infectious complications can range from local access-site infections to systemic illness, including bacteremia and sepsis. Although some institutions use prophylactic antibiotic therapy, no evidence supports its generalized use.[24]

Neurological injury can be multifactorial in critically ill patients but is commonly attributed to the migration of microemboli from the MCS device. Hemodynamically unstable patients often have associated cerebral hypoperfusion, hypoxia, or metabolic derangement that contribute to cerebrovascular events. The rate of stroke is similar in patients with an IABP, TandemHeart or Impella devices but is notably higher among those supported with ECMO.[25]

CARDIAC ARREST IN POISONED PATIENTS AND RESUSCITATION

As with any unstable patient, resuscitation of a poisoned patient should follow the advanced life support guidelines, with priority to ABC. This should also include the correction of reversible abnormalities such as hypoxia, hypotension, hypoglycemia, and electrolyte abnormalities. In advanced cardiac life support (ACLS) protocol, cardiopulmonary resuscitation (CPR) is terminated after 20–30 minutes unless there are signs of a viable central nervous system. However, more prolonged CPR is warranted in poisoned patients. Though cerebral blood flow drops dramatically with prolonged CPR, good neurological recovery has been reported in poisoned patients who received prolonged CPR.[26] This can be due to the marked vasodilatation associated with many types of severe poisonings.

Electrical cardioversion/defibrillation is appropriate for pulseless patients with drug-induced VT or VF. In case of sympathomimetic poisoning with refractory VF, high-dose epinephrine should be avoided during resuscitation. In conditions/poisoning associated with hypothermia, prolonged resuscitation and repeated cardioversion coupled with restoration of body temperature may help.

CONCLUSION

Poisoning has important cardiovascular implications, and all physicians should be aware of the common cardiac toxins, their effects, antidotes, and emergency resuscitative management to improve patient outcomes.

REFERENCES

1. Panchal AR, Bartos JA, Cabañas JG, Donnino MW, Drennan IR, Hirsch KG, et al. Part 3: Adult basic and advanced life support: 2020 American Heart Association Guidelines for Cardiopulmonary Resuscitation and Emergency Cardiovascular Care. Circulation. 2020;142:S366-468.
2. Mowry JB, Spyker DA, Brooks DE, McMillan N, Schauben JL. 2014 Annual Report of the American Association of Poison Control Centers' National Poison Data System (NPDS): 32nd Annual Report. Clin Toxicol (Philadelphia, Pa). 2015;53(10):962-1147.
3. Potts AJ, Thomas SHL. Cardiovascular complications of poisoning. Medicine. 2020;48(3):165-8.
4. Lange RA, Cigarroa RG, Yancy CW, Willard JE, Popma JJ, Sills MN, et al. Cocaine-induced coronary-artery vasoconstriction. N Engl J Med. 1989;321(23):1557-62.
5. Omar S, Zedan A, Nugent K. Cardiac vasoplegia syndrome: pathophysiology, risk factors and treatment. Am J Med Sci. 2015;349(1):80-8.
6. Gökdemir BN, Çekmen N. Vasoplegic syndrome and anaesthesia: a narrative review. Turk J Anaesthesiol Reanim. 2023;51(4):280-9.
7. Vernon DD, Banner W, Garrett JS, Dean JM. Efficacy of dopamine and norepinephrine for treatment of

hemodynamic compromise in amitriptyline intoxication. Crit Care Med. 1991;19(4):544-9.
8. Engebretsen KM, Kaczmarek KM, Morgan J, Holger JS. High-dose insulin therapy in beta-blocker and calcium channel-blocker poisoning. Clin Toxicol. 2011;49(4):277-83.
9. Cave G, Harvey M, Willers J, Uncles D, Meek T, Picard J, et al. LIPAEMIC report: Results of clinical use of intravenous lipid emulsion in drug toxicity reported to an online lipid registry. J Med Toxicol. 2014;10(2):133-42.
10. Thomas SHL, Behr ER. Pharmacological treatment of acquired QT prolongation and torsades de pointes. Br J Clin Pharmacol. 2015;81(3):420-7.
11. Thanacoody HR, Waring WS. Toxins that affect the cardiovascular system. Clin Med. 2008;8(1):92-5.
12. Shih RD, Hollander JE, Burstein JL, Nelson LS, Hoffmann RS, Quick AM. Clinical safety of lidocaine in patients with cocaine-associated myocardial infarction. Ann Emerg Med. 1995;26(6):702-6.
13. Guidelines 2000 for Cardiopulmonary Resuscitation and Emergency Cardiovascular Care. Part 8: Advanced challenges in resuscitation: section 1: life-threatening electrolyte abnormalities. The American Heart Association in collaboration with the International Liaison Committee on Resuscitation. Circulation. 2000;102(8 Suppl):I217-22.
14. Brown K. Tricyclic antidepressant overdosage. Clin Toxicol. 1976;9(2):255-72.
15. Siddaiah LM, Adhyapak SM, Jaydev SM, Shetty GG, Varghese K, Patil CB, et al. Intraaortic balloon pump in toxic myocarditis due to aluminum phosphide poisoning. J Med Toxicol. 2009;5(2):80-3.
16. Mehrpour O, Amouzeshi A, Dadpour B, Oghabian Z, Zamani N, Amini S, et al. Successful treatment of cardiogenic shock with an intraaortic balloon pump following aluminium phosphide poisoning. Arh Hig Rada Toksikol. 2014;65(1):121-6.
17. Bagheri-moghaddam A, Abbaspour H, Tajoddini S, Mohammadzadeh V, Moinipour A, Dadpour B. Using intraaortic balloon pump for management of cardiogenic shock following aluminum phosphide poisoning; Report of 3 cases. Emerg (Tehran) 2018;6(1):e3-3.
18. Parissis H, Graham V, Lampridis S, Lau M, Hooks G, Mhandu PC. IABP: History-evolution-pathophysiology-indications: what we need to know. J Cardiothorac Surg. 2016;11(1):122.
19. Burkhoff D, Sayer G, Doshi D, Uriel N. Hemodynamics of mechanical circulatory support. J Am Coll Cardiol. 2015;66(23):2663-74.
20. Naidu SS. Novel percutaneous cardiac assist devices. Circulation. 2011;123(5):533-43.
21. Thiha S, Robert CA, Zaidi ARZ. Ventricular assist devices and their usage as a bridge to recovery in patients with acute cardiotoxicity and cardiomyopathy. Cureus. 2020;12(10):e10915.
22. Chatterjee T, Salh O, Vo T, Patel M. A peculiar case of phosphine toxicity. Chest. 2017;152(4):A820.
23. Telukuntla KS, Estep JD. Acute mechanical circulatory support for cardiogenic shock. Methodist DeBakey Cardiovasc J. 2020;16(1):27.
24. Kapur NK, Esposito ML, Bader Y, Morine KJ, Kiernan MS, Pham DT, et al. Mechanical circulatory support devices for acute right ventricular failure. Circulation. 2017;136(3):314-26.
25. Tsangaris A, Alexy T, Kalra R, Kosmopoulos M, Elliott A, Bartos JA, et al. Overview of veno-arterial extracorporeal membrane oxygenation (VA-ECMO) support for the management of cardiogenic shock. Front Cardiovasc Med. 2021;8:686558.
26. Ramsay ID. Survival after imipramine poisoning. Lancet. 1967;290(7529):1308-9.

3.2 Ventilatory Support

Binila Chacko

INTRODUCTION

Ventilatory support may be necessary in severe poisoning or following exposure to toxic substances due to their direct or indirect impact on respiratory function. This support is aimed at maintaining adequate oxygenation and optimizing ventilation. The broad principles of ventilatory management in poisoning are not different from other situations. The specific approach, however, depends on the nature of the toxic exposure and the impact on the respiratory system.

MECHANISMS OF HYPOXIA AND HYPERCAPNIA IN TOXICOLOGY

Several factors contribute to compromise of airway and breathing and result in hypoxia without or without hypercapnia in toxicology **(Table 1)**.

TABLE 1: Factors contributing to compromise of airway and breathing in toxicology.

Airway component		
Inability to protect airway (reduced consciousness due to)	***Airway obstruction***	
	Intrinsic airway obstruction	***Extrinsic airway obstruction***
CNS suppressant effect of toxins	Intraluminal (secretions, blood, vomitus, foreign body)	Direct (e.g., trauma)
Co-ingestion of alcohol	Swelling of oral structures (e.g., tongue bite, hair dye, corrosives)	Indirect (subcutaneous emphysema)
Increased ICP (e.g., hypoxia, trauma)	Laryngeal edema (e.g., iatrogenic, Super Vasmol hair dye)	
Head injury (e.g., subdural hematoma)	Laryngeal muscle dysfunction (delayed OP manifestation)	
Seizures	Direct trauma	
Breathing component		
Mechanisms of hypoxia	Hypoxic hypoxia	Aspiration pneumonia, nosocomial infection
	Circulatory hypoxia	Myocardial dysfunction (e.g., dimethoate, beta blocker overdose)
	Histotoxic hypoxia	Cyanide overdose, alcohol-co-ingestion
Mechanisms of hypoventilation	CNS effects	*Direct* (e.g., OP, alcohol)
		Indirect (e.g., sedation, paralysis)
	Neuromuscular dysfunction	*Direct* (e.g., direct effect of OP)
		Consequential (e.g., CIP, metabolic problems like K, P)
	Increased work of breathing	Increased airway resistance (e.g., bronchospasm)
		Reduced compliance (e.g., aspiration, ARDS)

(ARDS: acute respiratory distress syndrome; CNS: central nervous system; CIP: critical illness polyneuropathy, ICP: Increased intracranial pressure; K: potassium; OP: organophosphorus compound; P: phosphate)

Hypoxia in poisoning can be due to:

- Ventilation-perfusion mismatch (type 1 respiratory failure) because of:
  - Inability to protect the airway, due to a reduced conscious state related to the toxin per se (e.g., alcohol) or secondary to head injury following a fall or due to hypotension, resulting in aspiration pneumonia
  - Airway obstruction due to edema of structures of the upper airway (tongue, epiglottis, and glottis), tongue falling back, or foreign body obstruction[1]
  - Direct alveolar or interstitial injury induced by the poison (e.g., paraquat)[2]
  - Flooding of the lungs due to increased secretions (e.g., cholinergic syndrome[3] in organophosphorus poisoning) or due to cardiac dysfunction secondary to cardiotoxic agents (e.g., beta blocker and calcium channel blocker overdose)[4] with resultant pulmonary edema
  - Atelectasis secondary to inspiratory muscle weakness (diaphragm, intercostals, and accessory muscles)
- Decreased oxygen delivery to the tissue due to:
  - Stagnant hypoxia due to decreased cardiac output secondary to cardiotoxic drug overdose[4]
  - Anemic hypoxia due to abnormal hemoglobins such as increased carboxyhemoglobin, sulf- or methemoglobin levels
  - Histotoxic hypoxia due to decreased tissue utilization of oxygen (e.g., cyanide poisoning)[5]

Hypercapnic respiratory failure can occur from either alveolar hypoventilation due to central nervous system depression; large airway compromise due to obstruction from foreign bodies (ref: Polythene predicament), oral structures (tongue falling back), laryngeal muscle dysfunction or laryngeal edema; and bronchospasm or neuromuscular involvement of the inspiratory muscles with drop in tidal volumes. Additionally, in patients with severe lung injury, there can be a compromise in carbon dioxide removal.

MANAGEMENT OF RESPIRATORY FAILURE IN TOXICOLOGY

The immediate management of a poisoned patient involves the assessment and optimization of the patient with regard to *a*irway, *b*reathing, *c*irculation, *d*isability, and *e*xposure (ABCDE).

In a patient with a compromised airway, standard techniques may be considered to keep the airway open and patent such as triple maneuver and the use of oral or nasopharyngeal airways. If specific antidotes are available for the relevant poison, it must be given in parallel since these may help avert endotracheal intubation. For example, naloxone or flumazenil can help reverse the effects of opioid or benzodiazepine overdose, respectively. In organophosphorus poisoning, atropine through its central effects on the brain, can help improve the Glasgow Coma Score (GCS) and through its effects on the respiratory secretions, atropine can clear the airway and improve respiratory function.[6] Furthermore, research has indicated that delaying the use of atropine in cases of organophosphorus poisoning may worsen the respiratory condition.

The patient may require an advanced airway device with an endotracheal tube either if the airway continues to remain compromised despite the above measures or if the patient has worsening type 1 or type 2 respiratory failure despite noninvasive ventilation (NIV). Strong evidence is, however, lacking to firmly guide the decision-making process when it comes to intubating unconscious poisoned patients.[7-9] While some studies suggest that early intubation and invasive ventilation may lower the risk of aspiration, others find no discernible difference in aspiration or death rates. Intensivists must also recognize the situations where poisoning can result in difficult airway situations, e.g., Corrosive substance (either acid or alkali) ingestion, paraquat[2] ingestion, and Super Vasmol hair dye ingestion which can cause life-threatening airway edema secondary to angioneurotic edema. Additionally, one may need to apply caution with the use of certain drugs for induction during intubation. For example, in organophosphorus poisoning, succinylcholine should be avoided for neuromuscular blockade during rapid-sequence intubation since clearance of this drug may be delayed due to acetylcholinesterase inhibition by the organophosphate compound.[10]

Ventilatory Support in Toxicology

Most patients with toxic overdose have either normal lungs or aspiration pneumonitis in patients with a depressed sensorium. There are, however, some toxins that are associated with the development of acute respiratory distress syndrome (ARDS). Paraquat can cause an acute alveolitis followed by a fibrotic phase: In this situation, the alveolitis gets aggravated by oxygen due to the formation of reactive oxygen species.[2] Other commonly encountered overdoses that are associated with ARDS are calcium channel blocker and opioid overdose.[11,12]

Broadly, ventilatory support may be provided for the management of hypoxia or hypercapnia through either NIV or invasive ventilation. The use of NIV is generally restricted to patients with respiratory failure not responding to conventional oxygen therapy or high-flow nasal cannula, as long as the GCS is >8 as for other situations in critical care. This strategy, however, has been questioned in poisoning, more so in patients with alcohol or sedative overdose where the effects can be reversed over a short period of time with or without antidotes. The recently published NICO (Noninvasive Airway Management of Comatose) trial, an unblinded multicenter randomized controlled trial,[13] examined whether delaying intubation in patients in a coma from acute poisoning would lead to better outcomes than standard care. The most common toxin in the participants was alcohol in two thirds of the group followed by benzodiazepines. In this study, among comatose patients with suspected acute poisoning, a cautious approach of postponing intubation was associated with a higher therapeutic benefit for the composite end point of in-hospital death, length of ICU stay, and length of hospital stay. Based on this evidence, it has been suggested that NIV can be considered in acute poisoning with respiratory failure even with a GCS < 8 as long as the airway is protected. While this strategy may be appropriate in poisoning due to short-acting toxins, this may not be appropriate for toxins with a prolonged effect.

In general, the principles and goals for invasive ventilation of the poisoned patient are the same as for any other critical care scenario where the focus is on ensuring safe ventilatory strategies targeting oxygen saturations of 92–96%.[14,15] In patients with ARDS, low tidal volume ventilation with tidal volumes of 4–8 mL/kg predicted body weight and maintaining safe pressure limits of plateau airway pressure <30 cm water[16] form the foundation of all ARDS guidelines. In patients without ARDS, the evidence on ventilatory management is, however, conflicting. While the PreVENT trial[17] demonstrated that a ventilation strategy using low tidal volume (6 mL/kg) was not more effective than a strategy using intermediate tidal volume (10 mL/kg) with respect to the number of ventilator-free days and alive at day 28, two prior studies[18,19] and an individual patient data meta-analysis have suggested that a lower tidal volume may shorten the time spent on the ventilator and duration of ICU stay in non-ARDS patients. It is important to note that the PreVENT study had several limitations, including an insufficient overall difference between the low and intermediate ventilation techniques after day 1, which can introduce the possibility of a beta error. Until more data contradicts the existing practice, clinicians will most likely continue to target lower (6–8 mL/kg) tidal volumes in patients without ARDS.

There are some situations that may warrant modification of ventilatory strategies or the goals of ventilation. For example, in individuals with tricyclic antidepressant overdose, raising arterial pH to ≥7.45 can reduce the amount of free drug accessible, thereby decreasing toxicity. This approach can be accomplished via mild hyperventilation and 8.4% sodium bicarbonate in 50 mmol aliquots. In paraquat poisoning, lower oxygen targets of 90%[20] are recommended as an increase in SpO_2 >90% was associated with increased mortality.

Are Weaning and Extubation Protocols Different in Patients with Poisoning?

The reasons for extubation failure are often due to factors that are seen in any mechanically ventilated patient that are related to the airway or nonairway causes.[21] In situations secondary to toxins that cause neuromuscular weakness, it is prudent to assess for "readiness for extubation" on at least two occasions, 6 hours apart, since neuromuscular weakness can be fluctuant. This is particularly important in organophosphorus poisoning where weakness may fluctuate within a matter of few hours.

CONCLUSION

Ventilatory care in poisoning, in general, follows the same guidelines as in other clinical situations. The results of the NICO trial may result in a possible revision of the intubation protocols in acute poisoning with toxins with short half-lives and who present with a low GCS.

REFERENCES

1. Jose R, Chacko B, Iyyadurai R, Peter JV. Polythene predicament. J Emerg Med. 2012;43(1):e31-3.
2. Gawarammana IB, Buckley NA. Medical management of paraquat ingestion. Br J Clin Pharmacol. 2011;72(5):745-57.
3. Peter JV, Sudarsan TI, Moran JL. Clinical features of organophosphate poisoning: a review of different classification systems and approaches. Indian J Crit Care Med. 2014;18(11):735-45.
4. Love JN, Howell JM, Litovitz TL, Klein-Schwartz W. Acute beta blocker overdose: factors associated with the development of cardiovascular morbidity. J Toxicol Clin Toxicol. 2000;38(3):275-81.
5. Nelson L. Acute cyanide toxicity: mechanisms and manifestations. J Emerg Nurs. 2006;32(4):S8-11.
6. Wadia RS, Sadagopan C, Amin RB, Sardesai HV. Neurological manifestations of organophosphorous insecticide poisoning. J Neurol Neurosurg Psychiatry. 1974;37(7):841-7.
7. Burket GA, Horowitz BZ, Hendrickson RG, Beauchamp GA. Endotracheal intubation in the pharmaceutical-poisoned patient: a narrative review of the literature. J Med Toxicol Off J Am Coll Med Toxicol. 2021;17(1):61-9.
8. Orso D, Vetrugno L, Federici N, D'Andrea N, Bove T. Endotracheal intubation to reduce aspiration events in acutely comatose patients: a systematic review. Scand J Trauma Resusc Emerg Med. 2020;28(1):116.
9. Eizadi-Mood N, Saghaei M, Alfred S, Zargarzadeh AH, Huynh C, Gheshlaghi F, et al. Comparative evaluation of Glasgow Coma Score and gag reflex in predicting aspiration pneumonitis in acute poisoning. J Crit Care. 2009;24(3):470.e9-15.
10. Sener EB, Ustun E, Kocamanoglu S, Tur A. Prolonged apnea following succinylcholine administration in undiagnosed acute organophosphate poisoning. Acta Anaesthesiol Scand. 2002;46(8):1046-8.
11. Lodhi FAK, Shogren SL, Vedre JG, Haque N, Reriani M, Ali R. Calcium channel blocker toxicity causing acute respiratory distress syndrome: a commonly used drug triggering a life-threatening condition. WMJ Off Publ State Med Soc Wis. 2020;119(1):66-8.
12. Bhardwaj H, Bhardwaj B, Awab A. Revisiting opioid overdose induced acute respiratory distress syndrome. Indian J Crit Care Med. 2014;18(2):119-20.
13. Freund Y, Viglino D, Cachanado M, Cassard C, Montassier E, Douay B, et al. Effect of noninvasive airway management of comatose patients with acute poisoning: a randomized clinical trial. JAMA. 2023;330(23):2267-74.
14. Barrot L, Asfar P, Mauny F, Winiszewski H, Montini F, Badie J, et al. Liberal or conservative oxygen therapy for acute respiratory distress syndrome. N Engl J Med. 2020;382(11):999-1008.
15. Schjørring OL, Klitgaard TL, Perner A, Wetterslev J, Lange T, Siegemund M, et al. Lower or higher oxygenation targets

for acute hypoxemic respiratory failure. N Engl J Med. 2021;384(14):1301-11.
16. Grasselli G, Calfee CS, Camporota L, Poole D, Amato MBP, Antonelli M, et al. ESICM guidelines on acute respiratory distress syndrome: definition, phenotyping and respiratory support strategies. Intensive Care Med. 2023;49(7):727-59.
17. Writing Group for the PReVENT Investigators, Simonis FD, Serpa Neto A, Binnekade JM, Braber A, Bruin KCM, et al. Effect of a low vs intermediate tidal volume strategy on ventilator-free days in intensive care unit patients without ARDS: a randomized clinical trial. JAMA. 2018;320(18):1872-80.
18. Rubenfeld GD, Shankar-Hari M. Lessons from ARDS for Non-ARDS research: remembrance of trials past. JAMA. 2018;320(18):1863-5.
19. Futier E, Constantin JM, Paugam-Burtz C, Pascal J, Eurin M, Neuschwander A, et al. A trial of intraoperative low-tidal-volume ventilation in abdominal surgery. N Engl J Med. 2013;369(5):428-37.
20. Lin XH, Pan HY, Cheng FJ, Huang KC, Li CJ, Chen CC, et al. Association between liberal oxygen therapy and mortality in patients with paraquat poisoning: a multi-center retrospective cohort study. PLoS One. 2021;16(1): e0245363.
21. Jaber S, Quintard H, Cinotti R, Asehnoune K, Arnal JM, Guitton C, et al. Risk factors and outcomes for airway failure versus nonairway failure in the intensive care unit: a multicenter observational study of 1514 extubation procedures. Crit Care Lond Engl. 2018;22(1):236.

3.3 Extracorporeal Elimination (Dialysis, Hemofiltration, Hemoperfusion)

Nita George, Kartik Ganesh, Thomas Sudarsan

INTRODUCTION

Extracorporeal elimination or detoxification, also known as extracorporeal treatment (ECTR), refers to a medical intervention used in cases of severe poisoning where toxic substances are removed from the blood stream by using a circuit outside the body [except for peritoneal dialysis (PD)]. Commonly used extracorporeal removal techniques include hemodialysis (HD), continuous renal replacement therapy (CRRT), hemoperfusion (HP), molecular adsorbent recirculating system (MARS), and plasma exchange.

Most poisonings can be managed with supportive care and corporal techniques for toxin elimination. Extracorporeal treatments are required only in 0.1% of poisonings.[1]

INDICATIONS FOR EXTRACORPOREAL TREATMENT

Indications for ECTR include evidence of severe toxicity wherein there is clinical deterioration despite supportive care, clinical evidence of severe toxicity (such as hypotension, coma, severe dysrhythmias, metabolic acidosis, heart failure, status epilepticus, or respiratory depression), impaired endogenous toxin clearance due to organ failure, and ingestion of a toxin with serious delayed effects which is amenable to removal by extracorporeal techniques.[2] The cost-benefit ratio of such a therapy should also be taken into consideration. The EXTRIP (*EX*tracorporeal *TR*eatment *I*n *P*oisoning; http://www.extrip-workgroup.org/) workgroup has published guidelines for the use of extracorporeal therapy in several poisons.

PRINCIPLES OF EXTRACORPOREAL TREATMENT

The choice of modality of ECTR depends on both toxin and ECTR technique-related factors.[3]

Poison-related Factors

- *Molecular size:* Low molecular weight poisons (<500 Da) are easily dialyzable. High efficiency and high flux filters are capable of clearing toxins in the middle molecular weight range (10,000–15,000 Da). Convective modalities such as continuous veno-venous hemofiltration (CVVH) and continuous veno-venous hemodiafiltration (CVVHDF) allow removal of molecules up to 40,000 Da. Poisons with large molecular sizes up to 40,000 Da can be removed by HP and those >100,000 Da can be removed by centrifugation and separation (therapeutic plasma exchange).

- *Volume of distribution (Vd):* This is the major determinant of a poison's potential for extracorporeal removal. Vd is calculated as the amount of drug in the body/concentration of drug in plasma. The more the presence of the drug in the intravascular space, the better its removal by extracorporeal techniques. This also explains why the efficacy of ECTR is time sensitive as a higher proportion of poison will be in the intravascular compartment in the first few hours after poisoning. Substances that are lipophilic have a high Vd and are poorly removed, whereas hydrophilic substances have prolonged intravascular presence and a low Vd and are more amenable to elimination by extracorporeal techniques. In general, substances with volumes of distribution >1–1.5 L/kg are poorly amenable to extracorporeal removal.
- *Plasma protein binding:* Substances that are highly plasma protein bound are not cleared by HD. The fraction of the substance that is not plasma protein bound is the amount cleared by dialysis. Substances with <80% protein binding are amenable to removal via HD. Some drugs, which are highly protein bound at therapeutic concentrations, saturate their binding sites at toxic levels and then become dialyzable when free drug levels rise (e.g., salicylates, valproic acid, carbamazepine, phenytoin).
- *Lipid solubility:* Lipid-soluble, highly protein-bound molecules that are not amenable to removal by dialysis modalities may be removed by HP. However, Vd is also an important factor as discussed previously.
- *Rebound effect:* Certain toxins exhibit slow transfer from tissue to plasma and may require prolonged or multiple sessions of dialysis. Such "rebound" effect can be seen in poisons such as lithium, metformin, methotrexate, and dabigatran.
- *Endogenous clearance:* ECTR will not be effective if endogenous clearance (via metabolism and native elimination) is far above that which can be obtained by ECTR. If any of these mechanisms are impaired, the relative contribution of ECTR in poison clearance might be greater.
- *Type of toxin:* Drugs such as calcium channel blockers, digoxin, tricyclic antidepressants, and isoniazid are not amenable to removal by ECTR.

Extracorporeal Treatment-related Factors

Extracorporeal treatment-related factors affecting poison clearance include the type of modality used, the characteristics of the filter used (porosity, surface area, material), blood flow rates, and dialysate flow rates. Optimization of extracorporeal removal of poisons depends primarily on increasing the volume of plasma filtered. This involves increasing the blood flow in HD and the dialysate flow in continuous therapies. However, these processes are not linear and difficult to quantify.

Modalities of extracorporeal elimination:[4]

- *Hemodialysis:* It involves the passage of blood through a dialyzer against the flow of a dialysate through a semipermeable membrane. This adjacent flow of different fluids facilitates exchange of substances between them by diffusion and convection. HD is the pre-eminently used modality of extracorporeal elimination. Substances with molecular weights up to 10,000 Da may be removed by this modality. In addition, benefits such as correction of metabolic parameters (acidosis, electrolyte abnormalities) as well as renal support in cases of renal failure can be provided.
- *Hemoperfusion:* This modality involves the passage of anticoagulated whole blood through a column that contains adsorbent particles. Toxins with higher molecular weights ranging from 100 to 40,000 Da bind to the particles and are removed as blood exits the column. Binding is through physical adsorption.
- *Continuous renal replacement therapy:* This modality has limited efficacy in toxin removal due to the low volume of blood filtered. Toxins with molecular weights of 15,000–20,000 Da may be removed.
- *High cutoff hemodialysis:* Removal of substances with high molecular weights (>50,000 Da) is possible. However, significant complications and poor availability limit the role of this modality.

CHOICE OF EXTRACORPOREAL REMOVAL IN POISONING

Table 1 shows the various modalities of extracorporeal methods and the various pharmacokinetic properties of the toxin which determine toxin clearance. The clinician, after determining the need for ECTR, must consider the various options available, keeping the patient's condition in mind as well as the toxicokinetic properties of the poison to be eliminated.

TABLE 1: Choice of extracorporeal removal in toxicology.

	Hemodialysis	*Hemofiltration/ CRRT*	*Hemoperfusion*	*MARS*	*Peritoneal dialysis*	*Exchange transfusion*	*Plasma exchange*
Mechanism of removal	Diffusion	Diffusion and convection	Adsorption	Diffusion/ convection	Diffusion	Separation	Centrifugal separation
Water/lipid soluble	Water soluble	Water soluble	Lipid soluble (Resin)	Water soluble and protein bound	Water	Protein bound	Protein bound and water soluble
Molecular weight. Mass of toxin in Daltons (Da)	*Low flux:* 1,000 Da; *high flux:* 10,000–15,000 Da; *HCO:* 50,000 Da	40,000 Da	5,000–10,000 Da	60,000–1,00,000 Da	<500 Da	No limit	13,00,000 Da
Protein binding	<80%	<80%	<90%	High	Low	Any	Any
Volume of distribution	Low Vd 1–2 L/kg		<1 L/kg		Very low Vd		<1 L/kg
Endogenous clearance	<4 mL/min/kg	<4 mL/min/kg	<4 mL/min/kg				
Poison examples	Acetaminophen, salicylates, toxic alcohols, lithium	Lithium (CVVHD), metformin (CVVHDF)	Paraquat, barbiturates, salicylates, theophylline, valproate, CBZ	Diltiazem, phenytoin, *Amanita*, *Galerina*, and *Lepiota* mushroom poisoning		Cyclosporine, tacrolimus	Monoclonal antibodies, arsine
Limitations	Hemodynamic instability, rebound	Limited availability, expensive	Limited role, hypocalcemia, clotting, cost, saturation of cartridge	Limited availability and role	Poor toxin clearance		Slow clearance

(CBZ: carbamazepine, CRRT: continuous renal replacement therapy, CVVHD: continuous veno-venous hemodialysis, CVVHDF: continuous veno-venous hemodiafiltration, HCO: high cutoff filter, MARS: molecular absorbent recirculating system, Vd: volume of distribution of toxin)

Hemodialysis

Among the modalities of ECTR, such as intermittent HD (IHD), HP, continuous methods (CRRT-CVVHD/CVVHDF), and plasma exchange (TPE), HD is most commonly applied to toxins which are suitable for extracorporeal removal, mainly in view of greater volume of plasma filtered. HD allows for good clearance of small molecules and concomitant correction of electrolyte and acid–base abnormalities. Although nonlinear, increasing blood flow rate, dialysate flow rate, dialyzer surface area, and time can help improve toxin removal. HD has the advantage of rapidity of clearance in situations where the toxidrome is life-threatening although it might be limited by hemodynamic instability in patients with shock.[5,6] Recent advances in HD with the use of high flux or high cutoff filters have improved their ability for clearance of large or protein-bound toxins such as carbamazepine and phenytoin and have overcome the need for other modalities such as HP.[7]

Toxic alcohols such as methanol and ethylene glycol and their metabolites are cleared by HD and are indicated in severe clinical toxidrome, central nervous system (CNS) or visual involvement, acute kidney injury (AKI), or metabolic acidosis or when refractory to treatment with alcohol dehydrogenase inhibitor, fomepizole. Early hemodialysis (HD) is warranted in cases of severe, refractory salicylate toxicity, particularly when levels exceed 100 mg/dL. Progressive toxicity, resulting from the uncoupling of oxidative phosphorylation, can present with hypoxemia and altered sensorium, often mimicking sepsis or seizures, necessitating prompt intervention. Severe neurotoxicity or arrhythmias with lithium levels >4.0 mEq/L are recommendations for HD as per the EXTRIP group and might require repeat sessions of HD or CRRT subsequently to prevent rebound. Metformin inhibits glycerophosphate dehydrogenase and causes lactic acidosis which carries a mortality of >50% and the recommendations are for HD in case of severe lactic acidosis and presence of concomitant organ failure even in the presence of shock.[8] Patients with poisoning may not have AKI, and typical dialysis solutions containing high bicarbonate and low potassium and phosphate may cause severe electrolyte abnormalities and they have to be monitored and corrected.

Continuous and Hybrid Methods

Continuous renal replacement therapy with CVVHD/CVVHDF is a modality of choice in cases where a more gradual and continuous removal of toxins is required although typically the rate of clearance of toxin is slower than HD. Certain toxins such as lithium, methotrexate, dabigatran, and metformin may exhibit "rebound" levels after HD due to slow transit along concentration gradients from tissue to plasma and hence may be amenable for sustained removal by continuous methods of dialysis. CRRT has the added advantage of maintaining hemodynamic stability in poisoned patients with shock and acute renal injury and, therefore, are integral life support systems in any patient with hemodynamic instability, multiple organ dysfunction syndrome (MODS), and compromised endogenous renal clearance.[9] Slow low-efficiency dialysis or prolonged intermittent RRT (SLED/PIRRT) differs from CRRT in the duration of treatment, the required flow of blood and dialysate, and the machine that is required. The presumed advantage of hemodynamic stability with increased clearance when compared to CRRT does not seem to provide any advantage over IHD when no net ultrafiltration is required. Although by its longer duration, PIRRT might conceptually be more appealing in toxins with rebound effect, their efficacy and role in toxicology are not well documented.[10]

Hemoperfusion

Hemoperfusion uses clearance of toxins by adsorption to charcoal or resins depending on their affinity and have previously been utilized in poisonings with lipid-soluble drugs such as barbiturates, salicylates, theophylline, valproate, and carbamazepine. Its use has come down and is now infrequently used only in the setting of paraquat poisoning in Asia, provided the time of presentation is early (within 2 hours).[11] The limited availability of HP filters and improvements in HD technique as well as various procedure-related complications such as filter clotting and hypocalcemia have contributed to the decline of use of HP in critical care. Valproate, which is highly protein bound and causes hemodynamic instability, hepatotoxicity, and metabolic acidosis, can be removed with a combination of HP and HD as its protein binding is saturable at toxic doses. Severe carbamazepine toxicity with hemodynamic compromise and neurological impairment can be effectively eliminated by HP or HD.[12]

Therapeutic Plasma Exchange

Apheresis or plasma exchange involves extracorporeal separation of plasma from the cellular components of blood, either by centrifugation or by filtration, both of which have equal efficacy. The discarded plasma is replaced with fresh plasma or albumin with saline. Technically, it has the capacity to remove large protein-bound toxins and the American Society of Apheresis recommends one to two plasma volume exchanges till clinical symptoms have improved and redistribution from tissue is not significant. Their role is limited to certain poisonings which have very low Vd but not amenable for removal by other extracorporeal methods. The slow rate of clearance when compared to HD leads to questioning the benefit of these techniques. Arsine, Amanita mushroom, monoclonal antibodies, vincristine, cisplatin, and thyroxine are possible toxins which can be removed by apheresis methods.[13]

Exchange transfusion, an apheresis method in which the patient's erythrocytes are separated from other blood components and replaced by fresh red blood cells (RBCs) with colloids, has been used in poisoning due to xenobiotics which have high affinity to erythrocytes such as cyclosporine, tacrolimus, and methemoglobinemia associated with toxic aniline dye or dapsone exposure. It is relatively simple to use in infants and in this population, it has been used for salicylate, theophylline, and barbiturate toxicities.

Albumin Dialysis Methods

Albumin dialysis methods including MARS and single pass albumin dialysis (SPAD) utilize CRRT with albumin added to the dialysate which is either removed or recycled depending on the method used. They have been theoretically postulated to remove protein-bound toxins such as phenytoin, diltiazem, and valproate. They may have an added benefit in these patients as extracorporeal liver-assisted devices (ELAD) in the setting of acute liver failure (ALF). The uncertain clinical benefit as per presently available data and the slower, inferior clearance of these toxins when compared to HD along with limited availability, technical difficulty, and cost of these methods have not been favorable to the universal application even in these toxicities.[14–16]

Peritoneal Dialysis

Peritoneal dialysis is rarely used for toxin removal. It involves diffusive clearance of small molecules across the peritoneal membrane and is dependent on various factors including patient's hemodynamic status and hence unreliable in the setting of poisoning. PD is not advocated in this context unless the patient is already receiving PD for ESRD, the poisoning effects are minimal, and no other treatment option is available. PD may be considered in small children in whom hemodialysis may be too difficult to perform.

Hemofiltration

The convective clearance methods of intermittent hemodiafiltration use solute clearance by solvent drag across a pressure gradient and subsequent replacement by ultrapure water. It can remove small and larger molecules, but the technical difficulties and limited availability have made them less appealing for clinical use.

Exchange Transfusion

Exchange transfusion involves removing a patient's blood in small aliquots and replacing it with donor blood. Its role in poisoning is uncertain but can be considered in the elimination of poisons which are tightly bound to erythrocytes such as tacrolimus and cyclosporine and those toxins which cause methemoglobinemia, e.g., propanil poisoning.[17] It can also be used in poison-induced hemolysis such as with exposure to dapsone, chromium, and sodium chlorate. It may also be considered in neonates where HD may be technically challenging and also in resource-poor settings.

PRACTICAL CLINICAL USE OF EXTRACORPOREAL TREATMENT IN POISONING (FLOWCHART 1)

The EXTRIP workgroup, comprised of experts from around the world representing various disciplines, conducted a comprehensive review of the literature on extracorporeal therapies for poisonings based on which a comprehensive set of recommendations for the treatment of poisonings using extracorporeal methods have been suggested **(Table 2)**, which can be accessed at www.extrip-workgroup.

Flowchart 1: Decision tree on choice of ECTR modality.

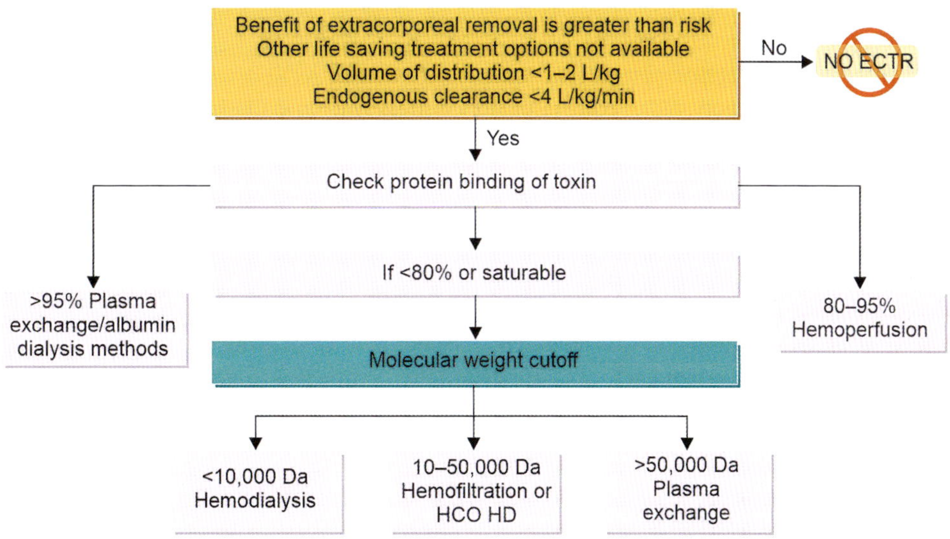

(ECTR: extracorporeal toxin removal; HCO: high cutoff filter; HD: hemodialysis)

TABLE 2: EXTRIP workgroup recommendations for ECTR in poisons amenable to extracorporeal.

Recommendation	*Poison*	*Poison concentration*	*Clinical indications*	*Choice of ECTR*
RECOMMENDED	Lithium	>4.0 mEq/L	Decreased LOC, seizures, dysrhythmias, impaired kidney function	HD > CRRT
RECOMMENDED	Barbiturates	Increasing or persisting	Coma, mechanical ventilation, shock	HD > HP/CRRT
RECOMMENDED	Metformin	Not specified	Shock, lactate >20 mmol/L, pH <7.0	HD > CRRT
RECOMMENDED	Dabigatran	Increasing or persisting	Active bleeding, coagulopathy	HD > CRRT
RECOMMENDED	Salicylates	>100 mg/dL	Altered mental status, ARDS, impaired renal function, pH ≤7.20	HD > HP > CRRT
RECOMMENDED	Ethylene glycol	>310 mg/dL (if antidote used)	Shock, coma, seizures, anion gap >24 mmol/L, AKI	HD > CRRT
RECOMMENDED	Methanol	• >70 mg/dL (w/fomepizole) • > 60 mg/dL (w/ethanol) • > 50 mg/dL (no antidote)	Coma, seizures, new vision deficits, pH ≤7.15, anion gap >24 mmol/L	HD > CRRT
RECOMMENDED	Theophylline	• >100 mg/L (acute) • >60 mg/L (chronic)	Seizures, dysrhythmias, shock	HD > HP > CRRT
RECOMMENDED	Valproic acid	>1,300 mg/L	Cerebral edema, coma, shock, acute hyperammonemia, pH ≤7.10, respiratory depression	HD > HP/CRRT
SUGGESTED	Acetaminophen	>1,000 mg/L	Metabolic acidosis, coma	HD > CRRT
SUGGESTED	Carbamazepine	Increasing or persisting	Refractory seizures, dysrhythmias, coma, respiratory depression	HD > HP/CRRT
NEUTRAL	Phenytoin			
NOT RECOMMENDED	• Tricyclics • Digoxin			

(AKI: acute kidney injury; ARDS: acute respiratory distress syndrome; CRRT: continuous renal replacement therapy; ECTR: extracorporeal toxin removal; EXTRIP: extracorporeal treatments in poisoning; HD: hemodialysis; HP: hemoperfusion; LOC: loss of consciousness)

org. In any given patient, the clinician intensivist must consider the patient's condition and complications (hemodynamics, other organ failure, and bleeding risk), availability of expertise related to the technique of ECTR, and timing and severity of the poisoning; each case must be individualized and decisions made in consultation with the clinical toxicologist and nephrologist.

FUTURE TRENDS AND RESEARCH

There are no randomized controlled trials (RCTs) comparing extracorporeal treatments with supportive care in poisoning for obvious reasons. Groups such as the EXTRIP workgroup are involved in developing and updating guidelines on ECTR based on best available evidence and play a major role in shaping the understanding and application of extracorporeal treatments in poisoning.

CONCLUSION

A vast majority of poisons can be managed conservatively with supportive care, corporeal techniques of toxin elimination, and antidotal therapy. The role ECTR in poisoning is a dynamic field that continues to evolve with advancements in medical technology. It is lifesaving in cases of severe poisoning, particularly when standard therapies are ineffective. The decision to employ ECTR should be individualized, based on careful consideration of factors such as type of toxin, its toxicokinetics and whether it is amenable to ECTR, severity of poisoning, the patient's clinical condition, timing, and availability of expertise. The successful application of ECTR often requires a multidisciplinary approach involving toxicologists, nephrologists, intensivists, and other healthcare professionals.

REFERENCES

1. Mowry JB, Spyker DA, Cantilena LR Jr, Bailey JE, Ford M. 2012 Annual Report of the American Association of poison control centers' national poison data system (NPDS): 30th annual report. Clin Toxicol (Phila). 2013;51:949.
2. de Pont AC. Extracorporeal treatment of intoxications. Curr Opin Crit Care. 2007;13(6):668-73.
3. Bouchard J, Roberts DM, Roy L, Ouellet G, Decker BS, Mueller BA, et al. Principles and operational parameters to optimize poison removal with extracorporeal treatments. Semin Dial. 2014;27:371-80.
4. King JD, Kern MH, Jaar BG. Extracorporeal removal of poisons and toxins. Clin J Am Soc Nephrol. 2019;14(9): 1408-15
5. Ouellet G, Bouchard J, Ghannoum M, Decker BS. Available extracorporeal treatments for poisoning: overview and limitations. Semin Dial. 2014;27:342-9.
6. Garlich FM, Goldfarb DS. Have advances in extracorporeal removal techniques changed the indications for their use in poisonings? Adv Chronic Kidney Dis. 2011;18:172-9.
7. Kirsch AH, Lyko R, Nilsson LG, Beck W, Amdahl M, Lechner P, et al. Performance of hemodialysis with novel medium cut-off dialyzers. Nephrol Dial Transplant. 2017;32: 165-72.
8. Lavergne V, Nolin TD, Hoffman RS, Roberts D, Gosselin S, Goldfarb DS, et al. The EXTRIP (extracorporeal treatments in poisoning) workgroup: guideline methodology. Clin Toxicol (Phila). 2012;50:403-13.
9. Kim Z, Goldfarb DS. Continuous renal replacement therapy does not have a clear role in the treatment of poisoning. Nephron Clin Pract. 2010;115:c1-6.
10. Bailey AR, Sathianathan VJ, Chiew AL, Paterson AD, Chan BS, Arora S. Comparison of intermittent hemodialysis, prolonged intermittent renal replacement therapy and continuous renal replacement hemofiltration for lithium toxicity: a case report. Crit Care Resusc. 2011;13:120-2.
11. Chen Ab, Li F, Di E-Mu, Zhang X, Zhao Q-Y, Wen J. Influence of strengthened hemoperfusion combined with continuous veno-venous hemofiltration on prognosis of patients with acute paraquat poisoning: SHP + CVVH improve prognosis of acute PQ patients. BMC Pharmacol Toxicol. 2020;21:49.
12. Gil HW, Kim SJ, Yang JO, Lee EY, Hong SY. Clinical outcome of hemoperfusion in poisoned patients. Blood Purif. 2010;30:84-8.
13. Jones JS, Dougherty J. Current status of plasmapheresis in toxicology. Ann Emerg Med. 1986;15:474-82.
14. Sen S, Ratnaraj N, Davies NA, Mookerjee RP, Cooper CE, Patsalos PN, et al. Treatment of phenytoin toxicity by the molecular adsorbents recirculating system (MARS). Epilepsia. 2003;44:265-7.
15. Askenazi DJ, Goldstein SL, Chang IF, Elenberg E, Feig DI. Management of a severe carbamazepine overdose using albumin-enhanced continuous veno-venous hemodialysis. Pediatrics. 2004;113:406-9.
16. Korsheed S, Selby NM, Fluck RJ. Treatment of severe theophylline poisoning with the molecular adsorbent recirculating system (MARS). Nephrol Dial Transplant. 2007;22:969-70.
17. Ranasinghe P, Dilrukshi SA, Atukorala I, Katulanda P, Gnanathasan A. Exchange transfusion can be life-saving in severe propanil poisoning: a case report. BMC Res Notes. 2014;7:700.

3.4 Extracorporeal Membrane Oxygenation

Vivek Gupta, Gurpreet S Wander

INTRODUCTION

The management of acute severe poisoning usually remains supportive and symptomatic with use of appropriate antidote if available. The clinical presentation depends on several factors including the intrinsic properties of toxic substance, quantity of ingestion, route of poison entry, and the presence of other additives with poison. Moreover, the patient-related factors such as age, co-morbidities, and underlying organ dysfunction also affect the survival of these acute severe intoxication victims.[1]

The supportive therapy may not be sufficient in cases of severe hemodynamic instability, cardiovascular collapse, cardiac arrest, or persistent life-threatening arrhythmias. Extracorporeal therapies are a heterogeneous group of therapies and have been used during acute severe poisoning ranging from enhancement of toxic substance elimination to supporting the failing vital organs to preventing cardiovascular collapse and death.[2] There is a significant increase in the use of extracorporeal membrane oxygenation (ECMO) in the recent past in general[3] and in life-threatening poisoning in particular with successful outcome. Patients with acute severe intoxication with cardiotoxic drugs or chemical substances affecting cardiovascular functions severely or producing life-threatening arrhythmia may be a candidate for venoarterial (VA) ECMO. VA ECMO helps in maintaining cardiac output, optimizing hemodynamic, and maintaining tissue perfusion till the myocardial function recovers. The use of venovenous (VV) ECMO may be helpful in patients developing severe acute respiratory distress syndrome (ARDS) after exposure to inhalational toxins. Though the current literature supports the use of ECMO in various poisoning situations, there is lack of evidence suggesting appropriate time for initiation of ECMO.[4]

WHAT KILLS IN SEVERE POISONING?

Acute severe poisoning may lead to death due to either hemodynamic instability or cardiovascular collapse or severe ARDS producing altered gas exchange in lungs as a primary event. The progressive metabolic derangements further worsen the myocardial dysfunction, hemodynamic instability, and rhythm disturbances as a secondary event leading to further clinical deterioration. The basic aim of tiding over the crisis in a severely poisoned patient includes airway management, mechanical ventilation, and supporting the hemodynamics with fluid and vasopressors.[5] Vasoactive drugs have proarrhythmic potential which can further worsen the myocardial function. Antiarrhythmic drugs due to their negative inotropic effect may cause myocardial depression and hemodynamic instability. The antiarrhythmic drugs may also cause arrhythmia, especially with existing metabolic acidosis and electrolyte imbalances.[5] The use of invasive hemodynamic monitoring for shock interpretation and guiding management has definitely improved the outcome in a severely poisoned patient.[6] The degree of hemodynamic instability and myocardial dysfunction after severe intoxication depends on the quantity, toxic potential, and type of ingested toxic substance. One of the common possibilities in cases of sudden cardiac arrest in young population without risk factors or co-morbidities may be severe intoxication.[5-8]

Substances with Life-threatening Potential for Cardiotoxicity or Respiratory Failure

Cardiotoxic Drugs

Cardiotoxic drugs have the potential to cause worsening of myocardial function after acute intoxication with symptoms of progressive heart failure. In severe cases, this myocardial dysfunction may lead to low cardiac output state, inadequate organ, or tissue perfusion which may progress to other organ dysfunction. Some of these drugs have arrhythmogenic potential in toxic doses and may produce refractory life-threatening arrhythmias. Drugs with cardiotoxic potential[9] are given in **Table 1**.

Pesticides

Acute severe pesticide intoxication[10] may cause multiorgan involvement with varying degrees of cardiac and/or respiratory involvement producing severe myocardial dysfunction, life-threatening arrhythmia (aluminum phosphide), or severe respiratory dysfunction progressing to pulmonary fibrosis (paraquet) **(Table 2)**.

Plant Toxins

Severe toxicity with plant toxin[11,12] may produce conduction disturbances including complete heart block, bradyarrhythmia, tachyarrhythmia, or life-threatening ventricular arrhythmia **(Table 3)**.

TABLE 1: Drugs with cardiotoxic potential.

Class	*Drugs*
Sympathomimetics	Amphetamines, cathinones, synthetic cannabinoid receptor agonist (recreational drugs)
Sodium channel blockers	Carbamazepine, cocaine, flecainide, lacosamide, quinidine, *Taxus* spp. (Yew), tricyclic and tetracyclic antidepressant, propafenone
Local anesthetics	Bupivacaine
Cardiac glycosides	Digoxin, digitoxin
Calcium channel blockers	Amlodipine
Beta-blockers	Metoprolol
Others	Cocaine

TABLE 2: Pesticides causing severe myocardial or respiratory dysfunction.

Class of agents	*Compounds*
Insecticides	Organophosphate, carbamate
Herbicides	Paraquet, diquat
Rodenticides	Aluminum phosphide, zinc phosphide, yellow phosphorus

TABLE 3: Plant toxins producing life-threatening arrhythmia.

Bioactive compounds	*Plants*
Aconite, quinidine, sodium channel activity	Monkshood, hellebore, rhododendron, death camas, cinchona
Cathinone, viscotoxins, synephrine belladonna alkaloids, tropine alkaloids, physostigmine: Autonomic dysfunction	Bitter orange, Mistletoe khat, belladonna, angel's chalice, jimsonweed, angel's trumpets, mandrake
Taxine alkaloids: Calcium channel activity	Yew
Cardiac glycosides: Na-K-ATPase activity	Foxglove, oleander, lily of the valley, *Cerbera odollam*

TABLE 4: Other poisons with cardiotoxic potential.

Mechanism of toxicity	*Compounds*
• Reduction in oxygen carrying capacity • Reduction in cardiac output with binding to myoglobin	Carbon monoxide
Cessation of aerobic metabolism	Cyanide

Miscellaneous

Carbon monoxide[13] is produced by cars and heating systems due to incomplete hydrocarbon combustion. Its toxicity may lead to tissue hypoxia, multiple-organ dysfunction, and cardiovascular collapse by rapidly binding to hemoglobin and form carboxyhemoglobin. Severe myocardial dysfunction and cardiogenic pulmonary edema may also occur due to inhibition of oxidative phosphorylation when carbon monoxide binds to myocardial myoglobin **(Table 4)**.

ROLE OF EXTRACORPOREAL MEMBRANE OXYGENATION IN SEVERE POISONING

Extracorporeal membrane oxygenation is indicated in severe intoxication leading to acute severe heart or lung failure once conventional therapy has failed with worsening of shock which increases the risk of mortality. The conventional dictum of extracorporeal life support organization (ELSO) for considering ECMO if the mortality risk is 50% and initiate ECMO if the mortality risk is 80%[14] is applicable for intoxicated patients as well. Moreover, a better outcome may be expected since these patients are usually of the younger age group and does not have comorbidities. The ECMO support may be required till the recovery of shock or improvement of gas exchange once toxin has been metabolized or eliminated.

Venoarterial ECMO helps in sustaining adequate cardiac output and improves organ and tissue perfusion, thus enhancing the metabolism and elimination of poison by improving hepatic and renal blood flow.[15]

Venovenous extracorporeal membrane oxygenation supports the lung function by proving that gas exchange may be helpful for inhalation or aspiration of toxins such as organic hydrocarbon (paint remover, thinner, etc.) leading to severe ARDS.

The current literature is limited with case reports and case series regarding the use of ECMO in severe poisoning, and there is no recommendation regarding an appropriate time for ECMO initiation in this group of patients. The patient selection for ECMO initiation should be on a case-to-case basis with thorough clinical evaluation and balanced judgment. However, a delay in ECMO initiation may be futile with poor outcome if irreversible end-organ damage occurs. The current scoring system may help to identify severe, most intoxicated patients (grades 3 and 4); however, its usefulness may be limited due to its subjective nature.[16]

Bridge to Complete Recovery

Cardiotoxic substances (drug overdose or chemicals) may be associated with fatal outcome in the most severe form even with aggressive conventional management. Cardiac function may be supported using VA ECMO in patients having severe left, right, or biventricular dysfunction; refractory life-threatening arrhythmias; or even cardiac arrest with severe metabolic derangements. VV ECMO may be required in toxin-induced severe lung injury to prevent further ventilator-induced lug injury (VILI) and maintain appropriate gas exchange. The duration of ECMO support depends on several factors such as poison severity, quantity and half-life of toxin, and organ dysfunction at the time of initiation of ECMO, which affect the recovery of cardiac or respiratory dysfunction.[17] VA ECMO support may be life saving in refractory cardiogenic shock with severe metabolic derangements even when toxic substance is unknown or there is severe intoxication with multiple substances. ECMO helps support organ function and maintain physiology while the body tries to get rid of the toxin naturally.

Bridge to Antidote and Recovery

The cardiovascular collapse may occur even with poison having specific antidotes due to delay in antidote administration, especially due to various reasons such as short shelf-life or cost. ECMO may be helpful for sustaining life till antidote administration and recovery from life-threatening arrhythmia or cardiovascular collapse. The best example is digoxin-specific antibodies fragments (Fab) which quickly restore the rhythm and improve from digitalis toxicity. But due to cost, limited shelf-life, and uncommon digoxin toxicity, availability is usually limited. The life-threatening arrhythmia may be addressed with VA ECMO support till the Fab administration and settling of arrhythmia.[18]

Bridge to Other Extracorporeal Therapies for Enhancing Toxin Elimination

Hemodialysis has been used successfully for removal of dialyzable toxins; around 140 poisons can be eliminated rapidly with dialysis which depends on several molecular properties such as molecular weight, protein-binding capability, and volume of distribution. Molecules with low molecular weight, lesser protein-binding capacity, and low volume of distribution can be easily removed with renal replacement therapy (RRT).

The ECMO support may be required in patients with refractory shock or severe ARDS till RRT is instituted for toxin removal in case of dialyzable toxin. However, the need of RRT may be used for managing AKI, fluid removal, and metabolic correction in case of nondialyzable toxins as well. The RRT may be initiated by attaching a circuit to ECMO circuit or may be started with separate venous access.

Various extracorporeal therapies are currently being used for toxin removal including hemodialysis, hemoperfusion, hemofiltration, and plasmapheresis with plasma exchange. The selection of therapy depends on the molecular properties of toxic substance and principle of extracorporeal therapy. For example, dialysis is a diffusive therapy through a semipermeable membrane for small molecular weight substances, while toxic substance adsorb on the surface of dialysis cartridge during hemoperfusion.[19] Similarly, solvent drag mechanism in hemofiltration helps in middle molecule removal. There may be need for combining more than one therapy to enhance the elimination. The plasmapheresis is helpful for high molecular weight toxins which are highly protein bound.[20] Continuous RRT (CRRT) and slow low efficiency dialysis (SLED) are suitable dialytic options in hemodynamically unstable patients during ECMO. Peritoneal dialysis may not be a suitable option for removal of toxins.

Bridge to Transplant

Certain poisoning substances may progress to irreversible lung fibrosis where the VV ECMO support maintains the gas exchange as a bridge till the availability of transplantable lung clearance of toxic metabolites from tissues to prevent fibrosis of the transplanted lung.[21] Similarly, VA ECMO may be helpful as a bridge prior to implantation of a long-term assist device in patients with persistent myocardial dysfunction.

HOW TO CHOOSE THE TYPE OF EXTRACORPOREAL MEMBRANE OXYGENATION?

The type of ECMO depends on return of blood through a cannula to either a major artery (VA ECMO) or a major vein (VV ECMO). VA ECMO is similar to cardiopulmonary bypass (CPB) with fundamental technical differences which allow prolonged and safe run minimizing the complications associated with CPB. Systemic arterial blood pressure is contributed by both native ejection of left ventricle and ECMO circuit flow. The adjustment of oxygen blender determines the gas exchange through the oxygenator, fraction of inspired oxygen (FiO_2) determines the oxygen tension, while the adjustment of sweep gas flow determines carbon dioxide (CO_2) tension or ventilation. The final systemic oxygen saturation depends on ECMO oxygenated blood and contribution of left ventricle ejected blood and mixing of native flow and ECMO flow in aorta.[22] In case of absent left ventricular (LV) ejections, the systemic oxygenation will completely depend on circuit oxygenation. A careful upper body oxygenation monitoring is important, especially when myocardial dysfunction is associated with severe ARDS where poorly oxygenated blood from heart is delivered to the proximal part of aorta during peripheral VA ECMO using the femoral artery. In spite of hypoxemia due to concomitant ARDS, arterial CO_2 may be controlled by adjusting sweep gas flow. VA ECMO helps by letting the heart rest while maintaining the hemodynamics. This type of ECMO support should be chosen for toxins having affinity for heart-like calcium channel blockers' toxicity, beta-blocker overdose, and aluminum phosphide, hydrogen sulfide, cardiac glycosides, and carbon monoxide poisoning.

During VV ECMO, the oxygenated blood is returned after gas exchange through a wide-bore cannula in close proximity to the right atrium (RA) where it mixes with the return from different parts of the body, and finally this mixed blood passes through the lungs and goes to systemic circulation. This mixing of oxygenated and deoxygenated blood does not allow normal arterial oxygenation when lung contribution is negligible due to severe ARDS.[23] The oxygen saturation of 86–92% is acceptable during VV ECMO; however, oxygen saturation below this may also be acceptable if tissue oxygenation is maintained.[24] In general, VV ECMO alone can maintain arterial oxygen saturation above 85% in severe ARDS with negligible gas exchange in the diseased lung. The primary indications would be in patients with toxic gas inhalations leading to ARDS (chlorine and ammonia) or in patients with drowning. Drowning in a poisoned patient may be a secondary event following intoxication but becomes an important contributor to mortality and morbidity. Severe ARDS secondary to aspiration would be another important indication.

CONTRAINDICATIONS FOR EXTRACORPOREAL MEMBRANE OXYGENATION[25-27]

The patient evaluation must include an assessment for contraindications. Patient with absolute contraindication should not be considered for ECMO support. Patients with relative contraindication must be evaluated on a case-to-case basis. An important contraindication is administration of lipid emulsion therapy as an antidote. Due to circulating large particles of lipid emulsion, the ECMO circuit is at a danger of getting blocked and the whole exercise of ECMO may become futile. If ECMO is an important consideration, it is important to reconsider the administration of lipid emulsion as an antidote.

Absolute

- Severe and irreversible neurologic injury, intracranial hemorrhage (ICH), severe immunosuppression, nonrecoverable multiorgan failure
- Prolonged cardiopulmonary resuscitation (CPR) or unwitnessed cardiac arrest, suboptimal CPR
- Aortic dissection or severe aortic regurgitation

Relative

- Untreatable malignancy
- *Prolonged mechanical ventilation* (>7 days) with high airway pressures and high ventilator settings in ARDS patients
- Age >70 years
- Morbid obesity
- Contraindications to anticoagulation administration

TIMING OF EXTRACORPOREAL MEMBRANE OXYGENATION INITIATION

The optimal timing for starting ECMO support in acute severe intoxication is not yet established, and further research may throw light upon this. This may be difficult due to multiple variables such as variety of toxic substances producing cardiovascular or respiratory dysfunction, diverse clinical spectra, quantity of toxin, and interval between poisoning and presentation to hospital. The recent literature supports that an early institution of ECMO may be associated with better outcome.[28,29]

The eligible patient should be evaluated by a trained clinical toxicologist or intensivist, on a case-to-case basis. Detailed clinical evaluation and criteria such as severe myocardial dysfunction, refractory life-threatening arrhythmia, severe metabolic derangements, and refractory shock may warrant the need of VA ECMO while a patient developing severe and refractory gas exchange abnormalities may be considered for VV ECMO. The early ECMO support may prevent further organ damage and support other organs as well by improving perfusion or oxygenation.[30] Another important factor is transfer of the patient from a peripheral facility to the ECMO-equipped unit. This should be taken up by experienced intensivists. The accompanying physician/intensivist should ensure hemodynamic stability during the transport. ECMO-equipped transport ambulances or aircraft may be needed for safe transport.

EXTRACORPOREAL MEMBRANE OXYGENATION SETUP AND EXTRACORPOREAL MEMBRANE OXYGENATION INITIATION

The most crucial step and prerequisite for ECMO initiation is securing vascular access to establish and ensure successful ECMO cannulation. Patients with acute severe intoxication, especially with severe myocardial dysfunction or arrhythmia, may deteriorate rapidly with risk of cardiac arrest requiring CPR prior to initiation or even CPR in progress during initiation. A quick evaluation of the patient for assessing the need of ECMO along with excluding contraindications before counseling the patient's relative for the need of ECMO is required **(Flowchart 1)**. The counseling should be balanced, including the destination of ECMO support, complications, and need of other organ support along with ethical dilemma in case of nonrecovery.

- *Criteria for VA ECMO initation:*[31]
  - Severe LV dysfunction [ejection fraction (EF) < 25%]
  - Severe metabolic acidosis
  - Lactic acidosis
  - Low cardiac output
  - Signs of hypoperfusion
  - Refractory life-threatening arrhythmia
  - High vasoactive drug requirement
- *Criteria for VV ECMO initiation:*[32] The usual presentation includes toxic fume inhalation-induced severe ARDS, airway obstruction, or aspiration syndrome
  - Murray score >3
  - PaO_2/FiO_2 <100 (mm Hg) despite high ventilator setting
  - Severe hypercapnia with $PaCO_2$ >80 or pH <7.20
  - *Other criteria:*
    - Intrapulmonary shunt (Qs/QT) right to left >30%
    - Poor lung compliance <30 mL/cmH_2O

COMPLICATIONS OF EXTRACORPOREAL MEMBRANE OXYGENATION

The advancement of technology, reduction in size of circuit and oxygenator, and better understanding of ECMO management have reduced the ECMO-associated complications. However, ECMO in an emergent situation always carries a high risk for complications at all stages including cannulation, during management, and even during weaning[33,34] **(Box 1)**. The common complications include bleeding, infection,[35] and vascular injuries. The complications may be general or specific to ECMO configuration. The complications range from minor to life-threatening situation or even death. The risk may be

Flowchart 1: Approach to acute severe poisoning for VA ECMO support.

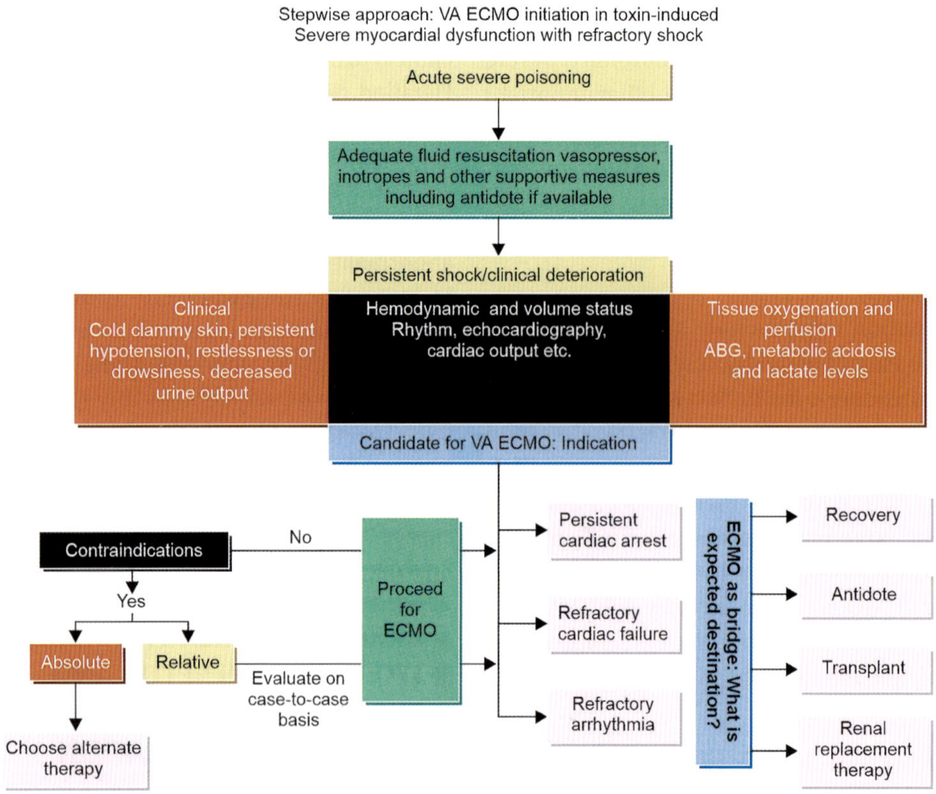

(ECMO: extracorporeal membrane oxygenation; VA: venoarterial)

BOX 1: Complications associated with ECMO.

- *Mechanical complications*:
  - Thrombus in circuit, cannula, or oxygenator
  - Distal limb ischemia (VA ECMO)
  - Perforation or dissection of target vessel
  - Inappropriate vessel cannulation/malposition
  - Air in circuit
  - Pump failure
  - Hemolysis
  - Accidental decannulation
- *Bleeding complications*:
  - Bleeding around cannula
  - Intracranial hemorrhage
  - Retroperitoneal hemorrhage and hematoma
  - Upper or lower gastrointestinal hemorrhage
  - Alveolar hemorrhage
- *Other complications*:
  - Thromboembolism (arterial or venous)
  - Stroke
  - Sepsis
  - North South syndrome (VA ECMO)
  - Hypoperfusion (end-organ injury including multiple organ failure)
  - Left ventricular thrombus and distension (VA ECMO)
  - Recirculation (VV ECMO)
  - Cannulation-site infection
  - Blood stream infection

minimized with vigilant monitoring and attention during ECMO run. The bleeding is attributed mainly to systemic anticoagulation.[36] Acute kidney injury due to pre-ECMO hemodynamic instability and systemic inflammatory response syndrome (SIRS) during ECMO may require RRT, especially during VA ECMO.[37]

CHALLENGES IN SUPPORTING SEVERE POISONING PATIENTS WITH EXTRACORPOREAL MEMBRANE OXYGENATION

The usual delay in obtaining medical help in case of intentional poisoning and rapid deterioration in clinical condition in severe poisoning is possibly create challenges[38] for shifting these patients to ECMO centers. This problem has partially been addressed by increasing the number of retrieval centers and safe ECMO transportation. Besides availability, the common reasons for not receiving of ECMO support in this group of patients are social, economic, and lack of awareness regarding usefulness of ECMO even in healthcare professionals. The major challenge for supporting severe poisoning patients with ECMO is lack of guidelines for use of ECMO in various poisoning. This was difficult in the past due to different toxin substances in different parts of world, variety of toxic substances, and lack of robust evidences in the form of case report and case series only. However, the last decade has witnessed increasing use of ECMO in different poison categories across the globe with successful outcome.

CONCLUSION

The management of acute severe intoxication may require ECMO support in cases of refractory cardiovascular collapse or refractory ARDS. This supportive therapy usually acts as a bridge to recovery; however, it may also be utilized as a bridge to other long-term bridge or transplant in cases of non-recovery of organ function. A careful patient evaluation and early initiation is essential to prevent irreversible organ damage. Since it is an extensive therapy with potential of several complications, a continuous vigilant monitoring is key to successful outcome.

REFERENCES

1. Nigussie S, Demeke F, Getachew M, Amare F. Treatment outcome and associated factors among patients admitted with acute poisoning in a tertiary hospital in Eastern Ethiopia: a cross-sectional study. SAGE Open Med. 2022;10:20503121221078155.
2. Ghannoum M, Hoffman RS, Gosselin S, Nolin TD, Lavergne V, Roberts DM. Use of extracorporeal treatments in the management of poisonings. Kidney Int. 2018;94:682-8.
3. Sauer CM, Yuh DD, Bonde P. Extracorporeal membrane oxygenation use has increased by 433% in adults in the United States from 2006 to 2011. ASAIO J. 2015;61:31-6.
4. Maier S, Rösner L, Saemann L, Sogl J, Beyersdorf F, Trummer G, et al. Extracorporeal membrane oxygenation in intoxication and overdoses: a systematic review. Thorac Cardiovasc Surg. 2024;72(04):288-95.
5. Jones AL, Dargan PI. Churchill's Pocket Book of Toxicology. London: Churchill Livingstone; 2001.
6. Antonelli M, Levy M, Andrews PJD, Chastre J, Hudson LD, Manthous C, et al. Hemodynamic monitoring in shock and implications for management. Intensive Care Med. 2007;33:575-90.
7. Clemessy JL, Taboulet P, Hoffman JR, Hantson P, Barriot P, Bismuth C, et al. Treatment of acute chloroquine poisoning: A 5-year experience. Crit Care Med. 1996;24:1189-95.
8. Huikuri HV, Castellanos A, Myerburg RJ. Sudden death due to cardiac arrhythmias. N Engl J Med. 2001;345:1473-82.
9. Mladěnka P, Applová L, Patočka J, Costa VM, Remiao F, Pourová J, et al. Comprehensive review of cardiovascular toxicity of drugs and related agents. Med Res Rev. 2018;38(4):1332-403.

10. El-Nahhal Y, El-Nahhal I. Cardiotoxicity of some pesticides and their amelioration. Environ Sci Pollut Res Int. 2021;28(33):44726-54.
11. Dickens P, Tai YT, But PP, Tomlinson B, Ng HK, Yan KW. Fatal accidental aconitine poisoning following ingestion of Chinese herbal medicine: a report of two cases. Forensic Sci Int. 1994;679(1):55-8.
12. Fuchs J, Rauber-Lüthy C, Kupferschmidt H, Kupper J, Kullak-Ublick GA, Ceschi A. Acute plant poisoning: analysis of clinical features and circumstances of exposure. Clin Toxicol. 2011;49:671-80.
13. Kalay N, Ozdogru I, Cetinkaya Y, Eryol NK, Dogan A, Gul I, et al. Cardiovascular effects of carbon monoxide poisoning. Am J Cardiol. 2007;99(3):322-4.
14. ELSO Guidelines for Cardiopulmonary Extracorporeal Life Support. Extracorporeal Life Support Organization, Version 1.4 August 2017. Ann Arbor, MI, USA. www.elso.org
15. Guglin M, Zucker MJ, Bazan VM, Bozkurt B, El Banayosy A, Estep JD, et al. Venoarterial ECMO for adults: JACC scientific expert panel. J Am Coll Cardiol. 2019;73(6):698-716.
16. Persson H, Sjöberg G, Haines J, de Garbino JP. Poisoning severity score: grading of acute poisoning. J Toxicol Clin Toxicol. 1998;36:205-13.
17. de Lange DW, Sikma MA, Meulenbelt J. Extracorporeal membrane oxygenation in the treatment of poisoned patients. Clin Toxicol (Phila). 2013;51(5):385-93.
18. Idialisoa R, Jouffroy R , Lamhaut L, Baud FJ, Carli P. Extra corporeal life support in life-threatening digoxin overdose: a bridge to antidote. Austin Emerg Med. 2016;2(5):1029.
19. Mahesh C, Nagalakshmi N, Karanam S, Nagaraj RD, Praveen N, Raja Amarendra N, et al. Hemoperfusion in the management of acute poisoning. J Dr. NTR Univ Health Sci. 2020;9(4):250-4.
20. Murat O, Yasemin O. The role of therapeutic plasma exchange in the treatment of childhood intoxication: a single-center experience. Pediatr Crit Care Med. 2020;21(11):e988-95.
21. Tang X, Sun B, He H, Li H, Hu B, Qui Z, et al. Successful extracorporeal membrane oxygenation therapy as a bridge to sequential bilateral lung transplantation for a patient after severe paraquat poisoning. Clin Toxicol. 2015;53(9): 908-13.
22. Choi MS, Sung K, Cho YH. Clinical pearls of venoarterial extracorporeal membrane oxygenation for cardiogenic shock. Korean Circ J. 2019;49(8):657-77.
23. Bartlett RH. Physiology of gas exchange during ECMO for respiratory failure. J Intensive Care Med. 2017;32(4):243-8.
24. Broman M, Frenckner B, Bjällmark A, Broomé M. Recirculation during veno-venous extra-corporeal membrane oxygenation—a simulation study. Int. J Artif Organs. 2015;38(1):23-30.
25. Terragni P, Faggiano C, Ranieri VM. Extracorporeal membrane oxygenation in adult patients with acute respiratory distress syndrome. Curr Opin Crit Care. 2014;20:86-91.
26. Saito S, Nakatani T, Kobayashi J, Tagusari O, Bando K, Niwaya K, et al. Is extracorporeal life support contraindicated in elderly patients? Ann Thorac Surg. 2007;83:140-5.
27. Kon ZN, Dahi S, Evans CF, Byrnes KA, Bittle GJ, Wehman B, et al. Class III obesity is not a contraindication to venovenous extracorporeal membrane oxygenation support. Ann Thorac Surg. 2015;100:1855-60.
28. Jentzer JC, Drakos SG, Selzman CH, Owyang C, Teran F, Tonna JE. Timing of initiation of extracorporeal membrane oxygenation support and outcomes among patients with cardiogenic shock. J Am Heart Assoc. 2024;13:e032288.
29. Soltaninejad K, Beyranvand MR, Momenzadeh S, Shadnia S. Early use of extracorporeal membrane oxygenation improves survival in acute aluminum phosphide poisoning. Indian J Crit Care Med. 2017;21(12):847-50.
30. Kiss B, Nagy B, Pál-Jakab Á, Lakatos B, Soltész Á, Osztheimer I, et al. Early application of ECMO after sudden cardiac arrest to prevent further deterioration: a review and case report. J Clin Med. 2023;12(13):4249.
31. Lorusso R, Shekar K, MacLaren G, Schmidt M, Pellegrino V, Meyns B, et al. ELSO interim guidelines for venoarterial extracorporeal membrane oxygenation in adult cardiac patients. ASAIO J. 2021;67(8):827-44.
32. Tonna JE, Abrams D, Brodie D, Greenwood JC, Mateo-Sidron JAR, Usman A, et al. Management of adult patients supported with venovenous extracorporeal membrane oxygenation (VV ECMO): Guideline from the Extracorporeal Life Support Organization (ELSO). ASAIO J 2021;67(6):601-10.
33. Zangrillo A, Landoni G, Biondi-Zoccai G, Greco M, Greco T, Frati G, et al. A meta-analysis of complications and mortality of extracorporeal membrane oxygenation. Crit Care Resusc. 2013;15:172-8.
34. Combes A, Leprince P, Luyt CE, Bonnet N, Trouillet J-L, Léger P, et al. Outcomes and long-term quality-of-life of patients supported by extracorporeal membrane oxygenation for refractory cardiogenic shock. Crit Care Med. 2008;36:1404-11.
35. Martínez-Martínez M, Nuvials FX, Riera J. Nosocomial infections during extracorporeal membrane oxygenation. Curr Opin Crit Care. 2022;28(5):480-5.
36. Mulder MM, Fawzy I, Lancé MD. ECMO and anticoagulation: A comprehensive review. Neth J Crit Care. 2018;26:6-13
37. Ostermann M, Lumlertgul N. Acute kidney injury in ECMO patients. Crit Care. 2021;25(1):313.
38. Jesslin J, Adepu R, Churi S. Assessment of prevalence and mortality incidences due to poisoning in a South Indian tertiary care teaching hospital. Indian J Pharm Sci. 2010;72(5):587-91.

3.5 Plasmapheresis in the Management of Acute Poisoning

Priyadarsini Jayachandran Arcot, Aarushi Sahni, Karan Kumar, Suchet Sachdev, Ashish Bhalla, Vijay Alexander

INTRODUCTION

Accidental or intentional poisoning with various substances is a challenge to manage in an emergency setup. In the early centuries, when the theories and concepts of poisoning were not scientifically understood, all kinds of remedies were tried blindly. Such methods included cauterization of wounds, ligature application, cold compresses, emetic oils, and application of vesicants.[1] In the 19th century, the toxicology concepts were better understood by scientists, and they started to develop specific treatments for specific poisons. The active compound in the poison is studied in detail for its absorption property and harmful effects on the human body, thereby initiating the search for an appropriate antidote. However, the challenge increased further with the discovery of newer drugs with newer side effects, thus expanding the horizon for the discovery of newer antidotes and management plans for the treatment of poisoning. Currently, the management of acute poisoning is a combined approach that includes initial airway–breathing–circulation stabilization, decontamination of the toxin from the body, antidote administration, removal of toxin, and supportive care.[2,3]

Removal of toxins from the body must be rapid and enhanced. Such methods include administration of multidose-activated charcoal, gastric irrigation, enhancing toxin excretion by acidification or alkalization of urine, and extracorporeal removal of toxin.[4] The extracorporeal methods to remove toxins have evolved largely in the past century with the advancement of medical science. In 1913, the first successful in vivo hemodialysis was performed to remove salicylates from poisoned animals.[5] Currently, extracorporeal treatments include hemodialysis, hemofiltration, continuous renal replacement therapy (CRRT), hemoperfusion, plasmapheresis, and exchange transfusion.[6] This chapter deals with the principle, indications, contraindications, and side effects of plasmapheresis.

PRINCIPLE OF PLASMAPHERESIS

Apheresis is a Greek word that means "to take away." Hence, plasmapheresis is a medical procedure in which plasma is selectively removed. The first plasmapheresis procedure was performed by Abel et al.[7] Plasmapheresis usually denotes low-volume plasma removal without replacement. When a high volume of plasma is removed from a patient's body and suitably replaced with fresh frozen plasma (FFP) or 5% human albumin or crystalloids or synthetic expanders, the procedure is termed therapeutic plasma exchange (TPE).[8] Apart from plasmapheresis, there are other apheresis procedures where only red cells (erythrocytapheresis) or platelets (thrombocytapheresis), or white blood cells (leukapheresis) can also be selectively removed. In some cases, the entire blood is exchanged (whole blood exchange) and replaced with an appropriate dose of red cell units, FFP, and platelets.

The apheresis procedure technique is based on either centrifugation or filtration. In the centrifugation technique, the blood drawn extracorporeal is separated into various components based on differences in specific gravity. Whereas in filtration, the extracorporeal blood is passed through a membranous filter, and various components are filtered based on their particle size.

Therapeutic plasma exchange by centrifugation technique: This method is carried out by an automated cell separator. The patient's blood is withdrawn and mixed with a citrate-based anticoagulant solution after which it is passed through a bowl which rotates at a fixed speed. The centrifugal force created by the rotating bowl separates whole blood into different blood components based on their specific gravity. Plasma has the least specific gravity as compared to red blood corpuscles, platelets, and white blood cells. Hence, the plasma is in the bottom-most part of the bowl. This plasma is removed in a separate sterile bag. The rest of the blood components are returned to the patient **(Fig. 1)**. The process of inlet and return of blood can occur either intermittently or simultaneously based on different cell separators available.

The advantage of this type of plasmapheresis is that it is faster. All particles in the plasma are removed irrespective of their molecular size. However, the main disadvantage

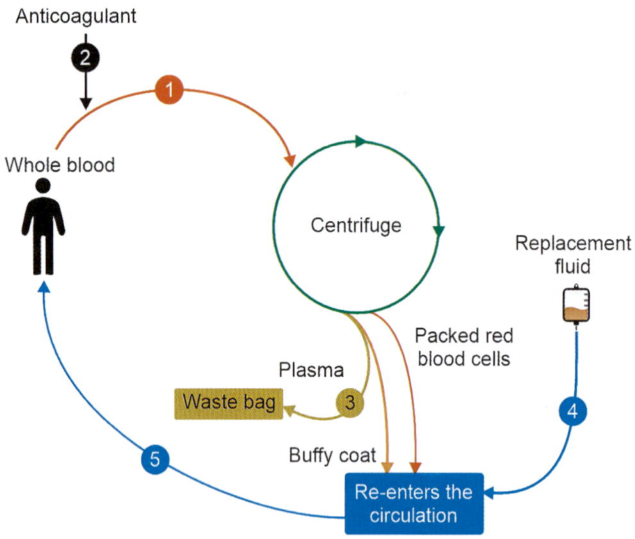

Fig. 1: Schematic representation of the process of TPE by centrifugation method. Whole blood is drawn into the disposable circuit by an inlet pump (1) and the anticoagulant solution is mixed with whole blood with the help of an AC pump (2). Further, whole blood enters the centrifuge where it is separated into different layers according to their specific gravity. Plasma is separated and collected into a waste bag by plasma pump (3) and remaining constituents like packed red cells and buffy coat are reinfused into circulation along with isosmotic replacement fluid via replacement pump (4). Return pump (5) pumps the reconstituted whole blood back to the patient. (TPE: therapeutic plasma exchange)

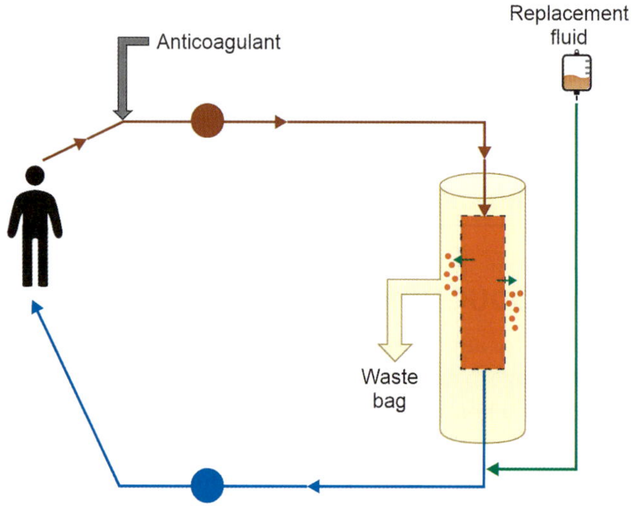

Fig. 2: Schematic representation of the process of therapeutic plasma exchange by centrifugation technique. Whole blood mixed with anticoagulant is pumped into the plasma filter. Smaller molecules like immunoglobulins, albumin, ions, etc., get filtered out through a semipermeable membrane and the cells are returned back to circulation along with replacement fluids.

with this method is that there is loss of some amount of platelets along with the removal of plasma.[9]

Therapeutic plasma exchange by membrane filtration technique: In this method, the patient's blood after mixing with an anticoagulant solution (heparin) is passed through a membrane that is made of hollow fibers and is permeable based on the size of the membranous pores **(Fig. 2)**. Usually, the pore diameter ranges from 0.2 to 0.5 µm. The mechanism of filtration is by applying pressure to transfer blood across the membrane. Although the plasma is filtered and removed from the patient's blood, not all particles can be removed from the blood. Particles with a size more than the pore diameter (like immune complexes, cryoglobulins, etc.) will be returned to the patient. Also, the rate of plasma extraction is lower as compared to the centrifugation method.[10] In this method, there is no platelet loss, but there is a chance of hemolysis when the procedure is conducted with a higher flow rate. The poisons with lower molecular weight are easily removed by membrane filtration.

Double-cascade TPEs: This method is a combination of the above techniques wherein after the initial separation of plasma from whole blood by centrifugation, the separated plasma is passed through a permeable membrane for removal of the specific substance. The advantage of this method is that it reduces the loss of albumin significantly.

INDICATIONS

Extracorporeal treatment for the management of poisoning is indicated when there is a chance of high mortality, nonavailability of corresponding antidote, nonavailability of drugs to prevent absorption/elimination, total clearance rate <4 mL/min/kg, and volume distribution <1–2 L/kg.[8,11]

The effectiveness of drug removal by plasma exchange depends on the pharmacokinetics and intrinsic properties of the poisonous substance, namely its distribution (volume and affinity), molecular weight, the tendency for plasma-protein binding, route of clearance, and in vivo half-life. TPE is mostly effective in the removal of substances in the intravascular compartment, with molecular weight >50,000 Da, low volume of distribution, and >95% bound to plasma protein.[12]

The indications of therapeutic plasma exchange are evidence-based and are updated regularly by the American Society for Apheresis (ASFA). Each disease/medical condition is designated a category and grade after thorough scrutiny of available literature. The category and grade definitions as per ASFA guidelines[13] are as follows:

Category I: Disorders for which apheresis is accepted as first-line therapy, either as a primary standalone treatment or in conjunction with other modes of treatment

Category II: Disorders for which apheresis is accepted as a second-line therapy, either as a standalone treatment or in conjunction with other modes of treatment

Category III: The optimum role of apheresis therapy is not established. Decision-making should be individualized.

Category IV: Disorders in which published evidence demonstrates or suggests apheresis to be ineffective or harmful. Institute research body/ethics committee approval is desirable if apheresis treatment is undertaken in these circumstances.

Grade 1A: Strong recommendation, high-quality evidence[a]

Grade 1B: Strong recommendation, moderate-quality evidence[b]

Grade 1C: Strong recommendation, low-quality or very-low-quality evidence[c]

Grade 2A: Weak recommendation, high-quality evidence[a]

Grade 2B: Weak recommendation, moderate-quality evidence[b]

Grade 2C: Weak recommendation, low-quality or very-low-quality evidence[c]

As per the ASFA guidelines, the role of TPE for the management of mushroom poisoning has been assigned category II (grade 2C). Since mushroom poisoning is associated with fulminant hepatic failure, which may need liver transplantation, plasmapheresis may mitigate the need or act as a "bridging therapy" before liver transplantation.

Envenomation (snakes, spiders, bees, etc.), drug overdose, and methemoglobinemia (red cell exchange) have been assigned category III (grade 2C). An important indication in envenomation is venom-induced microangiopathic hemolytic anemia (MAHA).[14] It is important to differentiate MAHA from disseminated intravascular coagulation before plasmapheresis is offered. There have been numerous reports in the literature, but no randomized controlled trials have been done. In a desperate situation, plasmapheresis may be offered in patients with envenomation with no definitive antivenom available.[15] Removal of the large protein-bound molecules of the venom may help in preventing ongoing tissue damage.

In severe methemoglobinemia, when the methemoglobinemia level is >10%, or in the presence of severe glucose-6-phosphate dehydrogenase (G6PD) deficiency, where methylene blue cannot be used, plasmapheresis may be tried.[16] Plasmapheresis has been lifesaving in patients with severe copper sulfate poisoning[17] and mild-to-moderate cyanide poisoning if the antidote is not available.[18]

For effective management, 1–2 total plasma volume (TPV) is to be removed daily until the patient improves symptomatically. The preferred replacement fluid is albumin, since it has a high protein content that binds effectively to the toxin and enhances its clearance.

Plasmapheresis can be offered, in certain pharmaceutical drug overdose **(Tables 1 and 2)**. In certain toxin compounds like propranolol, chlorpromazine, imipramine, quinidine, and dipyridamole which have more affinity to alpha-1-acid-glycoprotien, FFP is the preferred replacement fluid. In poisons that cause coagulopathy, FFP is the preferred choice as a replacement fluid.[13] In a meta-analysis to study the efficacy of combining plasma exchange and hemoperfusion in the management of organophosphorus poisoning, it was found that there was a decrease in mortality rate, duration for recovery, and hospital stay[19] but it is still not recommended as standard of care and should be performed if all the other options have been exhausted, taking into consideration the risk-benefit ratio.

A working group on extracorporeal treatments in poisoning (EXTRIP) has come up with guidelines on the use of extracorporeal treatments (ECTRs) in severe poisoning conditions.[20] A summary of their guidelines is listed in **Table 1**. It is important to note that intermittent hemodialysis is currently recommended in these guidelines, as more robust evidence is available for the same as compared to plasmapheresis[20] **(Table 1)**.

In none of the drug overdoses, plasma exchange is recommended as the first line of therapy; it has been used mainly as the second line or rescue therapy.[20] There is a

[a]*High-quality evidence:* Randomized controlled trials without important limitations or overwhelming evidence from observational studies.

[b]*Moderate-quality evidence:* Randomized controlled trials with important limitations.

[c]*Very-low-quality evidence:* Observational studies or case series.

paucity of published randomized controlled trials and good-quality evidence since the number of poisoning cases is also less. The indications of plasma exchange in toxins, other than medications and envenomation, are listed in **Table 2**.[8,13,21-30]

Certain novel approaches like poison-specific adsorption columns have been tried. Beta-2 microglobulin adsorption column has been proven to specifically absorb digoxin and may help in the management of digoxin poisoning.[31]

CONTRAINDICATIONS

Conditions like sepsis, hypocalcemia, unavailability of central/peripheral access, hemodynamically unstable, allergic to heparin/FFP/albumin, and consumption of angiotensin-converting enzyme (ACE) inhibitor in the last 24 hours are contraindications for TPE.

SIDE EFFECTS

Although TPE is tolerated well by patients, there are some side effects to the procedure reported as listed in

TABLE 1: Summary of EXTRIP working group's recommendation.

ECTR	*Drugs*
Recommended in severe poisoning (intermittent hemodialysis preferred)	• Acetaminophen • Baclofen • Barbiturates (long-acting) • Carbamazepine • Ethylene glycol • Isoniazid (seizure and refractory to GABAA receptor modulators) • Lithium • Methanol • Metformin (intermittent hemodialysis with bicarbonate buffer) • Phenytoin (prolonged coma, incapacitating asphyxia) • Salicylate • Thallium • Theophylline • Valproic acid
Not recommended	• Tricyclic antidepressants • Digoxin • Calcium channel blockers • Quinine/chloroquine/hydroxychloroquine • Gabapentin/pregabalin

(ECTR: extracorporeal treatments; EXTRIP: extracorporeal treatments in poisoning; GABA: gamma-aminobutyric acid type A)

TABLE 2: ECTR recommended in poisoning (other than medications) and envenomation.

Recommendation		*Poison/envenomation*
TPE	Adjuvant therapy	• *Organophosphates:* Replacement of cholinesterase by FFP[21,22] • Snakebite withcoagulopathy[15,23]
	Second-line therapy	• Mushroom poisoning[13] • *Cyanide:* Unavailable antidote kits/nonresponder to antidote/ concurrent intoxication[18] • *Iron:* Especially in pediatric patients[24] • Paraquat[8]
	Bridge between medical management and liver transplantation	Yellow phosphorus/rodenticides[25,26]
Red cell/whole blood exchange	Second-line therapy	• Aluminum phosphide (fumigant rodenticide/pesticide)[27] • Carbon monoxide[28] • Copper sulfate[29,30]

(ECTR: extracorporeal treatments; FFP: fresh frozen plasma; TPE: therapeutic plasma exchange)

TABLE 3: Side effects of TPE.

Side effects	*Clinical features*
Allergy and anaphylaxis	Urticaria and rash with redness, wheal, and flare indicate allergic reactions. This could be due to replacement fluid, anticoagulants, ethylene oxide, drugs, etc. Symptoms can seldom be severe leading to bronchospasm and breathlessness
Anxiety	The patient may experience uneasiness, sweating, tachycardia, dryness of mouth
Bleeding	Patients with coagulopathy may suffer bleeding during TPE, especially from central venous catheter insertion sites or hematoma at peripheral vascular access sites
Catheter-associated sepsis	Catheter-associated sepsis can occur due to improper handling of central venous catheters, repeated manipulation, and flushing due to flow problems during the procedure. If the patient has a fever within a few hours after TPE, bacterial cultures should be sent to identify catheter-associated sepsis
Hypocalcemia	Paresthesia in the form of perioral tingling, numbness, and tingling in feet are often observed. Dryness of mouth, epigastric pain, and prolongation of QTc interval in electrocardiogram may also be seen in severe cases
Hypotension	This may occur due to increased removal and decreased replenishment with fluids, resulting in an overall negative fluid balance thus lowering blood pressure
Transfusion reactions	Transfusion reaction to plasma used as replacement fluid or packed red blood cells used for priming the circuit. The severity of transfusion reactions may vary from mild allergic reaction, febrile nonhemolytic reaction to severe anaphylaxis and transfusion-associated lung injury (TRALI)
Transfusion transmissible infections	The use of multiple blood components during extracorporeal therapies imposes a risk of transfusion transmissible infections such as HIV, Hepatitis B, Hepatitis C, syphilis, and malaria
Vasovagal reaction	Patients may complain of uneasiness, light-headedness, and sweating and may show signs of tachycardia first followed by bradycardia and hypotension. Patients may suffer from sudden loss of consciousness as well

(HIV: human immunodeficiency virus, TPE: therapeutic plasma exchange)

Table 3. Most of them are mild or moderate which may require slight or no intervention. Around 5–12% of patients develop side effects to this procedure.[32] The most common side effects include hypocalcemic paresthesia, muscular cramps, and hypotension. Severe complications are seen in only 0.8% of the patients.[33] The risk of sepsis and serious side effects, in the presence of specific antidotes, may preclude the use of plasmapheresis as first-line therapy in many poisonings.

CONCLUSION

Therapeutic plasma exchange is one of the extracorporeal treatment modalities available for poisoning cases. However, it is recommended only as an adjunctive or a second-line mode of therapy for managing poisoning cases as per the current published literature. The decision to perform TPE is based on the pharmacokinetics and pharmacodynamics of the toxin in question. Patient affordability also plays a key role in the use of this treatment modality. Novel approaches like poison-specific adsorption columns may prove beneficial for the efficient removal of toxins from the plasma.

REFERENCES

1. Magowska A. The natural history of the concept of antidote. Toxicol Rep. 2021;8:1305-9.
2. Chandran J, Krishna B. Initial management of poisoned patient. Indian J Crit Care Med. 2019;23:S234-40.
3. Shannon MW, Borron SW, Bums MJ (Eds). Emergency management of poisoning. In: Haddad and Winchester's Clinical Management of Poisoning and Drug Overdose. Philadelphia: Elsevier; 2007. pp. 13-61.
4. National Health Mission Tamil Nadu. Handbook of poisoning management. [online] Available from https://www.nhm.tn.gov.in/en/node/6261. [Last accessed November, 2024].
5. Abel JJ, Rowntree LG, Turner BB. On the removal of diffusible substances from the circulating blood by dialysis. Trans Assoc Am Physicians. 1913;58:51-4.
6. Jha VK, Padmaprakash KV. Extracorporeal treatment in the management of acute poisoning: What an intensivist should know? Indian J Crit Care Med. 2018;22:862-9.

7. Abel IJ, Rowntree LG, Turner BB. Plasma removal with return of corpuscles (plasmapheresis). J Pharmacol Exp Ther. 1914;5:625-41.
8. Disel NR, Akpinar AA, Sebe A, Karakoç E, Sürer S, Turhan FT, et al. Therapeutic plasma exchange in poisoning: 8 years' experience of a university hospital. Am J Emerg Med. 2015;33:1391-5.
9. Filipov JJ, Zlatkov BK, Dimitrov EP. Plasma exchange in clinical practice. In: Tutar Y, Tutar L (Eds). Plasma Medicine: Concepts and Clinical Applications. 2018. [online] Available from: https://www.intechopen.com/chapters/60542. [Last accessed November, 2024].
10. Cervantes CE, Bloch EM, Sperati CJ. Therapeutic plasma exchange: Core curriculum 2023. Am J Kidney Dis. 2023;81:475-92.
11. Madore F. Plasmapheresis. Technical aspects and indications. Crit Care Clin. 2002;18:375-92.
12. Ghannoum M, Hoffman RS, Gosselin S, Nolin TD, Lavergne V, Roberts DM. Use of extracorporeal treatments in the management of poisonings. Kidney Int. 2018;94:682-8.
13. Smith LC, Alquist CR, Aqui NA, Hofmann JC, Klingel R, Onwuemene OA, et al. Guidelines on the use of therapeutic apheresis in clinical practice - evidence-based approach from the writing committee of the American Society for apheresis: The ninth special issue. J Clin Apher. 2023;38:77-278.
14. Mohan G, Guduri PR, Shastry S. Role of therapeutic plasma exchange in snake bite associated thrombotic microangiopathy: a case report with review of literature. J Clin Apher. 2019;34:507-9.
15. Yildirim C, Bayraktaroglu Z, Gunay N, Bozkurt S, Köse A, Yilmaz M. The use of therapeutic plasmapheresis in the treatment of poisoned and snake bite victims: an academic emergency department's experiences. J Clin Apher. 2006;21:219-23.
16. Shatila W, Verma A, Adam S. Plasmapheresis in severe methemoglobinemia following occupational exposure. Transfus Apher Sci. 2017;56:341-4.
17. Du Y, Mou Y. The role of plasmapheresis in treating lethal cupric sulfate poisoning. Am J Med Sci. 2019;357:338-42.
18. Esfahani NN, Zoofaghari S, Sigari AA, Dorooshi G. Plasmapheresis for the management of acute cyanide poisoning: a case report and review of literature. Clin Case Rep. 2021;9:e04228.
19. Yao ZY, Wang P, Fu Q, Song Q, Wang W, Liu A, et al. Efficacy and safety of plasma exchange combined with hemoperfusion in the treatment of organophosphorus poisoning: a meta-analysis. Blood Purif. 2023;52:578-90.
20. Ghaanoum M, Nolin TD, Lavergne V, Hoffman RS; EXTRIP workgroup. Blood purification in toxicology: nephrology's ugly duckling. Adv Chronic Kidney Dis. 2011;18:160-6.
21. Disel NR, Acikalin A, Kekec Z, Sebe A. Utilization of plasmapheresis for organophosphate intoxication: a case report. Turk J Emerg Med. 2016;16:69-71.
22. Ayyavoo A, Muthialu N, Ramachandran P. Plasmapheresis in organophosphorus poisoning - Intensive management and its successful use. J Clinic Toxicol. 2011;S1:002.
23. Rasulov AR, Berdymuradov DB. Intensive therapy in bites of poisonous snakes. Anesteziol Reanimatol. 1994;3:59-60.
24. Aslan N. A case of iron intoxication treated by plasmapheresis. Ind J Pediatrics. 2022;89:315.
25. Radhakrishnan K, Thokala RP, Anandan A, Rengan CR. Role of therapeutic plasma exchange in rat killer (yellow phosphorus) poisoning. Asian J Transfus Sci. 2023;17:74-8.
26. Angaraje S, Sekar M, Mishra B, Matcha J. Outcome of plasma exchange in acute liver failure due to yellow phosphorus poisoning: a single-center experience. Indian J Crit Care Med. 2021;25:1020-25.
27. Ozkale M, Ozkale Y, Kozanoglu I. Role of automated red blood cell exchange in the treatment of aluminium phosphide poisoning: a case report and review of the literature. J Clin Apher. 2022;37:320-5.
28. Zengin S, Yilmaz M, Al B, Yildirim C, Yavuz E, Akcali A. Therapeutic red cell exchange for severe carbon monoxide poisoning. J Clin Apher. 2013;28:337-40.
29. Banerjee P, Mohan AK, Baid H, Kaeley N, Khiamniungan CB, Prasanth V, et al. Off with the blues: therapeutic plasma exchange in case of copper sulphate poisoning. Transfus Apher Sci. 2023;62:103811.
30. Shankar JA, Kaur A, Tyagi L, Selvam S, Hans R, Pannu AK, et al. Severe copper sulphate poisoning: a case rescued with plasmapheresis. Trop Doct. 2023;53(2):327-8.
31. Tsuruoka S, Osono E, Nishiki K, Kawaguchi A, Arai T, Furuyoshi S, et al. Removal of digoxin by column for specific adsorption of beta (2)-microglobulin: a potential use for digoxin intoxication. Clin Pharmacol Ther. 2001;69:422-30.
32. Ruiz DD, Miguel FS, Molina FJG, Úbeda-Iglesias A, Pérez AN, Forés RJ. Plasmapheresis and other extracorporeal filtration techniques in critical patients. Med Intensiva. 2017;41:174-87.
33. Norda R, Stegmayr BG, Swedish Apheresis Group. Therapeutic apheresis in Sweden: update of epidemiology and adverse events. Transfus Apher Sci. 2003;29:159-66.

3.6 Exchange Transfusion and Therapeutic Plasma Exchanges

Lovely Thomas, CE Eapen

INTRODUCTION

Acute toxic hepatitis due to suicidal ingestion of poison—overdose of paracetamol in developed countries and of yellow phosphorus (contained in rodenticide) in parts of India and Iran—or due to accidental ingestion of poisonous mushrooms is seen worldwide. Recent reports document improved survival with plasma exchange (PLEX) to treat these patients.[1-3]

WHAT IS THERAPEUTIC PLASMA EXCHANGE?

Plasma exchange comprises two steps: Removing plasma from a patient with a disease condition ("plasmapheresis") and replacing this with another fluid (like fresh frozen plasma, albumin, or normal saline). As patients with liver failure are coagulopathic, the replacement fluid preferred is fresh frozen plasma.

WHAT ARE THE TYPES OF PLASMA EXCHANGE?

Types of PLEX can be classified on the basis of the technique used to separate plasma from blood cells and dose of plasma exchanged per session of PLEX.

Separation of plasma from blood cells can be done based on molecular density (by centrifugation) or molecular size (using a membrane filter). Centrifugal PLEX (cPLEX) allows much lower flow rates to process the blood (e.g., 30–50 mL/min) compared to membrane PLEX (mPLEX). In a critically ill patient, a slower flow rate to process blood in cPLEX may be associated with lesser hemodynamic fluxes, compared to mPLEX. Use of a membrane filter during mPLEX may activate blood cells more than with cPLEX.[4]

The plasma volume can be estimated using Kaplan's formula.[5] In patients with liver failure, different doses of PLEX—high, standard, and low volume PLEX (with 4 times, 1–2 times and 0.5–1 time the plasma volume exchanged per PLEX session, respectively)—provide survival benefit.[1,6,7] Low-volume PLEX (needs lesser resources, fewer complications)[8] maybe the preferred choice to treat these patients, especially in resource-constrained settings. Till date, there are no head-to-head studies comparing efficacy and complications of high-, standard-, and low-volume PLEX to treat liver failure.

DOES PLASMA EXCHANGE REMOVE POISON OR DAMPEN HOST IMMUNE RESPONSE TO POISON?

Plasma exchange was previously advocated as a modality to enhance removal of poison from the poisoned patient.[9]

In a landmark randomized controlled trial conducted in three European countries, 182 patients with acute liver failure (caused by paracetamol overdose in 59% of patients) were randomized to high-volume PLEX for 3 days or standard medical therapy.[1] Overall hospital survival was 59% in PLEX-treated patients and 48% in controls. PLEX-treated patients had higher reduction in systemic inflammatory response syndrome and sequential organ failure assessment (SOFA) scores compared to controls ($p < 0.001$). In conclusion, high-volume PLEX improved survival in acute liver failure, possibly by dampening innate immune activation and ameliorating multiorgan dysfunction.[1]

SPECTRUM OF ARTIFICIAL LIVER SUPPORT SYSTEMS TO TREAT PATIENTS WITH ACUTE LIVER FAILURE

In patients with liver failure, artificial liver support systems (blood cleansing) like molecular adsorbent recirculating system (MARS), fractionated plasma separation and adsorption, and PLEX are well tolerated. Both treatment modalities improve hemodynamic parameters and grade of hepatic encephalopathy. In randomized controlled trials in patients with acute liver failure, PLEX improved survival while MARS did not.[7,10]

PLASMA EXCHANGE OR CONTINUOUS RENAL REPLACEMENT THERAPY IN ACUTE LIVER FAILURE?

Hyperammonemia is associated with cerebral edema and death in acute liver failure. Continuous renal replacement therapy (CRRT) is shown to reduce ammonia levels and improve 21-day survival, without liver transplantation.[11]

In patients with cirrhosis and acute kidney injury, renal replacement therapy (RRT) is used extensively to treat life-threatening conditions not responding to medical treatment (like severe hyperkalemia, severe metabolic acidosis, pulmonary edema) and uremic complications like pericarditis or encephalopathy (i.e., "renal indications" for RRT).[12]

Plasma exchange has also been shown to cause significant reduction in ammonia levels compared to controls receiving no PLEX.[1,6] It is still not very clear if the survival benefit is related to ammonia removal at plasmapheresis or by the anti-inflammatory effect of PLEX, resulting in improved liver functions.

In acute toxic hepatitis patient without renal failure or encephalopathy, PLEX treatment is instituted, if clinically indicated. If the patient has acute kidney injury, requiring RRT (like refractory hyperkalemia), continuous RRT (continuous hemodialysis or hemofiltration or hemodiafiltration), hybrid RRT [sustained low-efficiency dialysis (SLED)], are better options to be considered. If the patient has encephalopathy in addition to toxic hepatitis and renal failure, ammonia-lowering treatment by PLEX alone or PLEX and continuous hemodialysis or continuous hemofiltration or SLED may be needed for improvement.

ACCESS TO URGENT PLASMA EXCHANGE TO TREAT RODENTICIDAL HEPATOTOXICITY ACROSS TAMIL NADU

In a restrospective study in Tamil Nadu (southern part of India) on acute toxic hepatitis, for each patient with paracetamol overdose, there were 75 patients with rodenticide ingestion (1:75). Of 450 rodenticide-related hepatotoxicity, 54% developed acute liver failure.[13] This study highlights a stark contrast between developed and low- and middle-income countries (LMICs). Rodenticides (especially yellow phosphorus) are a primary cause of acute liver failure in the southern part of India; however, the same pattern is not seen in northern or central India.

It is estimated that each year in India, only 50–75 patients undergo urgent liver transplantation for acute liver failure[14] and that in 2019 in Tamil Nadu alone, of 1,584 patients with rodenticide-related acute hepatotoxicity, 554 patients died due to severe hepatotoxicity.[13] Due to this urgent need, guidelines were issued by the government in consultation with specialists[15,16] focusing on affordable, available non-liver transplant therapies to reduce mortality from rodenticide ingestion **(Table 1)**. In the year 2022–2023, 1237 rodenticide hepatoxicity patients across Tamil Nadu were treated by low volume PLEX under the Tamilnadu Accident and Emergency Care Initiative (TAEI) of theNational Health Mission (NHM) program.[17]

LOW-VOLUME CENTRIFUGAL PLASMA EXCHANGE TO TREAT RODENTICIDAL HEPATOTOXICITY: THE VELLORE PROTOCOL[7,18]

The important protocol developed by a premier tertiary care institute includes standard supportive care (intravenous N-acetyl cysteine, anticerebral edema measures), and liver transplantation as a first-line option. Patients not able to access liver transplantation are offered PLEX.

Low-volume (0.5 times the plasma volume, replaced by an equal volume of synchronously transfused fresh frozen plasma) cPLEX has been developed as a low-cost model. Three PLEX sessions on consecutive days are provided. Patients are also administered low-dose steroid (oral prednisolone 10–20 mg once daily) in the peri-PLEX period.

In these patients with coagulopathy femoral PLEX port insertion is preferred. Regional citrate anticoagulation to

TABLE 1: "Hub and spoke" model to triage rodenticidal hepatotoxicity patients to provide access to urgent specialized care under Tamil Nadu Accident and Emergency Care Initiative–National Health Mission (TAEI–NHM).[16]

Time after poison ingestion	*Location*	*Treatment provided*
Immediately after	Nearby primary health center	Gastric lavage (to remove poison)
Next 5 days	Taluk hospital	Monitor for hepatotoxicity or any other complication
Patient who develops hepato-toxicity (3–5 days later)	District Government Medical College	Manage in a closely monitored area by specifically trained team. Urgent PLEX provided for patients who meet indications for the same

(PLEX: plasma exchange)

prevent clotting in extracorporeal PLEX circuit is preferred. Calcium is supplemented to prevent hypocalcemia due to citrate use.

TIMING OF PLASMA EXCHANGE IN ACUTE LIVER FAILURE

Overactive innate immune response is a characteristic feature of acute liver failure. Blood tests like serum ferritin, plasma von Willebrand factor (vWF), serum sCD163, and serum soluble mannose receptor, help assess degree of inate immune response.[19] These factors help in deciding when a poisoned patient needs PLEX. In addition, King's college criteria are used to identify patients who are unlikely to survive without urgent liver transplantation.[20] Improved survival with PLEX as stand alone therapy and as a bridge to liver transplantation is increasingly being reported now.[7]

SELECTION OF PATIENT WITH PHOSPHORUS POISON (RODENTICIDE) INGESTION FOR PLASMA EXCHANGE

As per the American Society for Apheresis, high-volume PLEX is a category 1 indication to treat acute liver failure, either as a stand—alone treatment or as an adjunct to other therapies; however, these guidelines do not state when to initiate PLEX.[21]

For patients with rodenticidal hepatotoxicity, guidelines[15,16] recommend initiating PLEX in patients with severe acute liver injury or acute liver failure **(Box 1)**. Hemodynamic instability is considered a relative contraindication for PLEX in these patients; however, we have noted that PLEX is well tolerated.[2]

A retrospective study analyzed the incidence of transfusion-related acute lung complications and found that <2% patients developed breathlessness within 12 hours after PLEX and <1% had circulatory overload. None of the patients had transfusion-related acute lung injury.[22] This indicates that the non-ventilated patient with acute toxic hepatitis are optimal candidates for PLEX.[22]

The short window (time period) for PLEX treatment opens from the onset of severe acute liver injury and closes with the onset of sepsis or more than two or three organ failure **(Table 2)**.

Daily clinical assessment, frequent (12 hourly) laboratory parameters, and blood tests of reticuloendothelial activation should be used to assess responsiveness to PLEX.

HOW DOES PLASMA EXCHANGE WORK IN A CRITICALLY ILL POISONED PATIENT?

It is not clear how PLEX has anti-inflammatory effects in patients with poison-induced acute liver failure; however, the following may provide some insights into this beneficial effect of PLEX:

- It is unlikely that a single molecule is driving inflammatory milieu in rodenticide-induced acute toxic hepatitis.[23] PLEX may remove as well as replenish a variety of molecules in this scenario.
- In patients with acute liver failure, in contrast to different RRT modalities that do not improve

BOX 1: Indications and contraindications for PLEX to treat patients with rodenticidal hepatotoxicity.[15,16]

Indications
- PT/INR ≥4
- Increase in serial PT/INR
- Encephalopathy

Relative contraindications
- Sepsis
- Hemodynamic instability

(PLEX: plasma exchange, PT/INR: prothrombin time/international normalized ratio)

TABLE 2: The window of opportunity to use PLEX to treat a patient with phosphorus poison (rodenticide) ingestion.

	Days after rodenticide (phosphorus) ingestion				
	Day 1	***Days 2–3***	***Day 4***	***Days 5–6***	***Day 7***
Clinical syndrome	May be asymptomatic	Asymptomatic	Acute liver injury	Acute liver failure	
Systemic involvement	GI symptoms	No	LFT abnormal, prolonged INR		
				Encephalopathy	
					Sepsis
PLEX	No	No	Yes	Yes	No

(INR: international normalized ratio; LFT: liver function tests; PLEX: plasma exchange) survival, PLEX improves survival. This suggests that macromolecules (>60 kDa molecular weight), which are too large to be removed at dialysis accumulating in the blood, may contribute to worsening of liver disease. These may be removed during PLEX.

One such macromolecule of interest is vWF.[24] vWF is cleared by macrophages (Kupffer cells) in liver sinusoids, and raised plasma vWF levels correlate with liver disease severity.[25-27] vWF—pheresis has been demonstrated during PLEX to treat liver failure patients and could be an important factor contributing to survival.[28]

- Ingress of inflammatory cells and debris, including macromolecules, may impede the perfusion in liver microcirculation and contribute to liver failure—"traffic jam in liver sinusoids" hypothesis.[29] This is a potentially reversible cause of acute liver failure.[7] PLEX and low-dose steroid may be helping to ameliorate the inflammation in the liver and reverse the organ function.
- Hepatocytes regenerate slowly (over 9 months). Spontaneous recovery over 3–7 days in the poisoned patient with acute liver failure is more likely explained by recovery of liver function as the perfusion in liver microcirculation returns when the "traffic jam" is unclogged. This short time frame does not fit in with hepatocyte regeneration as the predominant mechanism of recovery of liver function in this scenario. In animal models of hepatic regeneration, hepatic inflammation is an important difference between models of toxin-induced acute liver failure and of partial hepatectomy.[30]

FUTURE PERSPECTIVE

The improved survival with PLEX treatment of patients with acute toxic hepatitis suggests that PLEX may be useful to treat other causes of acute liver failure.[31] Recent reports of PLEX to treat patients with acute liver failure due to idiosyncratic drug-induced liver injury,[32] viral infections,[6] and acute fatty liver of pregnancy[33,34] indicate that PLEX is useful to treat acute liver failure of diverse etiologies.

CONCLUSION

Plasma exchange is now shown to improve survival in patients with acute toxic hepatitis. Selection of patients for PLEX treatment is still evolving. It appears that patients who are not critically ill may have better outcomes with PLEX treament.

REFERENCES

1. Larsen FS, Schmidt LE, Bernsmeier C, Rasmussen A, Isoniemi H, Patel VC, et al. High-volume plasma exchange in patients with acute liver failure: an open randomised controlled trial. J Hepatol. 2016;64:69-78.
2. Thomas L, Chandran J, Goel A, Jacob E, Chacko B, Subramani K, et al. Improving transplant-free survival with low-volume plasma exchange to treat children with rodenticide induced hepatotoxicity. J Clin Exp Hepatol. 2023;13:252-8.
3. Berber I, Cagin YF, Erdogan MA, Ataman E, Gozukara H, Erkurt MA, et al. Early therapeutic plasma exchange may improve treatment outcomes in severe acute toxic Hepatitis. Transfus Apher Sci. 2021;60(5):103250.
4. Kumar SE, Singh KA, Daniel D, Mammen J, Mammen J, David VG, et al. Therapeutic plasma exchange by centrifugal technique has survival benefit at 1 year over membranous technique in patients with severe alcoholic hepatitis. J Clin Exp Hepatol. 2022;12(suppl 2).
5. Kaplan AA. A simple and accurate method for prescribing plasma exchange. ASAIO Trans. 1990;36:M597-9:S14.
6. Maiwall R, Bajpai M, Singh A, Agarwal T, Kumar G, Bharadwaj A, et al. Standard-volume plasma exchange improves outcomes in patients with acute liver failure: a randomized controlled trial. Clin Gastroenterol Hepatol. 2022;20:e831-54.
7. Goel A, Zachariah U, Daniel D, Eapen CE. Growing evidence for survival benefit with plasma exchange to treat liver failure. J Clin Exp Hepatol. 2023;13(6):1061-73.
8. Larsen FS. Low volume plasma exchange to treat children with acute liver failure. J Clin Exp Hepatol. 2023;13:191-2.
9. Schutt RC, Ronco C, Rosner MH. The role of therapeutic plasma exchange in poisonings and intoxications. Semin Dial. 2012;25(2):201-6.
10. Larsen FS. Artificial liver support in acute and acute-on-chronic liver failure. Curr Opin Crit Care. 2019;25(2):187-91.
11. Cardoso FS, Gottfried M, Tujios S, Olson JC, Karvellas CJ, US Acute Liver Failure Study Group. Continuous renal replacement therapy is associated with reduced serum ammonia levels and mortality in acute liver failure. Hepatology. 2018;67(2):711-20.
12. Nadim MK, Garcia-Tsao G. Acute kidney injury in patients with cirrhosis. N Engl J Med. 2023;388(8):733-45.
13. Govindarajan R, Ramamoorthy G, Shanmugam RM, Bavanandam S, Murugesan M, Shanmugam C, et al. Rodenticide ingestion is an important cause of acute hepatotoxicity in Tamil Nadu, southern India. Indian J Gastroenterol. 2021;40(4):373-9.
14. Acharya SK. Acute liver failure: Indian perspective. Clin Liver Dis (Hoboken). 2021;18(3):143-9.

15. Eapen CE, Balasubramanian V, Ramamoorthy G, Venkataraman J, Malathi S, Natarajan M, et al. Management of rodenticide poisoning: Tamil Nadu chapter of Indian Society of gastroenterology guidelines. Gastroenterol Hepatol Endosc Pract. 2022;(2):1-6.
16. National Health Mission, Tamil Nadu. Handbook of Poisoning Management: Primary Care to Tertiary Care [online] Available from www.nhm.tn.gov.in/sites/default/files/2023-02/Hand%20book%20Poisoning%20management_1.pdf. [Last accessed November, 2024].
17. Satish SP, Narayanasamy K, Sambandam MT, Raghunanthan S, Johnson J, Mangaiyarkarasi A et al; Christian Medical College (CMC) Vellore Collaborative Group for PLEX to Treat Liver Failure. The "Hub and Spoke" model: a pathway for urgent plasma exchange to treat patients with rodenticide ingestion induced acute liver failure in Tamil Nadu, India. The Lancet Regional Health - Southeast Asia. 2024;25:100405. doi.org/10.1016/j.lansea.2024.100405
18. Alexander V, Zachariah U, Goel A, Kandasamy S, Chacko B, Punitha J, et al. Low-volume plasma exchange and low-dose steroid to treat secondary hemophagocytic lymphohistiocytosis: a potential treatment for severe COVID-19? Curr Med Issues. 2020;18(2):77-82.
19. Goel R, Eapen CE. Recognizing dysfunctional innate and adaptive immune responses contributing to liver damage in patients with cirrhosis. J Clin Exp Hepatol. 2022;12(3):993-1002.
20. O'Grady JG, Alexander GJ, Hayllar KM, Williams R. Early indicators of prognosis in fulminant hepatic failure. Gastroenterology. 1989;97(2):439-45.
21. Connelly-Smith L, Alquist CR, Aqui NA, Hofmann JC, Klingel R, Onwuemene OA, et al. Guidelines on the use of therapeutic apheresis in clinical practice - Evidence-based approach from the Writing Committee of the American Society for Apheresis: The Ninth Special Issue. J Clin Apher. 2023;38(2):77-278.
22. Alexander V, Rasalam JE, Kumar S, Daniel D, Nair SC, Subramani K, et al. Transfusion-related lung complications are uncommon in nonventilated liver failure patients undergoing low-volume plasma exchange. Indian J Gastroenterol. 2024;43(6):1220-22.
23. Vijayalekshmi B, Choudhary A, Alexander V, Prabhu SB, Sharma A, Balasubramanian KA, et al. Reticuloendothelial activation and phenotypic alteration of peripheral monocytes with enhanced liver recruitment drive liver injury secondary to yellow phosphorus. J Gastroenterol Hepatol. 2023;38(8):1408-15.
24. Stockschlaeder M, Schneppenheim R, Budde U. Update on von Willebrand factor multimers: focus on high-molecular-weight multimers and their role in hemostasis. Blood Coagul Fibrinolysis. 2014;25:206-16.
25. Eidelberg A, Kirubakaran R, Nair SC, Eapen CE, Elias E, Goel A. Systematic review: role of elevated plasma von-Willebrand factor as predictor of mortality in patients with chronic liver disease. Eur J Gastroenterol Hepatol. 2019;31(10):1184-91.
26. Sardar D, Mathews N, Mammen J, Nair SC, Jacob S, Patel L, et al. Rodenticidal hepatotoxicity: raised plasma Von Willebrand factor levels predict in-hospital survival and preliminary report of the outcome of Von Willebrand factor reducing management protocol. Indian J Gastroenterol. 2019;38(6):527-33.
27. Prasanna KS, Goel A, Amirtharaj GJ, Ramachandran A, Balasubramanian KA, Mackie I, et al. Plasma von Willebrand factor levels predict in-hospital survival in patients with acute-on-chronic liver failure. Indian J Gastroenterol. 2016;35(6):432-40.
28. Kumar SE, Goel A, Zachariah U, Nair SC, David VG, Varughese S, et al. Low volume plasma exchange and low dose steroid improve survival in patients with alcohol—related acute on chronic liver failure and severe alcoholic hepatitis—Preliminary experience. J Clin Exp Hepatol. 2022;12:372-8.
29. Zachariah U, Vijayalekshmi B, Matthai SM, Goel A, Eapen CE. Extra-corporeal non-liver transplant therapies for acute liver failure: focus on plasma exchange and continuous renal replacement therapy. Indian J Gastroenterol. 2024;43(2):338-48.
30. Gove CD, Hughes RD. Liver regeneration in relationship to acute liver failure. Gut. 1991;S92-6.
31. Zachariah U, Kumar SE, Alexander V, Patel L, Goel A, Eapen CE. Low-volume plasma exchange and low-dose steroid to treat severe liver injury. Gastroenterol Hepatol Endosc Pract. 2021;1:47-54.
32. Singh KA, Kumar SE, Zachariah UG, Daniel D, David V, Subramani K, et al. Single centre experience with low volume plasma exchange and low dose steroid to treat patients with idiosyncratic drug induced acute liver failure. J Clin Exp Hepatol. 2024;14(2):101303.
33. Li L, Huang D, Xu J, Li M, Zhao J, Shi Q, et al. The assessment in patients with acute fatty liver of pregnancy (AFLP) treated with plasma exchange: a cohort study of 298 patients. BMC Pregnancy Childbirth. 2023;23:(171).
34. Sithamparapillai K, Zachariah U, Eapen CE, Goel A. Plasma exchange improves survival in acute liver failure—An updated systematic review and meta-analysis focussed on comparing within single etiology. Indian J Gastroenterol. 2024;43(2):397-406.

3.7 Endoscopy and Colonoscopy

Gaurav Agrawal, Anupam Kumar Singh

INTRODUCTION

Acute poisoning is a significant global public health problem with 90% of the burden of fatal poisoning coming from developing countries. The World Health Organization (WHO) report estimated that 2 million lives and 53 million disability-adjusted life-years were lost in 2019 due to exposures to selected chemicals.[1] The exposure to these poisonous substances could be accidental (e.g., medication error and unsafe storage) or intentional (e.g., suicide and substance abuse). In developing countries like India, pesticides contribute to the majority of these poisoning cases.[2] Pesticide poisoning is common due to its widespread use for agricultural and household activities, contributing to 66% of the cases of adult poisoning.[2] The other common causes of poisoning include miscellaneous agents, drugs, venoms, and caustic substances. Diagnosis in most of these cases is established in history and clinical examination.

ROLE OF ENDOSCOPY IN ACUTE POISONING

The role of endoscopy in acute poisoning is limited to the cases of poisoning through the oral route, i.e., ingestion. However, different endoscopic devices can examine whole of the gastrointestinal (GI) tract. The benefit of endoscopy in acute poisoning is restricted to the upper GI tract and small bowel in selective situations. The role of endoscopy in acute poisoning could be categorized as (1) diagnostic, (2) prognostic, and (3) therapeutic. **Table 1** summarizes the various indications of endoscopy in different acute poisonings.

Diagnostic Role

The diagnostic role of endoscopy in acute poisoning is small. Endoscopy appearance does not discriminate against the type of poisoning, although in selective cases it is helpful. The color of the gastric mucosa or gastric residual substance can help in identifying the heavy metal toxins, e.g., blue-green color for copper compounds and reddish-brown for iron compounds. The injury to the esophagus in isolation with involvement of other organ systems points toward the liquid herbicide.[3] Also, the endoscopic-guided aspiration of the residual gastric content can help in identifying the type of poison.

TABLE 1: Different roles and indications of endoscopy in acute poisoning.

Role of endoscopy		*Poisons*
Diagnostic	• Identification of substance • Collection of residual poison from stomach	Heavy metals ingestion, paraquat ingestion, liquids, and solid drugs
Prognostic	• To assess the extent and severity of GI tract involvement • To predict the short- and long-term outcome	Caustic, paraquat, glyphosate, button-battery ingestion
Therapeutic	• Removal of residual substance from stomach • Removal of impacted substance • Placement of nasoduodenal or nasojejunal tube placement for nutritional support	Button-battery, caustic, drugs ingestion

(GI: gastrointestinal)

Prognostic Role

The plasma and urine concentrations obtained within the first 24 hours after ingestion are good predictors of outcome in certain acute poisoning.[4,5] However, these are not available at most of the centers. Endoscopic examination of the GI tract has been shown to predict the outcome in several poisonings. Zargar's grading is the most widely used endoscopic classification which was proposed for caustic ingestion though it was also used for other cases of poisoning, i.e., herbicide poisoning **(Fig. 1 and Table 2)**.[6] Several studies have shown the role of Zargar endoscopic grading in predicting the outcome in caustic ingestion.[7,8] A high grade of injury (Zargar grade ≥2b) is associated with

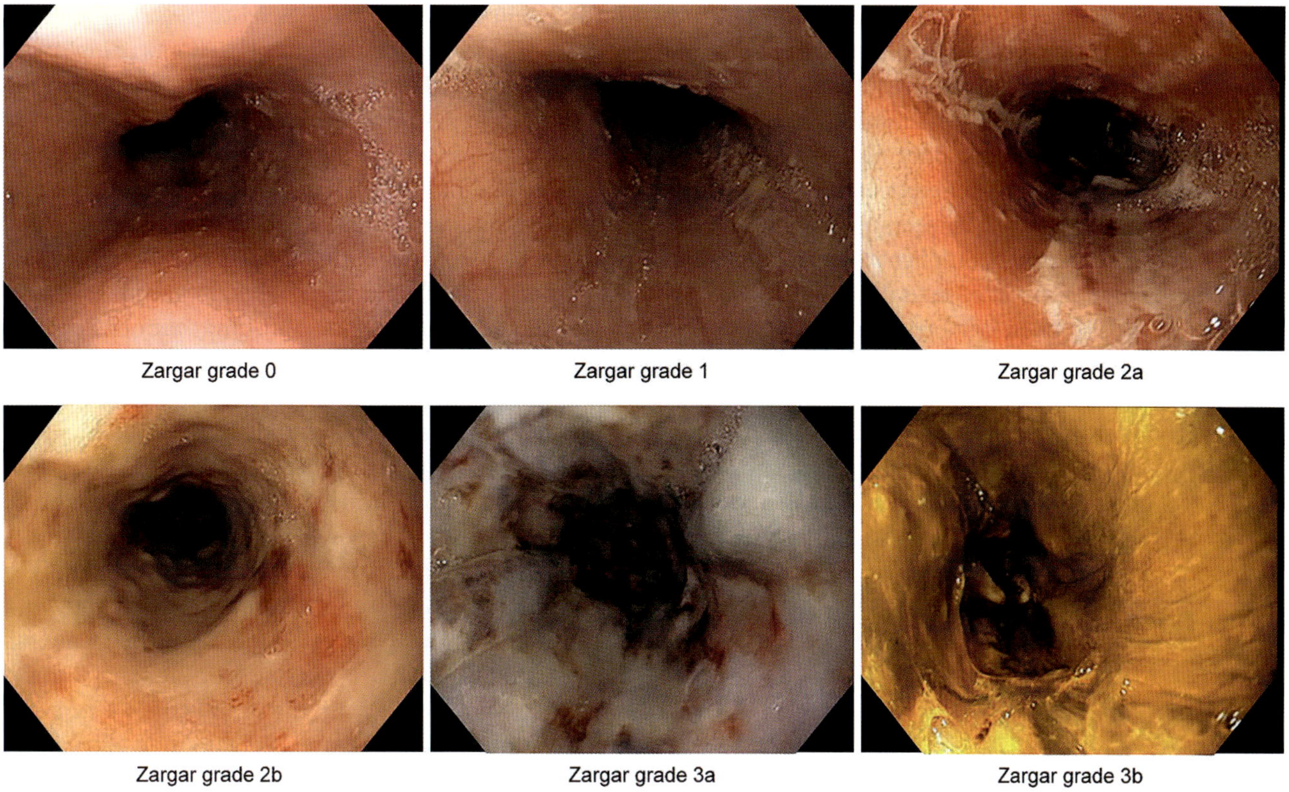

Fig. 1: Zargar grade of mucosal injury on endoscopy after caustic ingestion.

TABLE 2: Zargar's endoscopic grading of caustic-induced gastrointestinal injury.

Grade of injury	*Description of injury*
0	Normal mucosa
1	Edema and erythema of the mucosa
2a	Superficial localized ulcerations, blisters, friability, hemorrhage, or membranes over the mucosa
2b	Circumferential ulcerations or deep ulcerations (either discrete or circumferential), in addition to friability, hemorrhage, and superficial ulcerations
3a	Focal, scattered area of necrosis with deep gray or brownish-black discoloration
3b	Extensive area of necrosis involving most of the circumference with deep gray or brownish-black discoloration

the development of short- and long-term complications, prolonged hospital and intensive care unit (ICU) stay, and mortality.[7]

Similarly, the endoscopic grade of injury in paraquat or glyphosate ingestion predicts the poor outcome, systemic complications, and long hospital stay.[3] However, the predictive grade of poor outcome is not the same as for caustic substance. In paraquat or glyphosate ingestion, Zargar grade ≥2a is associated with poor outcome.[3,9,10] The role of endoscopy also extends to other poisoning like button battery ingestion. The presence of ulcers at the site of the battery reinforces the need for observation for subsequent GI tract perforation.

Therapeutic Role

Removal of residual substance from the stomach using endoscopy helps in identification of the substance as well as reduces the exposure to the poison. However, the benefit of endoscopy-guided aspiration or removal is proven only for solid substances.[11,12] Direct gastric lavage and decontamination carry the risk of aspiration and passage of substance in the small bowel; thus, endoscopic-guided aspiration is preferred.[13] Among patients with soluble toxic substance ingestion, variable time of presentation can affect the residual poison in the stomach. Endoscopic examination can identify such patients and facilitate the clearance of residual poison from the stomach by means of aspiration. Patients presenting in the initial 1–2 hours of ingestion are the best candidates for endoscopic removal of toxic substances.[13]

Endoscopic removal of toxic substances, e.g., button battery, solid drugs, and body packing drugs, also helps in reducing the subsequent complications. Endoscopic removal of the button battery is recommended in children for large batteries to avoid complications. The benefit of endoscopy-guided removal of solid drugs and poisonous substances has also been demonstrated in a number of cases by reducing the exposure.[12] Endoscopic removal of certain drugs also reduces the chronic complications of pharmacobezoar.[14] During follow-up of such patients, endoscopy can identify the luminal stricture which can easily be managed endoscopically. Such benefits are well established in high-grade caustic injuries on initial endoscopy.

TIMING OF ENDOSCOPY IN ACUTE POISONING

There is no consensus on the timing of endoscopy in acute poisoning. In general, the endoscopy should be done as early as possible when indicated. However, the exact timing of endoscopy depends on multiple factors including type of substance ingested, time of presentation, hemodynamic stability, etc. Endoscopy should be performed within 1–2 hours of ingestion for poisons which require decontamination and button-battery ingestion.[13,15] For caustic substance, the endoscopic examination should be performed within 24–48 hours of ingestion for assessing the extent and severity of GI tract injury. For the late presenters, endoscopy can be performed safely even after day 5. For other poisons, e.g., heavy metals and drugs, the timing of endoscopy should be individualized depending on the time of presentation and indication.

DIFFERENT POISONS AND ROLE OF ENDOSCOPY

Endoscopy has a potential role in a number of acute poisonings. However, a few are common in both developing and developed countries and are discussed in detail in the following text.

Acid and Alkali

Acid and alkali ingestion is a common and life-threatening emergency encountered in medicine. The endoscopic examination in caustic ingestion does not help in identifying the substance ingested but has a prognostic role. Early endoscopic examination, within 24–48 hours of ingestion, is the traditional method to assess the extent and severity of injury to the GI tract. Zargar's endoscopic grading is the most commonly used system to assess the severity of mucosal injury **(Fig. 1 and Table 2)**. Classification of Zargar's grading in low grade (grade ≤2a) and high grade (grade ≥2b) helps in identifying the patients who can be allowed orally with early discharge from hospital and also those who require long-term hospitalization. Kochhar et al. showed that patients with low-grade injury are less likely to develop complications and could be discharged with early oral feeding,[7] while patients with high-grade injury (Zargar grade ≥2b) require long-term hospitalization, ICU admission, and nutritional support and are more likely to develop long-term complications.

Endoscopic grading in caustic injury also identifies the appropriate patients for corticosteroid therapy and nutritional support. Usta et al. identified that patients with Zargar grade 2b are the one with beneficial effect for stricture prevention with the use of corticosteroids.[16] Also, patients with high grade (Zargar grade ≥2b) injury would require nutritional support due to a catabolic state. Such patients should be given nutritional support either through the enteral or the parenteral route. Endoscopy facilitates the placement of a nasoduodenal or nasojejunal tube for nutritional support during the same procedure.

Battery Ingestion

Ingestion of button batteries and foreign bodies (FB) is a commonly encountered emergency, especially among children below the age of 5 years. The mechanisms of battery-induced injury can be an alkaline electrolyte leak, electrical current production that hydrolyzes tissue fluids and creates hydroxide when it comes into contact with physiological solutions, and physical pressure necrosis on the surrounding tissues.[17] Damage to the esophageal mucosa itself can result in pneumothorax, pneumomediastinum, mediastinitis, or tracheoesophageal fistula formation and long-term scarring with esophageal stricture formation.

Early endoscopic removal of the button battery prevents the severity of mucosal damage and allows direct visualization of the extent of tissue injury. The current guideline recommends endoscopy in button-battery ingestion as early as possible and preferably within 2 hours of ingestion in high-risk patients (age <5 years or batteries >20 mm) over concerns for unrecognized

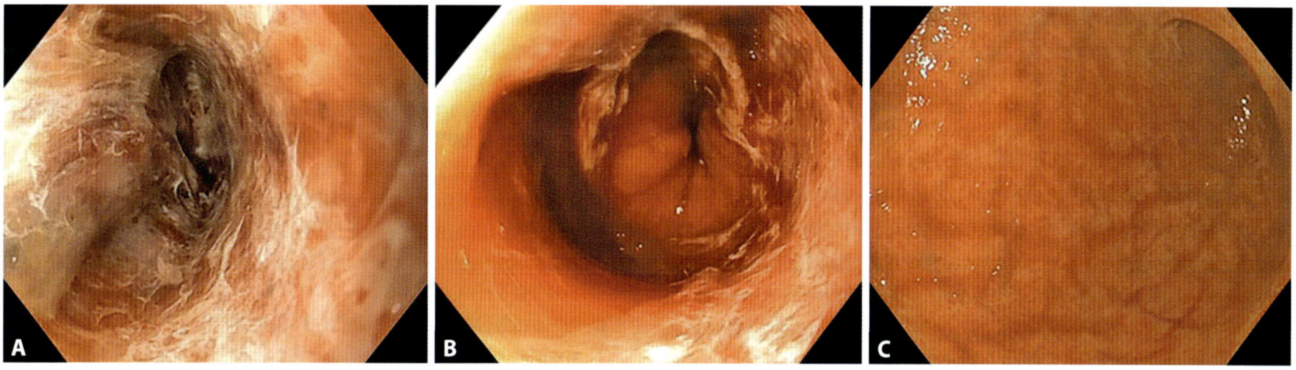

Figs. 2A to C: Upper gastrointestinal endoscopy in a paraquat poisoning showing: (A) Ulcers involving whole of circumference of esophagus with (B) demarcation at esophagogastric junction and (C) normal stomach.

esophageal injury during passage into the stomach.[18] The delayed presentation at emergency is no contraindication for deferring the endoscopy. However, the site of battery in abdomen and GI tract perforation should be ruled out with chest and abdominal X-ray before attempting the endoscopic removal.

Paraquat and Glyphosate

Paraquat (1,1′-dimethyl-4,4′-dipyridylium) and glyphosate are widely used liquid herbicides. Both are mild caustic agents although paraquat is more toxic than glyphosate. These substances produce mucosal injury due to their mild corrosive nature while the absorbed substance can lead to more hazardous outcomes with severe metabolic acidosis, hyperkalemia, and multiple organ failure.[3] Studies have suggested predominant involvement of esophagus sparing the stomach and duodenum.[3,19,20] These features of selective esophageal involvement with other organ system involvement can help in suspecting the paraquat poisoning **(Figs. 2A to C)**. Various hypotheses including the type of epithelium and presence of acid and mucus, etc., have been put forward to explain the relative sparing of stomach. However, the exact cause of gastric sparing and absence of gastric ulceration is unknown. Additionally, studies have also suggested the prognostic role of endoscopy in paraquat or glyphosate poisoning with a higher degree of esophageal injury (Zargar grade ≥2a) correlating with systemic complications, serious outcomes, and longer length of hospital stay.[4,10]

Body Backing/Stuffing

Body packing/stuffing is currently a huge healthcare and legal problem in many countries of the world. There is no consensus on the management of such cases, although a conservative approach and waiting for spontaneous packet expulsion are usually recommended. The endoscopic removal of these drug packets is highly controversial and has been attempted in body packers who have multilayered well-wrapped packets.[21] Endoscopic removal is safe when performed in a highly controlled setting, especially when a packet can be tested for strength against the snare.[22] However, in the case of body stuffers, the packet wrappings are loose and the risk of rupture will be high with endoscopic removal. Several case reports have shown successful removal using an endoscope and thus can be considered for the removal of packets that fail to pass the pylorus.

Other Poisons

Several other common poisoning cases present with GI manifestations. However, not all require endoscopic evaluation. Organophosphates are one such commonly encounter acute poisoning. These chemicals can cause erosive esophagitis and gastritis due to their mild corrosive effect. Concerns arise when such substances are consumed in large quantity. The endoscopic examination is indicated only when GI symptoms persist. Similarly, aluminum phosphide (Celphos) when taken in the tablet form can stuck in the esophagus and result in stricture and tracheoesophageal fistula as delayed complications.[23] All such patients should be evaluated with endoscopy in case of persistent GI symptoms.

CONCLUSION

Acute poisoning is a significant health problem with variable presentations, pesticides being the most common cause contributing to 66% of the cases. Endoscopy has a proven prognostic and therapeutic role in caustic injuries and button-battery ingestion. The role of endoscopic evaluation in other forms of poisoning is ambiguous. Limited studies suggest the prognostic and therapeutic role of endoscopy in paraquat poisoning, solid poisons, drug intake, and heavy metal toxicity. The timing of endoscopy should be individualized based on the characteristics of the poison and presentation, although early endoscopy is recommended. Endoscopic-guided aspiration can be considered in patients presenting within 1–2 hours of ingestion.

REFERENCES

1. Global Health Observatory (GHO) data. Poison centres: World directory of poison centres. Geneva: World Health Organization; 2020. [online] Available from: https://www.who.int/gho/phe/chemical_safety/poisons_centres/en/ [Last accessed November, 2024).
2. Pannu AK, Bhalla A, Vamshi V, Upadhyay MK, Sharma N, Kumar S. Changing spectrum of acute poisoning in North India: a hospital-based descriptive study. Turk J Emerg Med. 2022;22(4):192-9.
3. Chen HH, Lin JL, Huang WH, Weng CH, Lee SY, Hsu CW, et al. Spectrum of corrosive esophageal injury after intentional paraquat or glyphosate-surfactant herbicide ingestion. Int J Gen Med. 2013;6:677-83.
4. Proudfoot AT, Stewart MS, Levitt T, Widdop B. Paraquat poisoning: significance of plasma-paraquat concentrations. Lancet Lond Engl. 1979;2(8138):330-2.
5. Scherrmann JM, Houze P, Bismuth C, Bourdon R. Prognostic value of plasma and urine paraquat concentration. Hum Toxicol. 1987;6(1):91-3.
6. Zargar SA, Kochhar R, Mehta S, Mehta SK. The role of fiberoptic endoscopy in the management of corrosive ingestion and modified endoscopic classification of burns. Gastrointest Endosc. 1991;37(2):165-9.
7. Kochhar R, Ashat M, Reddy YR, Dhaka N, Manrai M, Sinha SK, et al. Relook endoscopy predicts the development of esophageal and antropyloric stenosis better than immediate endoscopy in patients with caustic ingestion. Endoscopy. 2017;49(7):643-50.
8. Park KS. Evaluation and management of caustic injuries from ingestion of acid or alkaline substances. Clin Endosc. 2014;47(4):301-7.
9. Chang CY, Peng YC, Hung DZ, Hu WH, Yang DY, Lin TJ. Clinical impact of upper gastrointestinal tract injuries in glyphosate-surfactant oral intoxication. Hum Exp Toxicol. 1999;18(8):475-8.
10. Yen TH, Lin JL, Lin-Tan DT, Hsu CW, Weng CH, Chen YH. Spectrum of corrosive esophageal injury after intentional paraquat ingestion. Am J Emerg Med. 2010;28(6):728-33.
11. Miyauchi M, Hayashida M, Hirata K, Hirata K, Yokota H. Gastric lavage guided by ultrathin transnasal esophagogastroduodenoscopy in a life-threatening case of tobacco extract poisoning: A case report. J Nippon Med Sch. 2013;80(4):307-11.
12. Miyauchi M, Hayashida M, Yokota H. Successful retrieval using ultrathin transnasal esophagogastroduodenoscopy of a significant amount of residual tricyclic antidepressant following serious toxicity: a case report. Int J Emerg Med. 2013;6(1):39.
13. Miyauchi M, Hayashida M, Yokota H. Evaluation of residual toxic substances in the stomach using upper gastrointestinal endoscopy for management of patients with oral drug overdose on admission: a prospective, observational study. Medicine (Baltimore). 2015;94(4):e463.
14. Jain SA, Agarwal L, Khyalia A, Chandolia P, Kaknale H. Pharmacobezoar – a rare case presented as gastric outlet obstruction. J Surg Case Rep. 2018;2018(5):rjy116.
15. Mubarak A, Benninga MA, Broekaert I, Dolinsek J, Homan M, Mas E, et al. Diagnosis, management, and prevention of button battery ingestion in childhood: a European Society for Paediatric Gastroenterology Hepatology and Nutrition Position Paper. J Pediatr Gastroenterol Nutr. 2021;73(1):129-36.
16. Usta M, Erkan T, Cokugras FC, Urganci N, Onal Z, et al. High doses of methylprednisolone in the management of caustic esophageal burns. Pediatrics. 2014;133(6):E1518-24.
17. Lampus H, Candy C, Rendy L, Rangan AA. Role of endoscopic procedure in foreign body (button battery) ingestion in children: a case report. Med Scope J. 2023;5(2):169-74.
18. Kramer RE, Lerner DG, Lin T, Manfredi M, Shah M, Stephen TC, et al. Management of ingested foreign bodies in children: a clinical report of the NASPGHAN Endoscopy Committee. J Pediatr Gastroenterol Nutr. 2015;60(4):562-74.
19. Chandel S, Dhibar DP, Singh V, Bhalla A, Sharma N. S3270 paraquat poisoning: esophageal injury spectrum at a tertiary care centre. Off J Am Coll Gastroenterol. 2021;116:S1347.
20. Ackrill P, Hasleton PS, Ralston AJ. Oesophageal perforation due to paraquat. Br Med J. 1978;1(6122):1252-3.
21. Choudhary AM, Taubin H, Gupta T, Roberts I. Endoscopic removal of a cocaine packet from the stomach. J Clin Gastroenterol. 1998;27(2):155.
22. Hoffman RS. Internal concealment of drugs of abuse (body packing). [online] Available from: https://www.uptodate.com/contents/internal-concealment-of-drugs-of-abuse-body-packing [Last accessed November, 2024].
23. Kochhar R, Dutta U, Poornachandra KS, Vaiphei K, Bhagat S, Nagi B, et al. Clinical profile and outcome of aluminum phosphide-induced esophageal strictures. J Med Toxicol. 2010;6(3):301-6.

4

SECTION

Antidotes

Section Editors: *Binila Chacko, Narendra Rungta, Syed Moied Ahmed*

4.1 Non-specific Binding: Activated Charcoal

Anusha Cherian, JV Peter

INTRODUCTION

Charcoal, also known as the universal antidote, is the most common agent used for gastrointestinal (GI) tract decontamination following acute ingestion of poison. The use of charcoal for decontamination dates to the 1800s when the French chemist, Michel Bertrand reportedly consumed 5 g of arsenic trioxide along with activated charcoal and did not suffer any adverse effects. Following this, several anecdotal reports appeared on the successful use of activated charcoal (AC) in acute ingestional poisoning without any reported side effects. The use of AC increased rapidly until the 1990s when it was the only known agent that served the dual action of enhanced elimination and rapid reduction in absorption. The steady advancement in the field of toxicology and improved clinical care and outcomes following poisoning led to a scientific approach to AC, especially with respect to its pharmacology and risk versus benefit. Reports of fatality following administration of AC in poisoning appeared in literature and the benefit of AC in these cases was questioned. A better understanding of AC, its limitations, and harmful effects, led to a decline in its use.[1] However, with the advent of newer chemicals with varying pharmacokinetic profiles such as sustained release and modified release formulations and the increased incidence of deliberate self-harm (DSH) with these preparations, there is a need to revisit the role of AC and its applications.

Activated Charcoal and Its Mechanism of Action

Charcoal is prepared from the thermal degradation of pulverized carbon containing materials such as coconut shell or peat. It is activated by exposing it to high heat from steam, carbon-dioxide, or air in the presence of low oxygen or by exposing it to an activating agent like phosphoric acid or zinc. Activation increases the surface area of adsorption by reducing the particle size and making it more porous by eroding its internal surface. The surface area of charcoal on activation can increase up to 3,500 m^2/g.[1] Weak intermolecular forces between the substance and charcoal help in the adsorption process.[2]

Substances that are ingested and stay in the stomach and passively diffuse out from the GI lumen, can be adsorbed by AC. Therefore, AC must be administered within 1–2 hours of exposure to have any benefit. As the time interval between ingestion and administration of AC increases, the bioavailability of the toxin increases. Substances that continue to remain within the lumen of the GI tract and have not been absorbed, and those that undergo enterohepatic or enteroenteric circulation or form bezoars in the stomach, which impair their elimination, benefit from the repeated administration of multidose AC (MDAC).

Charcoal adsorption depends on the equilibrium between the available AC–toxin complex and the free toxin. Therefore, an adequate dose of AC should be administered. Thus, MDAC may contribute to a more favorable AC–toxin complex when compared to single-dose AC (SDAC). Generally, a ratio of 10:1 to 40:1[3] is recommended. It must be recognized that it is often difficult to accurately estimate the dose of ingested toxin.[4] Several factors determine the capacity of AC to adsorb the toxin, and these are summarized in **Table 1**.

INDICATIONS AND CONTRAINDICATIONS

The decision to administer AC should be made after considering the risk versus benefit. Its use should be individualized for each patient. Bailey cites three factors to consider while choosing AC: Potential toxicity or hazard of poison, benefit of AC, and risks of administering AC. The indications and settings wherein AC can be considered for the purpose of GI decontamination are summarized in **Table 2**.

The clinical settings in which SDAC and MDAC can be considered are summarized in **Boxes 1 and 2**. The settings in which AC may not be helpful are summarized in **Box 3**. **Table 3** lists the contraindications for the use of AC.

TABLE 1: Factors that determine the capacity of AC to adsorb the toxin.

Factor	*Effect*
Size of the toxin	Molecular weight between 100 and 1,000 Da. Higher MW poorly adsorbed[5]
Solubility of the agent	Water-soluble agents (e.g., alcohols) are poorly absorbed; poorly soluble (e.g., fatty acids) are better adsorbed[6]
Ionization	Strongly dissociated ions are not adsorbed. Nonionized agents like iodine are better adsorbed[6]
pH	Adsorption is better at a pH at which the toxin is more nonionized (e.g., salicylates are more ionized at a lower pH)[6]
Presence of food in GI tract	Allows more time for AC to act, probably due to slow gastric movement[7]
Drugs causing gastric stasis (e.g., antimuscarinics, opioids)	
Drugs with prolonged elimination half-life	MDAC can accelerate elimination and shorten duration of action[5]
Volume of distribution	Small volumes of distribution may be better adsorbed, however, this characteristic has only a marginal influence
Dose of toxin	The recommended ratio of AC to toxin ranges from 10:1 to 40:1. (*Note*: It may not be possible to administer a high volume of AC to maintain this ratio in the event of very high dose ingestion.)

(AC: activated charcoal; GI: gastrointestinal; MDAC: multidose activated charcoal; MW: molecular weight)

EVIDENCE

A systematic review of all randomized controlled trials (RCTs) published in 2021 on AC revealed 296 human studies, 118 animal studies, and 142 in vitro studies. Among the human studies, the evidence from only 90 studies were graded as moderate or high quality while most of the other studies were of a very low-to-low in quality of evidence.[3]

- *Paracetamol*
  - *Clinical studies:* A large 12-year retrospective study on SDAC in paracetamol poisoning showed that the quantum of increase in liver enzymes was significantly lower in patients who were given acetylcysteine along with AC when compared to those who received only acetylcysteine, although the time between administering AC and poisoning was not reported.[10]

TABLE 2: Settings where activated charcoal may be considered for decontamination.

Setting or factor	*Basis*
Toxin	• Potential for adsorption by charcoal • Highly toxic poison (e.g., verapamil, colchicine) • High dose ingestion • Slow-release formulation • Nonavailability of an effective antidote
Circumstance	Presentation within 4 hours of ingestion
Patient related	• Severe poisoning (e.g., organ dysfunction, acid–base abnormalities) • Risk of life-threatening complications as assessed by a scoring system • GI tract is functional • Patient is maintaining airway and can self-administer AC or is intubated and AC can be given safely • Absence of contraindications

(AC: activated charcoal; GI: gastrointestinal)

BOX 1: Toxins for which single-dose-activated charcoal (SDAC) can be considered:[8]

Toxins for which SDAC is indicated:
- ACE inhibitors, amphetamines, antidepressants (not Lithium), aspirin, salicylates, atropine, barbiturates, benzodiazepines, beta blockers, Calcium channel blockers, quinine, digoxin, opiates, neurolepts, paracetamol, theophylline
- Colchicine, digitalis, nicotine, ergotamine, castor oil, taxanes

Ingestion of life-threatening amount of: Carbamazepine, dapsone, phenobarbital, quinine, theophylline

BOX 2: Toxins for which multi-dose activated charcoal (MDAC) can be considered:[8]

Toxins for which MDAC is indicated:
- *Enterohepatic circulation:* Carbamazepine, quinine, dapsone, phenobarbitone, digoxin
- *Bezoar formation:* Slow-release forms of quetiapine
- Amitriptyline, salicylates, phenytoin, sotalol, citalopram, venlafaxine, lamotrigine

BOX 3: Toxins for which activated charcoal is not helpful.[9]

P—Pesticides, petroleum distillates
H—Hydrocarbons, heavy metals
A—Acids, alkalis, alcohol
I—Iron
L—Lithium
S—Solvents

TABLE 3: Contraindications for activated charcoal use.	
Factor	***Clinical setting***
CNS related	• Patient not fully conscious • Unable to protect airway or airway not protected • Seizures or at risk for seizures
GI tract related	• GI bleeding • Non-functional GI tract • Suspected perforation • Swallowing disorders • Upper GI scopy planned • Recurrent vomiting
Patient related factors	Refusal by patient

(CNS: central nervous system; GI: gastrointestinal)

Another study showed that AC given within 2 hours had the most notable effect in decreasing subsequent levels of paracetamol after a dose of >10 g was ingested. A prospective observational study further showed that the odds ratio (OR) of developing hepatotoxicity was 0.12 when AC was administered within 4 hours as compared to those who did not receive it. Two other clinical studies demonstrated a reduction in absorption of paracetamol when the dose of paracetamol that was consumed was >5 g and AC was given within 4 hours.[11]

- *Human volunteer studies:*
  - *Timing:* All studies that reported on the timing of AC administration noted a rapid decline in its efficacy as the time to administer after poisoning increased. Most studies had administered AC within 2 hours.
  - *Dose:* AC dose ranged from 5 to 70 g and paracetamol from 960 g to 80 mg/kg in several studies and most often within 1 hour. In one study, AC to paracetamol was given in a ratio of 10:1. The reduction in absorption was 30–60% under various experimental conditions. The studies comparing MDAC and SDAC are of low grade of evidence with no significant difference reported in the clinical outcomes.[3]

- *Carbamazepine:* Human volunteer studies showed that a dose of AC between 8 and 50 g administered between 5 and 60 minutes after ingestion resulted in a significant decrease in the absorption of carbamazepine, although no studies have shown a significant difference in clinical outcomes. In a small study among overdosed comatose patients, administration of MDAC (50 g given 4th hourly) as compared to SDAC, led to a significant reduction in half life. The authors also reported a reduction in duration of mechanical ventilation and coma, although the evidence is low.[12]
- *Digoxin:* Experiments among healthy volunteers revealed that a dose of 50 g of AC given within 5–60 minutes of ingestion of 0.5 mg digoxin resulted in a 98% reduction in absorption.[13] The beneficial effect was significantly decreased if AC was administered beyond 1 hour of ingestion. MDAC of 20 g followed every 4th hourly by 20 g resulted in a decrease in half-life of intravenous digoxin by 26%; however, it did not increase digoxin clearance.[14] Another study reported a reduction by 41% when administered in a dose of 25 g every 4th hours with increase in digoxin clearance.[15]
- *Oleander:* A large study compared no AC, SDAC, and MDAC in patients presenting with oleander poisoning. This study did not show any difference in clinically significant patient outcomes in terms of requirement of pacing, atropine use and mortality when the mean time to first administration of AC was 4.2 hours. In a subset of patients, the authors found a significant reduction in elimination of half-life in the SDAC and MDAC groups.[16] The studies which showed a favorable outcome with SDAC or MDAC had multiple design flaws.[17]
- *Ethanol:* In a healthy volunteer study involving the ingestion of 88 g of ethanol and SDAC of 20 g did not show any difference in the peak concentration of ethanol when compared to those who did not receive SDAC.[18]
- *Salicylates:* Healthy volunteer studies involved ingestion of salicylates of a wide range from 30 mg to 3 g. Hence, the AC administered was also very different resulting in a wide range of reduction in absorption. Administration of AC within 1 hour and using higher surface area ACs resulted in a greater adsorption effect.[3,7,19] The effect of AC also depends on the pH. At lower pH, more nonionized form of salicylate is available; hence lesser amount of AC maybe required in an acidic pH when compared to an alkaline pH.
- *Theophylline:* Several human volunteer studies showed a significant decrease in half life and an increase in clearance.[20] However, the doses used were very varied and clinical trials were of poor quality. A total of

25–50 g MDAC given to volunteers every 4th hour after ingesting 600 mg of sustained release theophylline tablets showed a significant increase in elimination even when given at 6 hourly. Addition of sorbitol did not improve elimination.[21]

- *Tricyclic antidepressants (TCA):* Many factors affect the adsorption of TCA by AC. Adsorption is better at an alkaline pH and volume of distribution does not favor elimination by AC. Few studies on patients with TCA poisoning showed varied results following AC administration. Most studies did not show any significant reduction in elimination or clinical outcomes. There are no well-conducted studies to guide treatment with AC in poisoning with TCA.[22] Presently, it has a very low grade of recommendation to be used in poisoning with TCA.
- *Valproate:* An RCT among healthy volunteers reported a significant reduction in the peak concentration of valproate following a 500 mg dose of valproate, when 50 g of AC was given as compared to those who did not receive AC. The authors suggested that a poor aqueous solubility in gastric pH reduces the absorption of valproate and, therefore, delayed administration of AC can still be helpful.[23] No clinical data is available to guide treatment.
- *Phenobarbitone:* Studies among healthy volunteers revealed a reduction in the elimination half-life ($t_{1/2}$) when 30 g followed by 17 g every 6 hour of MDAC was given following the administration of 200 mg of intravenous phenobarbitone when compared with controls who received intravenous phenobarbitone without AC. Volunteer study on SDAC also showed a 97% reduction in absorption.[24] Despite evidence from several studies showing good adsorption by AC and a reduction in phenobarbitone elimination $t_{1/2}$ and decrease in the area under the curve (AUC) when AC was administered, there are no good quality studies supporting improvement in clinical outcomes and currently, its use in phenobarbitone poisoning is of doubtful value.
- *Direct Oral Anticoagulants: Rivaroxaban and Apixaban:* Healthy volunteer studies have shown a reduction in AUC and elimination $t_{1/2}$ of therapeutic doses of the oral anticoagulants when 50 g of charcoal was administered. This effect was sustained beyond 2 hours up to 6–8 hours of the study period although efficacy was reduced.[25,26]
- *Citalopram:* Healthy volunteer studies have shown a reduction in the incidence of torsades de pointes when 1,200 mg of citalopram was administered followed by 50 g of AC. The reduction was greatest within 1 hour and the effect of AC decreased progressively in the 4 hours that were studied where a 20% reduction in torsades des pointes was noted.[27]
- *Escitalopram:* Among healthy volunteers a dose of 50 g of AC given within 1.5–2.5 hours was found to reduce the absorption of escitalopram and decrease the incidence of QT abnormalities.[28]
- *Quetiapine:* In a study on 42 patients who had quetiapine poisoning, of whom 19 received 50 g of AC within a mean period of 3 hours, there was a 35% reduction in bioavailability of quetiapine. In another study, the requirement of intubation was found to be reduced by 7%.[29]

DOSING, TIMING, AND ADMINISTRATION OF AC

- *Timing:* A position paper published in 2005 recommended use of charcoal only if it can be given within the first hour of toxin exposure.[30] However, this was initially based on data from healthy volunteer studies and subsequently, based on a meta-analysis of published studies on the timing in healthy volunteers. The meta-analysis found that the efficacy of charcoal in reducing absorption and decreasing elimination $t_{1/2}$ continued up to 4 hours postexposure, although when given within the first hour, the effect seemed to be the maximum. It was also found in studies that evaluated efficacy using gastroscope that the ingested tablets continued to stay in the stomach beyond 4 hours. In case of sustained release tablets, they could be found even up to 13 hours after ingestion. The pharmacokinetic profile of newer drugs may thus further support the delayed administration of SDAC.[28,29] Another new development in drug pharmacology is the introduction of sustained or extended-release formulations. AC may be useful even if given beyond 4 hours of ingestion in these drugs. Further, for the active pharmaceutical ingredient (API) to be adsorbed onto AC, it must be in a liquid state. The disintegration and formation of liquid state are probably prolonged in sustained release formulations. Hence, the pharmacokinetics of newer sustained release formulation might influence the dosing and timing of AC which needs further evaluation.

- *Dosing:* There are no clear guidelines available on the dose of AC to be used in case of poisoning. Most of the doses described are arbitrary numbers, based on the weight of patients or the total dose of toxin taken.
    - *Single-dose AC:* The most common dose of SDAC that is recommended is in the range of 50–100 g (0.5–1 g/kg) in adults.[30] If the dose of toxin ingested is known, a 10–40 times dose of AC is given.
    - *Multidose AC:* Most studies used AC at a dose of 50–100 g followed by a dose equivalent to 12.5 g/hour given every 2–4 hours.[31] If toxin levels are measured in the plasma, AC can be given until the levels have reduced. It is usually never given beyond 24 hours.
- *Administration:* Activated charcoal is available in tablet (250 mg tablets) and powder and granulated (10–100 g) forms **(Fig. 1)**. It should be suspended in liquid to enhance adsorption. Water is preferred but yoghurt, or fruit juice can be used to make it more palatable while keeping in mind that the suspension fluid may affect adsorption. In patients who cannot consume it, it can be administered through nasogastric tube.

After decision to administer AC has been taken, these precautions are to be taken:

- Ensure that the patient can protect airway and self-administer AC
- Place a pliable, blunt tipped, cuffed endotracheal tube in the following patients and ensure correct placement.
    - Gag reflex absent or impaired
    - Drowsy or comatose patient
    - Central nervous system (CNS) depressant overdose
    - TCA overdose with significant systemic toxicity
    - Overdose of any drug that is likely to cause seizures
- If using a gastric tube to administer AC, ensure that it is in the stomach
- During charcoal administration
    - Minimize lavage pressures
    - Do not exceed 0.5 g/kg charcoal q 2 hour
    - Dilute charcoal with at least 8 mL of water per g of charcoal
    - Withhold AC if bowel sounds are absent or impaired
    - Avoid therapeutic agents that decrease gut motility
    - Withhold charcoal 4 hours prior to extubation
    - Aspirate stomach prior to extubation

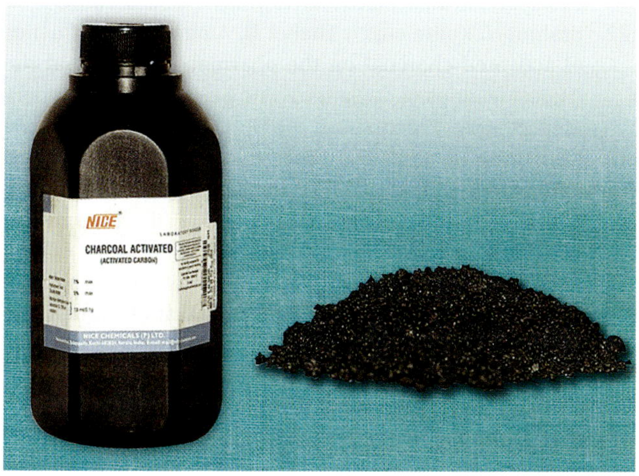

Fig. 1: Commercially available activated charcoal in India.
Source: Dr. Latif Rajesh Johnson, Department of Forensic Medicine, CMC, Vellore, Tamil Nadu, India

ADDITION OF CATHARTICS[31]

Cathartics are added to AC with the intention to hasten intestinal transit time, decrease absorption and help in elimination of drugs. There are four drugs that can be used along with AC and includes (1) Sorbitol, (2) Magnesium salts including magnesium sulfate and citrate, (3) Sodium salts that include sodium chloride, sulfate, and citrate, and (4) Polyethylene glycol.

Among studies done on healthy volunteers, the addition cathartics to AC did not result in any improvement in terms of further reduction in absorption or increase in elimination of the toxin as compared to AC administered alone. There are no clinical studies on patients comparing the effect of addition of cathartics to AC and AC alone in reducing the absorption and enhancing elimination of toxins.

Indications: There are currently no guidelines available to guide the use of cathartics in poisoned patients.

Contraindication: Bowel perforation, obstruction, trauma, or surgery on the GI tract, poisoning with corrosive substances, evidence of electrolyte imbalance, very young children. Magnesium salts are contraindicated in patients with renal failure.

Complications: Nausea, vomiting, abdominal pain, dehydration, electrolyte imbalance (hypermagnesemia and hypernatremia).

COMPLICATIONS AND ADVERSE EFFECTS OF ACTIVATED CHARCOAL

Activated charcoal is generally considered a safe agent. However, it is not risk free and can lead to fatal complications if adequate care is not taken while administering it.

The complications include gastrointestinal, pulmonary, eye complications, and electrolyte imbalances.

- *Gastrointestinal:* The most common side effects are constipation, abdominal fullness, nausea, vomiting, diarrhea, headache, and abdominal pain.
- *Pulmonary complications:* Aspiration of charcoal into the lungs is the most serious complication of charcoal administration and is often fatal.[32]

Aspiration of charcoal can result in rapid progression of lung injury to acute respiratory distress syndrome (ARDS) due to ongoing chemical irritation. There are also reports of charcoal empyema and bronchiolitis obliterans following aspiration.[33] The respiratory mucosa can get irritated, and charcoal can block and obstruct the airway, cause obstructive laryngitis and glottic edema. Pulmonary aspiration is commonly associated with inadequate airway management or administering it to an intoxicated and obtunded patient whose airway is not secured. The complication is, therefore, not attributed to the direct effect of charcoal itself. In a retrospective study of 4,462 patients, 71 developed aspiration. Vomiting, seizures, and alteration in sensorium, and delayed presentation of >24 hours were reported to be independent risk factors for aspiration and not the administration of AC [OR: 1.01, 95% confidence interval (CI): 0.63–1.7][34] The incidence of aspiration and regurgitation of charcoal in intubated patient has been reported to be around 4–25%.[32] Therefore, it should not be administered to a patient whose airway is not protected, or protective reflexes are obtunded. Before administering AC, the position of the nasogastric tube should be confirmed.

- *Eye complications:* Corneal abrasion following spill of charcoal has been reported.
- *Electrolyte imbalances:* Administration of cathartics could lead to hypernatremia, hypokalemia, hypermagnesemia, and metabolic acidosis.

CONCLUSION

The role of AC has undergone changes overtime. Although it started off as a go to remedy for poisonings in the 1800s when not much treatment was available for DSH with drugs and toxins, its use reduced with reports of complications and fatality with its use. Better understanding of its action and the limitations of its use in delayed presentations and complications resulted in a reduction in its use over the last few days. There has been resurgence in interest with newer formulations of medications that have delayed absorption. This needs to be studied scientifically to elucidate the current role of AC in drug and toxin overdose.

REFERENCES

1. Olson KR. Activated charcoal for acute poisoning: one toxicologist's journey. J Med Toxicol Off J Am Coll Med Toxicol. 2010;6(2):190-8.
2. Juurlink DN. Activated charcoal for acute overdose: a reappraisal. Br J Clin Pharmacol. 2016;81(3):482-7.
3. Hoegberg LCG, Shepherd G, Wood DM, Johnson J, Hoffman RS, Caravati EM, et al. Systematic review on the use of activated charcoal for gastrointestinal decontamination following acute oral overdose. Clin Toxicol. 2021;59(12):1196-227.
4. Silberman J, Galuska MA, Taylor A. Activated Charcoal. [Updated 2023 Apr 26]. In: StatPearls [Internet]. Treasure Island (FL): StatPearls Publishing; 2025 Jan-. Available from: https://www.ncbi.nlm.nih.gov/books/NBK482294/
5. Neuvonen PJ. Clinical pharmacokinetics of oral activated charcoal in acute intoxications. Clin Pharmacokinet. 1982;7(6):465-89.
6. Chacko B, Peter JV. Antidotes in poisoning. Indian J Crit Care Med. 2019;23(Suppl 4):S241-9.
7. Olkkola KT, Neuvonen PJ. Do gastric contents modify antidotal efficacy of oral activated charcoal? Br J Clin Pharmacol. 1984;18(5):663-9.
8. Zellner T, Prasa D, Färber E, Hoffmann-Walbeck P, Genser D, Eyer F. The use of activated charcoal to treat intoxications. Dtsch Arzteblatt Int. 2019;116(18):311-7.
9. Lapus RM. Activated charcoal for pediatric poisonings: The universal antidote? Curr Opin Pediatr. 2007;19(2):216-22.
10. Spiller HA, Sawyer TS. Impact of activated charcoal after acute acetaminophen overdoses treated with N-acetylcysteine. J Emerg Med. 2007;33(2):141-4.
11. Buckley NA, Whyte IM, O'Connell DL, Dawson AH. Activated charcoal reduces the need for N-acetylcysteine treatment after acetaminophen (paracetamol) overdose. J Toxicol Clin Toxicol. 1999;37(6):753-7.
12. Brahmi N, Kouraichi N, Thabet H, Amamou M. Influence of activated charcoal on the pharmacokinetics and the clinical features of carbamazepine poisoning. Am J Emerg Med. 2006;24(4):440-3.
13. Neuvonen PJ, Kivistö K, Hirvisalo EL. Effects of resins and activated charcoal on the absorption of digoxin, carbamazepine and frusemide. Br J Clin Pharmacol. 1988;25(2):229-33.
14. Park GD, Goldberg MJ, Spector R, Johnson GF, Feldman RD, Quee CK, et al. The effects of activated charcoal on digoxin and digitoxin clearance. Drug Intell Clin Pharm. 1985;19(12):937-41.
15. Lalonde RL, Deshpande R, Hamilton PP, McLean WM, Greenway DC. Acceleration of digoxin clearance by activated charcoal. Clin Pharmacol Ther. 1985;37(4):367-71.
16. Eddleston M, Juszczak E, Buckley NA, Senarathna L, Mohamed F, Dissanayake W, et al. Multiple-dose activated

charcoal in acute self-poisoning: a randomised controlled trial. Lancet Lond Engl. 2008;371(9612):579-87.
17. Roberts DM, Southcott E, Potter JM, Roberts MS, Eddleston M, Buckley NA. Pharmacokinetics of digoxin cross-reacting substances in patients with acute yellow Oleander (Thevetia peruviana) poisoning, including the effect of activated charcoal. Ther Drug Monit. 2006;28(6):784-92.
18. Hultén BA, Heath A, Mellstrand T, Hedner T. Does alcohol absorb to activated charcoal? Hum Toxicol. 1986;5(3):211-2.
19. Neuvonen PJ, Elfving SM, Elonen E. Reduction of absorption of digoxin, phenytoin and aspirin by activated charcoal in man. Eur J Clin Pharmacol. 1978;13(3):213-8.
20. Lapatto-Reiniluoto O, Kivistö KT, Neuvonen PJ. Activated charcoal alone and followed by whole-bowel irrigation in preventing the absorption of sustained-release drugs. Clin Pharmacol Ther. 2001;70(3):255-60.
21. Minton NA, Henry JA. Prevention of drug absorption in simulated theophylline overdose. J Toxicol Clin Toxicol. 1995;33(1):43-9.
22. Dargan PI, Colbridge MG, Jones AL. The management of tricyclic antidepressant poisoning: the role of gut decontamination, extracorporeal procedures and fab antibody fragments. Toxicol Rev. 2005;24(3):187-94.
23. Neuvonen PJ, Kannisto H, Hirvisalo EL. Effect of activated charcoal on absorption of tolbutamide and valproate in man. Eur J Clin Pharmacol. 1983;24(2):243-6.
24. Honda Y, Nakano M, Nakano NI. Prevention of gastrointestinal absorption of phenobarbital by activated carbon beads as an oral adsorbent. J Pharmacobiodyn. 1990;13(10):597-601.
25. Wang X, Mondal S, Wang J, Tirucherai G, Zhang D, Boyd RA, et al. Effect of activated charcoal on apixaban pharmacokinetics in healthy subjects. Am J Cardiovasc Drugs. 2014;14(2):147-54.
26. Ollier E, Hodin S, Lanoiselée J, Escal J, Accassat S, De Magalhaes E, et al. Effect of activated charcoal on rivaroxaban complex absorption. Clin Pharmacokinet. 2017;56(7):793-801.
27. Friberg LE, Isbister GK, Duffull SB. Pharmacokinetic-pharmacodynamic modelling of QT interval prolongation following citalopram overdoses. Br J Clin Pharmacol. 2006;61(2):177-90.
28. van Gorp F, Duffull S, Hackett LP, Isbister GK. Population pharmacokinetics and pharmacodynamics of escitalopram in overdose and the effect of activated charcoal. Br J Clin Pharmacol. 2012;73(3):402-10.
29. Isbister GK, Friberg LE, Hackett LP, Duffull SB. Pharmacokinetics of quetiapine in overdose and the effect of activated charcoal. Clin Pharmacol Ther. 2007;81(6):821-7.
30. Chyka PA, Seger D, Krenzelok EP, Vale JA, American Academy of Clinical Toxicology, European Association of Poisons Centres and Clinical Toxicologists. Position paper: single-dose activated charcoal. Clin Toxicol Phila Pa. 2005;43(2):61-87.
31. Position statement and practice guidelines on the use of multi-dose activated charcoal in the treatment of acute poisoning. American Academy of Clinical Toxicology; European Association of Poisons Centres and Clinical Toxicologists. J Toxicol Clin Toxicol. 1999;37(6):731-51.
32. Metheny NA, Clouse RE, Chang YH, Stewart BJ, Oliver DA, Kollef MH. Tracheobronchial aspiration of gastric contents in critically ill tube-fed patients: frequency, outcomes, and risk factors. Crit Care Med. 2006;34(4):1007-15.
33. Donoso A, Linares M, León J, Rojas G, Valverde C, Ramírez M, et al. Activated charcoal laryngitis in an intubated patient. Pediatr Emerg Care. 2003;19(6):420-1.
34. Isbister GK, Downes F, Sibbritt D, Dawson AH, Whyte IM. Aspiration pneumonitis in an overdose population: frequency, predictors, and outcomes. Crit Care Med. 2004;32(1):88-93.

4.2 Non-specific Binding: Intralipid

Jignesh Navinchandra Shah, Shivakumar Sankarnarayanan Iyer

INTRODUCTION

Poisoning is a common medical emergency and requires multimodal approach. Supportive care includes managing airway, breathing, and circulation. Diagnosis includes careful history taking and the use of toxidromes approach for identification of the poison. Treatment includes prevention of further absorption, removal of drugs or toxins, and specific antidotes if available.

Limited benefits of decontamination methods and absence of specific antidotes limit their effectiveness in managing various toxins/drug overdoses. Focus of interest, thus, remains on drug/toxin removal by methods such as hemodialysis and hemoperfusion using filters. This method of nonspecific drug bindings by the use of renal replacement therapies is evaluated for the drugs like lithium.

Lipid emulsion therapy or intravenous lipid emulsion (ILE) therapy is also a form of nonspecific binding modality used in certain cases of drug overdose and poisoning. This therapy involves the intravenous (IV) administration of a lipid-based solution, typically soybean oil-based emulsions, to counteract the toxic effects of certain drugs and toxins. It works on the principle of biodetoxification (drug scavenging) with nonspecific binding of lipophilic (fat-soluble) substances, reducing their circulation in the bloodstream and, consequently, their toxic effects on vital organs.

HISTORY

Intravenous lipid emulsion therapy was initially described for local anesthetic drug bupivacaine toxicity in experimental animal models of rats and dogs by Weinberg et al.[1,2] They hypothesized two possible reasons. The lipid emulsion creates a lipid pool that binds the lipid-soluble bupivacaine molecules from the plasma, thereby limiting the tissue toxicity. Alternate hypothesis was that the ILE diffuses directly into tissue and interacts with bupivacaine, preventing its toxicity. The first case of successful resuscitation in humans was reported by Rosenblatt et al.[3]

MECHANISM OF ACTION

The mechanism of action of lipid emulsion for the treatment effect of ILE in poisoning is not clear. One hypothesis is that ILE is thought to act as a "lipid sink," whereby lipid would bind the lipophilic drug in plasma pool and, hence, remove it from target tissue. Here, ILE acts as a "sponge" for lipophilic substances. They can encapsulate and bind to lipophilic toxins, effectively reducing their free concentration in the bloodstream.

Other hypothesis proposes ILE as "shuttles" for the lipophilic drug as in the case of local anesthetic from the heart and brain to the plasma pool, reducing its toxic effect at the organ site. Such IV sequestration of toxicant leads to redistribution to biologically inert site.

Other potential mechanisms suggested are ILE having direct cardiotonic effects involving sodium channels, fatty acid processing and mitochondrial uptake, inhibition of endothelial nitric oxide release, acceleration of hepatic shunting, and cytoprotective signaling.[4]

INDICATIONS

Lipid emulsion therapy is typically used in cases of severe or life-threatening toxicity from lipophilic drugs, such as local anesthetics (e.g., bupivacaine). However, ILE is being tried as an experimental therapy for other lipophilic drugs such as certain antidepressants, antiarrhythmic, anticonvulsants, antipsychotics, benzodiazepines and benzodiazepine agonists, calcium channel blockers, cocaine, and diuretics. Prerequisites for ILE intervention are lipophilicity, low volume of distribution, and low protein binding of a toxicant. The charged portion of ionized drugs interacts with the surface of lipid droplet from ILE, whereas uncharged portion sequesters within the triglyceride oil interior and phospholipid bilayer. The octanol/water partition coefficient (log P) of drug reflects lipophilicity in neutral form. Other proposed predictors for absorptive ability of ILE for a particular toxicant are distribution coefficient (logD) and drug accommodation capacity.[4]

EVIDENCE FOR LOCAL ANESTHETIC SYSTEMIC TOXICITY

Based on numerous case reports of successful resuscitation in case of cardiac arrest due to systemic toxicity of local anesthetic agent, guidelines from the American Society of Regional Anesthesia and Pain Medicine (ASRA), American Heart Association (AHA), and Association of Anaesthetists of Great Britain and Ireland (AAGBI)[5-7] recommend use of lipid emulsion concurrently as part of advanced cardiac life support (ACLS) if cardiac arrest is suspected to be as a result of local anesthetic systemic toxicity (LAST). Local anesthetic agents treated with lipid emulsion for LAST in this case reports/series are lidocaine, mepivacaine, ropivacaine, levobupivacaine, and bupivacaine.

Guidelines also recommend the administration of ILE for patients with LAST who do not have cardiac arrests but present as seizures and/or signs of cardiovascular toxicity such as arrhythmias and severe hypotension. Lipid emulsion should be used along with standard resuscitation measures such as vasoactive medications.

EVIDENCE FOR OTHER TOXICANTS

Gosselin et al.[8] through a systematic review and guideline development (GRADE) process gave clinical recommendations through consensus for the use of ILE in poisoning. This is primarily based on using ILE for cardiac arrest with ongoing ACLS, life-threatening toxicity if other treatments fail, and for nonlife-threatening conditions. These recommendations based on the lipid emulsion working group[9] are summarized in **Table 1**.

TABLE 1: Intravenous lipid emulsion (ILE) in poisoning.

Drug	Situation	Level of recommendation
Local anesthetics	• In cardiac arrest after standard ACLS • In life-threatening toxicity, as a part of treatment modality if other treatment fails • Nonlife-threatening toxicity	• Recommended (1D) • Suggested (1D) • Neutral (2D)
• Antidysrhythmics • Amitriptyline • Other tricyclics • Baclofen • Beta-blockers • Bupropion • Calcium-channel blockers • Cocaine • Lamotrigine • Olanzapine • Other antipsychotics • Selective serotonin reuptake inhibitors	• In cardiac arrest after standard ACLS • In life-threatening toxicity, as a part of treatment modality if other treatment fails • Nonlife-threatening toxicity	• Neutral (2D) • Neutral (2D) • Suggest not to use (2D)

TIMING OF ADMINISTRATION

Cardiac arrest occurs due to LAST or periarrest conditions such as arrhythmias or severe hypotension or seizures. Other toxicants indications are elaborated in **Table 1**.

Preparation

Intravenous lipid emulsions are sterile preparation of 200–600 nm sized droplets of triglyceride oil in water, which are stabilized with the surfactant phospholipid. The commonly available preparation of 20% lipid emulsion (e.g., intralipid) contains soybean oil and egg-yolk phospholipids and should not be used in patients with a history of allergies to egg or soybean. Lipid emulsion should be administered by IV infusion only, but intraosseous administration has been reported in a case where IV access was not possible.

Propofol (prepared in 10% lipid emulsion) is readily available in operating rooms but not a suitable alternative to 20% lipid emulsion because of its significant cardiovascular depressant effects, leading to hypotension.

Dose

Optimal dose of ILE for LAST is not determined through studies. Also, whether effect of ILE in LAST is dose related is not evaluated. The ASRA guideline[5] recommends a dose of 100 mL over 2–3 minutes for patients >70 kg and 1.5 mL/kg for patients <70 kg (lean body weight). This is followed by infusion at the rate of 0.25 mL/kg/min for at least 10 minutes after hemodynamic stability is achieved. A repeat bolus is recommended if there is persistent cardiovascular instability. Maximum total dose recommended is 12 mL/kg.

Though these dose recommendations are for bupivacaine, same dose is used for other local anesthetic agents. Peak levels of bupivacaine have been reported to occur up to 36 hours depending on injection site; extended infusions may be required if hemodynamic instability continues.

Administration

Lipid emulsion is administered intravenously. The specific dosing and rate of infusion depend on the patient's condition and toxic agent involved. Lipid emulsion is typically administered through a central venous catheter to minimize the risk of complications.

Monitoring

Patients receiving ILE therapy should be continuously monitored for their vital signs, cardiac rhythm, and the response to treatment.

ADVERSE EFFECTS

Dyslipidemias, allergic reactions, hyperlipidemia-induced pancreatitis, infections, thrombophlebitis with peripheral use, and fat embolism have been reported with prolonged lipid emulsion infusions. There are concerns of increased inflammation, oxidative stress, modulation of cell-mediated immunity, and acute respiratory distress syndrome (ARDS) with prolonged infusions of ILE.

Other issues with prolonged lipid emulsion infusions are preanalytical errors in laboratory samples and deposition in renal replacement therapy/extracorporeal membrane oxygenator circuits.

CONCLUSION

Despite physiological rationale, literature does not support the role of ILE as widely established treatment modality in cases of poisoning beyond its indication in LAST. It is important to note that ILE therapy is not a universal antidote for all poisonings and overdoses. The decision to use this therapy should be made on a case-by-case basis, considering the specific toxins involved, the patient's condition, and other treatment options.

REFERENCES

1. Weinberg GL, VadeBoncouer T, Ramaraju GA, Garcia-Amaro MF, Cwik M. Pretreatment or resuscitation with a lipid infusion shifts the dose-response to bupivacaine-induced asystole in rats. Anesthesiology. 1998;88:1071-5.
2. Weinberg G, Ripper R, Feinstein DL, Hoffman W. Lipid emulsion infusion rescues dogs from bupivacaine-induced cardiac toxicity. Reg Anesth Pain Med. 2003;28:198-202.
3. Rosenblatt MA, Abel M, Fischer GW, Itzkovich CJ, Eisenkraft JB. Successful use of a 20% lipid emulsion to resuscitate a patient after a presumed bupivacaine-related cardiac arrest. Anesthesiology. 2006;105(1):217-8.
4. Jaffal K, Chevillard L, Mégarbane B. Lipid emulsion to treat acute poisonings: mechanisms of action, indications, and controversies. Pharmaceutics. 2023;15(5):1396.
5. Neal JM, Bernards CM, Butterworth JF, Di Gregorio G, Drasner K, Hejtmanek MR, et al. ASRA Practice Advisory on Local Anesthetic Systemic Toxicity. Reg Anesth Pain Med. 2010;35:152-61.
6. Macfarlane AJR, Gitman M, Bornstein KJ, El-Boghdadly K, Weinberg G. Updates in our understanding of local anaesthetic systemic toxicity: a narrative review. Anaesthesia. 2021;76:27-39.
7. Christie LE, Picard J, Weinberg GL. Local anaesthetic systemic toxicity. BJA Education. 2014;15(3):136-42.
8. Gosselin S, Hoegberg LCG, Hoffman RS, Graudins A, Stork CM, Thomas SHL, et al. Evidence-based recommendations on the use of intravenous lipid emulsion therapy in poisoning. Clin Toxicol (Phila). 2016;54(10):899-923.
9. Levine M, Hoffman RS, Lavergne V, Stork CM, Graudins A, Chuang R, et al. Systematic review of the effect of intravenous lipid emulsion therapy for non-local anesthetics toxicity. Clin Toxicol (Phila). 2016;54(3):194-221.

4.3 Specific Binding: Chelating Agents–1 (Deferoxamine, EDTA)

Cynthia Habib, Tharwat El Zahran

INTRODUCTION

Exposure to heavy metal can be unintentional due to the use of contaminated groundwater, vegetables, meat, and seafood. Accidental exposure to metal fumes may also result in acute toxicity. Acute toxicity may occur due to intentional/unintentional exposure to a large amount; however, most of the cases are due to chronic low-dose exposure due to unintentional exposure. Removal from the source will suffice in many cases; however, some of the heavy metal poisonings need to be treated using specific antidotes. We discuss here two specific antidotes.

DEFEROXAMINE

Chemical and Biological Properties

Deferoxamine (DFO) or (desferrioxamine B) is a water-soluble hexadentate chelator with a molecular weight of 561 Da, available since 1960s. It is used to treat patients with acute iron overdose or those with transfusion-dependent anemias that lead to chronic iron overload.[1]

Ferrioxamine is a brownish compound made up of three trihydroxamic acid molecules and trivalent iron (ferric, Fe^{3+}) and is isolated from *Streptomyces pilosus*, a soil bacterium. When the trivalent iron is removed from ferrioxamine B, it results in the colorless compound deferoxamine. DFO works in treating iron toxicity by binding trivalent (ferric) iron (for which it has a strong affinity), forming ferrioxamine, a stable complex, which is eliminated via the kidneys.[1]

Iron Metabolism and Overload

Iron is essential for various metabolic processes in the human body, including oxygen transport, oxidative energy production, and immune system function. Excessive iron deposits can cause organ damage due to the generation of free oxygen radicals. Chronic iron overload can result from genetic mutations, such as in hemochromatosis, transfusion-related reactions, hemolytic reactions, or excessive dietary intake.

In these conditions, iron can accumulate in organs such as heart, liver, and endocrine glands, leading to end-organ damage.[2] Managing iron overdose is crucial for improving the quality of life of patient with acute overdose and those with inherited diseases. Normal plasma iron levels range between 12 and 25 μM/L. Maintaining appropriate dietary iron absorption is essential for regulating iron levels in the body.

In hereditary hemochromatosis, elevated plasma iron levels are linked to hepcidin production. The hereditary hemochromatosis protein regulates hepcidin production based on its binding to transferrin receptor 1 (TFR1). When TFR1 is bound, hepcidin production decreases, resulting in elevated serum iron levels.[2]

Whenever iron toxicity is suspected in chronic states, serum ferritin levels are measured rather than iron levels. A serum ferritin >300 ng/mL in males and >150–200 ng/mL in menstruating females raise suspicion for iron overload. Ferritin is also an acute phase reactant; therefore, the need to test other parameters such as total iron-binding capacity (TIBC) and serum transferrin percentage arises. A transferrin saturation >45% combined with high serum ferritin indicates a classic case of hemochromatosis.[2]

In acute iron toxicity, serum iron levels are most accurately measured at 4–6 hours postingestion or 6–8 hours if the tablets ingested are enterically coated or of sustained release. Iron is rapidly cleared from the bloodstream into the liver, so improper timing of the measurement may result in false negative results. Serum iron levels can indicate the severity of toxicity: Minimal (<350 μg/dL), moderate (350–500 μg/dL), or severe (>500 μg/dL).

Mechanism of Action

Its mechanism of action is crucial in patients with iron poisoning, as it chelates free iron during its transit between transferrin and ferritin. DFO does not directly affect the iron bound to transferrin, hemoglobin, or cytochromes. Ferritin stores iron and transfers it through the serum via transferrin. The human body does not physiologically excrete iron; instead, iron regulation is managed by the gastrointestinal (GI) system through the modification of hepcidin levels, which can prevent cell toxicity.

When iron stores are saturated, free iron disseminates in the human plasma.[3] The excess iron generates free radicals that damage deoxyribonucleic acid (DNA), causing cellular damage, and inhibit oxidative phosphorylation by inducing acidosis. The hexadentate formulation of DFO helps in iron toxicity by binding iron at 1:1 ratio. DFO binds Fe^{3+} at the 3NOH sites creating an octahedral iron complex. This binding targets the nontransferrin bound iron found in the plasma after transferrin saturation, benefiting patients with acute or chronic iron overdose.[1] In the acute phase, DFO binds and inactivates cytoplasmic and lysosomal iron through endocytosis, preventing further mitochondrial dysfunction. In the chronic phase, DFO slows the accumulation of iron in the hepatocytes, preventing hepatic fibrosis.[1] Iron bound to DFO is then excreted via urine or bile.[3]

Clinical Presentation

Patients with acute lead poisoning usually present with GI symptoms such as pain in abdomen and vomiting. A large overdose may result in encephalopathy. Patients presenting with GI symptoms or with signs of instability (hypotension, encephalopathy) are admitted in intensive care units for the appropriate treatment. Management of severe toxicity includes intravenous hydration and administration of a chelating agent such as DFO. Some patients may require whole bowel irrigation or gastric lavage if a large dose has been ingested, patient has reported early (within 1–2 hours), and a number of pills are visible on the abdominal X-ray.

Dosage and Administration

Deferoxamine is administered as a continuous infusion at a rate of 15 mg/kg/h for the first 24 hours, with a maximum rate reaching 35 mg/kg/h. One should not exceed a maximum daily dose of 6 g/24 h. Blood pressure should be monitored during the DFO infusion **(Table 1)**.[1]

Patients can be discharged if they remain asymptomatic for 6–12 hours or have only mild GI symptoms without any metabolic disturbances and serum iron levels below 350 μg/dL.[4] When DFO chelates with iron, it forms ferrioxamine, a water-soluble compound, which produces rose-colored urine. This can help detect the amount of DFO present in the patient's serum, indirectly indicating compliance. Another method for monitoring involves measuring the urine iron-to-creatinine ratio, which tracks the iron excretion into the urine while patients are on DFO therapy.[1]

Deferoxamine is also used for treating iron and aluminum toxicity, although its use in aluminum toxicity is currently off-label.[4]

TABLE 1: Dosage and indications.

Drug/chelator	*Indication*	*Dosage*	*IM/SC*	*IV*
EDTA ($CaNa_2EDTA$)	Lead poisoning	• Daily dose of 1,000 mg/m for 5 days • Repeat dose after 48–72 hours	Total dose divided in 3, given every 8 hours with lidocaine	• Total dose diluted in 5% dextrose or normal saline, concentration <0.5% • Given slowly, over 8–12 hours
DFO	Iron and aluminum	• 40–60 mg/kg/day is given for 4–5 days per week • Total dose should not exceed 2.5 g daily	10% DFO solution administered subcutaneously over 8–12 hours	Slow IV at a rate of not >15 mg/kg to a maximum of 80 mg/kg per 24 hours

(DFO: deferoxamine; EDTA: ethylenediaminetetraacetic acid; IV: intravenous; IM: intramuscular; SC: subcutaneous)

Aluminum is widely used by humans and in various industries, becoming a global health concern due its high toxicity, which can lead to lethal poisoning. Aluminum can be found in drinking water, medicines, food byproducts, deodorants, cosmetics, home appliances, buildings, industrial companies, and many equipment.

Chronic exposure to aluminum has multiple side effects, including disruption of DNA repair, inhibition of certain enzymes, alteration of protein synthesis, decreased activity of antioxidants, increased reactive oxygen species, and disruption of the cellular hemostasis of iron. Consequently, aluminum toxicity can cause multiorgan damage, affecting the blood, kidneys, liver, respiratory and nervous systems, and can be detected in urine, hair, nails, and sweat.[5] Aluminum enters the bloodstream through passive diffusion or active transport.

Deodorants containing aluminum deposit in the eccrine sweat glands, forming insoluble aluminum hydroxide, which blocks sweat secretion by loosening sweat plaques. Approximately 90% of aluminum in plasma is bound to transferrin, with 60% stored in bone (within the mitochondria of osteoblasts), 25% in the lungs, 10% in the muscles, and 3% in the liver. High levels of aluminum can be lethal, leading to multiorgan failure.[5]

Although aluminum is found in dialysis fluid, the safe level is yet to be determined due to the complexity of the physiochemistry of this mode of transfer.[6] The National Kidney Foundation Kidney Disease Outcomes Quality Initiative (NKF KDOQI) recommends using DFO in dialysis patients when aluminum concentrations reach 60–200 µg/L. In chronic dialysis patients, a 5 mg/kg dose of DFO is administered before their dialysis session. In acute toxicity, a dose of 15 mg/kg is given.[5]

Deferoxamine is the preferred chelating agents used to reduce aluminum toxicity. DFO binds aluminum deposited in tissues and plasma, forming aluminoxane, which is renally excreted. DFO can be administered intravenously, intramuscularly, or subcutaneously due to its low GI absorption. It is rarely given orally. The IV route is preferred in acute and life-threatening cases, while the subcutaneous route is favored in patients with chronic iron overload.[3] At very high levels of serum aluminum (<200 µg/L), administration of DFO may lead to mobilization from the tissues, resulting in very high serum aluminum levels causing neurotoxicity.[4]

Adverse Effects

Deferoxamine has multiple common side effects that range from GI disturbances to anaphylaxis to skin manifestations. DFO therapy should not be used for >24 hours due to its potential side effects, which are mostly observed within chronic use.

Sensorineural hearing loss and damage to the retinal epithelium have been reported with prolonged DFO therapy. Both hearing and vision loss are reversible if the drug is promptly discontinued. Children on chronic DFO therapy should be monitored for growth velocity,[4] as a study has reported growth retardation due to the toxic effects of unchelated DFO.[7] This usually happens in thalassemic patients; therefore, DFO should be initiated only when iron accumulation reaches a critical level.[7]

Deferoxamine can also increase the risk for bacterial and fungal infections, such as mucormycosis, *Yersinia*, and *Vibrio*. Additionally, DFO can also lead to acute respiratory distress syndrome when administered for >24 hours via an IV infusion. Therefore, administering <2.5 g of DFO daily and closely monitoring the therapeutic index are the safest ways to manage potential complications.[4] Increased risk of pulmonary complications following high-dose DFO therapy when administered in the presence of high concentrations of oxygen have been reported. It is attributed to the oxygen-free radical toxicity pathway.[1]

ETHYLENEDIAMINETETRAACETIC ACID

Introduction

Ethylenediaminetetraacetic acid (EDTA), also known as edetate calcium disodium or calcium disodium versenate, is a chelating agent that can bind to various metal ions such as calcium, magnesium, lead, or iron.[8] EDTA was synthesized in the mid-1930s to be used as a pharmacological or nonpharmacological chemical.

Chemistry

When used pharmacologically, EDTA is used as calcium disodium edetate, which prevents it from binding to calcium. When used as edetate disodium, it binds to calcium, preventing blood samples from clotting and making them ideal for testing by not distorting red blood cells. This form of EDTA poses a high risk of hypocalcemia, which can lead to serious seizures or cardiac arrest, making it less commonly used today.[9,10] In the industrial field, EDTA is used in cosmetic and food industries to chelate toxic metal ions and remove them from products. This application of EDTA is considered as nonpharmacological.[10]

Ethylenediaminetetraacetic acid, used as calcium disodium EDTA, is an ionic water-soluble compound with a molecular weight of 374.27 Da.[1] This form of EDTA is used as a chelator in severe lead poisoning in both adults and children. EDTA's complex molecular structure allows it to bind not only to lead but also to multiple other metals.

It was Food and Drug Administration (FDA) approved as lead chelator in the 1940s and is considered more effective than other chelators due to its ability to bind tightly with lead.[10] Edetate calcium disodium forms a stable ring compound wherein calcium is displaced by lead. The strong bonds formed with those metals prevent further toxicity until those metals are physiologically excreted from the body.[10] In addition to lead, EDTA can bind zinc, iron, manganese, copper, and mercury, with zinc being the most clinically significant binding. Lead chelates with EDTA primarily in the bones and is then eliminated through urine. Once chelation ends, lead can again be found in the brain, bones, and soft tissues.[2]

Mechanism of Action

When given orally, EDTA has a low absorption rate (<5%) and can lead to high lead concentrations in the GI system. The preferred route of administration for EDTA is IV, allowing it to rapidly move into the plasma and interstitial fluids. IV EDTA gets distributed though the extracellular compartment and gets excreted in the kidney without being metabolized. The half-life of EDTA is about 20–60 minutes, after which the kidneys filter out the drug, secreting it into the tubular lumen. This process leads to approximately 50% of the chelated lead being excreted into the urine within 1 hour and around 95% within the first 24 hours.[10]

Indications for Use

In addition to chelating lead in clinically significant lead toxicity, EDTA can also be utilized to detect lead levels in patients using the lead mobilization test. 2 g of EDTA are administered either intravenously or intramuscularly. A positive lead mobilization test is indicated when >6 g of lead are excreted in the urine within 24 hours.[10]

Due to its high affinity for divalent cations, some studies suggest that EDTA may be used in the treatment of cardiovascular diseases, especially atherosclerosis.[11] In atherosclerosis, fatty deposits rich in calcium get accumulated in the vascular system. Edetate disodium has high affinity for calcium that could potentially scavenge these calcium deposits from the atherosclerotic plaques.[10] However, it has never been tried or advocated as a treatment for atherosclerosis.

Heavy metals such as lead, cadmium, aluminum, nickel, and mercury are frequently detected in the serum of patients with neurodegenerative diseases.[12] These metals trigger an inflammatory cascade with detrimental effects on the nervous system. The cytokines and inflammatory markers released during this response lead to neurotoxicity. Some studies have explored the role of chelators such as EDTA in reducing the burden of toxicity by binding to these heavy metals;[10] however, chelation is not a standard of care in the absence of overtly high/toxic levels.

Ethylenediaminetetraacetic acid has been shown in some clinical trials to potentiate a synergistic effect with antimicrobial peptides against bacterial cell wall activity. As a divalent cation chelator, EDTA binds to metals found in the outer lipopolysaccharide membranes of bacteria, disrupting their outer membrane structure. Therefore, EDTA may be a promising bacteriostatic agent against both gram-negative and gram-positive bacteria. In a study, EDTA in combination with other antibiotics played an important role against resistant strains of *Pseudomonas aeruginosa*. This is due to EDTA's ability to cross the structural permeability barrier in conjunction with antibiotics that have otherwise become resistant;[13] however, it is not used clinically for the treatment of resistant bacteria.

Lead poisoning in adults is an important indication for using EDTA. Severe lead toxicity is indicated by blood concentrations >70 µg/dL. At concentrations between 45 and 70 µg/dL, succimer, a metal chelator, has replaced edetate calcium disodium due to the life-threatening hypocalcemic effect of EDTA, if not used at proper doses. If lead levels exceed 45 µg/dL and a patient is symptomatic, chelation by EDTA should be initiated. Symptoms of lead toxicity can vary widely and include GI complaints (abdominal pain and constipation), musculoskeletal complaints (myalgias and arthralgias), fatigue, sleep disturbance, decreased libido, neuropsychiatric complaints (headache, difficulty in concentration, deficits in short-term memory, irritability, depression), and hematological signs, such as anemia, which is usually a subacute effect.[14-16]

Dose and Duration

Ethylenediaminetetraacetic acid dosing is based on renal function and body surface area. In adults, for lead poisoning at levels between 20 and 70 µg/dL, 1,000 mg/m^2 is given daily either as intravenously or intramuscularly. At lead levels >70 µg/dL, EDTA is usually combined with dimercaprol at a dose of 1,500 mg/m^2/day with a maximum of 3,000 mg/day, administered IM or IV.

In patients with lead nephropathy, the dose should be reduced to 500 mg/m^2 every 24 hours for 5 days for creatinine levels of 2–3 mg/dL, 500 mg/m^2 every 48 hours for three doses for creatinine levels of 3–4 mg/dL, and 500 mg/m^2 weekly for creatinine levels above 4 mg/dL.

Pediatric populations are usually given the combination treatment of EDTA and dimercaprol, and lead levels >45 µg/dL should have prompt treatment. For lead levels between 45 and 70 µg/dL, 25 mg/kg/day of EDTA is administered over 5 days. If lead levels exceed 70 µg/dL, EDTA should be given intravenously at 50 mg/kg/day for six doses.

In children with cerebral edema due to lead toxicity, IV administration is withheld to avoid an increase in intracranial pressure, and EDTA is administered intramuscularly.[10]

Usually, a single dose suffices, but repeated courses may be needed. Repeat dosage should be administered after an interval of at least 2 weeks because lead may reaccumulate between the vasculature and extravascular storage sites.

Adverse Effects

Ethylenediaminetetraacetic acid, like all other chelators, has multiple side effects that depend on factors such as dosage, mode and frequency of administration, and renal function.

Renal toxicity is the most prominent side effect, manifesting as acute tubular necrosis, renal failure, anuria, and proteinuria. Although IV and IM routes are most effective, they have been shown to increase blood urea nitrogen (BUN) in >25% of patients. EDTA is contraindicated in patients with kidney disease or renal failure, as it is mainly excreted in the urine.

Other systemic side effects include fatigue, fever and chills, arthralgias, nausea and, at high levels, hypotension, cardiac arrhythmias, bone marrow suppression, anemia, and hypocalcemia. When administering edetate calcium disodium, serum calcium levels should be closely monitored to protect patients from potential life-threatening hypocalcemia. There have been reports of patients developing seizures and cardiac arrests secondary to hypocalcemia post-EDTA administration.

Calcium EDTA also has a high affinity for binding zinc, which may lead to loss of zinc and resultant zinc deficiency in patients. Monitoring zinc levels in patients treated with calcium EDTA should be included in routine laboratory studies.

Ethylenediaminetetraacetic acid is not only nephrotoxic but also hepatotoxic, so it should be avoided in patients with liver diseases. It is classified as category B drug, so it should be avoided in pregnant patients as well.

If patients develop signs and symptoms of EDTA toxicity, the drug should be discontinued. In cases of nephrotoxicity, hydration should be maintained, and urine output monitored after stopping the drug. In patients developing raised intracranial pressure (headache, visual blurring, and vomiting), osmotic agents can be administered to decrease intracranial pressure.[10]

CONCLUSION

Deferoxamine (DFO) is useful and safe chelating agent for iron and aluminum toxicity. Deferoxamine chelates non-transferrin bound iron and is approved to treat acute or chronic iron overload. While on therapy, monitoring the patient's iron stores is as important as regular screening for side effects of DFO. Eye, ear and kidney functions should be monitored frequently.

On the other hand, EDTA is widely used in food industry, paper manufacturing, cosmetics, medicine, and laboratories. Sodium calcium edetate is used as heavy metal chelator for systemic toxicity with iron, mercury, aluminum, cadmium, and lead. Treated patients must be carefully watched for development of renal, hepatic, and hematological toxicity.

REFERENCES

1. Hoffman RS, Nelson LS, Howland MA, Lewin NA, Smith SW, Goldfrank LR. Goldfrank's Toxicologic Emergencies, 11th edition. New York: McGraw-Hill Education; 2019.
2. McDowell LA, Kudaravalli P, Chen RJ, Sticco KL. Iron overload. In: StatPearls [Internet]. Treasure Island, FL: StatPearls Publishing; 2025.
3. Velasquez J, Wray AA. Deferoxamine. In: StatPearls [Internet]. Treasure Island, FL: StatPearls Publishing; 2025.
4. Yuen HW, Becker W. Iron toxicity. In: StatPearls [Internet]. Treasure Island, FL: StatPearls Publishing; 2025.
5. Rahimzadeh MR, Rahimzadeh MR, Kazemi S, Amiri RJ, Pirzadeh M, Moghadamnia AA. Aluminum poisoning with emphasis on its mechanism and treatment of intoxication. Emerg Med Int. 2022;2022:1480553.
6. Rahman H, Channon SM, Parkinson IS, Skillen AW, Ward MK, Kerr DN. Aluminum in the dialysis fluid. Clin Nephrol. 1985;24(Suppl 1):S78-83.
7. De Virgiliis S, Congia M, Frau F, Argiolu F, Diana G, Cucca F, et al. Deferoxamine-induced growth retardation in patients with thalassemia major. J Pediatr. 1988;113(4): 661-9.
8. National Cancer Institute. (2020). NCI Dictionary of Cancer Terms. [online] Available from www.cancer.gov/publications/dictionaries/cancer-terms/def/edta. [Last accessed January, 2025].
9. Shabnam I, S CD, C JB. Ethylenediaminetetraacetic acid (EDTA)—dependent pseudothrombocytopenia: a case report. J Clin Diagn Res. 2014;8(10):FL03-4.
10. George T, Brady MF. Ethylenediaminetetraacetic acid (EDTA). In: StatPearls [Internet]. Treasure Island, FL: StatPearls Publishing; 2025.
11. Ravalli F, Parada XV, Ujueta F, Pinotti R, Anstrom KJ, Lamas GA, et al. Chelation therapy in patients with cardiovascular disease: a systematic review. J Am Heart Assoc. 2022;11(6):e024648.
12. Ferrero ME. Neuron protection by EDTA may explain the successful outcomes of toxic metal chelation therapy in neurodegenerative diseases. Biomedicines. 2022;10(10):2476.
13. Umerska A, Strandh M, Cassisa V, Matougui N, Eveillard M, Saulnier P. Synergistic effect of combinations containing EDTA and the antimicrobial peptide AA230, an arenicin-3 derivative, on gram-negative bacteria. Biomolecules. 2018;8(4):122.
14. Hoffman RS, Gosselin S, Nelson LS, Howland MA, Lewin NA, Smith SW, Goldfrank, LR. Goldfrank's Clinical Manual of Toxicologic Emergencies, 2nd edition. New York: McGraw Hill Professional. 2023.
15. Safaee M, Malekzadeh M, Motamedi N, Sayadishahraki M, Eizadi-Mood N. (2023). Gastrointestinal manifestations of lead poisoning: a brief report. Iran J Med Sci. 2023;48(6):600-5.
16. UpToDate. (2024). Lead exposure, toxicity, and poisoning in adults. [online] Available from www.uptodate.com/contents/lead-exposure-toxicity-and-poisoning-in-adults?search=edta%20&source=search_result&selectedTitle=1%7E86&usage_type=default&display_rank=1#H6. [Last accessed January, 2025].

4.4 Specific Binding: Chelating Agents–2 (Dimercaprol, BAL, Succimer)

Indira M, Suneeth Kuriakose

INTRODUCTION

Chelating agents have a role as antidotes in medical toxicology. The term chelator is derived from the Greek word *chele* meaning claw. Deferoxamine, ethylenediaminetetraacetic acid (EDTA), dimercaprol/British anti-Lewisite (BAL), and succimer are used as chelating agents in various heavy metal poisoning.

DEFEROXAMINE

Deferoxamine (DFO) chelates free iron (nontransferrin bound), hemosiderin, ferritin, and aluminum.

Mechanism of Action

Deferoxamine has a high affinity to the ferric form of iron and binds to form a stable compound—feroxamine. DFO binds to iron in a 1:1 ratio.[1] DFO can bind to free plasma iron and bind iron after drawing iron from tissues to plasma including that from the myocardium, but will not bind to iron already bound to molecules such as transferrin, cytochrome, and hemoglobin.[2]

Deferoxamine will chelate aluminum in plasma and draw aluminum from tissues to plasma for chelation. The resultant aluminoxane is water-soluble and renally excreted or dialysable with a high flux membrane.

Kinetics

Deferoxamine is rapidly absorbed after the intravenous, intramuscular, and subcutaneous route of administration, but poorly absorbed after the oral route of administration.[3] The subcutaneous route is preferred for chronic iron overload and the intravenous route is for acute iron overdose, and life-threatening symptoms. DFO is poorly bound to plasma protein to less than 10%. DFO is metabolized by plasma enzymes and there is minimal hepatic metabolism. Iron bound from the liver will be excreted through bile, and iron bound from plasma and other tissues will be eliminated through the kidney.

Indications

Deferoxamine is a Food and Drug Administration (FDA)-approved drug to treat acute and chronic iron overload.

- *Acute overdosage:* Iron remains as a free form in the blood, and is distributed intracellularly where it causes damage. Removal of free iron from the blood and preventing its intracellular distribution is essential to treat iron toxicity. Intracellular damage once occurred cannot be reversed.

  The severity assessment of iron toxicity and need for DFO is done by three criteria—clinical features, dose of elemental iron ingested, and serum iron concentration.[4]
- Systemic toxicity of iron progresses through three stages—direct gastrointestinal toxicity in the initial 6 hours of ingestion, latent period 4–12 hours postingestion, and multiorgan failure 6–72 hours postingestion. DFO is indicated if the patient has consumed a toxic dose and should not wait for systemic toxicity to be established.
- Toxic dose of elemental iron is calculated as follows:
  - <10–20 mg/kg—nontoxic
  - 20–60 mg/kg—potentially toxic
  - 60–120 mg/kg—toxic but fatal outcome unlikely
  - 120 mg/kg—potentially fatal
- Serum iron concentration is a good guide to predicting prognosis and guide therapy. Serum iron should be tested before starting DFO therapy as falsely low levels may be shown in the presence of DFO, which interferes with the colorimetric or radioimmunoassay methods. Atomic absorption spectrophotometry is advised to measure serum iron in patients on DFO therapy.

  Deferoxamine therapy should be started with an iron level of >90 µmol/L (500 µg/dL) after 3–6 hours of ingestion, OR above 60 µmol/L with systemic toxicity. DFO therapy should be started when systemic toxicity like shock, altered mental status, gastrointestinal hemorrhage, and metabolic acidosis are present when serum iron level is not available.[5] Redistribution changes serum iron levels after 8 hours of ingestion and should not be used to guide the initiation of DFO. A change in urine color to wine red indicates but not mandatory evidence of iron chelation.

- *Transfusion-related iron overload:* Patients with hemolytic anemia, myelodysplastic syndrome, aplastic anemia, and chronic leukemia require frequent blood transfusions.[6] In such populations, iron chelation therapy should start after the first 10–20 transfusions or 2 years after starting transfusions whichever is earlier, serum ferritin level of >1,000 µg/L, or liver iron concentration is >3 mg Fe/gm.
- *Cardiotoxicity:* Iron overload with reduced cardiac T2 time in cardiac magnetic resonance imaging (MRI), which is associated with cardiomyopathy.[7] Cardiac T2 of <20 ms indicates excessive iron in cardiac nuclei.
- *Hemochromatosis:* Iron chelation therapy is not the first-line therapy in hemochromatosis, and it is advised when phlebotomy is contraindicated.[8]
- *Aluminum toxicity*: DFO chelation is used as an off-label therapy in aluminum toxicity, especially, in chronic kidney disease (CKD) patients. Chelation therapy is recommended with an aluminum level of more than 20 µg/L with clinical features of Al toxicity such as osteomalacia, anemia, hypercalcemia, and dialysis dementia.[9]

Administration and Dose

Deferoxamine mesylate is given intravenously at a rate of 5–15 mg/kg body weight/hour in acute iron overdose to a maximum of 6 g in 24 hours.[10,11] A dose reduction of up to 50% is warranted in severe renal impairment. Intravenous volume should be maintained for renal protection before starting DFO therapy by giving bolus IV fluid of 20 mL/kg normal saline. There are reports that higher doses of DFO up to 40 mg/kg/h is beneficial to patients with severe acute symptoms if the patient tolerates.[12]

The patient needs 6–8 hours of treatment usually and not more than 24 hours.[13] The dose can be adjusted according to the clinical status of the patient.[14] The decision to stop infusion is taken according to clinical improvement like reversal of metabolic acidosis, and recovery from shock. Serum levels should fall to <60 µg/L, but serum measurement gives false levels during DFO therapy. A change in the wine red color of urine is also not a good tool to stop therapy.[15] Normal urine color along with the stable clinical status of the patient and a possible serum level of <100 µg/L is an appropriate endpoint.

Deferoxamine infusion subcutaneously at 40–60 mg/kg over 8–12 hours is advised in transfusion-related iron overload. It is given 4 days a week, more adverse effects are seen with higher doses. Vitamin C mobilizes iron from iron stores, makes it available for chelation, and potentiates the action of DFO.[16] However, the free iron available can worsen the cardiac function. The FDA does not approve vitamin C supplementation in patients with cardiac failure and recommends starting vitamin C supplementation after the completion of 1 month of DFO therapy with close monitoring of cardiac function.

Adverse Effects

Acute side effects include anaphylaxis, nausea, vomiting, and urticaria.[17] ARDS is a fatal complication of intravenous infusion, especially, if given more than 24 hours.[17] Intermittent infusion with a 12-hour infusion-free period may reduce the risk of ARDS if a prolonged infusion is needed.[12] Hypotension is seen with a rapid infusion. Infusion causes renal failure in hypovolemic patients. DFO therapy increases the risk of infection with *Mucormycosis, Yersinia enterocolitica*, and vibrio.

The adverse effects of chronic chelation therapy include hearing loss and retinopathy.[18] Visual abnormalities include reduced visual acuity, field defects, and defective color vision. Hearing loss and visual defects are reversible if the drug is stopped early. Growth retardation is also reported in children receiving DFO.[19]

Contraindications

Contraindicated in patients with hypersensitivity to the drug previously. Otherwise, it is a safe drug. DFO is a category C drug in pregnancy and can be used if benefits outweigh risk.[20] During pregnancy, DFO is recommended in acute toxic ingestion of iron and cardiac involvement due to iron overload.

ETHYLENEDIAMINETETRAACETIC ACID

Ethylenediaminetetraacetic acid is a polyamino carboxylic acid. It is a colorless water-soluble solid and available as salts like calcium disodium EDTA (CaNa2EDTA) and disodium EDTA.[21] EDTA is an FDA-approved drug as a chelating agent in lead poisoning. It can chelate other heavy metals in the body like mercury, iron, zinc, and cadmium, though the FDA has not approved it as a treating agent in the mentioned heavy metal poisoning.[22]

There are reports that EDTA reduces coronary atherosclerosis by reducing the adverse effects of heavy metals on the cardiovascular system. Edetate disodium has a high affinity to calcium and removes Ca from atherosclerotic plaques.[23]

Heavy metals induce an inflammatory cascade and produce various cytokines and inflammatory mediators, which were shown to produce neurotoxicity. Calcium disodium edetate is proposed to reduce neurotoxicity by chelating heavy metals including iron and prevent further inflammatory cascade.[24]

Mechanism of Action

Ethylenediaminetetraacetic acid has a complex structure. It can bind to heavy metals through four carboxylate and two amine groups.[25] When calcium edetate is attached to a metal, calcium is replaced by the metal and the bond formed is so strong that further toxic effect of heavy metal is prevented.

Kinetics

Ethylenediaminetetraacetic acid has good absorption through the intravenous and intramuscular routes, but poorly through the oral route. It is rapidly distributed to plasma and interstitial fluid. It has extensive extracellular distribution, and its ionic form prevents it from entering the intracellular. It has a half-life of 20–60 minutes. Hence, it cannot bind heavy metals from tissues like the brain and liver. On binding to the heavy metal, a water-soluble compound is formed which is excreted through the kidney.[26]

Indications

Chelation therapy is rarely indicated in acute lead ingestion. In chronic exposure, chelation is indicated according to blood lead levels and the age of the patient.[27] CaNa2EDTA is used in combination with BAL (Dimercaprol) in lead encephalopathy and used alone in nonencephalopathic patients when Succimer is not available. The source of lead exposure should be removed to make chelation effective. Iron and zinc supplementation can be given after and not during chelation therapy. Periodic monitoring of lead level should be done after cessation of therapy as there will be a redistribution of lead from bone marrow stores into the blood, which warrants further dose of chelation.[28]

Pediatric Age

When the blood level of lead is >70 μg/dL or in the presence of encephalopathy, an intravenous infusion of calcium disodium edetate in combination with BAL is recommended. EDTA infusion is started with the second dose of BAL and should not be given alone.

Blood lead level <45 μg/dL—no chelation indicated

Blood lead level 46–70 μg/dL—EDTA is not the first choice as the chelating agent due to side effects.

Adults

Chelation therapy with EDTA is considered for acute severe symptoms of lead poisoning.[29,30]

Administration and Dose

CaNa2EDTA is given intramuscularly at 50–75 mg/kg/day in 2–4 divided doses deep IM. Alternatively, an intravenous infusion of 25 mg/kg/dose in 500 mL dextrose or normal saline over 2–6 hours every 12th hour for 5 days may be given, which is preferred over intramuscular administration due to the pain at the injection site. The dose is reduced in renal dysfunction. A gap of 3–7 days without treatment is given after the first course of therapy to allow redistribution of lead stores and to replenish Zn stores. Further treatment is decided by the clinical features and blood lead levels.[31]

Adverse Effects

- Renal toxicity—CaNa2EDTA-lead complex can cause dose-dependent and reversible acute tubular necrosis.[25]
- Syndrome of inappropriate antidiuretic hormone (SIADH)
- Deficiency of essential metals like Zn, Cu, and Mn[32]—Ca EDTA has a strong affinity to these metals and Zn deficiency is common in small children.
- Disodium edetate chelate calcium from the body and can cause life-threatening hypocalcemia.
- Lead encephalopathy when EDTA is used alone as it causes the accumulation of lead in brain tissue.
- Rebound blood lead levels from bone marrow stores following therapy.
- Fever, nausea, vomiting, pain at the injection site, tremors, and headache, transaminitis, glucosuria, mucocutaneous lesions are minor side effects.
- Bone marrow suppression
- Arrhythmia

Contraindications

Contraindicated in active renal disease or anuria, hypersensitivity to EDTA, and hepatitis.[33] It is a category B drug and may be given in pregnancy if indicated. Teratogenicity secondary to Zn deficiency is possible.

DIMERCAPROL

Dimercaprol (2,3-dimercapto-1-propanol) belongs to the chelating class of drugs; well known as BAL. Sir Rudolph Albert Peters' group at Oxford University developed this drug as an antidote to "Lewisite" the vesical arsenical biogas used during World War II. This drug is used to treat toxic exposure to metals like arsenic, lead, mercury, gold and bismuth.

Mechanism of Action and Pharmacokinetics

Dimercaprol is a dithiol, its sulfhydryl group chelates with heavy metals and forms stable mercaptides, neutralizing the metal and protecting the metal-bound enzymes. Dimercaprol is useful in acute metal toxicity as it is more effective in preventing enzyme inhibition than reactivation.[34] Dimercaprol metal complexes can be dissociated and oxidized in vivo. Nonchelated drug undergoes hepatic glucuronidation to form inactive metabolites. It is a clear colorless oily liquid with an unpleasant pungent mercaptan smell. Because of its lipophilic nature, it is not absorbed orally, it crosses intracellular space and gets distributed in all tissues.[35] It is readily absorbed through the skin. Due to its oily nature, it is administered by deep intramuscular injection. The metabolism and excretion are complete within the half-life of 4 hours,[36] peak plasma level reaches within 30–60 minutes of administration, and it is excreted in urine and bile. Tubular acidic urine dissociates the metal-sulfur complex thereby increasing the metal delivery to renal tissue hence, maintaining alkaline urine pH decreases renal toxicity. Because of the dose-dependent toxicity excessive plasma concentrations should be avoided, maintaining the plasma concentration for constant formation and excretion of BAL-metal 2:1 complex.

Indications

- *Acute exposure to arsenic*: The minimal lethal dose of arsenic trioxide is 1–3 mg/kg, and the fatal dose is 70–180 mg or 600 µg/kg/day; elevated urine arsenic concentrations >100 µg/L (after excluding prior seafood intake within 48 hours), arsenic-related skin injuries.
- Severe symptomatic lead poisoning with a whole blood lead concentration >100 µg/dL in adults and >70 µg/dL in children or lead encephalopathy. To prevent redistribution of lead to the brain, dimercaprol is given before calcium disodium edetate, another chelating agent.[37]
- Elemental mercury exposure acute or chronic with a whole blood or 24-hour urine mercury concentration of ≥100 µg/L. Acute poisoning of inorganic or metallic mercury with whole blood or 24-hour urine mercury concentration ≥100 µg/L.
- *Injectable gold salt*: Sodium aurothiomalate toxicity, gold-induced thrombocytopenia, and severe gold dermatitis.
- The metal poisoning where dimercaprol can be used are bismuth, nickel, and antimony.
- It was earlier used for copper chelation in Wilson's disease before the development of D-penicillamine.

Contraindications

- Iron, cadmium, and selenium poisoning are the contraindications as the resulting metal complexes are more toxic than the metal itself.[34]
- Dimercaprol is formulated in peanut oil solution, hence not to be used in patients with peanut allergy. No other FDA-approved solvent is currently available.
- *Chronic mercury poisoning:* The complex deposition in the brain causes more toxicity.
- Hepatic dysfunction except for arsenic-induced hepatitis
- G-6-PD deficiency—causes hemolysis.

Treatment Dosage and Schedule of Drug Administration

Dimercaprol is available as an intramuscular injection of 50 mg/mL solution in benzyl benzonate and peanut oil.

Administered as a deep IM injection in the upper outer quadrant of buttock, for multiple doses alternate between the right and left buttock 2 inches below previous shots.[38]

Arsenic and gold poisoning:

- *Day 1–2:* 10–12 mg/kg/dose divided q6h deep IM × 2 days
- *Day 3:* 5–6 mg/kg/day divided q12h deep IM × 1 day
- *Day 4–14:* 2.5–3 mg/kg/dose daily once × 11 days

Severe gold dermatitis: 2.5 mg/kg/dose q4h × 2 days, then BID × 1 week

Gold-induced thrombocytopenia: 100 mg IM BID × 15 days

Inorganic mercury poisoning: 5 mg/kg IM four hourly for days followed by once or twice daily for 7–10 days.[39]

Lead poisoning: 4 mg/kg q4h for 3 days and 2.5 mg/kg for 1–4 days; a combination of dimercaprol with calcium disodium edetate is administered. When given with calcium disodium edetate; dimercaprol is administered first, at a different site from calcium disodium edetate. If blood lead concentration rebounds to >45 μg/dL within 5–7 days, may repeat the course of treatment.

Renal Impairment

No renal adjustment is needed, but treatment-related acute kidney injury warrants discontinuation of dimercaprol. Contraindicated in hepatic impairment except arsenic-induced hepatic injury.

Adverse Effects and Drug Interactions

Local effects are painful injections and injection-site sterile abscesses. Redistribution of metal to the brain and testes occurs. Systemic effects are seen in 50% of individuals when the dose exceeds ≥5 mg/kg/dose, transient fever occurs in 30%. Tachycardia, systolic and diastolic hypertension, anxiety, conjunctivitis, blepharospasm, lacrimation, rhinorrhea, salivation, nausea, vomiting, headache, burning sensation in the mouth and throat, anginal pain, paresthesia of hands, a burning sensation in the penis, sweating, abdominal pain, and hepatotoxicity. Larger doses may induce convulsions and coma. Hemolysis occurs in patients with G6PD deficiency. No specific antidote is available, dose reduction and stopping the drug settles the effects after 2 hours. Dimercaprol-bound essential trace metals get excreted, resulting in a deficiency. Iron supplements should be given 24 hours or more after the last dose of dimercaprol. It should never be given at the same time as dimercaprol. Dimercaprol decreases insulin effectiveness by reducing disulfide bridges.

SUCCIMER

A meso isomer of 2, 3-dimercaptosuccinic acid (DMSA), first developed in the Soviet Union for mercury poisoning followed by treating tartar emetic (antimony) overdose. Approved by the FDA for the treatment of children with >45 μg/dL blood lead levels, followed by arsenic and mercury poisoning. The compound labeled with Technetium^{99m} is used for diagnostic imaging.

A dithiol similar to dimercaprol contains two carboxylic acids; which renders it hydrophilic and orally bioavailable; with an improved toxicity profile (does not mobilize metals to the brain or enter cells, hence the extracellular distribution is a major drawback). Essential metals like zinc, magnesium, calcium or iron are not chelated, however there is a reduction of serum copper after administration. Animal studies suggest that succimer may be effective as a chelator of cadmium.

Absorption is fast and variable, undergoes extensive hepatic metabolism, and 9% excreted in urine as succimer cysteine disulfide with t½ of 2 days.[40] The excreted metal complex in bile undergoes enterohepatic circulation. After exposure to inorganic mercury, an elevation of brain mercury after chelation occurred due to redistribution from extraneural sites.[41]

2,3-Dimercaptosuccinic acid 30 mg/kg/day increases urine lead elimination and significantly reduces blood lead concentrations, with a substantial individual response variation. Over a 5-day course, mean daily urine

TABLE 1: Common chelating agents and their adverse effects.

Chelating agent	*Used for chelating*	*Adverse effects*
BAL (British anti lewisite agent)	Arsenic, Lead, Mercury, Gold	Pain at injection site Allergic reaction
Dimercaptosuccinic acid (DMSA/Succimer)	Arsenic, Lead, Mercury, Tin, Cadmium, Silver, Copper	Allergic reactions, Transaminitis
Dimercaptopropane sulfonic acid (DMPS)	Cadmium, Silver, Copper, Zinc, Selenium, Magnesium, Zinc	Allergic reactions, Steven Johnson syndrome
Edetate calcium Sodium (EDTA)	Lead, Cadmium, Zinc	Renal failure, transaminitis, arrhythmia, bone marrow suppression
D Penicillamine	Copper, Arsenic, Lead, Mercury, Zinc	Allergic reaction, copper deficiency

lead excretion exceeds baseline by 5–20-fold, and blood lead concentrations fall to 50%, with individual variation. In severe poisoning, there can be a rebound increase in blood lead concentration by redistribution from bones and soft tissues later for which repeated 5-day courses are effective with a weekly drug-free period.[42]

2,3-Dimercaptosuccinic acid (DMSA) in pregnancy and the neonate: DMSA is not teratogenic but produces decreased weight gain in mothers and fetotoxicity when given in high doses (100–1,000 mg/kg/day) in experimental studies.

We can summarize all chelating agents and their adverse effects in the form of **Table 1**.

CONCLUSION

When we consider administering chelators despite of their effectiveness, these agents must be used cautiously due to potential side effects like kidney injuries, allergic reactions, and disruption of essential mineral homeostasis. The choice of chelating agent must be individualized considering the type of metal and its form, age of patient, and overall health. Continuous research is essential in this area to enhance their effectiveness and to improve their safety profile.

REFERENCES

1. Yuen HW, Gossman WG. Toxicity, Iron. 2017.
2. Aydinok Y, Kattamis A, Viprakasit V. Current approach to iron chelation in children. Br J Haematol. 2014;165(6):745-55.
3. Porter JB, Rafique R, Srichairatanakool S, Davis BA, Shah FT, Hair T, et al. Recent insights into interactions of deferoxamine with cellular and plasma iron pools: implications for clinical use. Ann NY Acad Sci. 2005;1054:155-68.
4. Madiwale T, Liebelt E. Iron: Not a benign therapeutic drug. Curr Opin Pediatr. 2006;18(2):174-9.
5. Perrone J. Iron. In: Goldfrank LR (Ed). Goldfrank's Toxicologic Emergencies, 10th edition. New York (NY): McGraw-Hill; 2015. 1882 p.
6. Brittenham GM, Griffith PM, Nienhuis AW, McLaren CE, Young NS, Tucker EE, et al. Efficacy of deferoxamine in preventing complications of iron overload in patients with thalassemia major. New England Journal of Medicine. 1994;331(9):567-73.
7. Oduor H, Minniti CP, Brofferio A, Gharib AM, Abd-Elmoniem KZ, Hsieh MM, et al. Severe cardiac iron toxicity in two adults with sickle cell disease. Transfusion. 2017;57(3):700-4.
8. Phatak PD, Brissot P, Bonkovsky H, Wurster M, Powell L, Niederau C, et al. A phase I/II, open-label, dose-escalation trial of once daily oral chelator deferasirox to treat iron overload in HFE-related hereditary hemochromatosis. Blood. 2010;114(22):1514.
9. Ackrill P, Ralston AJ, Day JP, Hodge KC. Successful removal of aluminium from patient with dialysis encephalopathy. Lancet. 1980;2(8196):692-3.
10. Howland MA. Antidotes in Depth: Deferoxamine. In: Goldfrank LR (Ed). Goldfrank's Toxicologic Emergencies. 10th edition. New York (NY): McGraw-Hill. 2015. 1904 p.
11. Cheney K, Gumbiner C, Benson B, Tenenbein M. Survival after a severe iron poisoning treated with intermittent infusions of deferoxamine. J Toxicol Clin Toxicol. 1995; 33(1):61-6.
12. Wright SW, Valento M, Mazor SS, Chen BC. Severe iron poisoning treated with prolonged deferoxamine infusion: a case report. Toxicology Communications. 2018;2(1):6-9.
13. Tenenbein M. Benefits of parenteral deferoxamine for acute iron poisoning. J Toxicol Clin Toxicol. 1996;34(5):485-9.
14. Sankar J, Shukla A, Khurana R, Dubey N. Near fatal iron intoxication managed conservatively. BMJ Case Rep. 2013;2013:bcr2012007670.
15. Baranwal AK, Singhi SC. Acute iron poisoning: management guidelines. Indian Pediatr. 2003;40(6):534-40.
16. Elalfy MS, Saber MM, Adly AA, Ismail EA, Tarif M, Ibrahim F, et al. Role of vitamin C as an adjuvant therapy to different iron chelators in young β-thalassemia major patients: efficacy and safety in relation to tissue iron overload. Eur J Haematol. 2016;96(3):318-26.
17. Poggiali E, Cassinerio E, Zanaboni L, Cappellini MD. an update on iron chelation therapy. Blood Transfus. 2012;10(4):411-22.
18. Taher AT, Weatherall DJ, Cappellini MD. Thalassaemia. The Lancet. 2018;391(10116):155-67.
19. Entezari S, Haghi SM, Norouzkhani N, Sahebnazar B, Vosoughian F, Akbarzadeh D, et al. Iron chelators in treatment of iron overload. J Toxicol. 2022;2022:4911205.
20. Singer ST, Vichinsky EP. Deferoxamine treatment during pregnancy: is it harmful? Am J Hematol. 1999;60(1):24-6.
21. Harris DC. Quantitative Chemical Analysis, 7th edition. New York: WH Freeman Company; 2007.
22. Wax PM. Current use of chelation in American Health Care. J Med Toxicol. 2013;9(4):303-7.
23. Lamas GA, Issa OM. Edetate disodium-based treatment for secondary prevention in post-myocardial infarction patients. Curr Cardiol Rep. 2016;18(2):20.
24. Fulgenzi A, Ferrero ME. EDTA chelation therapy for the treatment of neurotoxicity. Int J Mol Sci. 2019;20(5):1019.
25. Bradberry S, Vale A. A comparison of sodium calcium edetate (edetate calcium disodium) and succimer (DMSA) in the treatment of inorganic lead poisoning. Clin Toxicol (Phila). 2009;47(9):841-58.
26. Osterloh J, Becker CE. Pharmacokinetics of CaNa2EDTA and chelation of lead in renal failure. Clin Pharmacol Ther. 1986;40(6):686-93.

27. CDC. (2024). Childhood Lead Poisoning Prevention Program. Centers for Disease Control and Prevention. [online] Available from https://www.cdc.gov/lead-prevention/about/index.html#:~:text=Prevention-,The%20goal%20of%20CDC's%20Childhood%20Lead%20Poisoning%20Prevention%20Program%20(CLPPP,and%20prevention%20of%20lead%20exposure. [Last accessed February, 2025].
28. Rabinowitz MB. Toxicokinetics of bone lead. Environ Health Perspect. 1991;91:33-7.
29. Rae CE, Bell CN Jr, Elliott CE, Shannon M. Ten cases of acute lead intoxication among bridge workers in Louisiana. Ann Pharmacother. 1991;25:932-7.
30. Gordon JN, Taylor A, Bennett PN. Lead poisoning: Case studies. Br J Clin Pharmacol. 2002;53:451-8.
31. Roberts JR, Reigart JR, Ebeling M, Hulsey TC. Time required for blood lead levels to decline in nonchelated children. J Toxicol Clin Toxicol. 2001;39(2):153-60.
32. Flora SJS. Influence of simultaneous supplementation of zinc and copper during chelation of lead in rats. Hum Exp Toxicol. 1991;10:331-6.
33. Kosnett MJ, Wedeen RP, Rothenberg SJ, Hipkins KL, Materna BL, Schwartz BS, et al. Recommendations for medical management of adult lead exposure. Environ Health Perspect. 2007;115(3):463-71.
34. Allison K. Ehrlich. Environmental Toxicology. In: Laurence L. Brunton, Björn C. Knollmann (Eds). Goodman & Gilman's the Pharmacological Basis of Therapeutics, 14th edition. New York: McGraw Hill; 2022. pp. 1522-3.
35. Simpson SD, Young L. Biochemical studies of toxic agents; experiments with radioactive 2:3-dimercaptopropanol (British anti-lewisite). Biochem J. 1950;46(5):634-40.
36. Lars Gerhardsson, Jan Aaseth. Guidance for Clinical treatment of metal poisonings: use and misuse of chelating Agents. In: Jan Aaseth, Guido Crisponi, Ole Andersen (Eds). Chelation Therapy in the Treatment of Metal Intoxication. Philadelphia: Elsevier Inc.; 2016. pp. 313-41.
37. Dawn L, Whited L. Dimercaprol. In: StatPearls [Internet]. Treasure Island (FL): StatPearls Publishing; 2024. [online] Available from https://www.statpearls.com/nurse/ce/activity/101321. [Last accessed November, 2024].
38. Adefris Adal. Heavy Metal Toxicity. Medscape. 2023. [online] Available from https://emedicine.medscape.com/article/814960. [Last accessed November, 2024].
39. BAL in oil ampules. Drugs. Food and drug administration. 2007. p 5. https://www.accessdata.fda.gov/drugsatfda_docs/label/2007/005939s007lbl.pdf
40. JK Aronson (Ed). Succimer. Meyler's Side Effects of Drugs, 16th edition. Philadelphia: Elsevier; 2016. p. 537.
41. Ewan KB, Pamphlett R. Increased inorganic mercury in spinal motor neurons following chelating agents. Neurotoxicology.1996;17(2):343-9.
42. Bradberry S, Vale A. Dimercaptosuccinic acid (succimer; DMSA) in inorganic lead poisoning. Clin Toxicol (Phila). 2009;47(7):617-3.

4.5 Specific Binding: Bioscavenger Therapy (FFP, Albumin)

Syed Moied Ahmed, Maleha Ahmed, Ayushi Saxena

INTRODUCTION

Atropine and oximes are the two main antidotes used to counter the toxic effects of organophosphate (OP) since 1950s. Despite the free availability of these antidotes, the mortality rate remains as high as 10–20%.[1] Numerous studies have shown that atropine and oximes cannot prevent morbidity and mortality in poisoned patients.[2,3] The results of in vivo studies on humans are not proved yet, and there are no exhaustive meta-analyses to indicate oxime effectiveness.[4,5] Therefore, clinicians should be cautious in depending on oximes only, and other treatment modalities should be supplemented with the two antidotes.

Bioscavengers as a treatment have played an important role in ameliorating the damage caused by OPs.[6] These agents are supposed to thoroughly scavenge OPs and prevent them from reaching their target site, e.g., cells. These agents, thus, radically inhibit cellular damage, preventing organ dysfunction. Bioscavengers therapy includes utilizing enzymes, which are capable of blocking OP compounds or eliminating them before they reach their toxic threshold.[7] Fresh frozen plasma (FFP) has been investigated in human studies as a source of butyrylcholinesterase (BuChE) to treat organophosphorus poisoning.[8]

Basically, there are two generations of bioscavengers given as follows:

1. Stoichiometric enzyme-based bioscavengers [e.g., acetylcholinesterase (AChE)]
2. Catalytic enzyme-based bioscavengers [e.g., organophosphorus hydrolase (OPH)]

Of these, catalytic agents are more effective.

Bioscavengers must be extracted from enormous amounts of human plasma and administered in a concentrated regimen to counter nerve agent exposure. Harvesting bioscavengers from plasma is costly, inefficient, and impractical as a means of production. More efficient production methods, such as harvesting molecules from the milk of transgenic goats,[9] are currently under investigation. They have the potential to revolutionize the prevention of nerve agent poisoning. Bioscavengers may function as prophylactic agents, but this needs evaluation. Atropine and oximes, which are commonly used postexposure treatments for nerve agents, have limited efficacy. Damage to neuromuscular junctions only occurs in the presence of nerve agents. Thus, they are toxic if administered in the absence of nerve agents. Furthermore, they must be administered very shortly after nerve agent exposure to have any therapeutic effect. In other words, bioscavengers can eliminate the need for atropine and oximes while nullifying any chance of long-term neurologic damage.

MECHANISM OF ACTION

Organophosphate pesticides are fat-soluble macromolecular substances and bind to the proteins easily. This property is used to enable the formation of inert complexes by bioscavengers that bind to the toxin. These complexes are then eliminated from the body before the OP compounds reach target sites. This binding can be either specific or nonspecific. Specific binding occurs in the form of chelating agents for heavy metal poisoning, hydroxocobalamin for cyanide poisoning, or bioscavenger therapy (human BuChE) for organophosphorus poisoning.[10]

ALBUMIN

The serum albumin concentration has been studied as a predictor of mortality in seemingly healthy individuals of all ages for various reasons. First, hypoalbuminemia is a marker of poor nutritional status. Second, hypoalbuminemia correlates with the lack of crucial physiological functions of albumin, including maintaining oncotic pressure, transporting various ions and drugs, scavenging free oxygen radicals, and acting as an antioxidant, resulting in poor outcomes. Third, albumin is a negative acute-phase reactant whose synthesis decreases during inflammation. Other mechanisms involving the inflammatory state are the increased flux of albumin from the plasma to the extravascular space due to increased vascular permeability and the increased breakdown of albumin that has been oxidized or damaged due to its antioxidant and free radical scavenging activities.[11] Apart from the prognostic role of serum albumin level, albumin can also be used as bioscavengers, owing to the large number of amino acid residues in albumin that covalently bind OP molecules. Albumin displays a low esterase activity and slowly reacts with carbamoyl and phosphoryl esters. It appears to play a significant role in the detoxification of the carbaryl group of OP compounds, thus, may reduce the amount of OP available for reaction with AChE.

FRESH FROZEN PLASMA

Fresh frozen plasma is now being suggested as a useful therapy for clearing free OP, because it functions as a bioscavenger due to the presence of serum cholinesterase. When FFP is stored at 4°C, cholinesterase enzyme remains stable for a few weeks, but when it is dry and frozen, the enzyme activity may last for 2 years.[12] There is a potential for the use of frozen, dry plasma as a source of bioscavengers enzymes.

There are, however, some disadvantages to the large-scale pretreatment of individuals with significant quantities of protein. These include cost, possible immunogenicity, and the difficulties associated with pretreating at the appropriate time relative to anticipated exposure to toxic agent. This concept can still hold true for tentative exposure to nerve agents but may not work in self-harm cases.

INDICATION

Bioscavengers have been administered to patients presenting within 12 hours, with suppression of pseudocholinesterase activity to <1,000 U/L. 100 mL of 20% human albumin given four times a day over 3 days is the most recommended dosage.[13] Cholinesterase enzyme level in FFP is 90 mg in 11 packs of FFP. In other words, every two bags of FFP increase the serum cholinesterase by 461.7 ± 142.1 IU/L approximately. Many studies have, thus, used eight bags of FFP, 250 mL each, over 3 days in the treatment of OP poisoning.[14] The dosing can be potentially titrated according to the serum pseudocholinesterase levels.

CATALYTIC BIOSCAVENGERS

The stoichiometric neutralization of OPs needs the administration of huge amounts of costly biopharmaceuticals. Therefore, *catalytic bioscavengers* were introduced. As said earlier, the detoxification of OPs involves the hydrolysis of the phosphoester bond by organophosphorus acid anhydride hydrolases (OPAH), also called phosphotriesterases (PTEs), or oxidation to less toxic compounds by degrading their alkyl/aryl chain. These enzymes could be used as catalytic bioscavengers for prophylaxis and treatment of OP poisoning, for topical protection, and for the decontamination of skin, mucosa, and open wounds. Administered enzymes degrade toxic molecules before they reach their biological targets, thus providing protection against poisoning. The potential enzymes for the purpose are cholinesterases, phosphodiesterases, bacterial PTEs, and human paraoxonase 1 (PON1).[10]

The properties of an enzyme to be an efficient catalytic bioscavengers need to be studied in detail. There are certain prerequisites such as a wide spectrum of activity to counter OPs. The potential for mass production must be realizable at a reasonable cost. The enantioselectivity for toxin, bioavailability, biological stability, and immunotolerance are the other major issues.

FUTURE OF BIOSCAVENGERS

Secondary targets of OPs and other enzymes interacting with OPs are potential stoichiometric bioscavengers. The high number of amino acid residues in albumin that preferentially covalently bind OP molecules (five tyrosine and two serine) are important. The reactivity of tyrosine residues can be enhanced upon specific modification. Thus, modified human albumin could lead to a new generation of stoichiometric bioscavengers. Also, a low molecular stoichiometric scavengers could be an economic alternative to enzyme-based stoichiometric scavengers.

As discussed earlier, bioavailability and the biological stability of injected stoichiometric or catalytic bioscavengers are important issues. Increasing the size of the enzyme by polymerization, conjugation to albumin, reducing the microheterogeneity of glycans, and chemical modifications of solvent-exposed surfaces improve the biological life of injected bioscavengers. Fast clearance of glycoproteins is often due to glycosylation defects. These can be corrected by chemical modifications.

Targeted therapy with an aim to eliminate OP from a specific organ could be the future goal. An interesting animal study has elucidated that brain-targeted nanoreactor with a capacity to prevent OP-induced neurological damage is a real possibility now.[15] The nanoreactors were designed by integrating enzyme immobilization and erythrocyte-liposome hybrid membrane (E-Lipo) camouflage techniques based on a stoichiometric bioscavenger (RBC membrane-anchored AChE) and a catalytic bioscavenger [recombinant organophosphorus hydrolase (rOPH)].[15] The aim was to improve the detoxification efficiency and circulating stability of catalytic bioscavenger. It was shown to penetrate the blood–brain barrier (BBB), with an aim to get rid of the intracerebral OPs. This, in turn, led to the inhibition of oxidative stress, reduction of neuroinflammation, and a net effect on the reduction of neuronal apoptosis.[15] This is probably the first report of organ-specific (brain-targeted) nanoreactors aimed specifically at reducing OP-induced delayed neurological abnormalities.[15]

In the future, gene therapy could be considered for prophylaxis and treatment of nerve agents such as OPs.

CONCLUSION

Bioscavengers can radically eliminate OP compounds from the body by hydrolysis or other forms of metabolism. They can also block toxin (OP)–cell interactions. This results in the reduction in the toxin and reduced intracellular oxidative stress, including reactive oxygen species (ROS) production and abnormal antioxidants. They can also prevent direct mitochondrial as well as DNA damage. Damage-induced apoptosis was also blocked.

REFERENCES

1. Eddleston M, Chowdhury FR. Pharmacological treatment of organophosphorus insecticide poisoning: the old and the possible new. Br J Clin Pharmacol. 2016;81:462-70.
2. Johnson MK, Jacobsen D, Meredith TJ, Eyer P, Heath AJ, Ligtenstein DA, et al. Evaluation of antidotes for poisoning by organophosphorus pesticides. Emerg Med Australas. 2000;12:22-37.
3. Sudakin DL, Mullins ME, Horowitz BZ, Abshier V, Letzig L. Intermediate syndrome after malathion ingestion despite continuous infusion of pralidoxime. J Toxicol Clin Toxicol. 2000;38:47-50.
4. Pawar KS, Bhoite RR, Pillay CP, Chavan SC, Malshikare DS, Garad SG. Continuous pralidoxime infusion versus repeated bolus injection to treat organophosphorus

pesticide poisoning: a randomised controlled trial. Lancet. 2006;368:2136-41.
5. Peter JV, Moran JL, Graham P. Oxime therapy and outcomes in human organophosphate poisoning: an evaluation using meta-analytic techniques. Crit Care Med. 2006;34: 502-10.
6. Pichamuthu K, Jerobin J, Nair A, John G, Kamalesh J, Thomas K, et al. Bioscavenger therapy for organophosphate poisoning—an open-labeled pilot randomized trial comparing fresh frozen plasma or albumin with saline in acute organophosphate poisoning in humans. Clin Toxicol. 2010;48:813-9.
7. Cerasoli DM, Griffiths EM, Doctor BP, Saxena A, Fedorko JM, Greig NH, et al. In vitro and in vivo characterization of recombinant human butyrylcholinesterase (Protexia) as a potential nerve agent bioscavenger. Chem Biol Interact. 2005;157:363-5.
8. Gheshlaghi F, Savari MA, Nasiri R, Wong A, Feizi A, Maracy MR, et al. Efficacy of fresh frozen plasma transfusion in comparison with conventional regimen in organophosphate poisoning treatment: a meta-analysis study. Crit Rev Toxicol. 2020;50(8):677-84.
9. Denman J, Hayes M, O'Day C, Edmunds T, Bartlett C, Hirani S, et al. Transgenic expression of a variant of human tissue-type plasminogen activator in goat milk: purification and characterization of the recombinant enzyme. Biotechnology (N Y). 1991;9(9):839-43.
10. Masson P, Rochu D. Catalytic bioscavengers against toxic esters, an alternative approach for prophylaxis and treatments of poisonings. Acta Naturae. 2009;1(1): 68-79.
11. Noh E, Moon JM, Chun BJ, Cho YS, Ryu S, Kim D. The clinical role of serum albumin in organophosphate poisoning. Basic Clin Pharmacol Toxicol. 2021;128(4):605-14.
12. Pazooki S, Solhi H, Vishteh HR, Shadnia S, Beigi MJ. Effectiveness of fresh frozen plasma as supplementary treatment in organophosphate poisoning. Med J Malaysia. 2011;66(4):342-5.
13. Pichamuthu K, Jerobin J, Nair A, John G, Kamalesh J, Thomas K, et al. Bioscavenger therapy for organophosphate poisoning—an open-labeled pilot randomized trial comparing fresh frozen plasma or albumin with saline in acute organophosphate poisoning in humans. Clin Toxicol. 2010;48(8):813-9.
14. Dayananda VP, Bhaskara B, Pateel GN. A study of effectiveness of fresh frozen plasma in organophosphorus compound poisoning in reducing length of intensive care unit stay and in reducing need for tracheostomy. Anesth Essays Res. 2016;10(2):268-72.
15. Zou S, Wang Q, He Q, Liu G, Song J, Li J, et al. Brain-targeted nanoreactors prevent the development of organophosphate-induced delayed neurological damage. J Nanobiotechnol. 2023;21:256.

4.6 Specific Binding: Immunotherapy (Digibind)

Pankaj Soni, Manish Gupta

INTRODUCTION

The use of immunotherapy in the treatment of drug toxicity has been known for years (Colburn, 1980).[1] Antibodies have been produced in horses, rats, sheep, and goats against a lot of drugs such as aspirin, chloramphenicol, colchicine, strychnine, digoxin, imipramine, and nortriptyline.[2] But, only one product—digoxin-specific antibody fragments (DSFab)—is commercially available in the market since last 38 years. This immunotherapeutic antidote against digoxin poisoning has excellent record of efficacy and safety. DSFab are indicated for the management of patients with toxicity related to digoxin as well as oleander, squill, and cane toad poison (bufotoxin), which contain other cardioactive steroids.

HISTORY OF ANTIDIGOXIN FAB

Digoxin-specific antibody fragments are the definitive treatment for patients with severe digoxin poisoning. Treatment for cardiac glycoside toxicity was largely supportive[3] before availability of digoxin-specific antibodies. Butler and Chen[4] in 1967 suggested that purified antidigoxin antibodies with a high affinity and specificity should be developed to treat digoxin toxicity in humans. In 1976, Smith et al. first used antibody fragments (Digibind) successfully to treat a patient who ingested 22.5 mg of digoxin after failure of all conventional treatments,[5] and it became commercially available in 1986. Digibind, a relatively pure, very safe, and extremely effective Fab product, was produced. Another commercial

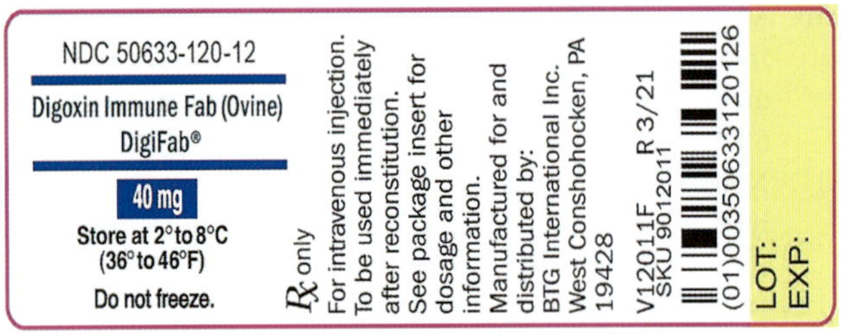

Fig. 1: DigiFab.

product, DigiFab **(Fig. 1)**, was approved by the US Food and Drug Administration (US FDA) in 2001. It is very similar to Digibind, except that it is prepared using a digoxin derivative (digoxin-dicarboxymethoxylamine) as the hapten. These antibodies remain highly effective, safe, and are widely used in clinical practice.[5,6]

DEFINITION OF FRAGMENT ANTIGEN-BINDING FRAGMENTS

Fragment antigen-binding (Fab) fragments consist of a variable domain and the first constant region each of heavy and light chains. They are purified preparations consisting of the Fab portion of immunoglobulin G (IgG) antidigoxin antibodies derived from immunized sheep. These Fab fragments bind free digoxin, thereby forming digoxin-immune fragment complexes.

Why Only Fragment Antigen-binding (FAB) Fragments?

Digoxin-specific Fab fragments are prepared after cleaving whole IgG antidigoxin antibodies with papain (papaya extract). When compared with whole IgG antibodies, the advantages of DSFab include a larger volume of distribution, more rapid onset of action, lesser risk of adverse immunologic effects, and more rapid elimination. Cleaving IgG into two separate antibody-binding fragments (Fab) and removing the Fc fragment change the pharmacokinetic profile without affecting its binding capacity (Colburn, 1980).[1] The smaller molecular weight (about 50,000) results in a larger volume of distribution. This explains the greater efficacy and faster onset of action of DSFab than intact digoxin-specific antibodies (Lloyd and Smith, 1978).[7] Fab fragments are mostly eliminated through the kidneys because of their small size. Elimination is more rapid than for whole immunoglobulin eliminated via the reticuloendothelial system (RES). One more advantage of Fab fragments is that the total amount of foreign protein administered to neutralize a given quantity of digoxin is reduced.[2]

PHARMACOKINETICS OF FRAGMENT ANTIGEN-BINDING FRAGMENTS

Fragment antigen-binding fragments are commercially available as Digibind.[8] It is derived from the Fab of ovine (sheep) antibodies specific for digoxin. Each DigiFab vial contains 40 mg of Fab fragments and binds 0.5 mg of digoxin approximately. Digibind has an elimination half-life of approximately 15–20 hours, but the half-life increases up to 10 times in patients with renal dysfunction. DigiFab has large volume of distribution (V_d)[8] 0.3 L/kg.

INDICATIONS OF ANTIDIGOXIN FAB

Fragment antigen-binding fragments should be given in all cases of severe digoxin poisoning, as there is no alternative therapy with comparable safety and efficacy.

- Hemodynamically unstable dysrhythmias (e.g., ventricular tachycardia, ventricular fibrillation, complete heart block, Mobitz II heart block, symptomatic bradycardia, asystole),[9] which are life-threatening
- Hyperkalemia (serum potassium levels > 5.5 mEq/L)
- Hypotension [systolic blood pressure (SBP) <100 mm Hg] and hypoperfusion with evidence of organ dysfunction (e.g., renal failure, hepatic failure, altered mental status)
- Based on serum digoxin concentration (SDC) at steady state (>10 ng/mL in acute and >4 ng/mL in chronic ingestion) or based on total digoxin dose ingested (>10 mg in adult and >4 mg in child)

MECHANISM OF ACTION (FIG. 2)

The binding affinity of Digibind for digoxin is much greater (10^9–10^{10} L/mol) than the affinity of digoxin for Na^+/K^+ ATPase pump receptor site. Immediately following intravenous (IV) administration, DSFab bind intravascular free (unbound) digoxin forming digoxin-immune fragment complexes. Uncomplexed Fab antibodies then diffuse into the interstitial space and bind free digoxin there. When free digoxin levels in plasma fall, the resulting concentration gradient pulls digoxin from intracellular site and facilitates digoxin dissociation from Na^+/K^+ ATPase pump. Digoxin–Digibind complexes are then renally excreted.

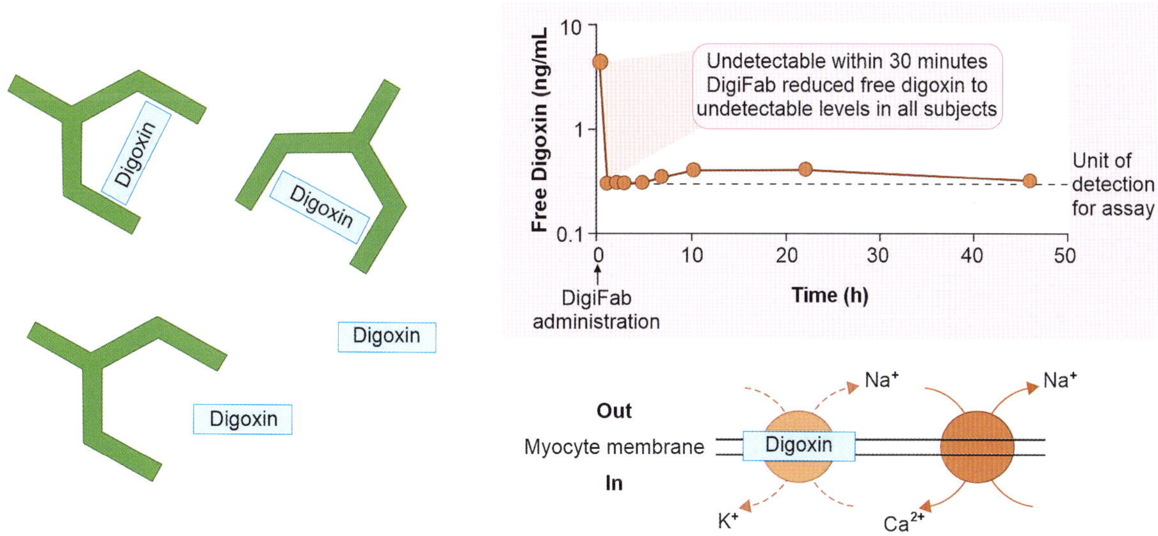

Fig. 2: Mechanism of action (MOA) of DigiFab.

DOSE CALCULATION OF ANTIDIGOXIN FAB (DIGIBIND)

The dose of digoxin immune Fab is calculated by either the amount of digoxin ingested or by SDC if the dose is not known. Now, there are three different clinical scenarios discussed here.

1. *Unknown serum digoxin levels and unknown amount of digoxin ingested:* In cases of severe digoxin toxicity with unknown amount of digoxin ingested, treatment consists of *empiric Fab fragments*. Dose depends upon following two clinical scenarios **(Flowchart 1)**:
   a. *Patient with relative hemodynamic stability*: Most patients with digoxin poisoning are relatively stable, and arrest is not imminent. In such patients, administer two vials of Fab fragments over 30 minutes.[9,10] If clinical response remains inadequate (i.e., a perfusing rhythm has not returned), then an additional one to two vials are administered.
   b. *Patient in cardiac arrest or cardiac arrest appears imminent*: The empiric dosing strategy of 10 vials of Fab fragments in adults or five vials in children administered by slow IV push is applied.[8] In case of inadequate clinical response, initial dose can be repeated.

   Note: In small children receiving empiric dosing, concern for volume overload must be considered.
2. *Known amount of digoxin ingested but unknown SDC:* The number of Fab fragment vials required in patients with an acute overdose, when only the amount ingested is known, is based upon the total body load (TBL).
   - *Step A: TBL calculation*: TBL for digoxin = Dose (in mg) ingested × 0.8 (0.8 reflects the digoxin oral bioavailability)
   - *Step B: Number of vials required*: = TBL/0.5

   The number of vials is rounded up to the nearest whole number **(Box 1)**.
3. *Steady-state SDC is known*: The number of Fab vials needed for treatment (i.e., full reversal of digoxin effects) when the SDC is known is calculated based upon the drug concentration and the patient's weight.

$$\text{Number of vials} = [\text{SDC (in ng/mL)} \times \text{patient's weight (in kg)}]/100$$

Many laboratories measure serum digoxin levels in nmol/L. The conversion factor is ng/mL × 1.28 = nmol/L.

The number of vials is rounded up to the nearest whole number **(Box 2)**. This formula provides a quick and accurate estimate of the antidote needed for treatment and is derived from a complex pharmacokinetic calculation incorporating apparent V_d of digoxin.[8]

Partial reversal of digoxin effects can be done by providing only half the calculated number of vials using the equation mentioned above. This approach is applied, mostly in chronic digoxin toxicity when there is concern that full reversal of digoxin therapeutic effect may precipitate an acute congestive heart failure (CHF) in patient with baseline reduced ejection fraction (EF) or loss of rate control in atrial fibrillation.

Flowchart 1: Treatment of digoxin toxicity with antidigoxin Fab.

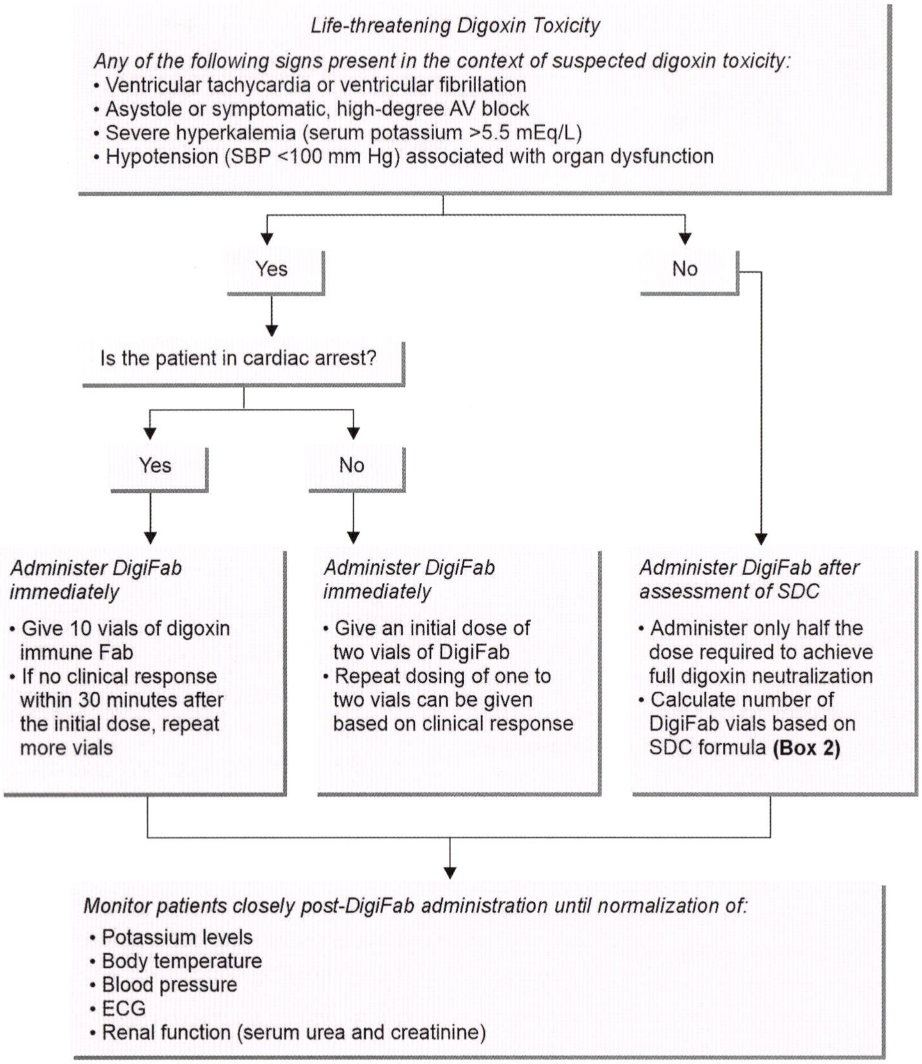

(AV: atrioventricular; ECG: electrocardiogram; SBP: systolic blood pressure; SDC: serum digoxin concentration)

BOX 1: DigiFab dose calculation based on digoxin dose.

- Adult weight = 70 kg
- Ingestion = 28 digoxin tablets (0.25 mg)
- So, ingested dose = 0.25 × 28 = 7 mg
- Absorbed dose = 7 × 0.8 = 5.6 mg (assume 80% is oral bioavailability)
- So, TBL for digoxin = 5.6 mg
- Number of DigiFab vials required = 5.6/0.5 = 11.2, which is rounded up to 12 vials

BOX 2: DigiFab dose calculation based on serum digoxin concentration.

- Weight = 75 kg
- SDC = 7.4 ng/mL
- Number of DigiFab vials required = 7.4 × 75/100 = 5.55, which is rounded up to 6 vials

DOSING OF DIGOXIN IMMUNE FAB IN RENAL DYSFUNCTION

The dose of DSFab needs not to be adjusted in patients with renal failure. The serum half-life of digoxin and DigiFab is similar. Both digoxin and Fab fragments and digoxin Fab immune complex are removed by the kidneys. While the duration of binding of digoxin immune Fab to free digoxin is unknown, case reports of patients with renal failure have found a rebound in serum digoxin levels 1–8 days after DigiFab administration,[11-13] suggesting that the DigiFab and digoxin have become unbound before

TABLE 1: Dosing of antidigoxin Fab depending on digoxin toxicity presentation.

Acute toxicity	*Acute-on-chronic toxicity*	*Chronic toxicity*
Digoxin overdose (intentional or accidental) in digoxin-naïve patient	Digoxin overdose (intentional or accidental) in a patient on regular digoxin	Subacute accumulation of toxic digoxin levels in a patient on regular digoxin who has a risk factor for digoxin toxicity (e.g., renal dysfunction/ hyperkalemia)
Give full calculated digoxin immune Fab dose over 30 minutes	Give full calculated dose if amount ingested is known	Give half the calculated dose over 30 minutes
Give repeat dose if inadequate clinical response after 2 hours	Give half dose if amount is unknown	Give the remaining dose if evidence of rebound toxicity occurs

excretion. There is no need to reduce dose of DigiFab in patients with renal dysfunction, but the monitoring period after Fab administration should be prolonged to treat any rebound toxicity if it happens. Cases of recurrent digoxin toxicity, including ventricular dysrhythmias, have been reported 72–90 hours after antidotal therapy. Thus, any patients with significant renal dysfunction who received Fab fragments should be closely monitored for a minimum period of 72 hours. Repeat serum digoxin levels should be measured 24–48 hours after DigiFab administration to detect any rebound in serum digoxin levels. It is important to note that total SDCs are not reliable after DigiFab administration as they represent free plus bound digoxin, but only free (unbound) digoxin levels are clinically useful **(Table 1)**.

AVAILABILITY AND ADMINISTRATION OF ANTIDIGOXIN FAB

Digoxin-specific antibody fragments are available as Digibind or DigiFab. It is available in vial in powder form and prepared with sterile water for injection (4 mL per vial) and then diluted in normal saline and given as IV injection over 3 minutes. Each vial contains approximately 38–40 mg of Fab fragments (Digibind 38 mg and DigiFab 40 mg). Each vial binds 0.5 mg of digoxin. Fab fragments should be given over 30 minutes, except in patients with cardiac arrest or in whom arrest is imminent. In such patients, the Fab fragments can be given as a slow IV push. The biggest difficulty to its extensive use is the high cost (US$ 750 per 40 mg vial) and nonavailability of the drug in many countries, including India.

ONSET OF RESPONSE AFTER ANTIDIGOXIN FAB

The antibody is utilized more often in the management of acute rather than chronic digoxin toxicity. It has been shown that the levels of free digoxin rapidly become negligible within a few minutes after Fab administration, with a time to reversal of digoxin toxicity within 30–45 minutes. Overall, the response to digoxin Fab has varied from 50% to 80–90% with better success rate in acute poisoning.[14,15] A possible explanation for this apparent poor efficacy of the antibody in chronic digoxin poisoning could be substantial comorbid illnesses such as cardiac or renal dysfunction and co-prescription of drugs such as angiotensin-converting enzyme inhibitors, calcium channel blockers, beta-blockers, or aldosterone antagonists.[16]

MONITORING POSTDIGOXIN IMMUNE FAB ADMINISTRATION

- Potassium levels should be monitored regularly, particularly during the first 6 hours post-treatment with DigiFab.
- Frequent electrocardiogram (ECG) monitoring is required to monitor cardiac side effects due to digoxin toxicity and potential worsening of preexisting cardiac disorders (due to withdrawal of digoxin therapeutic effect).
- Monitor renal function, including serum urea and creatinine as well as estimated glomerular filtration rate (eGFR)
- Continue monitoring till potassium levels, ECG, and renal function get "normalized."

ADVERSE EFFECTS

- Hypersensitivity reactions are the common adverse effects of DigiFab, as it is made from sheep antibodies, and it also contains papaya fruit extracts. Although uncommon, patients with highest risk are those with known allergies to sheep or hypersensitivity to papain/papaya extracts (used to cleave the whole IgG antibody).

- Use of DigiFab may result in complete reversal of digoxin therapeutic effects, precipitating an acute CHF (negative inotropy) or loss of rate control in patients with atrial fibrillation, leading to rapid ventricular rate.
- *Hypokalemia:* Hypokalemia associated with DigiFab administration generally resolves spontaneously in few hours, but potassium levels need to be monitored regularly, particularly during the first 6 hours after the treatment.

ANTIDIGOXIN FAB IN NONDIGOXIN CARDIAC GLYCOSIDES POISONING

Because Fab can bind to other cardiac glycosides also, it has been used in the management of poisoning with other nondigoxin cardiac glycosides, especially yellow oleander.[17] In a single-center study from Sri Lanka, 66 patients of yellow oleander poisoning with significant cardiac toxicity were randomized to receive either 1,200 mg of Fab or placebo.[16] Reversal of arrhythmias, increase in heart rate, and reduction in serum K^+ level were significantly higher in antibody-treated patients. Dose of antibody in yellow oleander toxicity is generally higher partly due to failure to quantify the toxin burden from history and in vitro assays and also due to lower cross-reactivity between Fab and other cardiac glycosides.[18]

CONCLUSION

Digoxin-specific antibody fragments have dramatically improved patient care with cardiac glycosides poisoning. In nearly 38 years since the commercial release of Digibind (DigiFab) in 1986, a fatal digoxin overdose has become easily clinically manageable. Digoxin immune Fab still remains an effective, rapid-acting, and potentially lifesaving treatment. Despite availability of highly effective treatment, nonavailability of antidigoxin Fab and high treatment cost have become biggest barrier to the delivery of this therapy mainly in developing countries, including India.

Following are the key points:

- Cardiac glycosides poisoning is common and includes digoxin and other plant toxins.
- Antidigoxin Fab is the treatment of choice for all potentially life-threatening toxic manifestations, including dysrhythmias, hyperkalemia, and hemodynamic instability, with high serum digoxin levels, but limited by cost and nonavailability in many countries, including India.
- Antidigoxin Fab dose can be calculated either by knowing the total digoxin dose ingested or steady-state serum digoxin levels.

REFERENCES

1. Colburn WA. Specific antibodies and Fab fragments to alter the pharmacokinetics and reverse pharmacologic/toxicologic effects of drugs. Drug Metab Rev. 1980;11(2):223-62.
2. Heath AJ. Immunotherapy for drug toxicity. In: Landon L, Chard T (Eds). Therapeutic Antibodies, 1st edition. London, UK: Springer-Verlag London Limited; 1995. pp. 89-106.
3. Bayer MJ. Recognition and management of digitalis intoxication: implications for emergency medicine. Am J Emerg Med 1991;9(2 Suppl 1):29-32.
4. Butler VP Jr, Chen JP. Digoxin-specific antibodies. Proc Natl Acad Sci U S A. 1967;57(1):71-78. doi:10.1073/pnas.57.1.71.
5. Smith TW, Haber E, Yeatman L, Butler VP. Reversal of advanced digoxin intoxication with Fab fragments of digoxin-specific antibodies. N Engl J Med. 1976;294(15):797-800.
6. Antman EM, Wenger TL, Butler VP, Haber E, Smith TW. Treatment of 150 cases of life-threatening digitalis intoxication with digoxin-specific Fab antibody fragments. Circulation. 1990;81(6):1744-52.
7. Lloyd BL, Smith TW. Contrasting rates of reversal of digoxin toxicity by digoxin-specific IgG and Fab fragments. Circulation. 1978;58(2):280-83.
8. Food and Drug Administration. (2017). DigiFab® Digoxin Immune Fab (Ovine). [online] Available from https://www.fda.gov/media/74693/download. [Last accessed February, 2025].
9. Al-Khatib SM, Stevenson WG, Ackerman MJ, Bryant WJ, Callans DJ, Curtis AB, et al. 2017 AHA/ACC/HRS guideline for management of patients with ventricular arrhythmias and the prevention of sudden cardiac death: a report of the American College of Cardiology/American Heart Association Task Force on clinical practice guidelines and the Heart Rhythm Society. J Am Coll Cardiol. 2018;72(14):e91-220.
10. Chan BS, Isbister GK, Chiew A, Isoardi K, Buckley NA. Clinical experience with titrating doses of digoxin antibodies in acute digoxin poisoning (ATOM-6). Clin Toxicol (Phila). 2022;60(4):433-9.
11. Ujhelyi MR, Robert S, Cummings DM, Colucci RD, Sailstad JM, Vlasses PH, et al. Disposition of digoxin immune Fab in patients with kidney failure. Clin Pharmacol Ther. 1993;54(4):388-94.
12. Allen NM, Dunham GD, Sailstad JM, Findlay JW. Clinical and pharmacokinetic profiles of digoxin immune Fab in four patients with renal impairment. DICP. 1991;25(12):1315-20.
13. Ujhelyi MR, Robert S, Cummings DM, Colucci RD, Green PJ, Sailstad JM, et al. Influence of digoxin immune Fab therapy and renal dysfunction on the disposition of total and free digoxin. Ann Intern Med. 1993;119(4):273-7.

14. Smith TW. Review of clinical experience with digoxin immune Fab (ovine). Am J Emerg Med. 1991;9(2 Suppl 1):1-6.
15. Protherics UK Limited DigiFab®. (2016). Summary of product characteristics. [online] Available from https://digifab.health/getmedia/6f38d7ed-1832-4b7d-863a-9c71905e4d02/SmPC_DigiFab_Dec17.pdf. [Last accessed February, 2025].
16. Eddleston M, Rajapakse S, Rajakanthan K, Jayalath S, Sjöström L, Santharaj W, et al. Anti-digoxin Fab fragments in cardiotoxicity induced by ingestion of yellow oleander: a randomised controlled trial. Lancet. 2000;355(9208):967-72.
17. Chan BSH, Buckley NA. Digoxin-specific antibody fragments in the treatment of digoxin toxicity. Clin Toxicol (Phila). 2014;52(8):824-36.
18. Chan BS, Isbister GK, O'Leary M, Chiew A, Buckley NA. Efficacy and effectiveness of anti-digoxin antibodies in chronic digoxin poisonings from the DORA study (ATOM-1). Clin Toxicol (Phila). 2016;54(6):488-94.

ANTIDOTES ACTING ON THE TOXIN BINDING SITE

4.7 Competitive Inhibition: Alcohols (Ethanol, Fomepizole)

Siju V Abraham

INTRODUCTION

Alcohols are hydrocarbons that contain a hydroxyl group. All alcohols are toxic causing inebriation and end-organ damage depending on their dose. However, alcohols that are not usually meant to be consumed orally even in minimal doses, such as methanol, ethylene glycol, and iso propranolol, are arbitrarily termed "toxic".

Toxic alcohol poisoning presents a significant clinical challenge due to the severe metabolic acidosis and organ damage caused by their metabolites. Effective treatment hinges on the use of antidotes such as ethanol and fomepizole. This chapter covers the metabolism of alcohols, role of alcohol dehydrogenase (ADH), mechanisms by which ethanol and fomepizole act, their administration routes and dosages, dose adjustments during hemodialysis, therapy end points, and potential side effects.

METABOLISM OF ALCOHOL AND ROLE OF ALCOHOL DEHYDROGENASE

Alcohol dehydrogenase is a critical enzyme in the metabolic processing of alcohols in the liver.[1] It catalyzes the conversion of alcohols into aldehydes, which are subsequently metabolized into other metabolites **(Flowchart 1)**. Ethanol is commonly metabolized by ADH into acetaldehyde and further into acetic acid, a relatively harmless substance that can be broken down into carbon dioxide and water.[2] However, for toxic alcohols such as methanol and ethylene glycol, the role of ADH becomes pivotal in the context of toxicity. Alcohols are rapidly absorbed postingestion but undergo metabolism by gastric ADH and hepatic ADH.[3] ADH is crucial in the metabolism of ethanol and toxic alcohols such as methanol, isopropanol, and ethylene glycol. ADH, primarily located in the liver, catalyzes the oxidation of alcohols to their respective aldehydes and ketones.

Ethanol Metabolism

Ethanol is rapidly absorbed from the gastrointestinal tract, primarily from the small intestine, with about 20% absorbed from the stomach under optimal conditions. Factors such as rapid gastric emptying and consumption without food can enhance this absorption, allowing 80–90% of an ingested dose to be absorbed within 60 minutes.

In the liver, ethanol metabolism is predominantly mediated by ADH in the cytosol of hepatocytes, converting ethanol to acetaldehyde, which is further metabolized to acetate by mitochondrial NAD^+-dependent aldehyde dehydrogenase (ALDH) into acetate.

The acetate is converted into acetyl-CoA, entering the Krebs cycle, and gets metabolized to carbon dioxide and water. A small portion, about 2–5%, of ethanol escapes metabolism and is excreted unchanged through urine, breath, and sweat.

Flowchart 1: Metabolism of alcohols.

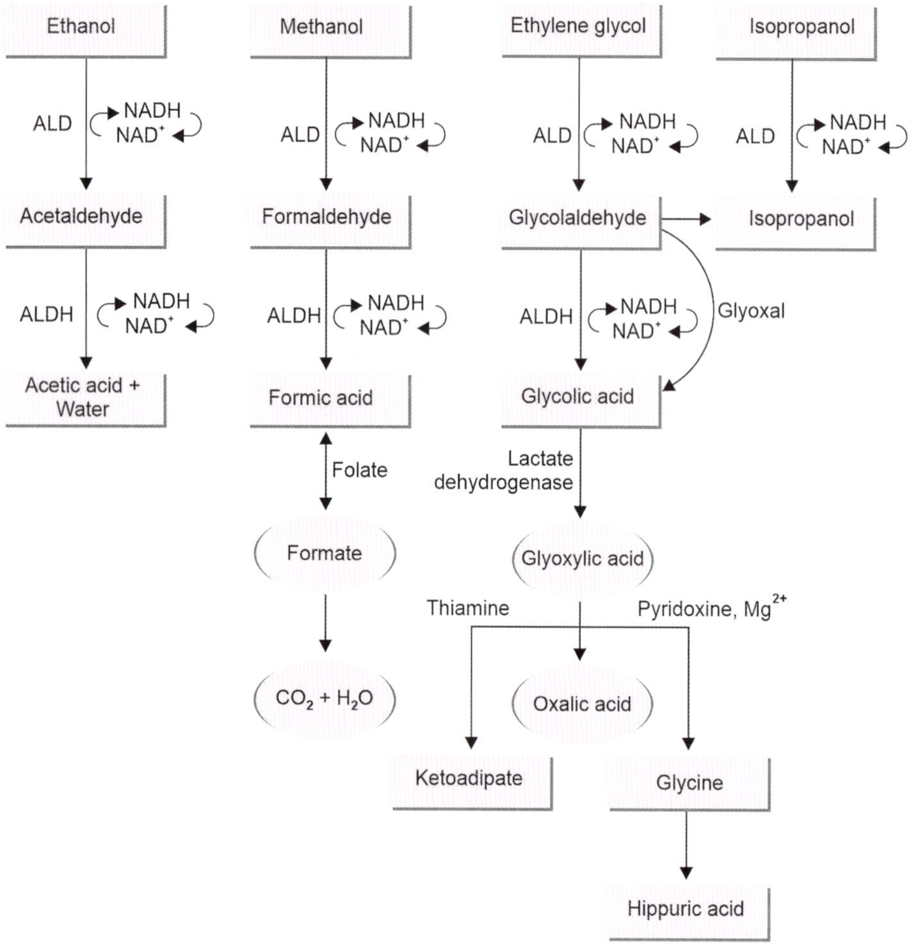

(ALDH: aldehyde dehydrogenase; NADH: nicotinamide-adenine dinucleotide hydrogen)

Methanol Metabolism

Methanol is initially metabolized by ADH to formaldehyde and subsequently to formic acid, which is associated with the toxicity symptoms of methanol poisoning, including metabolic acidosis and visual disturbances. The formate metabolite is then bound by tetrahydrofolate and metabolized by 10-formyltetrahydrofolate dehydrogenase into carbon dioxide and water. Methanol itself exhibits zero-order kinetics with a metabolic rate of approximately 8.5–10 mg/dL/h.[4,5] Methanol is primarily eliminated as a vapor in expired air, with minimal renal elimination—about 1% of the ingested dose in patients with intact hepatic metabolism. The half-life of methanol in the body is approximately 52–54 hours, which may extend at very high concentrations and when blocked by antidotes.[6,7]

Ethylene Glycol Metabolism

Ethylene glycol undergoes metabolism by ADH and ALDH, being oxidized to glycolaldehyde, glycolic acid, glyoxylic acid, and finally to oxalic acid, which are responsible for the renal toxicity and metabolic disturbances seen in ethylene glycol poisoning. Like methanol, its metabolism follows zero-order kinetics at a rate of about 10 mg/dL/h.[7]

In cases of normal kidney function, ethylene glycol is cleared with a half-life of approximately 17 hours. In patients with renal impairment, the half-life is significantly prolonged to about 34 hours on average.[8] Ethylene glycol is also metabolized to ketoadipate and glycine using thiamine and pyridoxine as cofactors, producing metabolites with lower toxicity. Enhancing these normally minor pathways can be beneficial in treating ethylene glycol poisoning.[9,10]

Flowchart 2: Metabolism of ethanol.

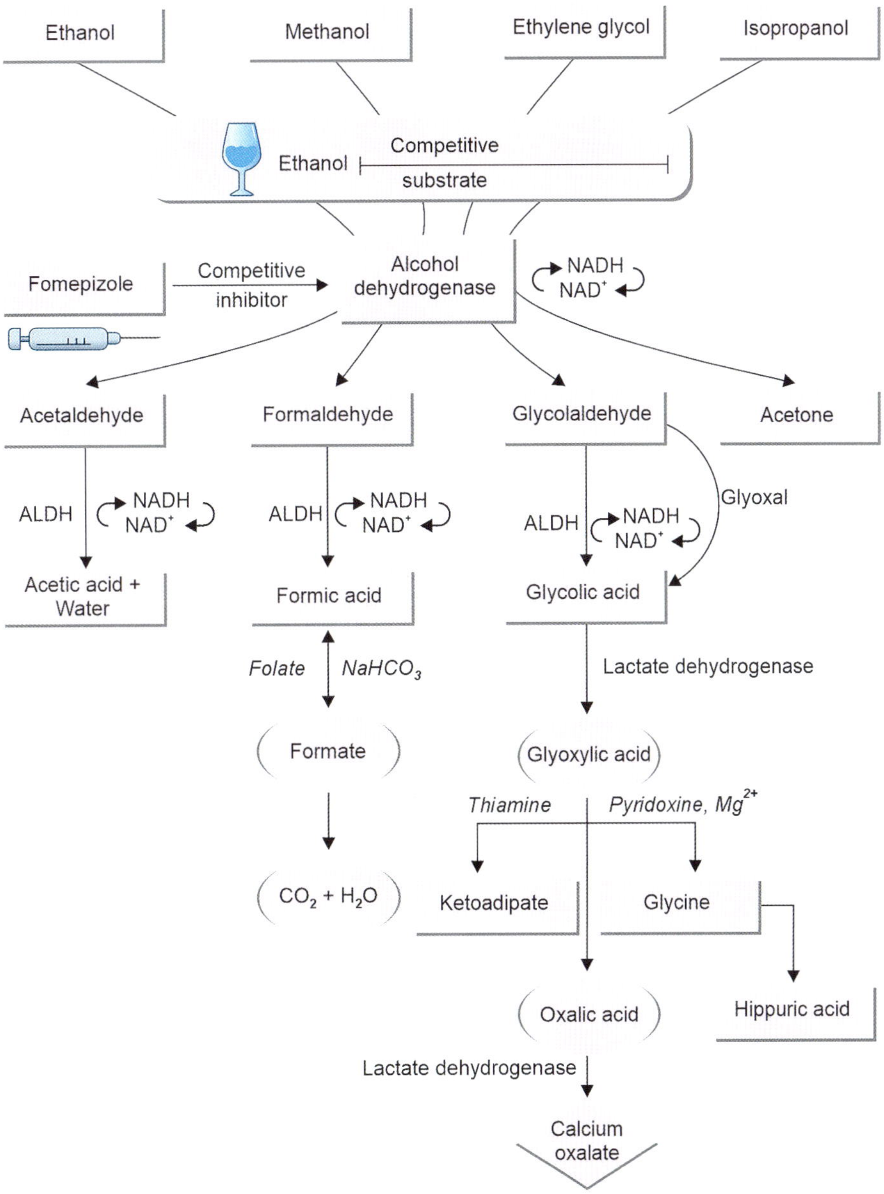

(ALDH: aldehyde dehydrogenase; NADH: nicotinamide-adenine dinucleotide hydrogen)

Alternate minor metabolic pathways, such as catalase, also exist for these alcohols. Isopropanol is metabolized by ADH to acetone, a ketone that cannot be further metabolized by ALDH, and is, thus, eliminated in the urine and expired air.

How Ethanol and Fomepizole Prevent Toxic Metabolite Generation?

Fomepizole (4-methylpyrazole) and ethanol both interact with ADH to prevent the metabolism of toxic alcohols into their harmful metabolites, though their mechanisms differ as fomepizole inhibits while ethanol competes **(Flowchart 2)**.

Fomepizole as a Competitive Inhibitor

Fomepizole is a potent competitive *inhibitor* of ADH, effectively blocking the conversion of methanol and ethylene glycol into their toxic metabolites—formaldehyde and glycolaldehyde, respectively, which in turn prevent production of more harmful compounds such as formic acid and oxalic acid.

Inhibition Constant

Measured in micromoles per liter (μmol/L), the inhibition constant (Ki) value for fomepizole indicates its efficacy in inhibiting ADH. Low Ki values demonstrate its strong inhibitory action, requiring only minimal concentrations to effectively block ADH. Clinical protocols recommend maintaining serum concentrations of fomepizole well above the Ki value to ensure the metabolism of toxic alcohols is inhibited.[11] The relative affinity of fomepizole for ADH is 80,000 times greater than that of methanol and ethylene glycol and 8,000 times greater than that of ethanol.[9,12,13]

Ethanol's Role as a Competitive *Substrate*

Unlike fomepizole, ethanol functions by competing with methanol and ethylene glycol for the active site of ADH. This competition reduces the rate at which these toxic alcohols are metabolized into their hazardous metabolites **(Table 1)**.

Michaelis Constant

The Michaelis constant (Km) value, expressed in millimoles per liter (mM), reflects the concentration of substrate at which ADH reaches half of its maximum activity. Lower the Km, more the affinity. Ethanol has a Km of 0.45 mM, much lower than that for methanol (7 mM) and ethylene glycol (30 mM), indicating a higher affinity of ethanol for ADH. This means that the molar affinity of ethanol for ADH is 67 times that of ethylene glycol and 15.5 times that of methanol. Using human ADH and a simulation model, the oxidation of 50 mM of methanol and ethylene glycol was inhibited by 20 mM (92 mg/dL) of ethanol and 50 mM (4 mg/dL) of fomepizole.[10]

TABLE 1: Comparing fomepizole and ethanol as an antidote for toxic alcohol poisoning.

Feature	*Fomepizole*	*Ethanol*
Mechanism of action	Inhibits alcohol dehydrogenase (ADH) directly, preventing the metabolism of toxic alcohols into harmful metabolites	Competes with methanol and ethylene glycol for ADH, reducing their metabolism into toxic metabolites
Affinity for ADH	High affinity, acting as a potent inhibitor	Lower affinity compared to fomepizole; functions as a competitive substrate
Usage	Used primarily when intravenous (IV) administration is possible and in settings where rapid control of toxic alcohol levels is critical	Commonly used in resource-limited and mass casualty settings
Dosage	Loading dose: 15 mg/kg IV, followed by 10 mg/kg every 12 hours up to 48 hours	• *Oral loading dose:* 0.8 g/kg; maintenance dose: 0.1 g/kg/h • *Intravenous:* 10% IV solution, 7.5 mL/kg over 30 minutes • *Maintenance dose:* 1.0–1.5 mL/kg/h of 10% ethanol solution to maintain a serum ethanol concentration of 100–150 mg/dL
Estimate for a 60 kg person	The loading dose is 900 mg IV, followed by a maintenance dose of 600 mg every 12 hours	• *Oral loading dose:* 52 g of 40% ethanol (approximately 130 mL of 40% ethanol), diluted with an equal volume of water (130 mL) to achieve a 20% ethanol solution, resulting in a total volume of 260 mL • *Maintenance dose:* 6.5 g/h of 40% ethanol (32.5 mL/h of 40% ethanol or 65 mL/h of 20% ethanol)
Side effects	Hypersensitivity reactions, headache, nausea, and transient liver enzyme elevations. Fewer side effects compared to ethanol	Can cause hypoglycemia, central nervous system (CNS) depression, gastric irritation, and electrolyte imbalances
Efficacy	Highly effective in inhibiting ADH and preventing the formation of toxic metabolites with minimal monitoring	Effective but requires close monitoring to maintain therapeutic serum concentrations and manage side effects
Therapeutic monitoring	Less frequent monitoring required due to more predictable pharmacokinetics	Requires regular monitoring of serum ethanol levels, especially during hemodialysis to maintain efficacy

ROUTE AND DOSE OF ADMINISTRATION OF ETHANOL IN TOXIC ALCOHOL POISONING

In India, where intravenous (IV) ethanol preparations are not available and procuring fomepizole is difficult to procure, oral ethanol serves as the primary treatment for toxic alcohol poisoning. There are several textbooks recommending sterile IV preparation making methods in the author's opinion that have a high risk of dosage errors and are best avoided.

A 20% ethanol concentration, administered orally or via a nasogastric tube, is recommended in most situations, except when oral administration is impractical (e.g., non-intact gastrointestinal tract or altered mental status).[5,7,14,15]

Oral Administration

The dosing regimen for oral ethanol administration is as follows:

- *Loading dose:* 0.8 g/kg of body weight of 40% ethanol (e.g., vodka and whiskey), diluted to 20% solution to minimize gastric irritation. This is approximately 4 mL/kg of 40% ethanol.
- *Maintenance dose:* 0.1 g/kg/h. This dose may need adjustment based on serum ethanol levels and the patient's metabolic rate.

Most strong spirits available in the market are 40% w/v alcohol and to make it more palatable and less gastric irritant, a 20% solution (or less) is recommended. To achieve that, we just need to dilute it with an equal amount of potable water.

So, in practice for a 65 kg individual: This would require 52 g of 40% ethanol (approximately 130 mL of 40% ethanol), diluted with an equal volume of water (130 mL) to achieve a 20% ethanol solution, resulting in a total volume of 260 mL and a maintenance dose: 6.5 g/h of 40% ethanol (approximately 32.5 mL/h of 40% ethanol).

So, for the loading dose: Mix 130 mL of 40% vodka with 130 mL of water to get 260 mL of 20% ethanol solution. Administer this mixture as the loading dose.

Maintenance dose: Administer 32.5 mL/h of 40% vodka, diluted with 32.5 mL of potable water, resulting in 65 mL/h of 20% ethanol solution.

Intravenous Administration

Intravenous administration provides more controlled and consistent plasma levels. However, plasma levels are not always available in demand.

The dosing regimen for IV ethanol is as follows:

- Loading dose: 10% ethanol solution, 7.5 mL/kg over 30 minutes.
- Maintenance dose: 1.0–1.5 mL/kg/h of 10% ethanol solution to maintain a serum ethanol concentration of 100–150 mg/dL.

During hemodialysis, the ethanol infusion rate should be increased to compensate for its removal by dialysis. Typically, the maintenance dose should be doubled during dialysis sessions to ensure that therapeutic levels are maintained.[5,14]

Consensus Recommendation

Hassanian-Moghaddam et al. provided consensus statements for managing methanol poisoning outbreaks, targeted at health professionals and government health authorities in various clinical and geographical settings.[14] These statements were developed with the input of 22 experts experienced in methanol poisoning outbreaks and clinical toxicology, and the discussions continued until no new themes emerged. The quality of evidence supporting the recommendations was graded from A (high-quality, well-conducted randomized controlled trials) to D (very low-quality, lesser data). The strength of the recommendations was classified into three levels: level 1 (strong recommendation), level 2 (weak recommendation), and level 3 (neutral recommendation/could not reach an agreement).

The consensus strongly recommends (level 1C) that patients with a high probability of methanol poisoning during an outbreak are promptly administered an antidote such as ethanol, while further assessment is undertaken. Additionally, it is recommended (level 1B) that antidote administration should occur in the prehospital setting wherever possible because early initiation of the antidote improves clinical outcomes.[14]

ROUTE AND ADMINISTRATION OF FOMEPIZOLE

Route of Administration

Intravenous Only

Fomepizole is administered solely via IV injection, ensuring rapid and controlled delivery into the bloodstream to effectively inhibit ADH.

Dosing and Administration

Loading Dose

The initial dose of fomepizole is 15 mg/kg IV. This is followed by a maintenance dose given every 12 hours (consensus recommendation: level 1D).[14]

Maintenance Dose

Initially, 10 mg/kg is administered every 12 hours for the first 48 hours. If further treatment is necessary, the dose is increased to 15 mg/kg every 12 hours.[16] Increased 15 mg/kg is to compensate for fomepizole-induced increased body clearance, resulting from autoinduction of the cytochrome P450 (CYP) drug-metabolizing enzyme.

CYP2E1 as recommended by drug manufacturers is questioned by some.[6,17] Dosing must also be adjusted during dialysis.

Special Considerations for Dialysis

For patients undergoing hemodialysis, fomepizole should be administered at the beginning of the dialysis session if >6 hours have passed since the last dose. After dialysis, the next scheduled dose should be administered if >3 hours have elapsed or half the dose if 1–3 hours have passed. Regular dosing resumes every 12 hours postdialysis.

Dilution and Infusion

Fomepizole must be diluted in 100 mL of 0.9% sodium chloride solution or 5% dextrose in water (D5W) before IV administration and then infused over 30 minutes to avoid venous irritation and thrombophlebitis.[18]

Continuation of Therapy

Fomepizole treatment should continue until toxic alcohol levels are reduced to safe concentrations (typically below 25 mg/dL) and any associated acid–base disturbances are resolved. The regimen may need to be adjusted based on the half-life of the toxic alcohol, which can be extended due to the interaction with fomepizole.

During hemodialysis, the dosing interval should be shortened to every 4 hours to account for the removal of fomepizole during dialysis.

Consensus Recommendation[14]

When both fomepizole and ethanol are available, it is recommended (level 1D) that patients with more severe poisoning receive fomepizole and those with lesser poisoning severity receive ethanol. Special priority for fomepizole is recommended (level 1D) for patients who are pregnant or younger than 14 years.

Dosing (Level 1D)

The published loading dose of fomepizole (15 mg/kg) is recommended for patients with the most severe poisonings (acidosis, visual disturbance, or coma).

High-risk Patients (Level 1D)

If sufficient fomepizole is available, patients at high risk of toxicity but without current acidosis or end-organ damage should receive fomepizole.

MODIFICATIONS IN DOSES IF EXTRACORPOREAL REMOVAL TECHNIQUE IS CONSIDERED

Toxic alcohols are readily removed by extracorporeal removal techniques (ECRTs), such as hemodialysis and continuous renal replacement therapy (CRRT).[8,19] The definitive treatment for toxic alcohol poisoning is hemodialysis.

Dialysis removes both the toxic alcohol and its toxic metabolites. Dialysis decreases the half-life of methanol to 2–3 hours and ethylene glycol to 3–4 hours.[20-22] However, hemodialysis significantly affects the pharmacokinetics of both ethanol and fomepizole, necessitating dose adjustments to maintain therapeutic levels.

Ethanol

During hemodialysis, the ethanol infusion rate must be increased to compensate for its removal by the dialysis process. The recommended adjustment is to increase the maintenance dose by two to three times the usual rate. Regular monitoring of serum ethanol levels is crucial to ensure that therapeutic concentrations are maintained.

Fomepizole

Fomepizole dosing during hemodialysis requires more frequent administration:

- *Intermittent hemodialysis (IHD):* Increase the maintenance dose to 10 mg/kg every 4 hours.
- *Continuous renal replacement therapy:* Administer 10 mg/kg every 8 hours.

These adjustments ensure that fomepizole maintains its inhibitory effect on ADH throughout the dialysis process.

Predialysis Dosing

If >6 hours have elapsed since the last fomepizole dose, administer a dose of fomepizole at the beginning of hemodialysis to ensure adequate levels throughout the procedure.

During dialysis, the manufacturer recommendation is to give one full dose every 4 hours the patient is on dialysis.

Postdialysis Dosing

At the completion of hemodialysis, administer the next scheduled dose if >3 hours have elapsed since the last dose.

If only 1–3 hours have passed, administer half of the next scheduled dose to compensate for the fomepizole removed during dialysis. If <1 hour, no additional doses are required.

Maintenance Dosing Posthemodialysis

Resume the regular dosing schedule of fomepizole every 12 hours following the completion of hemodialysis.

Considerations for Continuous Renal Replacement Therapies

For patients undergoing CRRTs such as continuous venovenous hemodialysis or continuous venovenous hemodiafiltration, the dosing of fomepizole may also need adjustment.

Increased Frequency of Dosing

While the exact dosing may vary based on the specific CRRT modality and rate of fomepizole removal, a reasonable approach would be to administer fomepizole every 8 hours during CRRT.

END POINTS OF DOSING

Antidote therapy should ideally be continued until the toxic alcohol is no longer present in sufficient concentrations to produce toxicity. However, in most clinical settings, the end points for dosing ethanol or fomepizole in toxic alcohol poisoning are based on clinical improvement and routine laboratory parameters.

Clinical Improvement

- *Resolution of metabolic acidosis:* Improvement in blood pH and bicarbonate levels
- *Improvement in visual symptoms:* Resolution of visual disturbances
- *Stabilization of vital signs:* Restoration of stable hemodynamics and normal respiratory function

Laboratory Parameters

- *Blood pH:* Normalization of pH (7.35–7.45)
- *Bicarbonate levels:* Restoration of normal bicarbonate levels (22–26 mEq/L)
- *Anion gap:* Reduction of the anion gap to normal levels (8–16 mEq/L)[19]

Methanol/Ethylene Glycol Levels

Monitoring the levels of methanol and ethylene glycol is ideal to guide the duration of therapy. Treatment can typically be discontinued when:

- *Methanol levels:* Fall below 20 mg/dL
- *Ethylene glycol levels:* Fall below 10 mg/dL

When fomepizole is used to treat methanol poisoning, it significantly extends the half-life of methanol in the body. The half-life for the systemic clearance of methanol has been reported to be 2.5–3 hours for doses <100 mg/kg body weight, increasing to 24 hours or longer for doses >1,000 mg/kg body weight. The half-life of methanol with fomepizole administration is approximately 54 hours, though it can range from 22 to 87 hours. In the case of ethylene glycol poisoning, the half-life ranges from 14 to 17 hours when kidney function is normal, extending to about 49 hours with impaired kidney function. This extended half-life underscores the impact of reduced renal function on the body's ability to eliminate ethylene glycol.[9,17,23,24]

The duration of fomepizole therapy should be adjusted based on these half-life estimates. Treatment should continue until blood levels of methanol or ethylene glycol decrease to safe levels, ensuring adequate time for metabolic clearance of the toxins. Monitoring of the patient's kidney function is crucial, as it influences the clearance rate of the toxic alcohols and, consequently, the necessary duration of fomepizole therapy. Without hemodialysis to accelerate the removal of toxic alcohols, reliance on fomepizole and the body's natural clearance mechanisms are essential. Therefore, therapy durations will be longer, particularly in patients with impaired kidney function.

Consensus Recommendation[14]

The guidelines recommend (level 1D) continuing the treatment until methanol or ethylene glycol levels fall below toxic levels, with additional recommendations on monitoring osmolality and other clinical parameters to guide therapy duration.

Optimal Treatment (Level 1D)

Patients requiring antidote treatment should also receive optimal treatment with bicarbonate, folic/folinic acid, and supportive treatment as necessary.

Laboratory Monitoring (Level 1D)

It is important to measure osmolality using a freezing point depression method, not a vapor pressure method, as the latter will not detect the increased osmolality caused by volatile alcohols and could give a false negative result.

SIDE EFFECTS

Fomepizole

- *Headache:* Reported by 14% of patients[25]
- *Nausea:* Gastrointestinal upset, including nausea, reported by 11% of patients[25]
- *Transient transaminitis:* Elevated liver enzymes, indicating transient liver stress, observed in some cases
- *Allergic reactions:* Rare hypersensitivity reactions
- *Other side effects:* Dizziness, increased drowsiness, dysgeusia (metallic taste), phlebitis, rash, fever, and eosinophilia.
- In clinical settings, fomepizole has been well tolerated even at higher doses; severe life-threatening adverse drug events were reported in 2% of cases.[25]

Ethanol

- *Hypoglycemia:* Ethanol can cause hypoglycemia, especially in children and malnourished individuals. Regular monitoring of blood glucose levels is essential.
- *Central nervous system (CNS) depression:* Causes sedation, inebriation, and CNS depression, complicating the clinical picture. CNS symptoms accounted for 48% of adverse drug events in ethanol-treated cases compared to 2% in fomepizole-treated cases.[25]
- *Gastric irritation:* Oral ethanol can cause gastric irritation and vomiting.
- *Electrolyte imbalances:* Diuresis from ethanol can lead to electrolyte imbalances such as hypokalemia and hyponatremia.
- In a retrospective review of records, toxicologists identified at least one adverse drug event in 57% of ethanol-treated cases, with 20% experiencing severe adverse drug events (e.g., coma, extreme agitation, cardiovascular issues) and 8% experiencing serious adverse drug events (e.g., respiratory depression, hypotension).

CONCLUSION

While both fomepizole and ethanol are effective antidotes for toxic alcohol poisoning, fomepizole is often preferred due to its efficacy and safety profile (adverse drug event rate of 0.93 events per treatment-day for ethanol compared to 0.13 events per treatment-day for fomepizole).[25] Ethanol, however, remains a vital alternative, particularly where fomepizole is unavailable.[15,26]

REFERENCES

1. Lutwak-Mann C. Alcohol dehydrogenase of animal tissues. Biochem J. 1938;32(8):1364-74.
2. Zakhari S. Overview: how is alcohol metabolized by the body? Alcohol Res Health. 2006;29(4):245-54.
3. Seitz HK, Oneta CM. Gastrointestinal alcohol dehydrogenase. Nutr Rev. 1998;56(2 Pt 1):52-60.
4. Clay KL, Murphy RC, Watkins WD. Experimental methanol toxicity in the primate: analysis of metabolic acidosis. Toxicol Appl Pharmacol. 1975;34(1):49-61.
5. Haffner HT, Wehner HD, Scheytt KD, Besserer K. The elimination kinetics of methanol and the influence of ethanol. Int J Legal Med. 1992;105(2):111-4.
6. Brent J, McMartin K, Phillips S, Aaron C, Kulig K. Fomepizole for the treatment of methanol poisoning. N Engl J Med. 2001;344(6):424-9.
7. Jacobsen D, McMartin KE. Antidotes for methanol and ethylene glycol poisoning. J Toxicol Clin Toxicol. 1997;35(2):127-43.
8. Ghannoum M, Gosselin S, Hoffman RS, Lavergne V, Mégarbane B, Hassanian-Moghaddam H, et al. Extracorporeal treatment for ethylene glycol poisoning: systematic review and recommendations from the EXTRIP workgroup. Crit Care. 2023;27:56.
9. Sivilotti MLA, Burns MJ, McMartin KE, Brent J. Toxicokinetics of ethylene glycol during fomepizole therapy: implications for management. Ann Emerg Med. 2000;36(2):114-25.
10. Lee SL, Shih HT, Chi YC, Li YP, Yin SJ. Oxidation of methanol, ethylene glycol, and isopropanol with human alcohol dehydrogenases and the inhibition by ethanol and 4-methylpyrazole. Chem Biol Interact. 2011;191(1-3):26-31.

11. McMartin K, Brent J. Analysis of fomepizole elimination in methanol- and ethylene glycol-poisoned patients. J Med Toxicol. 2022;18(1):19-29.
12. Pietruszko R. Human liver alcohol dehydrogenase—inhibition of methanol activity by pyrazole, 4-methylpyrazole, 4-hydroxymethylpyrazole and 4-carboxypyrazole. Biochem Pharmacol. 1975;24(17):1603-7.
13. Connally HE, Hamar DW, Thrall MA. Inhibition of canine and feline alcohol dehydrogenase activity by fomepizole. Am J Vet Res. 2000;61(4):450-5.
14. Hassanian-Moghaddam H, Zamani N, Roberts DM, Brent J, McMartin K, Aaron C, et al. Consensus statements on the approach to patients in a methanol poisoning outbreak. Clin Toxicol (Phila). 2019;57(12):1129-36.
15. Zakharov S, Pelclova D, Navratil T, Belacek J, Komarc M, Eddleston M, et al. Fomepizole versus ethanol in the treatment of acute methanol poisoning: comparison of clinical effectiveness in a mass poisoning outbreak. Clin Toxicol (Phila). 2015;53(8):797-806.
16. Food and Drug Administration. (2020). Fomepizole injection. Available from https://www.accessdata.fda.gov/drugsatfda_docs/label/2020/020696s006lbl.pdf. [Last accessed February, 2025].
17. Bestic M, Blackford M, Reed M. Fomepizole: a critical assessment of current dosing recommendations. J Clin Pharmacol. 2009;49(2):130-7.
18. McGraw-Hill Education. (2019). Antidotes in Depth. Available from https://accessemergencymedicine.mhmedical.com/content.aspx?sectionid=210256656&bookid=2569. [Last accessed February, 2025].
19. Roberts DM, Yates C, Megarbane B, Winchester JF, Maclaren R, Gosselin S, et al. Recommendations for the role of extracorporeal treatments in the management of acute methanol poisoning: a systematic review and consensus statement. Crit Care Med. 2015;43(2):461-72.
20. Lachance P, Mac-Way F, Desmeules S, de Serres SA, Julien AS, Douville P, et al. Prediction and validation of hemodialysis duration in acute methanol poisoning. Kidney Int. 2015;88(5):1170-7.
21. Iliuta IA, Lachance P, Ghannoum M, Bégin Y, Mac-Way F, Desmeules S, et al. Prediction and validation of the duration of hemodialysis sessions for the treatment of acute ethylene glycol poisoning. Kidney Int. 2017;92(2):453-60.
22. Kraut JA. Approach to the treatment of methanol intoxication. Am J Kidney Dis. 2016;68(1):161-7.
23. Leonard JB, Minhaj FS, Erickson K, King J. Fomepizole use reported to United States Poison Centers from 2010 to 2021. Clin Toxicol. 2024;62(2):120-5.
24. Beaulieu J, Roberts DM, Gosselin S, Hoffman RS, Lavergne V, Hovda KE, et al. Treating ethylene glycol poisoning with alcohol dehydrogenase inhibition, but without extracorporeal treatments: a systematic review. Clin Toxicol. 2022;60(7):784-97.
25. Lepik KJ, Levy AR, Sobolev BG, Purssell RA, DeWitt CR, Erhardt GD, et al. Adverse drug events associated with the antidotes for methanol and ethylene glycol poisoning: a comparison of ethanol and fomepizole. Ann Emerg Med. 2009;53(4):439-50.e10.
26. Rulisek J, Balik M, Polak F, Waldauf P, Pelclova D, Belohlavek J, et al. Cost-effectiveness of hospital treatment and outcomes of acute methanol poisoning during the Czech Republic mass poisoning outbreak. J Crit Care. 2017;39:190-8.

4.8 Drugs that Improve Enzyme Function (Oximes)

Vimal Krishnan S

INTRODUCTION

An *oxime* is an organic compound belonging to the imines. Oximes are usually generated by the reaction of hydroxylamine with aldehydes or ketones. Oximes are colorless and exist in the form of crystals or thick liquids. Oximes are poorly soluble in water. They get hydrolyzed by heating or by reacting with inorganic acids. The oximes then get converted into the corresponding ketones or aldehydes and hydroxylamines.

In 1951, Wilson demonstrated the key concept that cholinesterases inhibited by organic phosphorus (OP) compounds could be reactivated using hydroxylamine. Several hydroxylamine derivatives were studied and led to the design of pralidoxime (2-PAM), which American and British scientists independently synthesized as 2-PAM in 1955.[1,2] 2-PAM chloride is a quaternary pyridinium oxime with a molecular weight of 173 Da.

Pralidoxime has approval as an antidote for nerve agent poisoning and organophosphate-based pesticides. 2-PAM has also received approval to manage an overdose of acetylcholinesterase (AChE) drugs prescribed for myasthenia gravis, Alzheimer's disease, and dementia.

Obidoxime (Toxogonin, LuH-6) is an oxime that contains two active sites per molecule and is considered by some to be more effective than 2-PAM. On a molar basis, obidoxime is approximately 10–20 times more effective in reactivating AChE than 2-PAM.[3]

The H series of oximes (named after Hagedorn; HI-6, HIo-7) was developed to act against the chemical warfare nerve agents.[4] These oximes have superior effectiveness against sarin, VX, and certain types of newer pesticides (e.g., methyl fluorophosphonyl cholines).[3-7] Unfortunately, they are less efficacious for traditional OP insecticide poisoning, and their toxicity profile is inadequately defined.[3-10] In addition to reactivating AChEs, the Hagedorn oximes demonstrate direct central and peripheral anticholinergic effects at supratherapeutic concentrations[6] **(Figs. 1A and B)**.

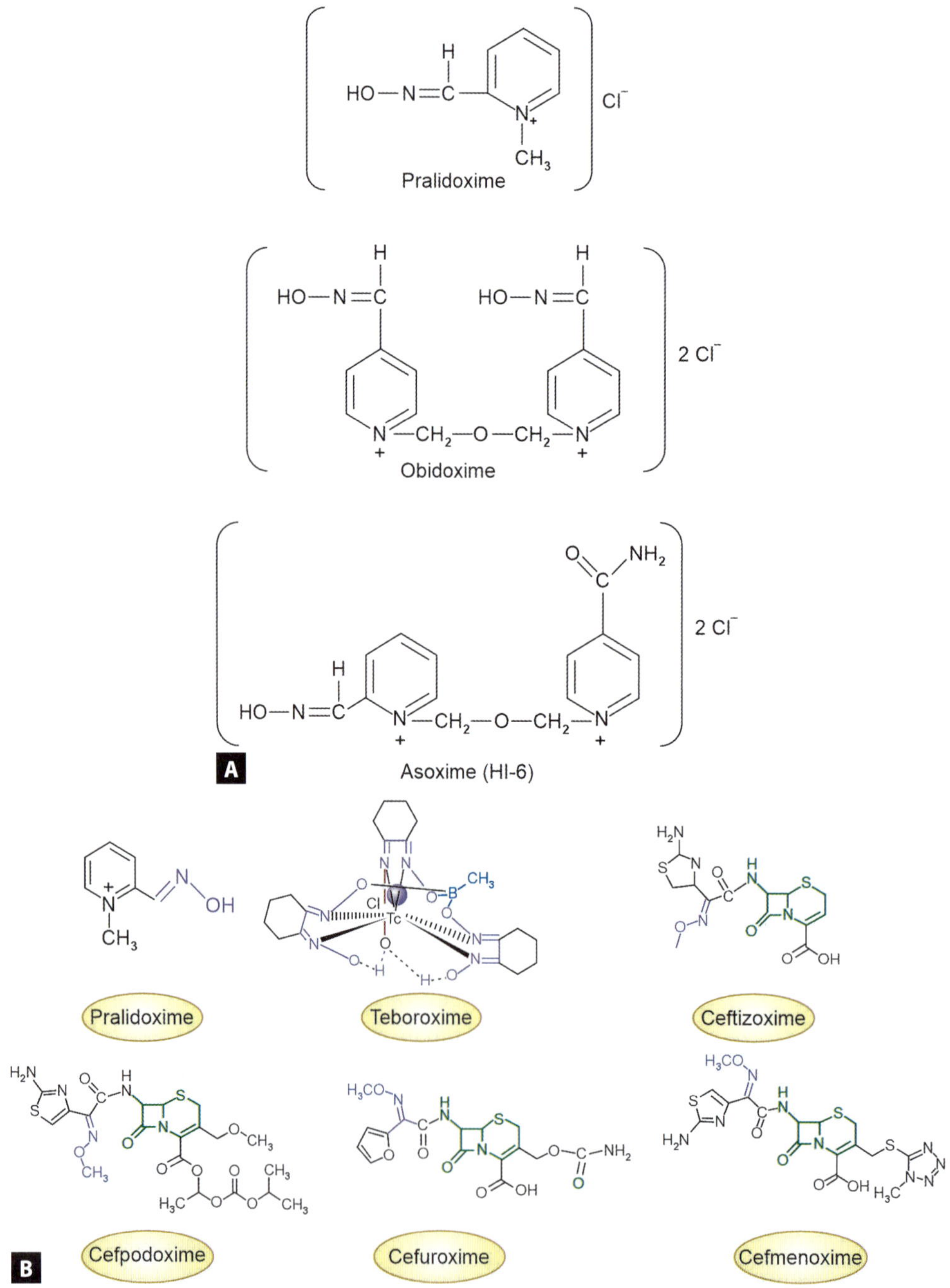

Figs. 1A and B: (A) Types of oximes and their structure; (B) Oxime's structure.[11]

MECHANISM OF ACTION

Organic phosphorus compounds are powerful inhibitors of carboxylic esterase enzymes, including AChE (true cholinesterase, found in red blood cells, nervous tissue, and skeletal muscle) and plasma cholinesterase or butyrylcholinesterase (BuChE) (found in plasma, liver, heart, pancreas, and brain).[12] The OP binds firmly to the serine-containing esteratic site on the enzyme, inactivating it by phosphorylation.[13-15] This reaction results in the accumulation of acetylcholine at muscarinic and nicotinic synapses in the peripheral and central nervous systems, leading to the clinical manifestations of OP poisoning. Following phosphorylation, the enzyme is inactivated by one of the three pathways given as follows:

1. Endogenous hydrolysis of the phosphorylated enzyme
2. Reactivation by a strong nucleophile, such as 2-PAM and the dealkylation of the inactivated phosphorylated enzyme
3. Aging, which involves biochemical changes that stabilize the inactivated phosphorylated molecule and render it incapable of reactivation by oximes.

Pathway 1 is very slow and, hence, not of much significance in case of OPs, but in case of carbamates, this process pathway is very significant.

The positively charged quaternary nitrogen of 2-PAM is attracted to the negatively charged anionic site on the phosphorylated enzyme, bringing it close to the phosphorus moiety. 2-PAM's primary action is restoring AChEs at nicotinic sites in the body, relieving symptoms such as muscle weakness, fasciculations, and paralysis. PAM has some muscarinic action too, but it is not clinically significant. 2-PAM then exerts a nucleophilic attack on the phosphate moiety, successfully releasing it from the AChE enzyme.[16] This action liberates the enzyme to a variable extent depending on the OP in question and restores enzymatic function.[17] The diethoxy OP compounds (e.g., chlorpyrifos, diazinon, ethyl parathion) take days to age ($t_{1/2}$, 33 hours to age) in comparison to hours ($t_{1/2}$, 3 hours to age) for the dimethoxy OP compounds (e.g., dimethoate, dichlorvos, fenthion, fenitrothion, malathion, monocrotophos) for 2-PAM to reactivate the phosphorylated AChE; it must be given within 4–8 hours of the OP ingestion. 2-PAM is, therefore, of limited or no effectiveness against organophosphates that form rapidly aging AChE complexes if given after the aging has been established **(Figs. 2A and B)**.

The action of oximes is most important at nicotinic sites where atropine is ineffective, most often typically improving muscle strength within 10–40 minutes after administration.[13,15] This effect is vital to maintaining the muscles of respiration. 2-PAM is also synergistic with atropine; it liberates cholinesterase enzyme, so that additional acetylcholine can be metabolized, while atropine inhibits the effects of acetylcholine at cholinergic receptors. This suggests that 2-PAM has a synergistic effect with atropine in compromised patients.[13]

Some OP compounds respond much better to 2-PAM than others. This response depends on many factors such as the affinity of 2-PAM for the particular type of phosphorylated enzyme, its reactivating ability, concentrations of both the oxime and OP, aging (rapid or slow), and OP redistribution from a depot site such as fat. There is no convincing evidence for any central nervous system (CNS) effect of 2-PAM. The reactivation of BuChE by 2-PAM is dependent on the concentration of 2-PAM, often has a flat dose response, is quite variable, and is susceptible to aging. Since there are many factors that can alter BuChE activation, it is not preferred agent for diagnosing or assessing response to 2-PAM in poisoned patients.

By contrast to the usefulness of 2-PAM in the management of the cholinergic syndrome, current understanding of the pathophysiology of the intermediate syndrome is inadequate to determine whether 2-PAM can prevent its development or improves the outcome once it has developed. The delayed neurotoxicity of OPs cannot be prevented or treated by 2-PAM.

INDICATIONS FOR OXIME TREATMENT[18]

In a selected group of patients defined by exposure to treatment interval of <4–6 hours, ingestion of diethyl OP compounds in large amounts presents to a center equipped with facilities of intensive monitoring, and mechanical ventilation, having symptoms of:

- Respiratory depression or failure, muscle fasciculations, seizures, dysrhythmias, and hemodynamic instability
- The use of large amounts or repeated doses of atropine to fail to completely control nicotinic signs and symptoms of organophosphate intoxication.

FACTORS AFFECTING EFFICACY

Sooner after exposure to an OP, more likely 2-PAM is to be effective. Timely administration reduces the likelihood

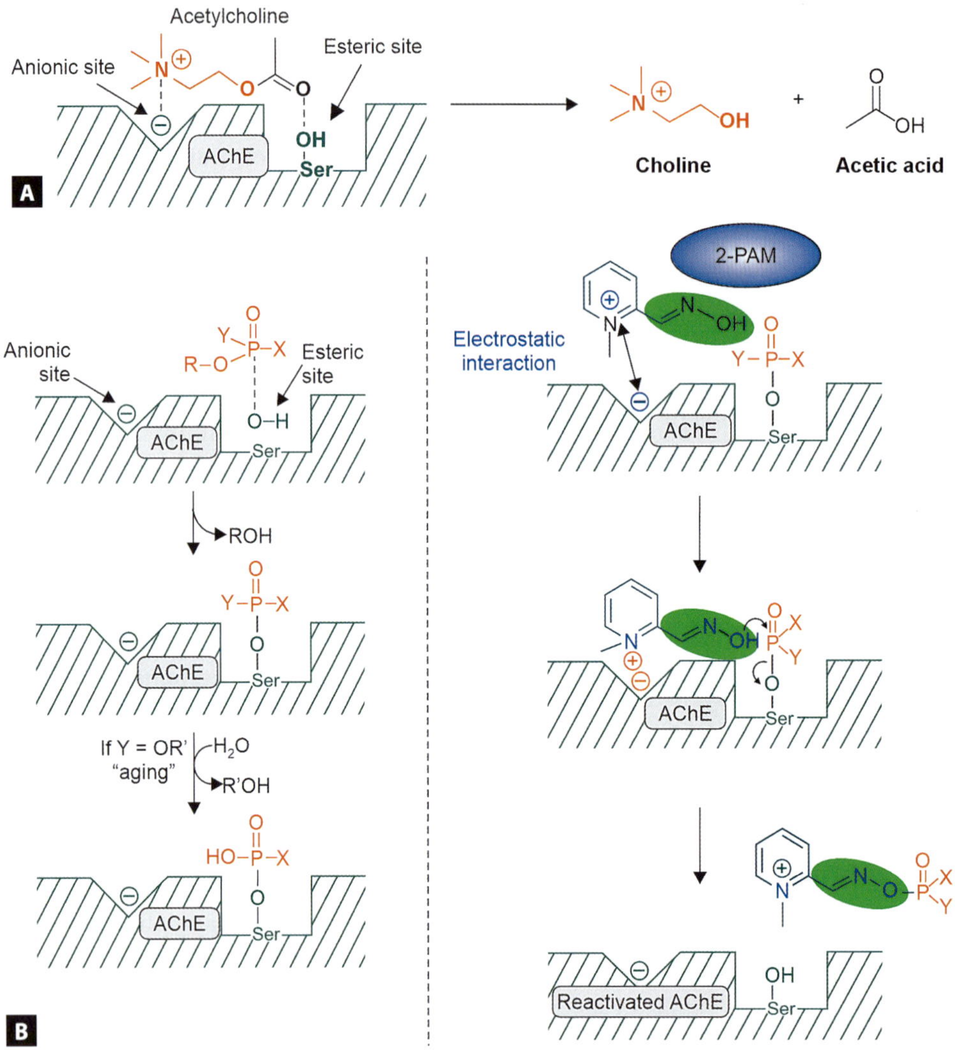

Figs. 2A and B: (A) AChE enzyme metabolism at neuromuscular (NM) junction; (B) Inhibition and reactivation of AChE. (i) Organophosphate compound poisoning and (ii) reactivation of AChE by 2-PAM.[11] (AChE: acetylcholinesterase; 2-PAM: pralidoxime)

that aging of the OP-AChE complex has occurred and is completed. There is no absolute time limitation on reactivation function, as long as the patient remains symptomatic.

The structure of the OP compound is important in the rates of aging and reactivation with 2-PAM. Fenitrothion and methyl parathion are both *o,o'*-dimethoxy OP compounds as are dichlorvos, dimethoate, fenthion, and malathion, whereas ethyl parathion is an *o,o'*-diethoxy OP compound as are chlorpyrifos and diazinon.[19] Some studies suggest that 2-PAM remains effective for >48 hours following exposure to diethyl OPs and to some fat-soluble OPs.[5,18,20-25]

As discussed above, phosphorylated AChE becomes aged and, therefore, unresponsive to oximes, at different rates according to the chemistry of the OP.[26] Oximes, therefore, are recommended early, within 3–4 hours of exposure, after dimethyl OP compound poisoning. In contrast, they can still be highly efficacious 48 hours after some of the diethyl OP compound poisoning, with some effect even when given several days after exposure. In cases of poisoning with highly fat-soluble OP insecticides, in which OP leaking out of fat stores can freshly inhibit AChE, oximes might be efficacious for longer period as well **(Table 1)**.

TABLE 1: Pharmacokinetic parameters of various oximes.[11]					
Oxime	***EC_{50} (mg/L)***	***T_{max} (min)***	***C_{max} (μM)***	***$T_{1/2}$ (min)***	***Status***
2-PAM[27]	4.67	10	37–132	37.6–55	Approved
Obidoxime[28-30]	57.0	4.5	78	28.4	Approved
HI-6[28,31,32]	304	5.8	138	25.7	Approved
RS194B[33]	ND	5	112	52	Candidate
K027[32,34]	229	5	586	60	Candidate
K203[35]	ND	22	242	101	Candidate

(C_{max}: maximum concentration in plasma; $T_{½}$: half-life; T_{max}: time to reach maximum concentration in plasma)

TABLE 2: Classification of nerve agents.			
Class	***Agents***	***DOC***	***Supportive care***
G series	• GA Tabun • GB Serine • GD Soman • GF Cycloserine	• Atropine • 2-PAM	• Airway • Breathing • Circulation
V series	• VE • VG • VM • VR • VX	• Atropine • 2-PAM	• Airway • Breathing • Circulation
Third generation	Novichok	• Atropine • 2-PAM	• Airway • Breathing • Circulation
Carbamates	• EA 1464 • EA 3990 • EA 4056	• Atropine • 2-PAM	• Airway • Breathing • Circulation

(2-PAM: pralidoxime)
Atropine: 1–3 mg every 5 minutes.
2-PAM: 30 mg/kg bolus followed by 8 mg/kg/h for 24–48 hours.

OXIMES FOR NERVE AGENTS

Major nerve agents used as chemical weapons are Sarin, VX, VR, Soman, and Tabun. Sarin and VX are odorless; Tabun has fruity odor, while Soman smells like camphor.[1] These are rapidly acting agents, result in cholinergic crisis. Their action starts within 30 seconds.[1] The major cause of mortality is pulmonary (asphyxiation) and cardiac events (arrhythmia/arrest). The treatment needs to be initiated as soon as the exposure is suspected, and it consists of autoinjectors containing atropine and 2-PAM.[18] Some countries use obidoxime instead of 2-PAM in autoinjectors **(Table 2)**.

In a recent animal study, where 2-PAM, obidoxime, HLo-7 DMS, and MMB4 DMS were compared after exposure to VX, VR, and phorate oxone, it was established that maximum benefit was obtained with MMB4 DMS. These are important results, which may guide further modification into treatment protocols for nerve agents.

OXIMES FOR CARBAMATES

Pralidoxime is rarely indicated for carbamate poisoning, but it is not contraindicated as previously suggested. This erroneous conclusion was based solely on data regarding a single carbamate, carbaryl, and inappropriately applied to all carbamates.

Thus, 2-PAM should never be withheld in a seriously poisoned patient out of concern that a cholinergic xenobiotic is a carbamate.[36] 2-PAM should always be used in conjunction with atropine (primary drug) and rarely as the sole therapy in OP or carbamate poisoning.

DOSING AND DURATION

General consensus by experts suggests a loading dose of 2-PAM chloride of 30 mg/kg (up to 2 g) over 15–30 minutes, followed by a maintenance infusion of 8–10 mg/kg/h for adults (up to 650 mg/h) and 10–20 mg/kg/h for children (up to 650 mg/h).[18,37] This is the dosing schedule recommended by the World Health Organization (WHO).

The addition of 20 mL of sterile water for injection to the 1-g vial of 2-PAM chloride results in a 5% solution (50 mg/mL). Following reconstitution, the 2-PAM should be used within a couple of hours. This solution can be further diluted to a volume of 100 mL of 0.9% sodium chloride solution for IV infusion or a concentration of

10–20 mg/mL. The loading dose can be infused over 15–30 minutes. If pulmonary edema is present, the 1 g of 2-PAM in 20 mL can be infused slowly over not <5 minutes.[25]

The BMJ best practice guidelines[18] recommend the following dose of 2-PAM: 1,000–2,000 mg intravenously initially, followed by 250–500 mg/h continuous infusion for 48 hours.[18]

The duration of 2-PAM therapy is variable, dependent on the particular OP and dose ingested, and different for each patient. A reasonable approach would be to discontinue the 2-PAM when the patient has improved and no longer requires atropine. The general recommendation is not to exceed 48 hours, if initiated. The patient must be observed carefully for recrudescence of toxicity potentially from a fat-soluble long-acting OP. If symptoms return, therapy with 2-PAM and atropine should be continued for at least an additional 24–48 hours. There is no definitive evidence that 2-PAM helps in reversing intermediate syndrome.[18]

ADVERSE EFFECTS

At therapeutic doses of 2-PAM in humans, adverse effects are minimal.[12,13,38-42] Transient dizziness, blurred vision, and elevations in diastolic blood pressure appear to be related to the rate of administration.[43,44] Doses of 45 mg/kg produce blood pressure elevations that persist for several hours but are reversed with IV phentolamine.

Rapid IV administration has produced sudden cardiac and respiratory arrest as a result of laryngospasm and muscle rigidity,[45,46] whereas intramuscular (IM) administration in volunteers produced diplopia, dizziness, headache, drowsiness, nausea, tachycardia, increased systolic blood pressure, hyperventilation, decreased kidney function, muscular weakness, and pain at the injection site.

Pralidoxime is Food and Drug Administration (FDA) pregnancy risk category C. Reproduction studies have not been done, and human case reports are limited. However, considering the maternal benefit of 2-PAM, it should be used as clinically indicated to protect the maternal fetal dyad. The use of 2-PAM should not be withheld because of pregnancy.[47] It is unknown whether 2-PAM is excreted into breast milk.

CURRENT EVIDENCE ON OXIMES

There is conflicting evidence regarding the efficacy of oximes in the management of organophosphate poisoning. A study by Pawar et al.[48] in a subset of patients arriving early to a peripheral center showed benefit, when given in a loading dose of 2 g stat, followed by hourly infusion of 1 g for 48 hours; however, another study by Eddelston et al.[49] did not find any benefit of the oxime administration in a peripheral center in Sri Lanka, in spite of a definitive improvement in levels of RBC cholinesterase. In one of the meta-analysis of the various randomized controlled trials (RCTs) that investigated the efficacy of oximes in OP poisoning cases, they did not find any significant positive impact induced by oximes.[50]

Another recent double-blinded RCT[51] from India could not find any benefit for the add-on oxime therapy suggested by the WHO over conventional atropine monotherapy; however, they did not find any increased mortality with 2-PAM use as well. Similar experiences from some other centers have also shown that a good supportive therapy and early, complete atropinization are the keys to survival in organophosphate compound poisoning. Considering the cost involved and no harm, the authors suggest to avoid oxime therapy in all OP poisoning cases. The WHO recommendations still endorse oximes for the management of organophosphate poisoning; however, the recent BMJ practice guidelines suggest a cautious approach to administration of oximes, to be decided on case-to-case basis.

CONCLUSION

The exact role of oximes is currently unclear. Several consensus guidelines, based more on expert consensus rather than hard evidence, suggest that oximes should be given as soon as possible after exposure to organophosphate compounds to increase the chance of benefit. The duration of intervention postexposure is also not very clear; however, most researchers believe that the maximum benefit may be achieved if oximes are administered within first 4–6 hours of exposure. The exact duration is also not clear, but most researchers believe that once initiated, it should be continued for 48 hours.

Oximes should only be administered in a setting where intensive monitoring is possible with an ability to provide critical respiratory support and care to reduce the risk of serious complications. The duration of use is unclear. It is reasonable to stop oxime administration when atropine is no longer clinically required or 48 hours whichever is early. The decision to administer oximes should be tailored to the type of compound ingested, clinical condition of the patient, and interval between exposure to presentation. Beyond 4–6 hours, intensive supportive care is needed.

REFERENCES

1. Petroianu GA. The history of pyridinium oximes as nerve gas antidotes: the British contribution. Pharmazie. 2013;68:916-8.
2. Wilson IB, Ginsburg B. A powerful reactivator of alkylphosphate-inhibited acetylcholinesterase. Biochim Biophys Acta. 1955;18:168-70.
3. Worek F, Bäcker M, Thiermann H, Szinicz L, Mast U, Klimmek R, et al. Reappraisal of indications and limitations of oxime therapy in organophosphate poisoning. Hum Exp Toxicol. 1997;16:466-72.
4. Bokowjić D, Jovanović D, Jokanović M, Maksimović M. Protective effects of oximes HI-6, and PAM 2, applied by osmotic minipumps in quinalphos poisoned rats. Arch Int Pharmacodyn Ther. 1987;288:309-18.
5. Lundy PM, Hansen AS, Hand BT, Boulet CA. Comparison of several oximes against poisoning by soman, tabun and GF. Toxicology. 1992;72:99-105.
6. Rousseaux CG, Du AK. Pharmacology of HI-6, an H-series oxime. Can J Physiol Pharmacol. 1989;67:1183-9.
7. Worek F, Thiermann H, Szinicz L. Reactivation and aging kinetics of human acetylcholinesterase inhibited by organophosphonylcholines. Arch Toxicol. 2004;78:212-7.
8. Clement JG, Bailey DG, Madill HD, Tran LT, Spence JD. The acetylcholinesterase oxime reactivator HI-6, in man: pharmacokinetics and tolerability in combination with atropine. Biopharm Drug Dispos. 1995;16:415-25.
9. Kassa J, Cabal J. A comparison of the efficacy of a new asymmetric bispyridinium oxime BI-6, with currently available oximes and H oximes against soman in in vitro and in vivo methods. Toxicology. 1999;132:111-8.
10. Kusic R, Jovanović D, Randjelović S, Joksović D, Todorovic V, Bosković B, et al. HI-6, in man: efficacy of the oxime in poisoning by organophosphorus insecticides. Hum Exp Toxicol. 1991;10:113-8.
11. Dhuguru J, Zviagin E, Skouta R. FDA-approved oximes and their significance in medicinal chemistry. Pharmaceuticals (Basel). 2022;15(1):66.
12. Namba T, Hiraki K. PAM (pyridine-2-aldoxime methiodide) therapy for alkyl-phosphate poisoning. JAMA. 1958;166:1834-9.
13. Namba T, Nolte CT, Jackrel J, Grob D. Poisoning due to organophosphate insecticides: acute and chronic manifestations. Am J Med. 1971;50:475-92.
14. Karczmar A. Invited review. Anticholinesterases: dramatic aspects of their use and misuse. Neurochem Int. 1998;32:401-11.
15. Taylor P. Anticholinesterase agents. In: Hardman JG (Ed). Goodman and Gilman's The Pharmacological Basis of Therapeutics, 9th edition. New York, NY: Macmillan; 1996. pp. 100-19.
16. Willems JL, Langenberg JP, Verstraete AG, De Loose M, Vanhaesebroeck B, Goethals G, et al. Plasma concentrations of pralidoxime methyl sulfate in organophosphorus poisoned patients. Arch Toxicol. 1992;66:260-6.
17. Luo C, Saxena A, Smith M, Garcia G, Radić Z, Taylor P, et al. Phosphoryl oxime inhibition of acetylcholinesterase during oxime reactivation is prevented by edrophonium. Biochemistry. 1999;38:9937-47.
18. Buckley N. Organophosphate poisoning. BMJ Best Practice, 2024.
19. Uehara S, Hiromori T, Suzuki T, Kato T, Miyamoto J. Studies on the therapeutic effect of 2-pyridine aldoxime methiodide (2-PAM) in mammals following organophosphorus compound (OP)-poisoning (report II): aging of OP-inhibited mammalian cholinesterase. J Toxicol Sci. 1993;18: 179-83.
20. Amos WC, Hall A. Malathion poisoning treated with Protopam. Ann Intern Med. 1965;62:1013-6.
21. Bowls BJ, Freeman JM, Luna JA, Meggs WJ. Oral treatment of organophosphate poisoning in mice. Acad Emerg Med. 2003;10:286-8.
22. Davies DR, Green AL. The kinetics of reactivation, by oximes, of cholinesterase inhibited by organophosphorus compounds. Biochemistry. 1956;63:529-35.
23. Eyer P. The role of oximes in the management of organophosphorus pesticide poisoning. Toxicol Rev. 2003;22:166-90.
24. Merrill D, Mihm F. Prolonged toxicity of organophosphate poisoning. Crit Care Med. 1982;10:550-1.
25. Food and Drug Administration. (2010). Protopam chloride (pralidoxime chloride) for injection. [online] Available from https://www.accessdata.fda.gov/drugsatfda_docs/label/2010/014134s022lbl.pdf. [Last accessed February, 2025].
26. Uehara S, Hiromori T, Suzuki T, Kato T. Studies on the therapeutic effect of 2-pyridine aldoxime methiodide (2-PAM) in mammals following organophosphorus compound (OP)-poisoning (report III): distribution and antidotal effect of 2-PAM in rats. J Toxicol. 1993;18:265-75.
27. De Boer D, Nguyen N, Mao J, Moore J, Sorin EJ. A Comprehensive review of cholinesterase modeling and simulation. Biomolecules 2021;11(4):580.
28. Chambers JE, Meek EC. Novel centrally active oxime reactivators of acetylcholinesterase inhibited by surrogates of sarin and VX. Neurobiol Dis. 2020;133:104487.
29. Gorecki L, Korabecny J, Musilek K, Nepovimova E, Malinak D, Kucera T, et al., Progress in acetylcholinesterase reactivators and in the treatment of organophosphorus

intoxication: a patent review (2006–2016). Expert Opin Ther Pat. 2017;27(9):971-85.
30. Kuca K, Musilek K, Jun D, Zdarova-Karasova J, Nepovimova E. Soukup O. et al. A newly developed oxime k203 is the most effective reactivator of tabun-inhibited acetylcholinesterase. BMC Pharmacol Toxicol. 2018 Feb 21;19(1):8.
31. NATO Advanced Study Institute on Toxicology of Pesticides; Costa LG, Gall, CL, Murphy SD, North Atlantic Treaty Organization; Scientific Affairs Division. Toxicology of Pesticides: Experimental, Clinical, and Regulatory Perspectives; Springer: Berlin/Heidelberg, Germany, 1987.
32. Lorke DE, Nurulain SM, Hasan MY, Kuča K, Petroianu GA. Oximes as pretreatment before acute exposure to paraoxon. J Appl Toxicol. 2019 Nov;39(11):1506-15.
33. Sakurada K, Ohta H. No promising antidote 25 years after the Tokyo subway sarin attack: A review.Leg Med (Tokyo). 2020;47:101761.
34. Faiz Norrrahim MN, Idayu Abdul Razak MA, Ahmad Shah NA, Kasim H, Wan Yusoff WY, Halim NA, et al. recent developments on oximes to improve the blood brain barrier penetration for the treatment of organophosphorus poisoning: a review. RSC Adv. 2020;10(8):4465-89.
35. Jaćević V, Nepovimova E, Kuča K. Interspecies and intergender differences in acute toxicity of k-oximes drug candidates. Chem Biol Interact. 2019;308:312-16.
36. Lifshitz M, Rotenberg M, Sofer S, Tamiri T, Shahak E, Almog S. Carbamate poisoning and oxime treatment in children: a clinical and laboratory study. Pediatrics. 1994;93: 652-5.
37. Nelson LS, Howland MA, Lewin NA, Smith SW, Goldfrank LR, Hoffman RS. Goldfrank's Toxicologic Emergencies,11th edition. United States: McGraw-Hill Education; 2011.
38. Grob D, Jones RJ. Use of oximes in the treatment of intoxication by anticholinesterase compounds in normal subjects. Am J Med. 1958;24:497-511.
39. Hagerstrom-Portnoy G, Jones R, Adams AJ, Jampolsky A. Effects of atropine and 2-PAM chloride on vision and performance in humans. Aviat Space Environ Med. 1987;10:47-53.
40. Namba T. Diagnosis and treatment of organophosphate insecticide poisoning. Med Times. 1972;100:100-26.
41. Quimby G. Further therapeutic experience with pralidoximes in organic phosphorus poisoning. JAMA. 1963;187:202-6.
42. Thompson DF, Thompson GD, Greenwood RB, Trammel HL. Therapeutic dosing of pralidoxime chloride. Drug Intell Clin Pharm. 1987;21:1590-3.
43. Jager BV, Staff GN. Toxicity of diacetyl monoxime and of pyridine-2-aldoxime methiodide in man. Bull Johns Hopkins Hosp. 1958;102:203-11.
44. Medicis JJ, Stork CM, Howland MA, Hoffman RS, Goldfrank LR. Pharmacokinetics following a loading plus a continuous infusion of pralidoxime compared with the traditional short infusion regimen in human volunteers. J Toxicol Clin Toxicol. 1996;34:289-95.
45. Jeong TO. Respiratory arrest caused by accidental rapid pralidoxime infusion. Clin Toxicol. 2015;53:412.
46. Pickering EN. Organic phosphate insecticide poisoning. Can J Med Technol. 1966;28:174-9.
47. Briggs GG. Drugs in Pregnancy and Lactation. Philadelphia, PA: Lippincott Williams & Wilkins; 2011.
48 Pawar KS, Bhoite RR, Pillay CP, Chavan SC, Malshikare DS, Garad SG. Continuous pralidoxime infusion versus repeated bolus injection to treat organophosphorus pesticide poisoning: a randomised controlled trial. The Lancet. 2006;368(9553):2136-41.
49 Eddleston M, Eyer P, Worek F, Juszczak E, Alder N, Mohamed F, et al., Pralidoxime in acute organophosphorus insecticide poisoning—a randomised controlled trial. PLoS medicine. 2009;6(6):e1000104.
50. Kharel H, Pokhrel NB, Ghimire R. The efficacy of pralidoxime in the treatment of organophosphate poisoning in humans: a systematic review and meta-analysis of randomized trials. Cureus. 2020;12(3):e7174.
51. Syed S, Gurcoo SA, Farooqui AK, Nisa W, Sofi K, Wani TM. Is the World Health Organization-recommended dose of pralidoxime effective in the treatment of organophosphorus poisoning? A randomized, double-blinded and placebo-controlled trial. Saudi J Anaesth. 2015;9(1):49-54.

4.9 Competitive Receptor Blockade (Naloxone, Flumazenil)

Ashish Kumar Kakkar, Tarun Sharma

INTRODUCTION

Competitive receptor blockade is an important strategy in the management of poisonings, where specific antidotes or receptor antagonists are used to counteract the effects of toxic substances. This approach involves the administration of a substance that competes with the toxin for binding to a specific receptor, thereby preventing or reversing the toxic effects. This method is used for various poisons, including opioids, and benzodiazepines, that will be dealt with in this chapter.

NALOXONE

INTRODUCTION

Naloxone is N-alylnor-oxymorphone and a pure competitive antagonist of all opioid receptors, particularly affinity for μ receptors. It fully reverses all the effects of opioids, including respiratory depression, sedation, miosis, and analgesia. Naloxone is lipid soluble and has excellent central nervous system (CNS) penetration after systemic delivery under ordinary circumstances. It produces few effects in the absence of exogenous agonists. On the other way around in the presence of shock when endogenous opioid systems are activated, the administration of naloxone alone may have a positive effect on the hemodynamic system.

PHARMACODYNAMICS

Being a competitive antagonist of all types of opioid receptors, naloxone blocks μ receptors in much lower doses than those needed to block kappa and delta receptors. No subjective or autonomic effects are produced in individuals who have not received an opioid. A number of studies have suggested that agents such as naloxone may attenuate the analgesic effects of placebo medications and acupuncture. The administration of naloxone increases the secretion of gonadotropin-releasing hormone (GnRH) and corticotropin-releasing hormone (CRH) and elevates the plasma concentration of luteinizing hormone (LH), follicle-stimulating hormone (FSH), and adrenocorticotropic hormone (ACTH) as well as the steroid hormones produced by the target hormones. It stimulates the prolactin in women. Short-term administration of naloxone reduces food intake in lean and obese individuals. Long-term administration of naloxone increases the opioid receptors in the brain and causes a temporary exaggeration of responses to subsequent administration of opioid agonists. The antagonistic effect of naloxone is often accompanied by an overshoot phenomenon; respiratory rate depression by opioids transiently becomes higher than before the period of depression.[1] Rebound release of catecholamines may cause hypertension, tachycardia, and ventricular arrhythmia. Pulmonary enema has also been seen after naloxone administration.

PHARMACOKINETICS

Small doses (0.4–0.8 mg) of naloxone given intramuscular or intravenous (IV) promptly reverse the effects of receptor agonists. Subcutaneous doses of naloxone up to 12 mg produce no discernible effects in humans, and 24 mg may cause slight drowsiness or hyperalgesia. 1 mg of naloxone IV completely blocks the effect of 25 mg of heroine. In patients with respiratory depression, an increase in respiratory rate is seen within 2–3 minutes. Sedative effects are reversed, and hypotension returns to normal. At higher doses of 10–15 mg, it reverses the psychotomimetic and diaphoretic effects of pentazocine. The duration of the antagonistic effect is 1–4 hours but depends on the dose of opioid taken. The elimination half-life of naloxone is 60–90 minutes, but the duration of action is as short as 20 minutes if a large amount of opioid agonist is present. In opioid-dependent patients, a small subcutaneous dose of naloxone (0.5 mg) precipitates a moderate-to-severe withdrawal syndrome that is similar to that seen in abrupt stoppage of opioids, except that it appears within minutes and subsides in 2 hours.[2]

PROTOCOL FOR ADMINISTRATION

Naloxone should be started at a low dose to avoid withdrawal. Start with 0.04 mg IV in opioid-dependent

TABLE 1: Classification

Drug	Route	Dose	Onset of action (minutes)	Duration of action (hours)
Naloxone	IV	• Start with 0.04 mg in case of opioid chronic user • 0.4 mg in opioid-naïve patient • 2 mg in apnea or cyanosis	1–2	1–2
	IM/SC	2 mg	5–6	
	Intranasal	1 mg in each nostril	6–8	
	Nebulized	2 mg in 3 mL normal saline	5	

patients who present with mental status depression and respiratory depression. An initial dose of 0.4 mg IV naloxone is recommended in nonopioid-dependent patients who present with respiratory and mental status depression. Then, same doses are administered every 2–3 minutes IV until the desired effect is reached.[3] For patients presenting with apnea or near apnea and cyanosis, larger starting doses of naloxone 2 mg IV every 3 minutes are recommended until 10 mg IV is reached or respiratory depression is reversed. In neonates, the initial dose is 10 µg/kg IV, intramuscular or subcutaneous **(Table 1)**.

INDICATIONS

Naloxone is a drug of choice for morphine poisoning and for reversing neonatal asphyxia due to opioid use during labor (10 µg/kg in cord). Naloxone should be given to any person who shows signs of an opioid overdose or when an overdose is suspected. It can be given as a nasal spray or can be injected into the muscle, under the skin, or into the veins. The effectiveness of naloxone depends on the dose administered and the amount of opioids taken. Withdrawal should be avoided. Toxicity from leaking opioid body packets in gut may require larger doses of naloxone. The duration of action of naloxone may be shorter than that of ingested opioids, so naloxone infusion can be given. This is especially helpful in long-acting opioids such as buprenorphine and methadone. A continuous infusion should only be considered when the patient responds to initial naloxone bolus.[4] To calculate the naloxone infusion dose, calculate the wakeup dose and administer two-thirds of that dose per hour by infusion. Infusion dose needs titration by seeing the response. The patient should be continuously monitored during the infusion. Naloxone has a very good safety profile.[5]

ADVERSE EFFECTS

The most common adverse effects are anxiety, nausea, vomiting, diarrhea, abdominal cramps, and piloerection. Yawning and rhinorrhea are the common symptoms of opioid withdrawal. A rise in blood pressure and pulmonary edema may occur and need to be monitored.

CONTRAINDICATIONS

Naloxone has been found to elevate blood pressure in endotoxic or hypovolemic shock, stroke, and spinal injury. Opioid peptides are implicated for these adverse effects if morphine is used in these conditions. The use of naloxone in these conditions to reverse the effects of morphine is uncertain if it has been inadvertently used.[6]

Naloxone is being used more by laypersons, police personnel, emergency medical technicians, and nonemergency first responders than before. The American Heart Association (AHA) has also included naloxone in its advanced cardiac life support (ACLS) protocol for respiratory depression. In most instances, people who are at risk or who know someone at risk for an opioid overdose can be trained on how to give naloxone. Families can ask their healthcare provider how to use the naloxone pens or spray.

ALGORITHM BY THE AMERICAN HEART ASSOCIATION FOR SUSPECTED OPIOID OVERDOSE

The algorithms in **Flowcharts 1 and 2** should be followed by rescuers coming to the aid of a person known or strongly suspected to be under the influence of opioid drugs:[7]

- Check for responsiveness. Shake and shout at the victim, if necessary.
- If you are the lone rescuer, use a cell phone to call for help, if one is available.
- If more than one rescuer is available, use a cell phone to call for help, retrieve naloxone, and an automated external defibrillator (AED).
- Check breathing and pulse for no >10 seconds.
- Perform rescue breathing on victims with a pulse and inadequate breathing. Perform cardiopulmonary

Flowchart 1: Opioid-associated emergency for lay responders algorithm.

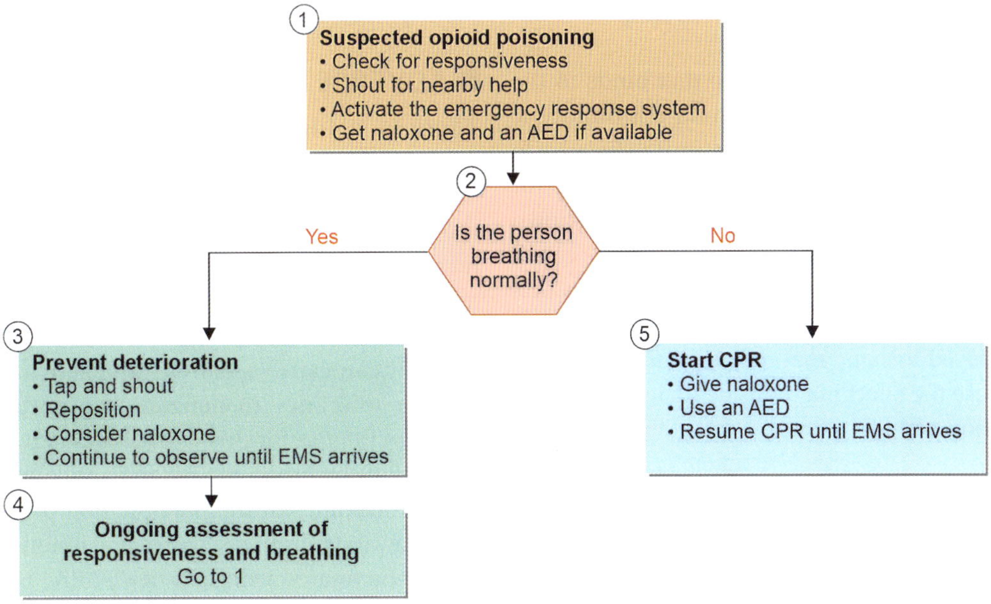

Flowchart 2: Opioid-associated emergency for healthcare providers algorithm.

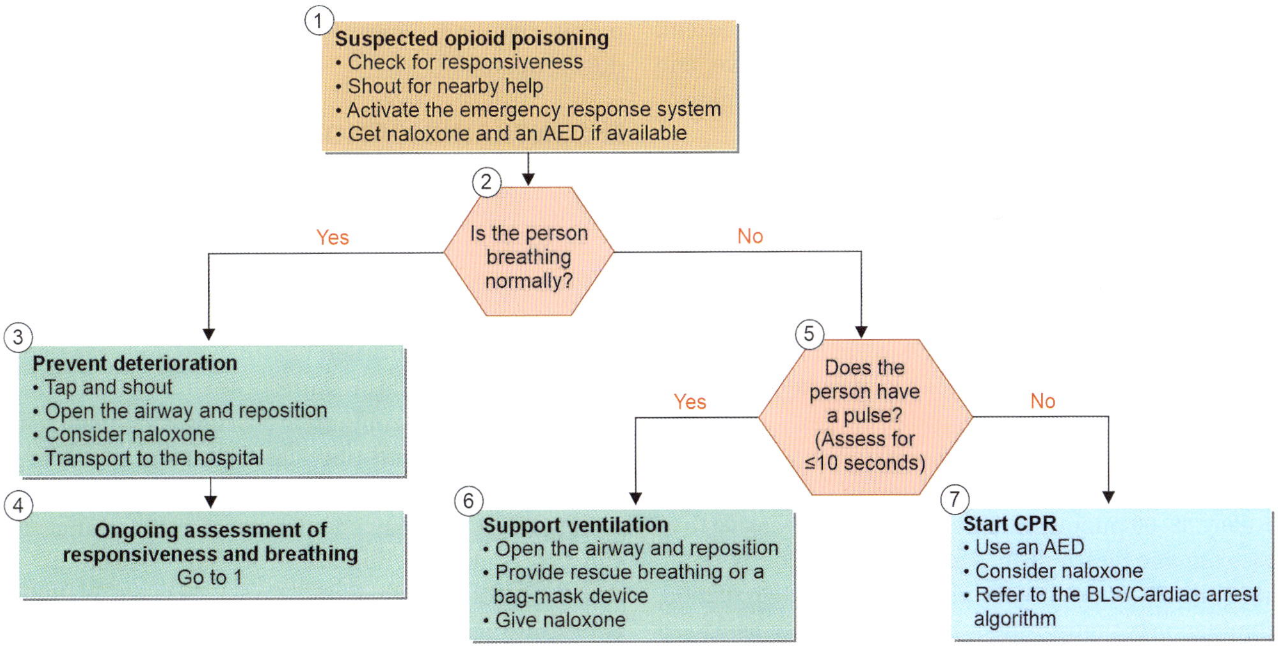

resuscitation (CPR) on victims without a pulse and inadequate breathing. If you are the lone rescuer, perform rescue breathing and/or CPR for 2 minutes before leaving the victim to get help and supplies (naloxone, AED).

- Administer naloxone when available. In an out-of-hospital setting, naloxone can be administered via spray in the nose (2 mg) or with a needle into the arm (0.4 mg). Always follow local dosing and administration protocols.
- If the victim responds, continue to monitor and stimulate the victim (sternal chest rubs, voice commands). If the victim fails to respond or again loses consciousness, resume CPR. You may administer additional doses of naloxone every 4 minutes.

FLUMAZENIL

INTRODUCTION

Flumazenil is imidazobenzodiazepine that binds to the benzodiazepine-binding site on gamma-aminobutyric acid ($GABA_A$) receptors with high affinity. Its use in benzodiazepine toxicity may obviate the need for tracheal intubation. However, some studies have shown that flumazenil has a limited role in the emergency department; it is useful mainly in reversing the effects of short-acting benzodiazepines used in diagnostic and therapeutic procedures and that may also not require an antidote because the effect may subside on its own after a short observation period.

PHARMACODYNAMICS

Flumazenil competitively antagonizes the binding and allosteric effects of benzodiazepine and other ligands. It antagonizes both electrophysiological and behavioral effects of agonists and inverse agonists benzodiazepines and beta-carbolines. It has little intrinsic activity and has practically no effect on normal subjects. Flumazenil abolishes the hypnogenic, psychomotor, cognitive, and electroencephalogram (EEG) effects of benzodiazepines.

PHARMACOKINETICS

Flumazenil is available for IV administration. A series of small injections are preferred to a single bolus dose. A dose of 0.2 mg of flumazenil over 3–5 minutes is given and a total dose of 3 mg is given. Empirical administration of flumazenil should not be used freely. Approximately 3 mg of flumazenil is sufficient to reverse the effects of therapeutic doses of benzodiazepines. If sedation reappears, additional doses of flumazenil may be required within 20–30 minutes. The duration of clinical effect is usually 30–60 minutes. Flumazenil has an extensive first-pass hepatic metabolism. The oral absorption is rapid, but only 25% of drug is absorbed in systemic circulation. Elimination is almost entirely by hepatic metabolism to an inactive form, which has a half-life of 1 hour. The plasma elimination half-life is approximately 1 hour, and the duration of action is variable.

INDICATIONS

The primary use of flumazenil is management of suspected benzodiazepine overdose and reversal of sedative effects produced by benzodiazepine. It is not effective in single-drug overdose of either benzodiazepine or tricyclic antidepressants (TCAs).

ADVERSE EFFECTS

There is a high incidence of side effects if given empirically. If taken orally, it can cause headache or dizziness. Other side effects included with IV dose are agitation, nausea, vomiting and abdominal pain, fearfulness, and coldness. Recurrent benzodiazepine toxicity may result once the effect of flumazenil has worn off. If used in the settings of either benzodiazepine or TCAs, it can cause seizures, especially in patients with TCA or tolerance to benzodiazepine has developed. The explanation for this convulsive activity is either the reversal of cerebroprotective and anticonvulsive effects of benzodiazepines or the precipitation of benzodiazepine withdrawal syndrome. Seizures precipitated by flumazenil should be treated with another $GABA_A$ receptor agonist because the benzodiazepine site on the receptor is antagonized. In such cases, phenobarbitone or propofol is recommended in the treatment of seizures. Careful monitoring and securing of respirations are required during treatment.

CONTRAINDICATIONS

- Overdose of an unknown compound or a mixture of compounds
- Physical dependence on benzodiazepines
- Suspected TCA overdose
- Coingestion of substances that may induce seizures
- Known seizure disorder
- Raised intracranial pressure

Since benzodiazepines are drugs responsible for aborting seizures and physical dependence, unknown substance overdose/suspected TCA poisoning may lead to seizures or enhanced toxicity of other coingested substances. Use of flumazenil in "coma cocktails" is, therefore, not recommended. Coma cocktails, including IV dextrose and naloxone, can still be used in select patient population.[8,9]

CONCLUSION

Competitive receptor blockade is a crucial strategy in managing opioid and benzodiazepine toxicity. Naloxone rapidly reverses opioid-induced respiratory depression but requires careful dosing and monitoring due to its short duration of action. Flumazenil effectively reverses benzodiazepine sedation but must be used cautiously due to the risk of withdrawal seizures. The timely and appropriate use of these antagonists can be lifesaving, emphasizing the need for clinical vigilance and tailored administration based on individual patient factors.

REFERENCES

1. Brunton LL, Hilal-Dandan R, Knollmann BC. Goodman & Gilman's: The Pharmacological Basis of Therapeutics, 13th edition. United States: McGraw-Hill Education; 2017.
2. Love JS, Perrone J. Opioids. In: Tintinalli JE, Ma O, Yealy DM, Meckler GD, Stapczynski J, Cline DM, Thomas SH. (Eds). Tintinalli's Emergency Medicine: A Comprehensive Study Guide, Ninth Edition. McGraw-Hill Education; 2020.
3. An H, Godwin J. Flumazenil in benzodiazepine overdose. CMAJ. 2016;188(17-18):E537.
4. Wermeling DP. Review of naloxone safety for opioid overdose: practical considerations for new technology and expanded public access. Ther Adv Drug Saf. 2015;6(1):20-31.
5. Goodrich PM. Naloxone hydrochloride: a review. AANA J. 1990;58(1):14-6.
6. Arpino PA, Thompson BT. Safety of enteral naloxone for the reversal of opiate-induced constipation in the intensive care unit. J Clin Pharm Ther. 2009;34(2):171-5.
7. Clarke SF, Dargan PI, Jones AL. Naloxone in opioid poisoning: walking the tightrope. Emerg Med J. 2005;22(9):612-6.
8. Brogden RN, Goa KL. Flumazenil. A preliminary review of its benzodiazepine antagonist properties, intrinsic activity and therapeutic use. Drugs. 1988;35(4):448-67.
9. American Heart Association. (2020). Guidelines for CPR and ECC. [online] Available from https://cpr.heart.org/-/media/cpr-files/cpr-guidelines-files/highlights/hghlghts_2020_ecc_guidelines_english.pdf. [Last accessed January, 2025].

ANTIDOTES THAT DECREASE TOXIC METABOLITES

4.10 N-Acetyl Cysteine

Alisha Chaudhury, Banambar Ray

INTRODUCTION

N-acetylcysteine (NAC) is a chemical that was discovered in the 1960s but first used in clinical practice in 1967.[1] It was an important drug with mucolytic properties that led to its rampant use in cystic fibrosis. Since then, the use has been expanded to other chronic lung diseases and paracetamol overdose.

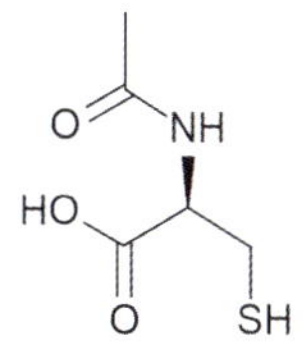

Fig. 1: Chemical structure of N-acetylcysteine.

PROPERTIES

N-acetylcysteine is an acetylated form of the amino acid L-cysteine. It contains many thiol (sulfhydryl) groups, which confer antioxidant effects that reduce free radicals **(Fig. 1)**.

It is essentially insoluble in ether and chloroform but soluble in water and alcohol. It is a white crystalline powder with minimal odor.[2]

Oral NAC has a documented bioavailability of 6–10% in humans. Research utilizing doses of <1,200 mg/day has not provided any discernible benefit.[3] NAC has a half-life of 6.25 hours, and both renal and nonrenal systems are involved in its clearance.[4]

MECHANISM OF ACTION[2] (FLOWCHART 1)

- N-acetylcysteine is converted to L-cysteine after ingestion, which, in turn, is converted into glutathione in the liver. Since glutathione is a powerful antioxidant, administration of NAC replenishes glutathione stores and scavenges free radicals.
- Cross-linking of the cysteine sulfide molecules aids in DNA repair and protection.
- It works as a good mucolytic as it splits the disulfide bonds in mucoproteins in the respiratory system, lowering the viscosity of the secretions.
- It exerts anti-inflammatory action by reducing the levels of proinflammatory cytokines.

- The thiols are good binding sites for metals, helpful for chelating activity in overdose.

PREPARATION

N-acetylcysteine comes in 30 mL vials with a 20% concentration, and before intravenous (IV) use, it must be diluted as per protocol. Oral NAC comes in 10-mL bottles of 10% and 20% concentrations, which also need to be diluted to 5% before use.[5]

USE IN TOXICOLOGY

Acetaminophen Overdose

It is generally known that NAC can be used to prevent acute liver failure caused by acetaminophen overdose. By the middle of the 1980s, it had gained increasing acceptance as an antidote after being initially proposed in 1977 as one.[6] It produces its therapeutic effects through various mechanisms.

Acetaminophen, once ingested, is rapidly absorbed from the gut with peak concentrations achieved within 90 minutes after a therapeutic dose. The half-life of acetaminophen is 2.0–2.5 hours. The half-life is extended to >4 hours in cases of hepatic injury. The recommended maximum therapeutic dosages of acetaminophen are 4 g daily in an adult and 50–75 mg/kg/day in children.[7]

Acetaminophen undergoes extensive hepatic metabolism. Approximately 85% of the dose undergoes conjugation to sulfated and glucuronidated metabolites, which are renally eliminated. Of these two processes, sulfation predominates in children under the age of 12 years, while glucuronidation predominates in adults. But the rest 10–15% undergoes oxidation, which is cytochrome P450 mediated, to form an intermediate compound called N-acetyl-para-benzoquinone imine (NAPQI).[8] Usually, this NAPQI gets conjugated with glutathione to nontoxic cysteine and mercapturate metabolites **(Flowchart 2)**.

In cases of overdose (>4 g/day), the sulfate conjugation pathway becomes saturated with the diversion of the drug to the oxidation pathway and increased production of NAPQI.[9] In toxic doses of acetaminophen, this continued production of NAPQI eventually results in the depletion of glutathione stores, and once these stores are reduced to <70%, NAPQI binds to cellular proteins and leads to cell injury.[10]

Flowchart 1: Mechanism of action of N-acetylcysteine.

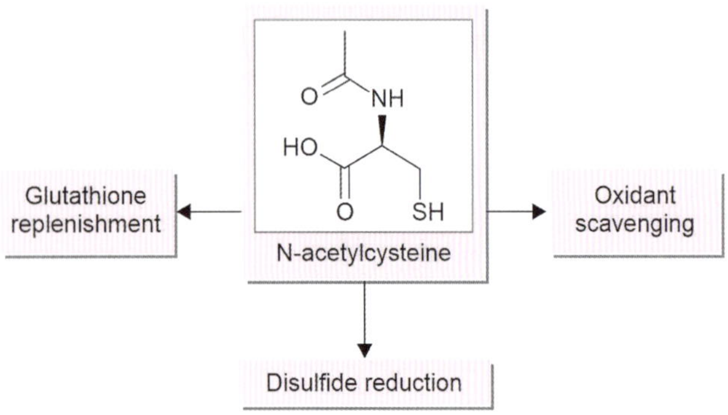

Treatment

N-acetylcysteine is an effective antidote for acetaminophen poisoning. When administered early, it provides cysteine for the replenishment and maintenance of hepatic glutathione stores, enhances the sulfation pathway of elimination, and may directly reduce NAPQI back to acetaminophen. In patients who receive NAC within the first 8 hours after an acute overdose, the risk

Flowchart 2: Metabolism of acetaminophen.

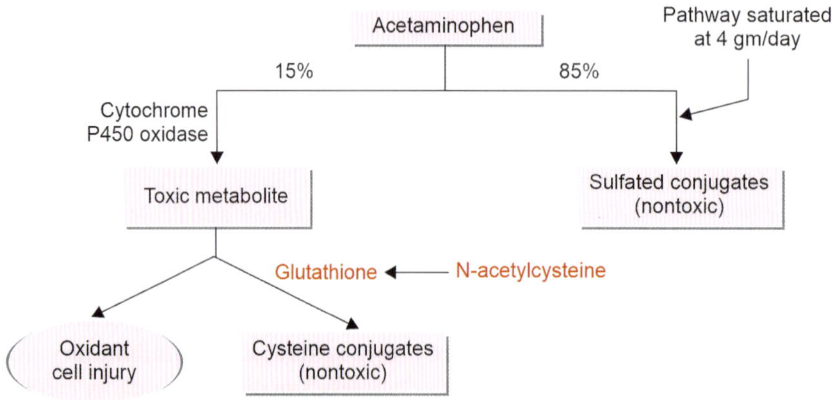

BOX 1: Dosing schedule of N-acetylcysteine for acetaminophen overdose.

Intravenous regimen:
- *Loading dose*: 150 mg/kg in 200 mL dextrose 5% water over 60 minutes
- *Second (maintenance) dose*: 50 mg/kg in 500 mL dextrose 5% water over 4 hours
- *Third dose*: 100 mg/kg in 1,000 mL dextrose 5% water over 16 hours
- *Total dose*: 300 mg/kg over 21 hours

Oral regimen:
- *Loading dose*: 140 mg/kg orally
- *Maintenance dose*: 70 mg/kg should be given every 4 hours for 17 doses
- *Total dose*: 1,330 mg/kg over 72 hours
- Solution should be diluted to 5% and mixed with a soft drink or juice (2:1)
- Any vomited doses should be readministered

of hepatotoxicity is <5%, whereas delays beyond 10 hours are associated with an increased risk of hepatic injury. Despite this, NAC should be continued in cases where liver injury has set in as the benefit has been documented.[10] It improves hepatic perfusion, scavenges reactive oxygen species, and improves mitochondrial energy production. There are two dosing schedules **(Box 1)**:

1. 21-hour IV protocol
2. 72-hour oral NAC protocol

There are no clear guidelines as to when NAC should be discontinued. However, clinical improvement along with decreasing aminotransferase levels with normal prothrombin time/international normalized ratio (INR) and no acidosis on the blood gas could be the end points to discontinuing the therapy.[10]

Nonacetaminophen-induced Acute Liver Failure

Viruses, toxins from mushrooms, autoimmune hepatitis, and drugs (both herbal and conventional) are other important etiological factors causing acute liver failure. Treatment in these cases will be removal of the causative agent along with supportive therapy for organ involvement. NAC seems to have some benefit in nonacetaminophen-induced acute liver failure (NAI-ALF), which may be due to its mechanism of action (anti-inflammatory, antioxidant, and vasodilator effects), which has been confirmed based on evidence from the literature. Sanabria-Cabrera et al. conducted a systematic review that looked at the benefits and safety of NAC in drug-induced liver injury (DILI).[11] They quoted randomized double-blinded trials by Lee et al.[12] and Stravitz et al.,[13] which reported that use of NAC in DILI led to overall survival in both the NAC and placebo groups, but transplant-free survival was higher in the NAC group. In addition, liver transplantation was lower in the NAC cohort. The DILI patients also showed improved outcomes compared with those of other etiologies.

Use as Chelator for Metal Toxicity

N-acetylcysteine has been found to chelate harmful metals such as mercury, lead, and arsenic without affecting the levels of essential minerals in our body important for day-to-day functioning. Few studies have reported that NAC was effective in safely lowering chromium levels in the blood, which are frequently raised by hip prostheses.[14] Case studies have been published about NAC, preventing the harmful effects of arsenic-induced hepatotoxicity in rats. In a case report of acute ingestion of a potentially fatal overdose of sodium arsenate poison, IV NAC prevented the expected clinical outcome of death.[15]

Chloroform Overdose

Chloroform ($CHCl_3$), also known as trichloromethane, is a halogenated hydrocarbon that causes central nervous system depression, cardiac arrhythmias, and hepatotoxicity. Ingestion or inhalation of 5–10 mL of either of these can be lethal to an adult.[16]

Chloroform toxicity occurs most commonly due to inhalation, which leads to the production of an important metabolite called phosgene ($COCl_2$), which utilizes glutathione to form diglutathionyl dithiocarbonate. This compound attaches to cell macromolecules and results in tissue necrosis.[17] The use of NAC is to replete the glutathione stores and scavenge free radicals.

Paraquat Ingestion

Despite reports of NAC having beneficial effects secondary to its scavenging action, replenishing glutathione stores, and anti-inflammatory action, the role in cases of human poisoning has been minimally studied.[18]

SIDE EFFECTS

Gastroesophageal reflux disease (GERD), nausea, vomiting, diarrhea, and flatulence are all potential side effects of oral NAC. Up to 18% of patients receiving IV NAC may experience infusion-related anaphylactoid responses; this is not a concern when taking NAC orally.[19]

Up to 33% of those who take NAC orally may complain of vomiting. There may be worries about causing gastrointestinal (GI) bleeding in patients who already have GI ulcers or varices by using oral NAC.

The majority of anaphylactoid events are mild (6%) to moderate (10%), with severe reactions such as bronchospasm and hypotension being rare (1%). Patients with preexisting reactive airway illnesses, such as asthma, are more likely to experience bronchospasm. Treatment for these patients with bronchodilators is successful.

When an anaphylactoid reaction occurs, NAC should be stopped right away, and the patient should be given antihistamine medication (such as diphenhydramine) and IV fluids to address hypotension.[20] Typically, vasopressors are not required. After the response has subsided, NAC therapy may be resumed more slowly. Oral NAC should be the alternative treatment if there is a persistent response.[21]

CONCLUSION

N Acetyl Cysteine is considered the antidote for Acetaminophen overdose and if administered within four hours of ingestion, it replenishes the glutathion stores in the liver and neutralizes the toxic metabolites of acetaminophen. Its role in non-acetaminophen substance overdose is yet to be established.

REFERENCES

1. Lillibridge CB, Docter JM, Eidelman S. Oral administration of n-acetyl cysteine in the prophylaxis of "meconium ileus equivalent". J Pediatr. 1967;71(6):887-9.
2. Schwalfenberg GK. N-acetylcysteine: a review of clinical usefulness (an old drug with new tricks). J Nutr Metab. 2021;2021 (13):9949453.
3. Borgström L, Kågedal B, Paulsen O. Pharmacokinetics of N-acetylcysteine in man. Eur J Clin Pharmacol. 1986;31(2):217-22.
4. Holdiness MR. Clinical pharmacokinetics of N-acetylcysteine. Clin Pharmacokinet. 1991;20(2):123-34.
5. Keays R, Harrison PM, Wendon JA, Forbes A, Gove C, Alexander GJ, et al. Intravenous acetylcysteine in paracetamol induced fulminant hepatic failure: a prospective controlled trial. BMJ. 1991;303(6809):1026-9.
6. Prescott LF, Illingworth RN, Critchley JA, Stewart MJ, Adam RD, Proudfoot AT. Intravenous N-acetylcystine: the treatment of choice for paracetamol poisoning. Br Med J. 1979;2(6198):1097-100.
7. Prescott LF, Roscoe P, Wright N, Brown SS. Plasma-paracetamol half-life and hepatic necrosis in patients with paracetamol overdosage. Lancet. 1971;1(7698):519-22.
8. Forrest JA, Clements JA, Prescott LF. Clinical pharmacokinetics of paracetamol. Clin Pharmacokinet. 1982;7(2):93-107.
9. Hodgman MJ, Garrard AR. A review of acetaminophen poisoning. Crit Care Clin. 2012;28(4):499-516.
10. Green JL, Heard KJ, Reynolds KM, Albert D. Oral and intravenous acetylcysteine for treatment of acetaminophen toxicity: a systematic review and meta-analysis. West J Emerg Med. 2013;14(3):218-26.
11. Sanabria-Cabrera J, Tabbai S, Niu H, Alvarez-Alvarez I, Licata A, Björnsson E, et al. N-acetylcysteine for the management of non-acetaminophen drug-induced liver injury in adults: a systematic review. Front Pharmacol. 2022;13:868-76.
12. Lee WM, Hynan LS, Rossaro L, Fontana RJ, Stravitz RT, Larson AM, et al. Intravenous N-acetylcysteine improves transplant-free survival in early stage non-acetaminophen acute liver failure. Gastroenterology. 2009;137:856-64.
13. Stravitz RT, Sanyal AJ, Reisch J, Bajaj JS, Mirshahi F, Cheng J, et al. Effects of N-acetylcysteine on cytokines in non-acetaminophen acute liver failure: potential mechanism of improvement in transplant-free survival. Liver Int. 2013;33:1324-31.
14. Giampreti A, Lonati D, Ragghianti B, Ronchi A, Petrolini VM, Vecchio S, et al. N-acetyl-cysteine as effective and safe chelating agent in metal-on metal hip-implanted patients: two cases. Case Rep Orthop. 2016;2016:8682737.
15. Martin DS, Willis SE, Cline DM. N-acetylcysteine in the treatment of human arsenic poisoning. J Am Board Fam Pract. 1990;3(4):293-6.
16. Dell'Aglio DM, Sutter ME, Schwartz MD, Koch DD, Algren DA, Morgan BW. Acute chloroform ingestion successfully treated with intravenously administered N-acetylcysteine. J Med Toxicol. 2010;6(2):143-6.
17. Dreisbach RH, Robertson C. Handbook of Poisoning: Prevention, Diagnosis and Treatment, 12th edition. Norwalk, CT: Appleton & Lange; 1987. pp. 148-50.
18. Flanagan RJ. The role of acetylcysteine in clinical toxicology. Med Toxicol. 1987;2:93-104.
19. Kerr F, Dawson A, Whyte IM, Buckley N, Murray L, Graudins A, et al. The Australasian Clinical Toxicology Investigators collaboration randomized trial of different loading infusion rates of N-acetylcysteine. Ann Emerg Med. 2005;45(4):402-8.
20. Waring WS, Stephen AF, Robinson OD, Dow MA, Pettie JM. Lower incidence of anaphylactoid reactions to N-acetylcysteine in patients with high acetaminophen concentrations after overdose. Clin Toxicol (Phila). 2008;46(6):496-500.
21. Yip L, Dart RC. A 20-hour treatment for acute acetaminophen overdose. N Engl J Med. 2003;348(24):2471-2.

4.11 Sodium Thiosulphate

Kushal Rajeev Kalvit, Atul Prabhakar Kulkarni

INTRODUCTION

Sodium thiosulfate ($Na_2S_2O_3$) is a well-known antidote that forms a pentahydrate complex and is highly water soluble in nature. Its use in the field of toxicology has been exploited since more than 100 years ago when Lang studied its use in reversing the toxicity of hydrocyanic acid.[1] There are multiple reports of its successful intravenous use for treating poisoning with arsenic, bismuth, lead, and mercury in humans and cattle. Though the intravenous use improved outcomes, oral administration did not.[2] Since then, several animal studies in different species have proven its usefulness as an antidote for cyanide toxicity[3,4] and other medical conditions.

INDICATIONS FOR USE

- Antidote for cyanide toxicity (including sodium nitroprusside-induced cyanide toxicity)
- Cisplatin-induced nephrotoxicity
- Calciphylaxis (calcific uremic arteriolopathy)
- Extravasation of cisplatin and bendamustine

MECHANISM OF ACTION IN CYANIDE TOXICITY

Cyanide enters the body via inhalation, ingestion, intravenous medications, or dermal exposure. It rapidly enters the intracellular space and subsequently binds to the inner mitochondrial membrane. It specifically inhibits the cytochrome oxidase a3, which is a crucial part of the electron transport chain (ETC) for aerobic respiration. This inhibition leads to cellular respiratory arrest and can cause serious clinical manifestations within minutes to hours depending on the exposure. Cyanide is metabolized in the body via enzymes such as rhodanese (cyanide sulfurtransferase) or mercaptopyruvate sulfurtransferase. These enzymes are ubiquitous and catalyze the transfer of sulfur to cyanide, leading to the formation of thiocyanate. Thiocyanate is water soluble and readily excreted by the kidneys. However, if the magnitude of cyanide exposure is large enough to overwhelm this detoxification system, toxicity ensues.[5]

The exact mechanism of action of sodium thiosulfate is still a matter of debate. However, it is believed that sodium thiosulfate acts as a sulfur donor and enhances the formation of thiocyanate and its subsequent excretion. The only caveat to this theory is that the enzyme rhodanese is mainly located inside the mitochondria in the liver and skeletal muscles. Hence, it is more likely that rhodanese and mercaptopyruvate sulfurtransferase extract the sulfur moiety from sodium thiosulfate, and albumin carries it via blood to all organs. The moiety is then released by albumin if it encounters cyanide, and the detoxification reaction proceeds.[6]

OTHER MECHANISM OF ACTION

Sodium thiosulfate, when used for calciphylaxis, is effective owing to its antioxidant, vasodilatory, and calcium-chelating properties where it acts to increase the solubility of the deposited calcium.[7]

Cisplatin-induced nephrotoxicity and ototoxicity are well-known adverse effects of this chemotherapeutic agent. Sodium thiosulfate can interact with cisplatin and form inactive platinum species. It can also enter the cells via sodium–sulfate cotransporter and increase the antioxidant activity intracellularly. The cytoprotective and nephroprotective effects of sodium thiosulfate have been demonstrated in patients treated with cisplatin.[8]

PHARMACOKINETICS

Oral sodium thiosulfate is poorly absorbed and has a bioavailability of <10%. It has to be administered intravenously with or without sodium nitrite. Once infused, it gets rapidly distributed in the extracellular space with a volume of distribution around 0.15 L/kg. However, owing to its water solubility, it does not cross membranes easily and is slow to get transported inside the cells and mitochondria. The distribution half-life is around 20 minutes, while the elimination half-life is around 3 hours in which 50% of the drug is excreted unchanged in the urine. The renal excretion is partly dependent on the baseline serum levels of thiosulfate.

If the baseline levels are low, thiosulfate is reabsorbed in the renal tubules and vice versa. Exogenous administration of sodium thiosulfate increases the serum levels manifold, leading to filtration and secretion by the renal tubules. Starved patients and children have higher thiosulfate levels at baseline presumably due to high protein catabolism. On the other hand, thiocyanate formed after binding with cyanide is excreted renally with a half-life of around 3 days and has a volume of distribution of 0.25 L/kg.[9-11]

DOSE AND ADMINISTRATION

- *Cyanide toxicity:* Sodium thiosulfate is administered intravenously at a dose of 12.5 g (50 mL of a 25% solution) once. It has to be administered immediately after the completion of sodium nitrite infusion. The same intravenous cannula and/or needle can be used for the dilution and administration as the two drugs are compatible. If the symptoms/signs of cyanide intoxication persist after an hour, half of the initial dose can be administered again. No dosage adjustment is necessary in patients with renal failure or hepatic failure. However, it should be kept in mind that patients with renal failure will eliminate thiocyanate at a much slower rate.[12]
- *Calciphylaxis:* A dose of 5–25 g is administered IV during the last hour or immediately after the hemodialysis session and repeated thrice weekly till the condition resolves. Extreme caution needs to be exercised while administering higher doses, as the patient may develop severe metabolic acidosis with the accumulation of thiosulfate in renal failure.[13]

OTHER POSSIBLE USE IN THE FUTURE

Neuroprotective Properties

Literature suggests that sodium thiosulfate has significant and potent neuroprotective effects.[14,15] The pathogenesis of parkinsonism, Alzheimer's, and other neurogenerative disorders involves chronic neuroinflammatory processes. Studies suggest that patients taking anti-inflammatory drugs for disorders unrelated to the central nervous system (CNS), such as arthritis, have less severe manifestations of concurrent neurogenerative disorders.[16] Use of sodium thiosulfate may prove beneficial in these patients. Further studies of sodium thiosulfate in these patients are warranted.

ADVERSE EFFECTS AND PRECAUTIONS

Although sodium thiosulfate administration is safe in most cases of cyanide toxicity, it comes with its own set of problems. Sodium thiosulfate has a slow onset of action as it cannot cross membranes easily. Hence, it has to be administered with sodium nitrite always. Sodium nitrite is a rapid and short-acting antidote that converts cyanide into cyanmethemoglobin. Cyanide binds reversibly to the ferric ions in the cytochrome oxidase enzyme. However, the affinity of cyanide for the ferric ions in sodium nitrite is greater and leads to a reaction that drives the cyanide out of the cells. This carries a risk of increasing levels of methemoglobin in the blood and its attendant effects. Consequently, sodium nitrite administration should be avoided if the risk of methemoglobinemia is high as in the cases of concurrent carbon monoxide toxicity or other dyshemoglobinemias. Sodium thiosulfate as a monotherapy is effective only in mild-to-moderate cases of cyanide toxicity. It is always preferable to use hydroxocobalamin as the first-line antidote and it can be used with or without sodium thiosulfate. It should be borne in mind that hydroxocobalamin and sodium thiosulfate should be administered via different IV lines as the two are incompatible with each other.[17,18]

Sodium thiosulfate may accumulate in patients with renal failure and may rarely lead to severe high anion gap metabolic acidosis with lethal consequences. Hence, the anion gap and/or acid–base status should be monitored in patients receiving multiple doses or large doses of sodium thiosulfate, especially in the presence of renal dysfunction.

Sodium thiosulfate has a pregnancy category C status. It is not known if the drug is secreted in the breast milk. However, the manufacturer recommends not to continue breastfeeding if the mother is being treated with the drug. Sodium thiosulfate crosses the placenta. However, its administration, if indicated, should not be withheld in pregnant women, as cyanide toxicity can be lethal for both the mother and the fetus.[19]

CONCLUSION

Sodium thiosulfate is an effective antidote against cyanide poisoning when given in conjunction with sodium nitrite. Its use is safe in most cases and should be considered as first-line therapy if hydroxocobalamin is not available. Newer drugs such as sulfanegen and next-generation sulfane sulfur donors are under research and may be more effective and safer than sodium thiosulfate.[20]

REFERENCES

1. Lang S. Über Entgiftung der Blausäure. Arch f Exp Pathol u Pharmakol. 1895;36:75-99.
2. McGeer PL, McGeer EG, Lee M. Medical uses of sodium thiosulfate. J Neurol Neuromed. 2016;1(3):28-30.
3. Chen KK, Rose CL. Nitrite and thiosulfate therapy in cyanide poisoning. J Am Med Assoc. 1952;149(2):113-9.
4. Chen KK, Rose CL, Clowers GHA. Methylene blue, nitrites, and sodium thiosulphate against cyanide poisoning. Proc Soc Exp Biol Med. 1933;31:250-2.
5. Westley J. Mammalian cyanide detoxification with sulphane sulphur. Ciba Found Symp. 1988;140:201-18.
6. Way JL. Cyanide intoxication and its mechanism of antagonism. Annu Rev Pharmacol Toxicol. 1984;24:451-81.
7. Peng T, Zhuo L, Wang Y, Jun M, Li G, Wang L, et al. Systematic review of sodium thiosulfate in treating calciphylaxis in chronic kidney disease patients. Nephrology (Carlton). 2018;23(7):669-75.
8. Hazlitt RA, Min J, Zuo J. Progress in the development of preventative drugs for cisplatin-induced hearing loss. J Med Chem. 2018;61(13):5512-24.
9. Farese S, Stauffer E, Kalicki R, Hildebrandt T, Frey BM, Frey FJ, et al. Sodium thiosulfate pharmacokinetics in hemodialysis patients and healthy volunteers. Clin J Am Soc Nephrol. 2011;6(6):1447-55.
10. Ivankovich AD, Braverman B, Stephens TS, Shulman M, Heyman HJ. Sodium thiosulfate disposition in humans: relation to sodium nitroprusside toxicity. Anesthesiology. 1983;58(1):11-7.
11. Foulks J, Brazeau P, Koelle ES, Gilman A. Renal secretion of thiosulfate in the dog. Am J Physiol. 1952;168(1):77-85.
12. Hope Pharmaceuticals. (2018). Sodium Thiosulfate Injection. [online] Available from https://hopepharm.com/wp-content/uploads/2018/07/Sodium-Thiosulfate-Prescribing-Information-2018.pdf. [Last accessed January, 2025].
13. Lee M, McGeer EG, McGeer PL. Sodium thiosulfate attenuates glial-mediated neuroinflammation in degenerative neurological diseases. J Neuroinflammation. 2016;13:32.
14. Zhang MY, Dugbartey GJ, Juriasingani S, Sener A. Hydrogen sulfide metabolite, sodium thiosulfate: clinical applications and underlying molecular mechanisms. Int J Mol Sci. 2021;22(12):6452.
15. McGeer PL, Schulzer M, McGeer EG. Arthritis and anti-inflammatory agents as negative risk factors for Alzheimer disease: a review of seventeen epidemiological studies. Neurology. 1996;47:425-32.
16. Generali JA, Cada DJ. Sodium thiosulfate: calciphylaxis. Hosp Pharm. 2015;50(11):975-7.
17. Meredith TJ. Antidotes for Poisoning by Cyanide. New York, NY: Cambridge Press; 1993.
18. Moore SJ, Norris JC, Walsh DA, Hume AS. Antidotal use of methemoglobin forming cyanide antagonists in concurrent carbon monoxide/cyanide intoxication. J Pharmacol Exp Ther. 1987;242(1):70-3.
19. Culnan DM, Craft-Coffman B, Bitz GH, Capek KD, Tu Y, Lineaweaver WC, et al. Carbon monoxide and cyanide poisoning in the burned pregnant patient: an indication for hyperbaric oxygen therapy. Ann Plast Surg. 2018; 80(3 Suppl 2):S106-12.
20. Petrikovics I, Budai M, Kovacs K, Thompson DE. Past, present and future of cyanide antagonism research: from the early remedies to the current therapies. World J Methodol. 2015;5(2):88-100.

ANTIDOTES THAT COUNTERACT TOXIC EFFECTS

4.12 Anticholinergic Agents (Atropine, Glycopyrrolate, Scopolamine)

Harsha Vardhini CP, Bhuvana Krishna

INTRODUCTION

Atropine is a prototypical agent belonging to the class of anticholinergic substances. This group of agents is also called antimuscarinics, as they act by competitively inhibiting the action of acetylcholine at muscarinic receptors. In the 17th century, they were used by inhaling atropine after burning plants to relieve obstructed airways. The role of atropine to counter the cholinergic crisis of organophosphorus is proven beyond doubt.[1,2]

CHEMISTRY

Chemically, these compounds are extensively extracted from plant sources of the Solanaceae family. Atropine is an alkaloid derived from the plant *Atropa belladonna* **(Fig. 1)**. It is well known for its various toxic effects. It derives its name from the Greek word "Atropas" meaning Greek goddess of fate and "Belladonna" an Italian word meaning "beautiful woman," as Italian women used the mydriatic effect of this alkaloid to enhance their esthetic beauty.[3]

Atropine and scopolamine are tropane alkaloids with tertiary amine compounds that cross the blood-brain barrier. Glycopyrrolate, ipratropium, and tiotropium are synthetic quaternary amine compounds with action like atropine but due to chemical structure, they fail to cross the blood-brain barrier[3] **(Fig. 2)**.

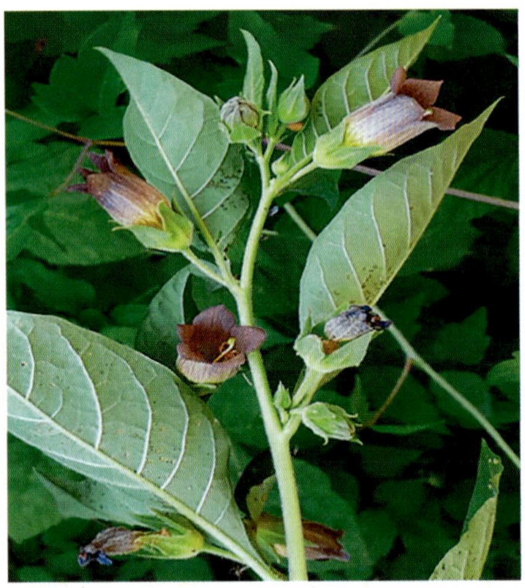

Fig. 1: *Atropa belladonna*: "Deadly nightshade."[22]

Atropine was the first tropane alkaloid to be isolated from the leaves and roots of *A. belladonna* by Mein in 1832. A year later, Geiger and Hesse[23] published the isolation of atropine from *A. belladonna.*[1,3]

PHARMACOLOGY

The anticholinergic agents act by competitively inhibiting acetylcholine-mediated responses at muscarinic receptors in the central and peripheral nervous system. The muscarinic receptors are G protein-coupled receptors. They have five types, namely M1, M2, M3, M4, and M5. The M1 receptors are present abundantly in the cerebral cortex and regulate memory and learning. Smooth muscle, cardiac muscle, ciliary muscle, salivary glands, and sympathetic ganglia are the other nonneurological sites of distribution[3] **(Table 1 and Fig. 3)**

Atropine and scopolamine are nonselective antagonists, with atropine having maximum affinity for M1 > M2 and least for M4–M5. Scopolamine, on the other hand, has a high affinity for M4–M5 receptors. Atropine has additional phosphodiesterase 4 inhibitor activity, which increases cardiac contraction following β stimulation. On the other hand, glycopyrrolate has more affinity for M1–M4 receptors and has actions twice as potent as atropine but lacks the central nervous system (CNS) effects.[4,5]

CLINICAL INDICATIONS IN TOXICOLOGY

Atropine and glycopyrrolate have been widely used as a preoperative medication to inhibit salivary gland and respiratory secretions. Anticholinergics have a profound antisialagogue effect. They also have sedative and amnesic effects. They are also used to prevent reflex bradycardia and treat symptomatic bradyarrhythmia.

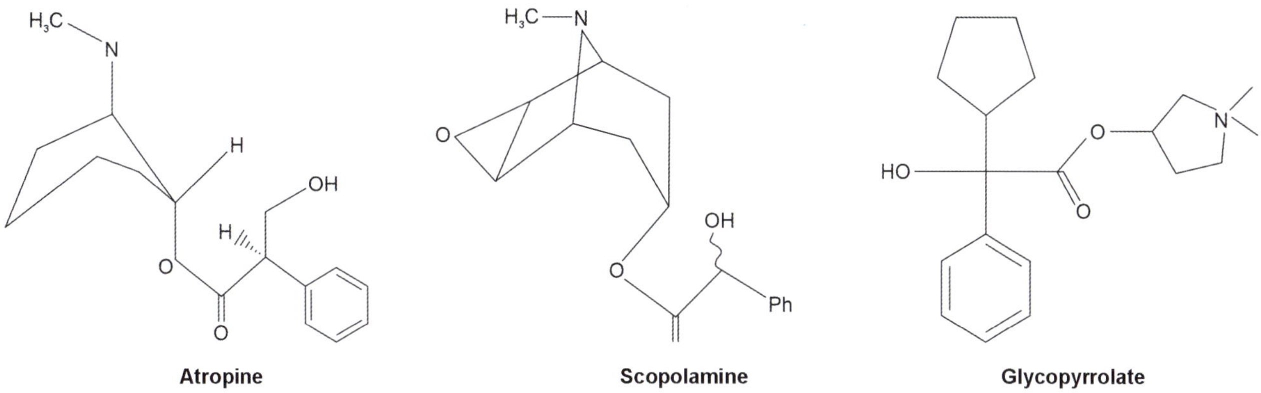

Fig. 2: Chemical structures.[22]

TABLE 1: Muscarinic receptors in the body.	
M1	Brain: Hippocampus, cortex, sympathetic ganglia, salivary glands, and enteric nerves
M2	Heart, hindbrain, and smooth muscle
M3	Smooth muscle, glands, and brain
M4	*Brain:* Forebrain and striatum
M5	*Brain:* Substantia nigra and eye

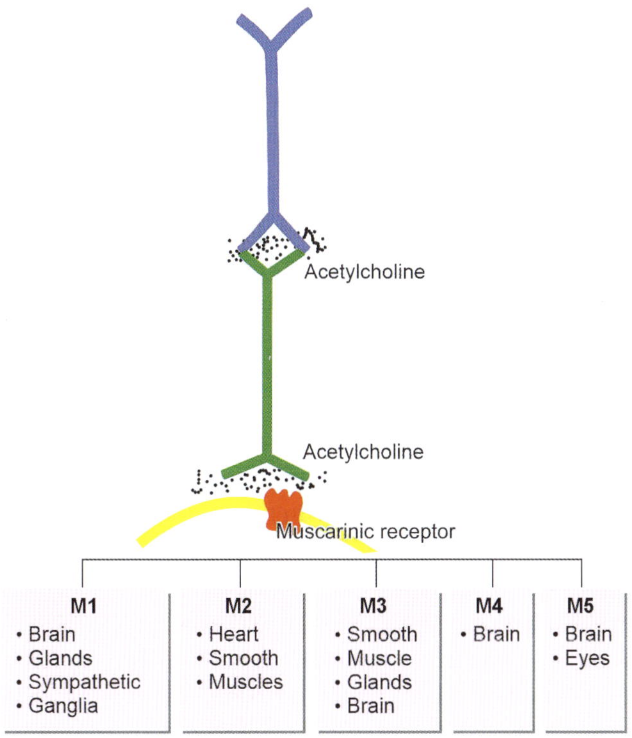

Fig. 3: Muscarinic receptors and their actions.[22]

Loenic and Navratil[24] had elicited the acetylcholine inhibitor property of atropine by 1926.[6] But, it was much earlier in 1864 that atropine was known to antagonize the miotic effects of pyridostigmine.[6] It has been the drug of choice to reverse the cholinergic crisis associated with organophosphorus compounds [organophosphate (OP)]. However, atropine lacks activity against nicotinic receptor-mediated toxicity, i.e., neuromuscular dysfunction of organophosphorus agents.

Common events noted with atropine use are tachycardia, tachypnea, hyperthermia, and CNS stimulation, resulting in restlessness, confusion, psychotic reactions, delirium, and seizures. Severe overdose may result in neuronal depression, coma, and cardiorespiratory failure, leading to death.[7]

To overcome the neural stimulatory effect of atropine, glycopyrrolate with lack of penetration to the CNS and prolonged duration of action was used in organophosphorus toxicity. Also, this agent will not cross the placental barrier and, therefore, can be used safely in pregnant females.[7-10] However, they fail to antagonize central neurologic symptoms of OP toxicity. In spite of the clinical evidence of similar effects, glycopyrrolate has a limited role in the management of OP poisoning. It may be used when atropine-induced CNS effects are pronounced, limiting the dosage administered. Ipratropium is another synthetic antimuscarinic that has shown some beneficial effects as an adjunct therapy for recurrent bronchospasm and bronchorrhea in these patients **(Table 2)**.

Apart from organophosphorus toxicity, anti-cholinergics can also be used in severe mushroom toxicity with muscarinic symptoms (*Amanita muscaria*) and nerve agent toxicity.

TABLE 2: Pharmacology and uses.

	Atropine	*Scopolamine*	*Glycopyrrolate*
Pharmacology	• Nonselective anticholinergic • CNS stimulant	• Nonselective anticholinergic • CNS depressant	• Quaternary compound • No CNS effects
Uses	• Symptomatic bradycardia • Cholinergic toxicity • Nerve agent toxicity • Mushroom poisoning (*Amanita muscaria*) • Preanesthetic medication	• Motion sickness • Antispasmodic	• Hyperhidrosis • Antisialagogue • Cholinergic toxicity

(CNS: central nervous system)

They have also been used in poisoning causing symptomatic bradycardia (beta-blockers, calcium channel blockers, and plant poisons as supportive therapy).

ADMINISTRATION

Atropine can be administered in a small dose through all routes, such as intramuscular, intravenous, as well as intratracheal. For symptomatic bradycardia, 1 mg initial dose may be sufficient but may be increased if the patient does not respond. The dosage can be increased for many toxins. For cholinergic poisoning, atropine is initiated at a dose of 1–3 mg. Depending on the severity of toxicity of organophosphorus compounds, the initial dose may be more. Multiple bolus doses can be continued at fixed intervals or incremental doses every 5 minutes are given to achieve complete "atropinization" relatively early.[11,12] As little as 1–2 mg and as high as 11,000 mg have been required to achieve target atropinization. Therefore, the initial dose requirement is decided based on the cardiorespiratory goals of atropinization and not a fixed value. The current recommendations/practices for OP poisoning are to double the dose of atropine every 3–5 minutes till the lungs are dry.[13,14]

The target for atropinization is the resolution of bronchorrhea, bronchospasm, systolic blood pressure >90 mm Hg, and heart rate >80 beats/min. Pupillary size and absence of sweating are no longer used to titrate atropine therapy in cholinergic poisoning. Once the targets are reached, 10–20% of the total dose should be continued as an infusion, every hour for the next 24 hours. This can be titrated and needed for quite a long time depending on patient clinical symptoms to avoid delayed cholinergic crisis.[15,16]

With the development of agitation and restlessness, delirium atropine needs to be stopped or the dose needs to be decreased by 50%. If the CNS symptoms persist, glycopyrrolate may be used as a substitute for atropine. The dose is 1–2 mg bolus given and can be repeated at intervals as per the patient's need.[15]

Other CNS-active antimuscarinic agents such as scopolamine were tried to substitute atropine. Few studies showed the use of scopolamine for seizures induced due to nerve gas agent exposures. Although more potent than atropine, there was increased permeability across the blood–brain barrier, and the risk of delirium escalated with their use.[16] Ipratropium and other agents have been studied as antidotes, but they have not been used in clinical practice.[17]

Atropine bolus doses were compared with incremental doses in an open-label randomized controlled trial and showed significant improvement with incremental dosing in relation to death and intermediate syndrome.[12,18,19] There were studies that compared atropine with glycopyrrolate; although there was a mortality benefit, atropine-induced delirium was not reduced.[14,20] Few studies have also compared atropine alone versus a combination of atropine and pralidoxime. They did not show any added benefit in terms of mortality when two drugs were used.[15,16]

Glycopyrrolate is available as 0.2 mg/mL solution for injection. Intramuscular or intravenous administration requires no dilution and should be used at 0.2 mg over 1–2 minutes **(Flowchart 1)**. The dose may be repeated every few minutes till respiratory secretions are dry.[21]

ADVERSE EFFECTS

Atropine administration may precipitate acute glaucoma and convert partial organic pyloric stenosis into complete obstruction. Therefore, it is important to observe, especially in elderly patients, the development of abdominal distension and headaches. Since atropine

Flowchart 1: Doubling dose versus bolus dose of atropine.

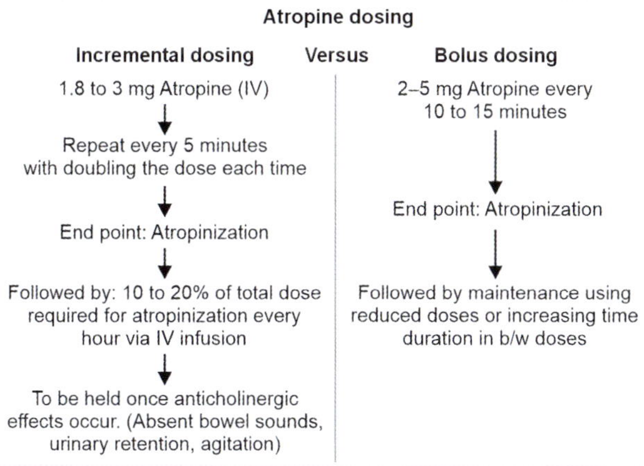

causes pupillary dilatation, difficulty/distortion in vision is commonly reported. Atropine may also lead to complete urinary retention in patients with prostatic hypertrophy. This may lead to incontinence. Thickening of bronchial secretions and formation of viscid plugs in patients, especially with chronic lung disease, may be responsible for obstruction and collapse of lung.

The half-life of atropine ranges from 2 to 4 hours. In geriatric patients (65–75 years old), intravenous atropine has a longer half-life (10 hours). In the presence of an adverse event, just stopping the drug will lead to clearance of toxicity; however, at times, benzodiazepines may be needed to control the agitation/restlessness in patients.[7]

Adverse reactions after glycopyrrolate administration are similar to anticholinergic symptoms as atropine (mydriasis, hyperthermia, tachycardia, and cardiac arrhythmia). Constipation, dry mouth, dry skin, flushing, photophobia, urinary retention, and xerophthalmia are also reported.[21] Dose needs to be altered in the presence of renal and hepatic dysfunction. Closed-angle glaucoma, pyloric obstruction, cardiac tachyarrhythmia, and prostatic hyperplasia are contraindications.[21] Since the half-life is 50 minutes, stoppage of the drug can ameliorate toxicity. Neostigmine may be used to reverse life-threatening side effects.

CONCLUSION

Atropine is an important, lifesaving antidote and is recommended as an essential drug in the World Health Organization (WHO) drug list. It remains the drug of choice for acute symptomatic bradycardia and toxicity of organophosphorus compounds. Incremental doses of atropine may be required to achieve the desired effect. Glycopyrrolate can be used as a substitute when a patient develops atropine-related delirium. The cost of glycopyrrolate is an important consideration when using it as an antidote for cholinergic poisoning. There is no added benefit to adding glycopyrrolate to atropine as a combination therapy. The role of scopolamine as an antidote is yet unproven.

REFERENCES

1. Kohnen-Johannsen KL, Kayser O. Tropane alkaloids: chemistry, pharmacology, biosynthesis and production. Molecules. 2019;24(4):796.
2. Grynkiewicz G, Gadzikowska M. Tropane alkaloids as medicinally useful natural products and their synthetic derivatives as new drugs. Pharmacol Rep. 2008;60(4):439-43.
3. Shim KH, Kang MJ, Sharma N, An SS. Beauty of the beast: anticholinergic tropane alkaloids in therapeutics. Nat Prod Bioprospect. 2022;12(1):33.
4. Berizzi AE, Gentry PR, Rueda P, den Hoedt S, Sexton PM, Langmead CJ, et al. Molecular mechanisms of action of m5 muscarinic acetylcholine receptor allosteric modulators. Mol Pharmacol. 2016;90(4):427-36.
5. Dulawa SC, Janowsky DS. Cholinergic regulation of mood: from basic and clinical studies to emerging therapeutics. Mol Psychiatry. 2019;24(5):694-709.
6. Costa LG. Organophosphorus compounds at 80: some old and new issues. Toxicol Sci. 2017;162(1):24-35.
7. Robenshtok E, Luria S, Tashma Z, Hourvitz A. Adverse reaction to atropine and the treatment of organophosphate intoxication. Isr Med Assoc J. 2002;4(7):535-9.
8. Sovell P. Organophosphate poisoning: grading the severity and comparing the treatment between atropine and glycopyrrolate. Ann Emerg Med. 1991;20(4):435-6.
9. Mirakhur RK, Dundee JW. Glycopyrrolate: pharmacology and clinical use. Anaesthesia. 1983;38(12):1195-204.
10. Eddleston M, Buckley NA, Checketts H, Senarathna L, Mohamed F, Sheriff MR, et al. Speed of initial atropinisation in significant organophosphorus pesticide poisoning—a systematic comparison of recommended regimens. J Toxicol Clin Toxicol. 2004;42(6):865-75.
11. Abedin MJ, Sayeed AA, Basher A, Maude RJ, Hoque G, Faiz MA. Open-label randomized clinical trial of atropine bolus injection versus incremental boluses plus infusion for organophosphate poisoning in Bangladesh. J Med Toxicol. 2012;8:108-17.
12. Hopmann G, Wanke H. Maximum dose atropine treatment in severe organophosphate poisoning. Dtsch Med Wochenschr. 1974;99(42):2106-8.
13. Blain PG. Organophosphorus poisoning (acute). BMJ Clin Evid. 2011;2102.
14. Chugh SN, Aggarwal N, Dabla S, Chhabra B. Comparative evaluation of atropine alone and atropine with pralidoxime

(PAM) in the management of organophosphorus poisoning. J Indian Acad Clin Med. 2005;6(1):33-7.
15. Afzali S. The comparison of atropine and atropine + oxime in organophosphate poisoning with muscarinic signs. Avic J Clin Med. 2002;9(3).
16. Kventsel I, Berkovitch M, Reiss A, Bulkowstein M, Kozer E. Scopolamine treatment for severe extra-pyramidal signs following organophosphate (chlorpyrifos) ingestion. Clin Toxicol. 2005;43(7):877-9.
17. Shemesh I, Bourvin A, Gold D, Kutscherowsky M. Chlorpyrifos poisoning treated with ipratropium and dantrolene: a case report. J Toxicol Clin Toxicol. 1988;26(7):495-8.
18. Connors NJ, Harnett ZH, Hoffman RS. Comparison of current recommended regimens of atropinization in organophosphate poisoning. J Med Toxicol. 2014;10(2):143-7.
19. Bardin PG, van Eeden SF. Organophosphate poisoning: grading the severity and comparing treatment between atropine and glycopyrrolate. Crit Care Med. 1990;18(9):956-60.
20. Cimanga RK, Mukenyi PN, Kambu OK, Tona GL, Apers S, Totté J, et al. The spasmolytic activity of extracts and some isolated compounds from the leaves of Morinda morindoides (Baker) Milne-Redh (Rubiaceae). J Ethnopharmacol. 2010;127(2):215-20.
21. Chabicovsky M, Winkler S, Soeberdt M, Kilic A, Masur C, Abels C. Pharmacology, toxicology and clinical safety of glycopyrrolate. Toxicol Appl Pharmacol. 2019;370:154-69.
22. Wikimedia Foundation. (2023). Atropa belladonna. [online] Available from https://commons.wikimedia.org/wiki/File:Atropa_belladonna_L._longipedicellate_flower.jpg.z. [Last accessed January, 2025]
23. Geiger PL, Hesse O. Ueber das Atropin und das Hyoscyamin. Ann Pharm. 1833;7:189-208.
24. Loewi O, Navratil E. Über humorale Übertragbarkeit der Herznervenwirkung. Pflügers Arch. 1926;214:678-88.

4.13 High Dose Insulin Euglycemic Therapy

Ashish Bhalla

INTRODUCTION

Insulin has been the most important medication, which has revolutionized the patient care, especially the care of diabetic patients. It has impacted the morbidity and mortality associated with one of the most important noncommunicable diseases in the world. It was recognized as having a positive inotropic effect in the early 1900s.[1]

INSULIN: HOW DOES IT WORK?

The exact molecular mechanisms of insulin action are a complex mixture of metabolic effects and direct effects on cells. It is also important to know that insulin primarily is neither a vasopressor nor a specific antidote for any toxin **(Fig. 1)**.[2]

In stress, cardiac myocytes switch their metabolism from free fatty acids (FFA) to glucose. Insulin helps in promoting glucose uptake in cardiac myocytes. This allows the heart to overcome the "metabolic starvation" induced by certain toxins **(Fig. 2)**.[2]

Insulin increases cardiac output by working on cardiac myocytes as a strong inotrope.[3] Insulin does this by switching cardiac myocyte cell metabolism from fatty acids to carbohydrates. Insulin helps in restoring calcium flux into the cells and improves cardiac contractility. The inotropic effect of insulin is independent of catecholamines; therefore, any condition or pharmaceutical agents blocking catecholamine action do not affect insulin's action.[4]

Insulin also activates the phosphoinositide 3-kinase (PI3K) pathway, which in turn causes enhancement of endothelial nitric oxide synthase (eNOS). This leads to vasodilation, resulting in a drop in systemic vascular resistance.[2] The increase in cardiac output and the vasodilatory effect lead to increased capillary perfusion. The enhanced perfusion ameliorates microvascular dysfunction and organ damage seen with cardiogenic shock.[5]

Way back in 1993, in an animal model, insulin was compared to epinephrine and glucagon as a novel treatment for cardiac toxicity from verapamil. Due to its positive inotropic effects that are independent of cyclic AMP, insulin was found to be superior to inotropes and glucagon in verapamil-induced cardiac dysfunction.[6] This laid the foundation for the use of insulin as an antidote in calcium channel blocker (CCB) toxicity.

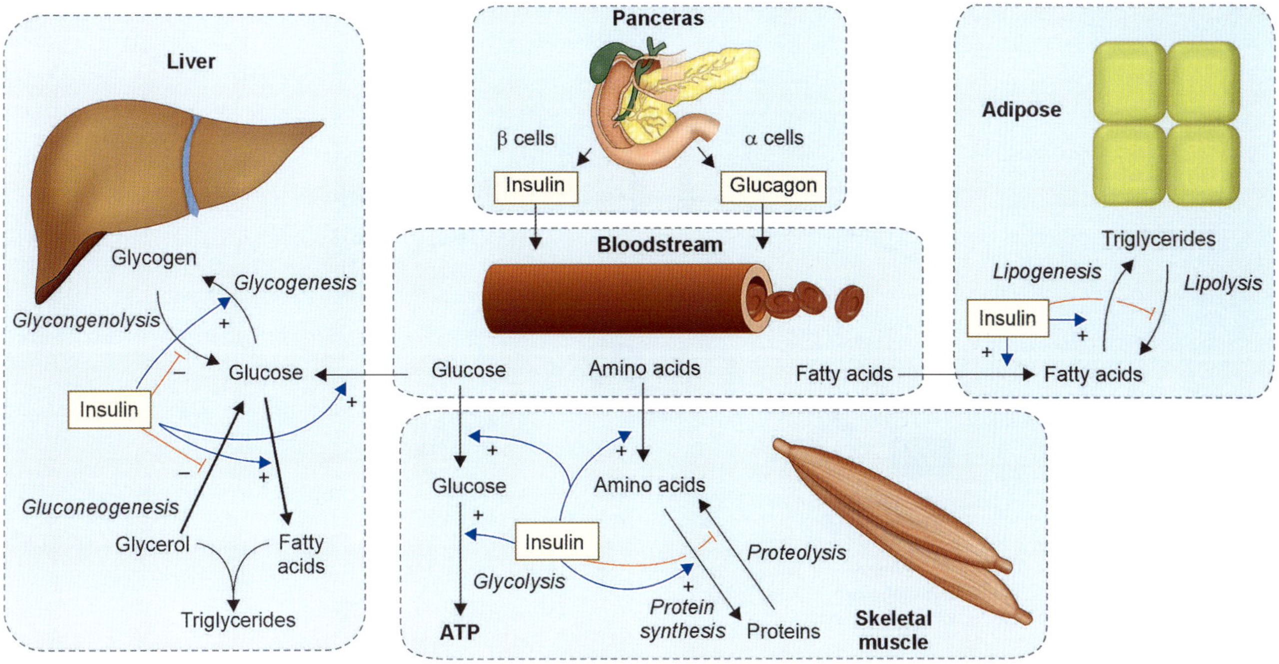

Fig. 1: Insulin action in the body. (ATP: adenosine triphosphate)

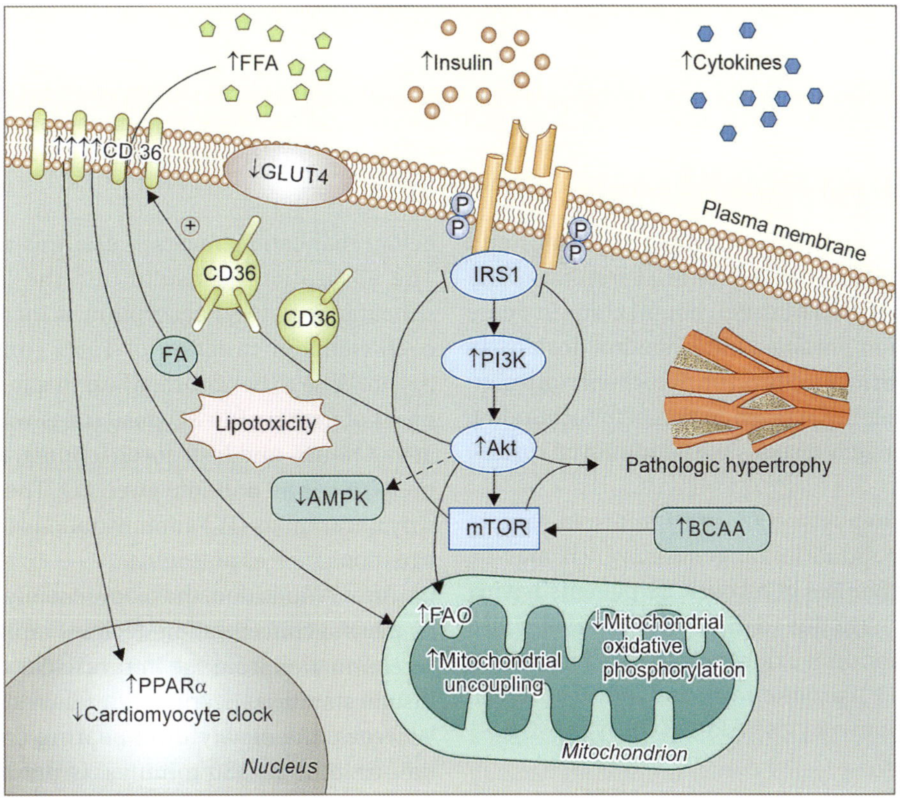

Fig. 2: Insulin signaling in cardiac myocyte. [Akt/PKB: serine/threonine kinase/protein kinase B; BCAA: branched-chain amino acids; cAMP: cyclic adenosine monophosphate; eNOS: endothelial nitric oxide; FAO: fatty acid oxidation; FFA: free fatty acids; GLUT-4: glucose transporter protein 4; IGF-1: insulin-like growth factor-1; IGF-2: insulin-like growth factor-2; IR: insulin receptor; IRS-1/2: insulin receptor substrate 1/2; mTOR: mammalian target of rapamycin (protein kinase); PI3K: phosphoinositide 3-kinase; PPAR: peroxisome proliferator-activated receptor α]

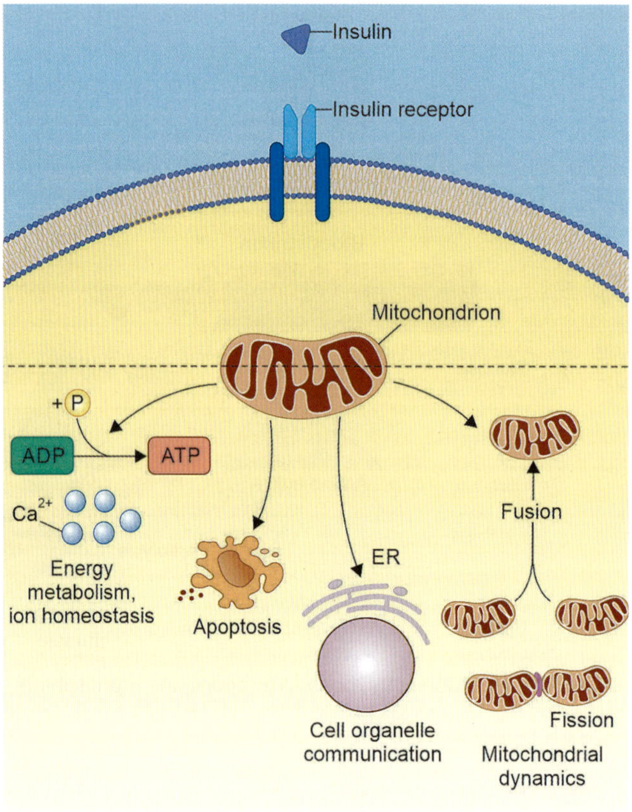

Fig. 3: Insulin effect on mitochondrial dynamics. (ADP: adenosine diphosphate; ATP: adenosine triphosphate; ER: endoplasmic reticulum)

Certain toxins such as phosphine, cyanide, and hydrogen sulfide disrupt mitochondrial respiration by knocking out mitochondria. Insulin cannot act and increase glucose utilization in poisoned mitochondria. Insulin, in high doses, is known to directly act on mitochondrial fusion and fission, thus helping in regeneration of mitochondria, which may be ultimately responsible for improved cardiac function **(Fig. 3)**.[7]

Hypoxia and hypoglycemia are important factors upregulating mitochondrial biogenesis, which may be an important mechanism of recovery in patients having mitochondrial damage due to direct toxins. Insulin also stimulates mitochondrial oxidative capacity [adenosine triphosphate (ATP) production] and mitochondrial function in cardiomyocytes (Akt-mTOR-NFκB-Opa-1 signaling pathway).[7]

PHARMACOKINETICS

Only regular insulin/short-acting insulin has been used as an antidote till date. The rationale is to have a quick action that can be reversed easily as and when needed. The absorption of insulin into the bloodstream after subcutaneous (SQ) absorption is inconsistent with the coefficients of variation of T50% (time for 50% of the insulin dose to be absorbed) varying from 15 to 30%.[8] The onset of action after SQ dose starts within 1 hour, peaks at 2–4 hours, and lasts for 5–6 hours, therefore, it is not preferred as an antidote given SQ. These are the reasons why intravenous (IV) administration is preferred in acute situations such as poisoning.

After IV injection, the bioavailability is immediate, and its plasma concentration declines rapidly initially due to its elimination from the intravascular space. Levels of IV insulin start disappearing with a half-time of 2.4 minutes.[2] Whereas, the slowly disappearing component, with a half-time of 50–130 minutes, is due to its elimination from the interstitial fluid and tissues. Total clearance of insulin, which is the result of metabolic degradation, ranges between 700 and 800 mL/min.[2] Since the sites of degradation of IV insulin are primarily the liver and kidneys, its disposal depends on the function of these organs. Exogenous IV insulin is degraded in the kidney (30%) and liver (~60%).[9]

Dose: There are two main regimens for insulin use as an antidote. The basic principle and the dose are quite similar, but there are finer differences between the two.

High-dose Insulin Regimen

There is wide variation in the dosage of insulin used as an antidote; however, the consensus is to give 0.5–1 U/kg/h. For high-dose insulin (HDI) therapy, it is recommended to give a bolus dose of 1 U/kg followed by an infusion at the rate of 0.5–1 U/kg/h. It is important to titrate the dose according to the response; therefore, starting with 0.5 U/kg/h is the preferred option after the bolus. In various studies, very high insulin doses—up to 10 U/kg/h—have been used.[10] A bolus dose of insulin (1 or >1 U/kg) should be given only if the blood sugar is >200 mg/dL at the time of initiation of therapy. If blood sugar is <200 mg/dL, lesser dose as bolus may be given.

Insulin can lead to gross shift of glucose into cells, thereby causing hypoglycemia; therefore, it is important to administer a dextrose bolus of 0.5 g/kg. This should be done only if the blood sugar is <200 mg/dL at the time of initiation of therapy. It is desirable to start simultaneously a dextrose infusion (0.5 g/kg/h).[11] Any concentration of dextrose can be used, but it is preferred to use highly concentrated solution of dextrose to prevent volume overload. It is also advisable to administer concentrated dextrose solution through a central venous catheter.[11] It is also advisable to frequently monitor blood sugar and give additional boluses if the blood sugar falls between 110 and 150 mg/dL, to maintain euglycemia.

Glucose–Insulin–Potassium Infusion

Glucose-insulin-potassium (GIK) is a simple and very effective insulin delivery algorithm. The rationale is that an average-built 70 kg person would require 5–10 g of dextrose per hour to maintain metabolic homeostasis in the body. On average, one unit of insulin is expected to lower blood glucose by 25–30 mg/dL and also is responsible for pushing potassium into the cells. In an individual who is not accepting anything orally, the aim is to maintain capillary blood sugar around 80–110 mg/dL and serum potassium level between 3.5 and 4.5 mEq/dL. The GIK infusion can maintain normal homeostasis.[12]

This combination has been used in the management of acute myocardial infarction and postcardiac surgery with variable results.[12,13] It has also been used in critically ill patients and patients with sepsis as well, with variable results.[14] By adding glucose to insulin, the protein catabolism to meet gluconeogenic needs in the body reduces significantly. This leads to reduced or less negative nitrogen balance in critically ill patients. GIK regimen has been used/tried in cardiotoxic poisons with good results.[15]

Glucose-insulin-potassium has been used in metal phosphide (aluminum and zinc) poisoning.[16] Studies have implicated hyperglycemia as one of the parameters responsible for adverse outcomes in metal phosphide poisoning, therefore the need to correct/control it.[17]

The conventional "Alberti's regimen" for GIK infusion was first described in 1979, and it can be easily remembered as the rule of 10.[18] This comprises 10% dextrose 500 mL mixed with 10 U of short-acting (regular) insulin and 10 mEq KCl. This is usually instituted at a rate of 100 mL/h (i.e., 2 U/h of insulin and 10 g of dextrose). This regimen is generally recommended for blood glucose levels up to 10 mmol (180 mg/dL) with an aim to maintain target blood glucose of around 100 mg/dL during the period of surgery. Modifications to this have been done over time.[19] These regimens are effective when used in perioperative setting in patients needing dextrose as an energy source and insulin as a metabolic driving force.[18,19]

When insulin is used as an antidote, GIK infusion is prepared using 100 mL of 10% dextrose, with 100 U of insulin and 40 mEq of potassium added. The infusion can be started at 0.25–0.5 mL/kg/h with hourly monitoring of capillary blood sugar and serum potassium, continuous electrocardiogram, and hemodynamic monitoring.[20] This is preceded by a bolus of 0.5–1 U/kg regular insulin bolus. This insulin regimen is more intense than Alberti's regimen. This should be instituted only when blood sugar is >200; if it is less than that, the bolus dose of insulin may be reduced by 50% or bolus of dextrose may be administered at the same time. In this setting, it is advisable to initiate GIK infusion at a lower dose of insulin per hour. It is preferred to have more frequent capillary blood glucose measurements during the first hour (every 20 or 30 minutes).[20]

Another insulin antidote regimen is the Western Australian regimen **(Box 1)**.[21] In this regimen, dextrose bolus of 50 mL of 50%, if blood sugar is <200 mg/dL, is followed by 1 U/kg regular insulin bolus to saturate insulin receptors. This can be followed by adding

BOX 1: Western Australian antidote regimen.

Once a decision to initiate HDI therapy is taken, give:
- Glucose 25 g (50 mL of 50% solution) IV bolus, unless marked hyperglycemia (blood glucose > 22 mmol/L) is present
- Short-acting insulin 1 IU/kg bolus to maximally saturate insulin receptors

HDI therapy is to be continued with:
- Short-acting insulin infusion starting at 0.5 IU/kg/h and titrated every 30 minutes to a maximum of 5 IU/kg/h*
- 50% dextrose at 25 g/h IV infusion titrated to maintain euglycemia (blood glucose 80–200 g/dL)

Strictly monitor:
- Glucose—every 20 minutes for first hour, then every 1 hour
- Potassium—replace only if < 2.5 mmol/L and there is a source of potassium loss

End points:
- Improvement in myocardial ejection fraction (>50%)
- Increased BP (systolic BP >90 mm Hg in adults)
- Heart rate (>60 beats/min)
- Resolution of acidemia with euglycemia
- Adequate urine output (1–2 mL/kg/h)
- Reversal of cardiac conduction abnormalities (QRS interval <120 ms)
- Improvement in mentation

It is important to continue therapy till weaning/withdrawal of other vasopressors. Dextrose is to be continued after cessation of insulin with monitoring

*The maximum safe and effective rate of infusion is unknown but may be even higher than 5 IU/kg/h. Up to 10 IU/kg/h is safely used.
(BP: blood pressure; HDI: high-dose insulin; IV: intravenous)
Source: Adapted from Nickson CP, Little M.[21]

100 IU of regular insulin to 100 mL of 50% dextrose and 40 mEq of potassium, to be started at a rate to give insulin 0.5 IU/kg/h. Since this is a concentrated dextrose solution, central venous access is needed for it. Frequent blood glucose monitoring every 20–30 minutes may be needed.[21] The target is to keep capillary blood glucose around 100 mg/dL while using this regimen. The infusion rate can be titrated according to capillary glucose levels. If needed, an additional bolus of 25% dextrose can be given if the blood sugar is <100 mg/dL, and potassium can be added if the serum potassium level is <4 mEq/dL. The difference between the GIK regimen for acute poisoning and Alberti's regimen is that the amount of insulin used is much more, additional dextrose boluses may be needed, and HDI will require prophylactic administration of potassium.[21]

Insulin in Calcium Channel Blocker Overdose

Calcium channel blockers are very commonly prescribed, very effective antihypertensive agents.[15,22] A large number of patients are prescribed these agents, and they usually tend to buy the antihypertensive medication in amounts that can last them a month or two. Frequent prescriptions, easy availability over the counter, and bulk dispensing make these agents easily accessible for self-harm purposes. CCBs along with beta-blockers (BBs), antiepileptic agents, and paracetamol are commonly used pharmaceutical preparations used for self-harm purposes.[22]

CCB overdoses can result in:[15]
- Hypoinsulinemia, as insulin release is dependent on calcium influx into islet beta cells. CCBs block this influx through L-type calcium channels into islets, leading to impaired release.
- CCBs impair the heart muscle's adaptive response in stress. During stress, normal cardiac myocytes shift from FFA as substrate for energy production to carbohydrates, due to:
  - Impaired uptake of glucose and FFA
  - Inhibited glucose catabolism in the cells, an action dependent on calcium channels

A workgroup of experts involved in the care of poisoned patients developed evidence-based recommendations to guide the in-hospital management of CCB poisoning.[23]

They recommend the use of HDI in symptomatic patients as a first-line therapy if evidence of myocardial dysfunction is present. The workgroup has endorsed an HDI regimen, which includes a bolus of 1 U/kg followed by an infusion of 1 U/kg/h with maintenance of euglycemia with a dextrose infusion as needed. For the therapy of patients in refractory shock or periarrest, the workgroup recommends rescue treatment with incremental doses of HDI (up to 10 U/kg/h) if evidence of myocardial dysfunction is present; however, the level of evidence is low.[23]

The experts caution that HDI should be avoided if there is evidence of hypertrophic obstructive cardiomyopathy or ischemic cardiomyopathy with low ejection fraction.[24,25] Therefore, it is always a good idea to rule out these conditions by history and bedside echocardiography before initiating HDI therapy. The patient most likely to benefit from HDI is one with a heart that has a baseline normal ejection fraction that now has drug-induced cardiogenic shock.[24]

Treatment of CCB overdose comprises multiple interventions simultaneously (i.e., IV calcium, HDI, vasopressors); therefore, the effect of a single intervention is difficult to study or interpret.[23] It has been emphasized that first-line treatments need to be prioritized. This can be based on the desired effect needed upfront in the symptomatic patient.[26]

Calcium channel blockers are categorized into three different classes based on selectivity for cardiac or vascular channels.[20] These are dihydropyridines (e.g., nifedipine and amlodipine), phenylalkylamines (verapamil), and benzothiazepines (diltiazem). Dihydropyridines have a dominant effect on vascular smooth muscle cells than cardiac myocytes. Dihydropyridines are very potent antihypertension medications. Their overdose would most certainly lead to vasoplegic shock.[21]

Nondihydropyridines (verapamil and diltiazem) have a dominant effect on the myocardium. They are important antiarrhythmic and antianginal drugs. Their overdose is likely to cause bradycardia and conduction disturbances leading to myocardial dysfunction and cardiogenic shock.[21] In severe CCB poisoning, this selectivity gets altered profoundly, making the clinical effects less predictable.[5]

When HDI is used to treat amlodipine overdose, there could be synergistic vasodilation; therefore, despite increasing cardiac output, there may be low systemic pressures and regional hypoperfusion.[25]

Vasopressor in Calcium Channel Blocker Overdose[27]

Vasopressor selection should be guided by the type of shock. The use of norepinephrine is recommended in vasoplegic shock or if myocardial function has not yet been assessed. Alternately, epinephrine may also be used to increase contractility and heart rate.[23] In the presence of myocardial dysfunction (low ejection fraction), dobutamine may be used.[23]

Calcium channel blocker overdose may require very high doses of vasopressors and inotropes, and HDI may help in bringing them down.[28] Other potential benefits of adding HDI to vasopressors are better cerebral perfusion and lesser requirement of IV fluid transfusion. This fluid resuscitation strategy is known to be better for survival in critically ill poisoned patients and may hold true in CCB toxicity too.[29]

Beta-blocker Overdose

Beta-blockers are also very important cardiovascular drugs used routinely and have the potential to be used for self-harm purposes.[22,30]

There are three distinct types of beta receptors. Beta-1 receptors are present in the heart and mediate cardiac activity. Beta-2 receptors are present in many organ systems. They control many aspects of metabolic activity and relax smooth muscle. Beta-3 receptors induce the breakdown of fat cells.[15]

Beta-blockers are commonly indicated for the treatment of hypertension, myocardial infarction/coronary artery disease, congestive heart failure, cardiac arrhythmias, hyperthyroidism, migraine, and essential tremor. They are also used to lower pressure in patients with aortic dissection and portal hypertension. They have a potent anxiolytic effect. In high doses, BBs impair lipolysis, glycogenolysis, and insulin release from beta cells.[31] BBs are available in three forms: Oral, IV, and ophthalmic. For self-harm purposes, oral BBs are implicated, and IV BBs overdose may be accidental/prescription error.

The clinical presentation is in the form of severe myocardial depression and to some extent vasoplegia leading to severe hypotension and compromised organ perfusion. This may be persistent in case of using long-acting preparations, which may have prolonged half-life.[15]

Treatment of Overdose

All the patients must be admitted to intensive care units for continuous monitoring of vitals and cardiac rhythm. First-line therapy for BB overdose involves supportive care with IV fluids and atropine to reverse hypotension and bradycardia.[31] Point-of-care ultrasound (POCUS) may guide therapy as dilated left ventricle with low ejection fraction will not improve with fluid bolus and inotropes will be needed.[31] Other options for therapy are vasopressors, glucagon, HDI, or lipid emulsion therapy. Choosing therapy is very simple, if hypotension is due to vasodilation (normal left ventricular ejection fraction), vasopressors are needed. For myocardial depression presenting with cardiogenic shock (low ejection fraction), inotropic agents, HDI, lipid emulsion therapy, or extracorporeal membrane oxygenation (ECMO) may be needed.

High-dose Insulin in Beta-blocker Overdose

Insulin acts as a positive inotrope. In BB poisoning, insulin acts by switching cell metabolism from fatty acids to carbohydrates in cardiac myocytes. It also restores calcium fluxes and improves cardiac contractility.[24]

The utility of HDI was first proven in a swine model of propranolol toxicity; pigs treated with vasopressors alone died within 20 minutes while those treated with HDI survived for 2–3 hours.[32] HDI in BB toxicity has shown to improve survival. The dose and the protocols for administration are the same as discussed earlier for CCB toxicity.[24]

Metal Phosphide Poisoning

Metal phosphides are the most common agent responsible for rodenticide poisoning in India. The details about their mechanism of action have been discussed in the chapter on rodenticides.

Phosphine, the toxic gas released when metal phosphides come in contact with moisture, is a protoplasmic poison. It acts like cyanide and disrupts the electron transport chain in mitochondria.[33] This results in cellular hypoxia, and the most important organs affected are the heart and brain.[34] Cardiac myocyte hypoxia results in left ventricular dysfunction, arrhythmia, and subsequent renal injury.[33] Cerebral hypoxia results in alteration in sensorium. Severe metabolic acidosis and fluid refractory hypotension are the hallmarks of metal phosphide toxicity.[33,34] The changes observed in organs demonstrate the primary damage to the heart and brain, while kidneys, gastrointestinal tract (GIT), and liver are involved due to organ hypoperfusion.[35]

Insulin has been tried as a part of GIK infusion in multiple studies and has been found to be effective.[20,36] The exact mechanism of the action of insulin as an antidote in this poisoning is not completely understood. It has been proposed that insulin acts as an inotrope. It shifts the cardiac myocyte energy source from FFA to glucose, thereby improving cardiac function. This improvement in cardiac myocyte function is reflected in improved blood pressure and reduced requirement of inotropes, and mechanical cardiovascular support.[36] This stands true for CCB and BB overdose where the cardiac myocytes have normal functioning mitochondria.

Unlike normal mitochondria in CCB and BB overdose, in metal phosphide overdose the mitochondria are diseased, due to abnormalities in the electron transport chain.[37] This would lead to disruption of the electron transport chain and the mitochondria will not be able to utilize either glucose, pyruvate, lactate, or FFA. This effect would persist till the time the toxin persists or the mitochondrial regeneration takes place.[37]

Insulin is supposed to regulate the metabolism in the cells by changing the substrate (FFA to glucose/lactate), and it has been shown to have a significant effect on mitophagy.[7,38]

Insulin also mediates mitochondrial biogenesis and function by affecting the SIRT1/PGC1α pathway. The actual effect of HDI or GIK infusion in metal phosphide poisoning may be changes in mitochondrial biogenesis and mitophagy rather than changing the substrate utilization in cardiac myocytes with diseased mitochondria.[38]

Different protocols for administration have been discussed in the chapter earlier and any one of them may be used. We recommend using 100 mL 10% dextrose with 100 U insulin, and 40 mEq of potassium as GIK infusion.[20,36]

Adverse Effects of Insulin

Insulin is a very potent antidiabetic drug, having great ability to alter the metabolic homeostasis in the body. Its overdose may be accidental (inadvertent injection of highly potent insulin containing 100 U in 1 mL) or intentional (HDI and GIK therapy).

The most common and most feared side effects with insulin therapy are hypoglycemia and hypokalemia in any clinical situation.[39] In spite of significant beneficial effects of HDI in the management of toxin-mediated myocardial dysfunction, there is significant metabolic disruption. Both glucose and electrolyte homeostasis get severely compromised and may be detrimental.[39] Hypoglycemia is the most common adverse effect, and it could be severe (<2.5 mmol/L).[39]

Hypoglycemia was noted not only during HDI therapy but also after HDI is discontinued. Hypokalemia is the most important and most feared complication of IV insulin therapy but is usually mild even with higher doses used. Rebound hyperkalemia may be noted in a small subset of patients after stoppage of high doses of insulin. All the patients receiving IV insulin therapy should be monitored either by electrocardiogram or frequent electrolyte measurements.[39]

The other common electrolyte abnormalities noted are hypomagnesemia and hypophosphatemia. Surprisingly, no direct relationship could be observed in a study between insulin dose and the severity of these metabolic alterations.[39] The need for frequent, close monitoring of metabolic alterations cannot be stressed more. Volume overload is another significant concern when IV insulin therapy is used as an antidote. This may manifest as pulmonary edema, peripheral edema, or hyponatremia.[40]

The incidence of hypoglycemia and volume overload decreases significantly when concentrated maintenance dextrose infusions are used along with insulin infusion.[24]

After insulin infusion is discontinued, it is advisable to continue glucose supplementation for a longer duration. Large doses of glucose administered along with IV insulin stimulates endogenous insulin secretion, which may be responsible for hypoglycemia even after insulin infusion is stopped.[39,41] Too early discontinuation of insulin therapy could result in recurrent hypotension, especially in patients with sustained release toxins overdose. This may require restarting or reinstitution of antidote.[42,43] It is therefore recommended to have intensive monitoring while using insulin as an antidote. Many physicians are unfamiliar with or even may be afraid to use high doses needed for IV insulin to act as an antidote, which is also difficult to prepare and institute by someone not used to handle it.[44] It is desirable that physicians and intensivists are sensitized to this useful and easily available antidote.

CONCLUSION

Insulin is a potent antidote and can be safely used as an adjunct therapy to treat cardiotoxic poisons. A better understanding of the pathophysiology of the toxin and its effects on the heart and blood vessels will guide you to choose antidotes wisely. HDI administration requires intensive, frequent monitoring of cardiovascular status and metabolic profile in critically ill poisoned patients. When used as an antidote, clinicians must be prepared to anticipate and treat metabolic alterations.

REFERENCES

1. Krenz JR, Kaakeh Y. An overview of hyperinsulinemic-euglycemic therapy in calcium channel blocker and beta-blocker overdose. Pharmacotherapy. 2018;38(11):1130-42.
2. Mayer JP, Zhang F, DiMarchi RD. Insulin structure and function. Biopolymers. 2007;88(5):687-713.
3. Visscher MB, Muller EA. The influence of insulin upon the mammalian heart. J Physiol. 1927;62(4):341-8.
4. Kline JA, Raymond RM, Leonova ED, Williams TC, Watts JA. Insulin improves heart function and metabolism during non-ischemic cardiogenic shock in awake canines. Cardiovasc Res. 1997;34:289-98.
5. Stellpflug S, Kerns R. High dose insulin. In: Nelson L, Howland M, Lewin N, Smith S, Goldfrank L, Hoffman R (Eds). Goldfrank's Toxicologic Emergencies, 11th edition. New York: McGraw-Hill Education; 2020. pp. 953-8.
6. Kline JA, Tomaszewski CA, Schroeder JD, Raymond RM. Insulin is a superior antidote for cardiovascular toxicity induced by verapamil in the anesthetized canine. J Pharmacol Exp Ther. 1993;267(2):744-50.
7. Schell M, Wardelmann K, Kleinridders A. Untangling the effect of insulin action on brain mitochondria and metabolism. J Neuroendocrinol. 2021;33(7):e12932.
8. Gradel AKJ, Porsgaard T, Lykkesfeldt J, Seested T, Gram-Nielsen S, Kristensen NR, et al. Factors affecting the absorption of subcutaneously administered insulin: effect on variability. J Diabetes Res. 2018;2018:1205121.
9. Turnheim K, Waldhäusl WK. Essentials of insulin pharmacokinetics. Wien Klin Wochenschr. 1988;100(3):65-72.
10. Holger JS, Stellpflug SJ, Cole JB, Harris CR, Engebretsen KM. High-dose insulin: a consecutive case series in toxin-induced cardiogenic shock. Clin Toxicol. 2011;49:653-8.
11. Engebretsen KM, Kaczmarek KM, Morgan J, Holger JS. High-dose insulin therapy in beta-blocker and calcium channel blocker poisoning. Clin Toxicol (Phila). 2011;49:277-83.
12. Oh TJ, Kook J, Jung SY, Kim DW, Choi SH, Kim HB, et al. A standardized glucose-insulin-potassium infusion protocol in surgical patients: use of real clinical data from a clinical data warehouse. Diabetes Res Clin Pract. 2021;174:108756.
13. Mantle JA, Rogers WJ, Smith LR, McDaniel HG, Papapietro SE, Russell RO Jr, et al. Clinical effects of glucose-insulin-potassium on left ventricular function in acute myocardial infarction: results from a randomized clinical trial. Am Heart J. 1981;102(3):313-24.
14. Puskarich MA, Runyon MS, Trzeciak S, Kline JA, Jones AE. Effect of glucose-insulin-potassium infusion on mortality in critical care settings: a systematic review and meta-analysis. J Clin Pharmacol. 2009;49(7):758-67.
15. Mégarbane B, Karyo S, Baud FJ. The role of insulin and glucose hyperinsulinaemia/euglycaemia therapy in acute calcium channel antagonist and beta-blocker poisoning. Toxicol Rev. 2004;23:215-22.
16. Abstracts of the 2008 North American Congress of Clinical Toxicology Annual Meeting, September 11–16, 2008, Toronto, Canada. Clin Toxicol (Phila). 2008;46(7):591-645.
17. Mehrpour O, Alfred S, Shadnia S, Keyler DE, Soltaninejad K, Chalaki N, et al. Hyperglycemia in acute aluminum phosphide poisoning as a potential prognostic factor. Hum Exp Toxicol. 2008;27(8):591-5.
18. Alberti KG, Thomas DJB. The management of diabetes during surgery. Br J Anaesth. 1979;51(7):693-710.
19. Miriam A, Korula G. A simple glucose insulin regimen for perioperative blood glucose control: the Vellore regimen. Anesth Analg. 2004;99(3):598-602.
20. Hassanian H, Zamani N. Therapeutic role of hyperinsulinemia/euglycemia in aluminum phosphide poisoning. Medicine (Baltimore). 2016;95(31):e4349.
21. Nickson CP, Little M. Early use of high-dose insulin euglycaemic therapy for verapamil toxicity. Med J Aust. 2009;191(6):350-2.

22. Pannu AK, Bhalla A, Vamshi V, Upadhyay MK, Sharma N, Kumar S. Changing spectrum of acute poisoning in North India: a hospital-based descriptive study. Turk J Emerg Med. 2022;22(4):192-9.
23. St-Onge M, Anseeuw K, Cantrell FL, Gilchrist IC, Hantson P, Bailey B, et al. Experts consensus recommendations for the management of calcium channel blocker poisoning in adults. Crit Care Med. 2017;45(3):e306-15.
24. Cole JB, Arens AM, Laes JR, Klein LR, Bangh SA, Olives TD. High dose insulin for beta-blocker and calcium channel-blocker poisoning. Am J Emerg Med. 2018;36(10):1817-24.
25. Stellpflug SJ, Fritzlar SJ, Cole JB, Engebretsen KM, Holger JS. Cardiotoxic overdose treated with intravenous fat emulsion and high-dose insulin in the setting of hypertrophic cardiomyopathy. J Med Toxicol. 2011;7(2):151-3.
26. Greene SL, Gawarammana I, Wood DM, Jones AL, Dargan PI. Relative safety of hyperinsulinaemia/euglycaemia therapy in the management of calcium channel blocker overdose: a prospective observational study. Intensive Care Med. 2007;33 (11):2019-24.
27. Bailey B. Glucagon in beta-blocker and calcium channel blocker overdoses: a systematic review. J Toxicol Clin Toxicol. 2003;41(6):595-602.
28. Levine M, Curry SC, Padilla-Jones A, Ruha AM. Critical care management of verapamil and diltiazem overdose with a focus on vasopressors: a 25-year experience at a single center. Ann Emerg Med. 2013;62(3):252-8.
29. Messmer AS, Zingg C, Muller M, Gerber JL, Schefold JC, Pfortmueller CA. Fluid overload and mortality in adult critical care patients: a systematic review and meta-analysis of observational studies. Crit Care Med. 2020;48(12):1862-70.
30. Gummin DD, Mowry JB, Beuhler MC, Spyker DA, Bronstein AC, Rivers LJ, et al. 2020 Annual Report of the American Association of Poison Control Centers' National Poison Data System (NPDS): 38th annual report. Clin Toxicol (Phila). 2021;59(12):1282-501.
31. Kerns W. Management of beta-adrenergic blocker and calcium channel antagonist toxicity. Emerg Med Clin N Am. 2007;25(2):309-31.
32. Krukenkamp I, Sorlie D, Silverman N, Pridjian A, Levitsky S. Direct effect of high-dose insulin on the depressed heart after beta-blockade or ischemia. Thorac Cardiovasc Surg. 1986;34:305-9.
33. Singh S, Bhalla A. Aluminum phosphide poisoning. J Mahatma Gandhi Inst Med Sci. 2015;20:15-9.
34. Sivvach SB, Yadav DR, Arora BB, Dalal S, Jagdish. Acute aluminium phosphide poisoning. An epidemiological, clinical and histopathological study. J Assoc Phys India. 1988;36:594-6.
35. Mehrpour O, Dolati M, Soltaninejad K, Shadnia S, Nazparvar B. Evaluation of histopathological changes in fatal aluminum phosphide poisoning. Indian J Forensic Med Toxicol. 2008;2(2):34-6.
36. Pannu AK, Bhalla A, Gantala J, Sharma N, Kumar S, Dhibar DP. Glucose-insulin-potassium infusion for the treatment of acute aluminium phosphide poisoning: an open-label pilot study. Clin Toxicol (Phila). 2020;58(10):1004-9.
37. Anand R, Kumari P, Kaushal A, Bal A, Wani WY, Sunkaria A, et al. Effect of aluminium phosphide exposure on rats: a biochemical and histological correlation. Toxicol Lett. 2012;215(1):62-9.
38. Cheng Z, Tseng Y, White MF. Insulin signalling meets mitochondria in metabolism. Trends Endocrinol Metab. 2010;21(10):589-98.
39. Page CB, Ryan NM, Isbister GK. The safety of high-dose insulin euglycemia therapy in toxin-induced cardiac toxicity. Clin Toxicol (Phila). 2018;56(6):389-96.
40. Schult RF, Nacca N, Grannell TL, Jorgensen RM, Acquisto NM. Evaluation of high-dose insulin/euglycemia therapy for suspected β-blocker or calcium channel blocker overdose following guideline implementation. Am J Health-Syst Pharm. 2022;79(7):547-55.
41. Corcoran JN, Jacoby KJ, Olives TD, Bangh SA, Cole JB. Persistent hyperinsulinemia following high-dose insulin therapy: a case report. J Med Toxicol. 2020;16(4):465-9.
42. Woodward C, Pourmand A, Mazer-Amirshahi M. High dose insulin therapy, an evidence-based approach to beta-blocker/calcium channel blocker toxicity. Daru. 2014;22(1):36.
43. Yuan TH, Kerns WP, Tomaszewski CA, Ford MD, Kline JA. Insulin-glucose as adjunctive therapy for severe calcium channel antagonist poisoning. Clin Toxicol (Phila). 1999;37(4):463-74.
44. Koliastasis L, Lampadakis I, Milkas A, Strempelas P, Sourides V, Kakava K, et al. Refractory shock from amlodipine overdose overcomed with hyperinsulinemia. Cardiovasc Toxicol. 2022;22(1):63-6.

4.14 Methylene Blue

Prashant Kumar, Manisha Manohar, Sumedha Vashishth

INTRODUCTION

Methylthioninium chloride, commonly known as methylene blue (MB), is a phenothiazine-derived synthetic dye. Heinrich Caro first synthesized the compound in 1876.[1] The medicinal properties of this textile dye were revealed much later when it demonstrated efficacy in the treatment of malaria. It subsequently became an important treatment modality in methemoglobinemia, cyanide poisoning, ifosfamide poisoning, and refractory vasoplegic shock.

Like most pharmacologic agents, MB offers a spectrum of benefits, but it is important to recognize that the compound carries potential risks that can at times lead to toxicity. Its use to identify the parathyroid gland intraoperatively was found to be associated with central nervous system toxicity. Noncompliance to prescribed dosage can lead to toxicity, underscoring the need for caution while dealing with this drug. In the light of increasing prevalence of the use of antidepressants,[2] the interaction between MB and selective serotonin reuptake inhibitors (SSRIs) is of importance for clinicians. This chapter will explore the clinical uses of MB and its toxicity with special emphasis on etiology, underlying mechanism, clinical features, management, and prevention.

METHYLENE BLUE OVERVIEW

Historical Background

Methylene blue was first prepared by Heinrich Caro in 1876 for use as a cotton dye. It was found not only to stain but also to kill the malarial parasite, making it the first synthetic dye to be used to treat malaria by Paul Ehrlich in 1891. The metamorphosis of MB from a dyeing agent to an important pharmacological agent illustrates how a compound application can transform and expand through the clinical need and integration of concepts of diverse fields of study.

Medical Uses

Methemoglobinemia

Oxidative stress in erythrocytes leads to the formation of ferrihemoglobin ($HbFe^{3+}$), which is the nonoxygen-carrying hemoglobin. However, the formation of methemoglobin (metHb) is normally counteracted by cytochrome b5 reductase (major pathway) and nicotinamide adenine dinucleotide phosphate (NADPH) metHb reductase, maintaining the metHb levels at the physiologic level of 0–2%.[3]

Cytochrome b5 reductase uses NADH to reduce metHb to functional hemoglobin.[4] NADPH is generated through glucose-6-phosphate dehydrogenase (G6PD) in hexose monophosphate shunt. NADPH-metHb reductase uses this NADPH as reducing agent to restore the functional hemoglobin form.[5] When these protective mechanisms are overwhelmed either due to congenital (enzymatic defects, genetic)[5] or acquired processes (oxidizing drugs: Benzocaine, prilocaine, aniline, nitrates, and dapsone),[6] the concentration of metHb increases, leading to congenital or acquired methemoglobinemia **(Table 1)**. The hemoglobin molecule is unable to carry oxygen due to the conversion of the ferrous part of the heme molecule to the ferric state.

TABLE 1: Agents inducing methemoglobinemia.

Amyl nitrite	Metoclopramide
Aminophenol	Naphthalene
Aniline dye and its derivatives	Nitrobenzene
Chlorates	Nitroglycerin
Chloroquine and primaquine	Nitroprusside
Copper sulfate	Oxides of nitrogen
Lidocaine, benzocaine	Phenacetin
Local anesthetic agent	Phenazopyridine
	Sulfonamide

Methylene blue: While methylene blue is a known treatment for methemoglobinemia, it also induces oxidation and worsens the clinical status of individuals with an underlying glucose-6-phosphate dehydrogenase (G6PD) deficiency. In these patients, it may induce acute hemolysis that can further decrease oxygen delivery to the tissues. In high doses, methylene blue can paradoxically increase methemoglobinemia

Rasburicase: Risk of methemoglobinemia with rasburicase is especially high in individuals with G6PD deficiency; rasburicase should be avoided in these individuals

TABLE 2: Clinical features of methemoglobinemia.

Methemoglobin concentration (%)	*Clinical features*
0–3	Asymptomatic
3–15	Mild symptoms/may be asymptomatic
15–20	Cyanosis with gray-brown hue, *unresponsive* to O_2
20–50	Dyspnea, headache, fatigue, syncope, weakness, dizziness, and tachycardia
50–70	Tachypnea, hypoxia, metabolic acidosis, seizure, arrhythmia, CNS depression, and bradycardia
>70	Hemolytic anemia, renal failure, coma, and death

(CNS: central nervous system; O_2: oxygen)

The clinical pictures vary from mild to severe symptoms. Patients without any coexisting abnormalities usually become symptomatic at levels exceeding 15%,[7] while those with concomitant hematologic, cardiovascular, and pulmonary diseases may become symptomatic at lower levels **(Table 2)**. Dyspnea, cyanosis, and hypoxemia; refractory to oxygen administration; and the presence of chocolate-colored brown blood should alert the physician to the presence of methemoglobinemia. Co-oximetry is a sensitive, less expensive, and noninvasive test that should be ordered in patient suspected of methemoglobinemia.

Methylene blue is an effective antidote for methemoglobinemia due to its inherent oxidizing properties. Although no randomized clinical trials evaluating its role are available, the observational data and case reports demonstrate its favorable role in managing methemoglobinemia. Intravenous (IV) MB oxidizes and metabolizes to leukomethylene blue that acts as a reducing agent converting metHb to hemoglobin, leading to the restoration of oxygen-carrying capacity. MB is approved by the Food and Drug Administration (FDA) for the treatment of methemoglobinemia. While mild methemoglobinemia is treated with supplemental oxygen, moderate-to-severe cases would require IV administration of 1% MB at the dose of 1–2 mg/kg body weight slowly over 5 minutes.

Vasoplegic Shock

Hypotension despite normal or increased cardiac output and decreased systemic vascular resistance is called vasoplegic shock. MB administration for the treatment of vasoplegic syndrome results in an improvement of mean arterial pressure with a compensatory increase in systemic vascular resistance and a reduction in requirement of vasopressors.[8] MB acts via the inhibition of nitric oxide (NO) cyclic guanosine monophosphate (cGMP) pathways, which are responsible for systemic vasodilation. Although it is not yet approved by FDA for use in the settings of vasoplegic shock, its early administration is shown to provide better outcomes that improve the survival in cardiac surgery patients[8] and reduce the incidence of postoperative renal failure. It has been used for the treatment of vasoplegic shock after cardiopulmonary bypass. NO production in septic shock manifests as hypotension, cardiodepression, and vascular hyporeactivity.[9] As an inhibitor of NO production, MB probably modulates the inflammatory responses. Moreover, critically ill patients with shock have depleted levels of antioxidants. MB is also an antioxidant. In critically ill patients with shock, IV administration of MB is reported to reduce 28-day mortality.[10] For vasoplegic shock, IV MB can be infused for 20 minutes at a dose of 2 mg/kg. This may be given preoperatively and postoperatively to reduce mortality.

Refractory Anaphylaxis

The inhibition of smooth muscle relaxation and vasodilation with MB has led to its use in refractory anaphylaxis unresponsive to standard treatment. Protamine-induced anaphylaxis[11] and anaphylaxis without hypotension[12] have been successfully managed with MB. However, cases implicating MB as the cause of anaphylaxis have also been reported;[13] hence, well-designed trials are needed to establish the role of MB in anaphylaxis.

Hepatopulmonary Syndrome

Widespread pulmonary vasodilatation due to increased cGMP results in hypoxemia in patients with hepatopulmonary syndrome. By inhibiting guanylyl cyclase enzymes, MB decreases cGMP and vascular smooth muscle relaxation and improves partial pressure of arterial oxygen (PaO_2). The dose same as vasoplegic shock may be used.

Staining in Medical Procedures

Methylene blue is lipophilic compound, which allows the easy penetration and distribution across the cell membranes. This leads to temporary accumulation of the dye inside cells. This property of MB serves as several purposes in medical procedures such as endoscopic diagnostics,[14] delineation of parathyroid gland during surgery,[15] diagnosis of intragastric balloon rupture, and detection of surgical leaks. A dose of 2 and 5 mL of a 1% solution given intraparenchymal is usually enough.

Ifosfamide Neurotoxicity

Ifosfamide is an alkylating agent used in the treatment of sarcomas, lymphomas, and germinal tumors. However, this chemotherapeutic agent is associated with neurotoxicity in 10–40% of the patients. Choloroacetaldehyde, a metabolite of ifosfamide, is believed to be responsible for central nervous system toxicity. MB is used in the treatment and prevention of ifosfamide neurotoxicity (IFN). For ifosfamide-induced encephalopathy, MB is given intravenously at a dose of 50 mg every 4 hours until asymptomatic.

Disinfectant

Methylene blue in combination with sunlight offers a solution for disinfecting surgical masks and personal protective equipment.[16]

METHYLENE BLUE TOXICITY

Most MB toxicity cases are documented following its IV administration, either during parathyroid surgeries to aid in parathyroid gland identification or management of vasoplegic shock in patients undergoing cardiopulmonary bypass. These cases typically result in intensive care unit admissions. Most of the patients are usually receiving SSRI medications preoperatively and are admitted to intensive care units after the intraoperative use of MB.

Most common adverse effects of MB are the bluish-green discoloration of urine. Another common adverse effect is limb pain following IV administration. MB can cause dizziness, confusion, and headaches. In neonates, it may cause hyperbilirubinemia, respiratory depression, pulmonary edema, phototoxicity, and hemolytic anemia. In G6PD-deficient patients, worsening of anemia may be seen due to hemolysis. In elective situations, it is better to evaluate the patient for G6PD deficiency before administering MB.

Methylene Blue-induced Serotonin Toxicity

Once regarded to be an inert compound, years of clinical experience with MB have revealed a compelling association with serotonin syndrome,[17,18] especially in patients who are on SSRIs such as fluoxetine, citalopram, fluvoxamine, olanzapine, and paroxetine and serotonin-norepinephrine reuptake inhibitors (SNRIs) such as duloxetine, sibutramine, and venlafaxine.[19,20]

Serotonin syndrome is a potentially life-threatening complication generally associated with intentional self-poisoning and medications such as tryptophan, amphetamine, cocaine, mirtazapine, lithium, fentanyl, linezolid, and tramadol. MB is shown to be a potent reversible monoamine oxidase inhibitor (MAOI).[21] IV administration results in partial inhibition of MAOB and complete inhibition of MAOA. Even small doses of MB ranging from 0.7 to 1 mg/kg can lead to significant inhibition of the enzyme MAOA, leading to increased serotonin levels in patients on SSRI, which manifests as serotonin toxicity (ST). With a substantial increase in the use of antidepressants and multiple clinical uses of MB, the incidence of MB toxicity would likely to increase in the near future.

Clinical Presentation

The diagnosis of serotonin syndrome is based on clinical presentation. A triad of autonomic dysfunction, neuromuscular excitation, and altered mental status in the setting of suspected pharmacological agents should alert the clinician. The triad symptoms may not present simultaneously, and the spectrum can vary from mild to severe life threatening symptoms. Neuromuscular excitation may present as hyperreflexia, tremor, twitching opisthotonus, myoclonus, spontaneous or inducible clonus, rigidity, respiratory failure, and tonic-clonic seizures. Central nervous system signs include anxiety, restlessness, insomnia, agitation, coma, delirium, and confusion. Autonomic hyperactivity manifests as diaphoresis, mydriasis, tachycardia, hypertension, hyperthermia, hyperactive bowel sounds, diarrhea, nausea, vomiting, and hypersalivation. Hunter criteria[22] is the recommended clinical tool for the diagnosis of ST. History of administration/intake of serotonergic drug and presence of at least one of the following signs on physical examination would point toward a diagnosis of ST:

- Spontaneous clonus
- Inducible clonus with agitation or diaphoresis
- Oral clonus plus agitation or diaphoresis
- Inducible clonus or ocular clonus plus hypertonia and hyperthermia
- Tremor and hyperreflexia

Severe ST is a life-threatening condition that can lead to multiorgan failure within hours. Patients develop severe muscle rigidity and body temperature as high as 40°C. Serum serotonin level is an unreliable indicator of toxicity. Laboratory workup would reveal and help rule out the alternate diagnosis and evaluate the complications of serotonin syndrome. Nonspecific laboratory findings would include leukocytosis, lactic acidosis, elevated creatinine kinases, deranged renal and liver functions, and dyselectrolytemia. Electroencephalography can rule out any epileptic foci, and noncontrast computed tomography (NCCT) of head would rule any acute intracranial event.

Differential Diagnosis

Serotonin syndrome mimics other clinical conditions such as neuroleptic malignant syndrome, ischemic brainstem infarction, epileptic insults, anticholinergic toxicity, malignant hyperthermia, and sepsis, which should be ruled out.

TREATMENT

Most of the cases of serotonin syndrome can be managed by stopping the drugs and ensuring high-quality supportive care by ensuring the following:

- Adequate hydration
- Standard cooling measures for hyperthermia
- *Adequate sedation:*
    - Benzodiazepines: Diazepam in a dose of 5 mg IV can be administered to provide anxiolysis. It is preferred in patients with seizures. It controls agitation and prevents excessive muscular activity that can lead to an increase in body temperature. It also acts by blunting the hyperadrenergic symptoms of serotonin syndrome. Any physical restraints should be avoided.
    - Dexmedetomidine: It causes sedation and reduces the sympathetic tone by stimulating alpha-2A receptors in the prefrontal cortex and locus coeruleus. It has given better results compared to midazolam in animal studies. There is not yet conclusive evidence to establish it as a frontline IV sedative in serotonin syndrome; however, case reports suggest that it should be used in patient's refractory to the standard treatment.[23,24] Dexmedetomidine can achieve symptom control and potentially obviate intubation, especially in patients who have not experienced seizures and do not necessitate intubation but require sedation.
- *Hyperthermia:* Core temperature monitoring should be done. Active measures to control hyperthermia through physical cooling techniques should be started as soon as possible. Mitigating agitation is imperative to control heightened muscular activity that worsens hyperthermia. Since the high temperature is not hypothalamic mediated, antipyretics administration has no therapeutic role in managing hyperthermia. Dantrolene may be of additive value since it acts on both the peripheral and central ryanodine receptors. The central action modulates the dopaminergic system, which might be involved in the pathogenesis of some central-mediated hyperthermic syndromes.[25]
- *Serotonin receptor antagonists*: Cyproheptadine is a potent 5-HT2A antagonist, available as an enteral preparation that is to be administered via nasogastric tube at an initial dose of 12 mg, followed by 2 mg every 2 hours if symptoms do not resolve. Chlorpromazine is a 5-HT1A and 5-HT2A antagonist that can be administered parenterally.
- For ongoing hypertension, esmolol or nitroglycerin (NTG) infusion can be used. Short-acting agents are preferred to deal with labile hemodynamics, whereas managing severe ST treatment should focus on airway, breathing, and circulation. The two primary life-threatening concerns are rigidity and hyperthermia (temperature 104°F), which need to be managed at the earliest. Patients with profound hyperthermia, uncontrollable agitation, status epilepticus, and severe chest wall rigidity should be sedated, paralyzed, and mechanically ventilated. The neuromuscular blockade will prevent the worsening of hyperthermia resulting from muscle rigidity. Succinylcholine should be avoided due to the risk of exacerbation of rhabdomyolysis and hyperkalemia. Nondepolarizing agent such as vecuronium is preferred. For sedation benzodiazepines, dexmedetomidine[23,26] and propofol may be used. Fentanyl should be avoided due to the propensity to increase serotonin levels.

PREVENTION OF METHYLENE BLUE TOXICITY

- Avoid concomitant use of MB with SSRI, MAOI, and SNRI

- Alternative to MB should be considered for identification of parathyroid glands such as high-resolution ultrasound and preoperative radionuclide scanning.
- Clinicians should exercise extreme caution while administering MB to treat vasoplegic shock in patients already receiving SSRI. A detailed drug history about the intake of medications cannot be overemphasized.
- In cases where the use of MB cannot be avoided, the dose should be minimized, and the patient should be monitored for symptoms.
- *Glucose-6-phosphate dehydrogenase deficiency*: Administering MB to patients with known or suspected G6PD deficiency is a relative contraindication.[26] Inadequate NADPH levels in these patients are ineffective for the reduction of MB to leukomethylene blue. This cohort is also prone to MB-induced hemolysis.[27] In the presence of hemolysis, high doses of MB can lead to paradoxical metHb formation.[28]
- *Avoid in patients with renal impairment*: MB is excreted mainly via the urine, primarily as leukomethylene blue. MB is contraindicated in patients with severe renal impairment. Caution should be exercised when administering MB to patients with mild-to-moderate renal impairment.
- *Anaphylaxis*: MB is generally considered a very safe drug and despite being a treatment option for refractory anaphylaxis, MB itself is known to cause rare but life-threatening anaphylactic reactions. Cases have been reported after sentinel lymph node procedures in adults[29,30] as well as in pediatric patients.[13]

  It should be avoided in the pediatric age group as MB administration in neonates is reported to induce hemolytic anemia.[31,32] The clinical picture includes skin, urine discoloration, jaundice, mixed hyperbilirubinemia, and respiratory distress. Blood film can reveal irregularly contracted cells, blister cells, and ghost cells. The hemolytic process can continue up to 10 days after the administration of MB.

CONCLUSION

The clinical applications of MB continue to broaden across all specialties. The understanding of the pharmacodynamics of this MAOI, particularly in the context of antidepressants, is imperative for clinicians. Given the absence of an antidote for MB toxicity, early recognition and intervention with high-quality supportive treatment can avert mortality and morbidity in such cases.

REFERENCES

1. Wiklund L, Basu S, Miclescu A, Wiklund P, Ronquist G, Sharma HS. Neuro- and cardioprotective effects of blockade of nitric oxide action by administration of methylene blue. Ann N Y Acad Sci. 2007;1122:231-44.
2. Brody DJ, Gu Q. (2020). Antidepressants use among adults: United States, 2015-2018. National Centre for Health Statistics Data Brief No. 377. [online] Available from www.cdc.gov/nchs/products/databriefs/db377.htm#:~:text=Key%20findings,-Data%20from%20the&text=During%202015%E2%80%932018%2C%2013.2%25,60%20and%20over%20(24.3%25). [Last accessed February, 2025].
3. Yawata Y, Ding L, Tanishima K, Tomoda A. New variant of cytochrome b5 reductase deficiency (b5RKurashiki) in red cells, platelets, lymphocytes, and cultured fibroblasts with congenital methemoglobinemia, mental and neurological retardation, and skeletal anomalies. Am J Hematol. 1992;40(4):299-305.
4. Skold A, Cosco DL, Klein R. Methemoglobinemia: pathogenesis, diagnosis, and management. South Med J. 2011;104(11):757-61.
5. Curry S. Methemoglobinemia. Ann Emerg Med. 1982; 11(4):214-21.
6. Bradberry SM. Occupational methaemoglobinaemia. Mechanisms of production, features, diagnosis and management including the use of methylene blue. Toxicol Rev. 2003;22(1):13-27.
7. Jaffé ER. Methemoglobin pathophysiology. Prog Clin Biol Res. 1981;51:133-51.
8. Mehaffey JH, Johnston LE, Hawkins RB, Charles EJ, Yarboro L, Kern JA, et al. Methylene blue for vasoplegic syndrome after cardiac operation: early administration improves survival. Ann Thorac Surg. 2017;104(1):36-41.
9. Kirkebøen KA, Strand OA. The role of nitric oxide in sepsis—an overview. Acta Anaesthesiol Scand. 1999;43(3): 275-88.
10. Sari-Yavuz S, Heck-Swain KL, Keller M, Magunia H, Feng YS, Haeberle HA, et al. Methylene blue dosing strategies in critically ill adults with shock—a retrospective cohort study. Front Med (Lausanne). 2022;9:1014276.
11. Sheth SS, Duca DD, Ergina P, Clarke AE. Methylene blue as a treatment for refractory anaphylaxis. J Aller Clin Immunol. 2007;119(1 Suppl):S33.
12. Bauer CS, Vadas P, Kelly KJ. Methylene blue for the treatment of refractory anaphylaxis without hypotension. Am J Emerg Med. 2013;31(1):264.e3-5.
13. Dewachter P, Mouton-Faivre C, Tréchot P, Lleu JC, Mertes PM. Severe anaphylactic shock with methylene blue instillation. Anesth Analg. 2005;101(1):149-50.
14. Bruno MJ. Magnification endoscopy, high resolution endoscopy, and chromoscopy; towards a better optical diagnosis. Gut. 2003:52(Suppl 4):iv7-11.

15. Dudley NE. Methylene blue for rapid identification of the parathyroids. Br Med J. 1971;3(5776):680-1.
16. Vos KA, Gordon PMK, Heyne B. Methylene blue in combination with sunlight as a low cost and effective disinfection method for coronavirus-contaminated PPE. Am J Infect Control. 2022;50(8):906-8.
17. Basta MN. Postoperative serotonin syndrome following methylene blue administration for vasoplegia after cardiac surgery: a case report and review of the literature. Semin Cardiothorac Vasc Anesth. 2021;25(1):51-6.
18. Venkatesh S, Rubachandran M, Michael B, Najmosama N. Serotonin syndrome secondary to methylene blue interaction with SSRI in the context of drug shortage. Crit Care Med. 2019;47(1):659.
19. Stanford SC, Stanford BJ, Gillman PK. Risk of severe serotonin toxicity following co-administration of methylene blue and serotonin reuptake inhibitors: an update on a case report of post-operative delirium. J Psychopharmacol. 2010;24(10):1433-8.
20. Gillman PK. Methylene blue and serotonin toxicity: definite causal link. Psychosomatics. 2010;51(5):448-9.
21. Ramsay RR, Dunford C, Gillman PK. Methylene blue and serotonin toxicity: inhibition of monoamine oxidase A (MAO A) confirms a theoretical prediction. Br J Pharmacol. 2007;152(6):946-51.
22. Dunkley EJC, Isbister GK, Sibbritt D, Dawson AH, Whyte IM. The Hunter serotonin toxicity criteria: simple and accurate diagnostic decision rules for serotonin toxicity. QJM. 2003;96(9):635-42.
23. Rushton WF, Charlton NP. Dexmedetomidine in the treatment of serotonin syndrome. Ann Pharmacother. 2014;48(12):1651-4.
24. Akingbola OA, Singh D. Dexmedetomidine to treat lisdexamfetamine overdose and serotonin toxidrome in a 6-year-old girl. Am J Crit Care. 2012;21(6):456-9.
25. Oyamada T, Hayashi T, Kagaya A, Yokota N, Yamawaki S. Effect of dantrolene on K(+)- and caffeine-induced dopamine release in rat striatum assessed by in vivo microdialysis. Neurochem Int. 1998;32(2):171-6.
26. Sikka P, Bindra VK, Kapoor S, Jain V, Saxena KK. Blue cures blue but be cautious. J Pharm Bioallied Sci. 2011;3(4): 543-5.
27. Liao YP, Hung DZ, Yang DY. Hemolytic anemia after methylene blue therapy for aniline-induced methemoglobinemia. Vet Hum Toxicol. 2002;44(1): 19-21.
28. Wright RO, Lewander WJ, Woolf AD. Methemoglobinemia: etiology, pharmacology, and clinical management. Ann Emerg Med. 1999;34(5):646-56.
29. Jangjoo A, Forghani MN, Mehrabibahar M, Sadeghi R. Anaphylaxis reaction of a breast cancer patient to methylene blue during breast surgery with sentinel node mapping. Acta Oncol. 2010;49(6):877-8.
30. Oomah S, Dembinski T, Becker A, Kalicinsky C. Prolonged elevation of serum tryptase resulting from intraoperative anaphylaxis to methylene blue. Allergy Asthma Clin Immunol. 2010;6(Suppl 2):P29.
31. Vanhinsbergh L, Uthaya S, Bain BJ. Methylene blue-induced Heinz body hemolytic anemia in a premature neonate. Am J Hematol. 2018;93(5):716-7.
32. Kirsch IR, Cohen HJ. Heinz body hemolytic anemia from the use of methylene blue in neonates. J Pediatr. 1980;96(2):276-8.

4.15 Vitamins that Counteract Toxic Effects (Pyridoxine, Vitamin K, Folinic Acid, Hydroxocobalamin)

Riyaz Sogiawalla, Firoze Sogiawalla

INTRODUCTION

The term "antidote" comes from the Greek word ἀντίδοτον (antídoton), derived from ἀντί (antí, "against") and δίδωμι (dídomi, "I give"). Tradition attributes its invention to Mithridates VI (135–63 BC), the king of Pontus, but this is an oversimplification.[1]

CONCEPT OF A UNIVERSAL ANTIDOTE

The first universal antidote was mithridate.[2] In the 1st century AD, its composition was modified by Andromachus the Elder, Nero's physician.[3] Theriaca Andromachi, the first antivenom antidote, was used for people bitten by snakes and other wild animals in the Roman Empire.[4]

For Paracelsus (1493–1541), a Swiss physician, philosopher, and alchemist, the concept of a universal antidote was the starting point for the theory of the ubiquity of poisons, including potent poisons.[5,6] "All things are poison and nothing is without poison, only the dose permits something not to be poison" matched the dual nature of the Colchis concentrate.[2]

CONCEPT OF A SPECIFIC ANTIDOTE

The first use of antidotes for the bites of poisonous snakes and rabid dogs were *Belladonna*, datura, and strychnine, alone or combined together.[7,8] Later, the extracts of some of these plants were used.[9] Over the years, with the advent of newer, more toxic chemical and pharmaceutical agents, demand for specific antidotes surged.

In theory, two chemical compounds binding to each other to produce a less toxic product, which can be safely excreted from the body, explains how a specific antidote is supposed to work. The classical example is cyanide binding to hydroxocobalamin rather than cytochrome oxidase and forming cyanocobalamin, a nontoxic compound, which is renally excreted.[10]

REVIVAL OF THE CONCEPT OF A UNIVERSAL ANTIDOTE

There have been changes, which have resulted in revival of the concept of a universal antidote, but we are still far away from it. Activated charcoal, a chemical reagent, in aqueous suspension, is known to absorb many medications, for example, vitamin K antagonists, alkaloids, but it fails miserably to adsorb many chemicals such as pesticides, mineral oils, heavy metals, and corrosives.[11] The dream of finding a universal antidote still remains a dream. As chemical sciences have progressed, the concepts of a specific chemical antidote have been proposed such as monospecific antivenom and monoclonal antibodies to toxins and venoms. The thrust now is to find antidotes that act at the molecular level.[12]

CLASSIFICATION OF VITAMINS

Vitamins are vital organic compounds required in small quantities for numerous physiological functions.[13] They are broadly classified into:

- *Fat-soluble vitamins*: A, D, E, and K
- *Water-soluble vitamins*: C and B complex (B_1, B_2, B_3, B_5, B_6, B_7, B_9, and B_{12})

TABLE 1: Sources and roles.

Vitamins	*Sources*	*Roles*
A	Liver, fish oils, milk	Vision, immune function, skin health
D	Sunlight, fortified dairy	Bone health, calcium regulation
E	Vegetable oils, nuts	Antioxidant, cell protection
K	Green vegetables, fish	Blood clotting, bone metabolism
C	Citrus fruits, broccoli	Collagen synthesis, antioxidant
B_1	Whole grains, pork	Energy metabolism, nerve function
B_2	Eggs, green vegetables	Energy production, cellular function
B_3	Poultry, fish	DNA repair, metabolism, skin health
B_5	Avocados, eggs	Coenzyme A synthesis
B_6	Poultry, potatoes	Amino acid metabolism, neurotransmission
B_7	Eggs, nuts	Fatty acid synthesis, glucose metabolism
B_9	Green leafy vegetables, beans	DNA synthesis, cell division
B_{12}	Meat, dairy	Red blood cell formation, neurological function

Vitamin deficiency and overdose: Optimal intake of vitamins is crucial to prevent deficiencies that can lead to significant health issues and to avoid toxicities due to excessive intake **(Tables 1 and 2)**.

VITAMINS AS ANTIDOTES

While many antidotes are synthetic drugs specifically developed for the purpose of neutralizing toxic substances, certain vitamins also possess potent antidote properties. Vitamins play critical roles in metabolic processes, enzyme function, and cellular repair. When administered in therapeutic doses, some vitamins can counteract the toxic effects of specific agents. In this chapter, we explore the use of pyridoxine (vitamin B_6), vitamin K, folinic acid, and hydroxocobalamin as antidotes. These vitamins are chosen for their established efficacy in reversing the toxicities associated with various poisons and drugs.

TABLE 2: Deficiency and overdose.

Vitamins	Deficiency symptoms	Overdose symptoms
A	Night blindness, xerophthalmia	Liver damage, nausea
D	Rickets, osteomalacia	Hypercalcemia, kidney stones
E	Neurological problems	Increased bleeding risk
K	Increased bleeding tendency	May affect anticoagulant medications
C	Scurvy, anemia	Gastrointestinal disturbances
B_1	Beriberi, Wernicke–Korsakoff syndrome	Rare
B_2	Ariboflavinosis	None reported
B_3	Pellagra	Liver damage, flushing
B_5	Dermatitis, alopecia	No known toxicity
B_6	Anemia, neuropathy	Sensory neuropathy
B_7	Dermatitis, neurological symptoms	No known toxicity
B_9	Megaloblastic anemia	Can mask B_{12} deficiency
B_{12}	Pernicious anemia	No known toxicity

Pyridoxine (Vitamin B_6)[14]

First used in the mid-20th century to treat isoniazid poisoning, pyridoxine's role as an antidote is well documented. Its absorption is rapid and efficient, with peak plasma levels reached within hours, a wide distribution, including the central nervous system, and excretion primarily via the kidneys. Its half-life allows for sustained levels conducive to treating acute exposures.

Synonyms

Vitamin B6, vitamin B6 Streuli

Dose Formulations

Pyridoxine, available as tablets (20 and 100 mg) and injectable forms (various strengths)

Synthesis and Biological Action

Vitamin B_6 has three natural forms: (1) Pyridoxine (PN), (2) pyridoxal (PL), and (3) pyridoxamine (PM), all of which transform into its active forms in the body, which is the coenzyme pyridoxal 5-phosphate.[15] Pyridoxine is converted to pyridoxal phosphate, a coenzyme vital for amino acid metabolism, neurotransmitter synthesis, and hemoglobin production. Vitamin B_6 is also involved in glycogenolysis and gluconeogenesis.[16]

Absorption and Pharmacokinetics[16]

- *Absorption:* Well absorbed orally; also available in intravenous (IV) and intramuscular (IM) forms
- *Distribution*: Widely distributed in tissues, especially liver, muscle, and brain
- *Metabolism*: Metabolized in the liver
- *Elimination*: Excreted in urine
- *Half-life*: Approximately 15–20 days

Indications[17]

- In cases of its deficiency, which may be due to poor renal function, autoimmune diseases, and increased alcohol intake.
- Deficiency is due to intake of isoniazid, cycloserine, valproic acid, phenytoin, carbamazepine, primidone, hydralazine, and theophylline therapy.
- Pyridoxine is indicated in the treatment of isoniazid overdose, false morel (*Gyromitra*) mushroom poisoning, hydrazine exposure, ethylene glycol toxicity, and crimidine toxicity. It is the drug of choice for the management of convulsions caused by isoniazid poisoning.[14]

Dosage

- *Adult:* 1 g IV per gram of isoniazid ingested (maximum 5 g). If the dose of isoniazid is unknown, administer 5 g IV. Infuse at 0.5 g/min in 5% dextrose. If convulsions are controlled before full dose is given, administer the remaining dose as a slow IV infusion over 1–2 hours. Repeat if convulsions persist.
- *Pediatric:* 70 mg/kg (maximum 5 g). Administer as for adults. If a parenteral preparation is unavailable, tablets may be crushed and given orally or via a nasogastric tube.

Contraindications

Contraindications include hypersensitivity to pyridoxine or its components

Side Effects

Administration of high doses (>1 g/day) may rarely cause sensory neuropathy.[18]

Vitamin K_1 (Phytomenadione)

Poisoning with oral anticoagulants (warfarin), leading to symptomatic bleeding, is a real threat compared to intentional overdose. Accidental overdose is likely in patients chronically on anticoagulants and in children; however, underlying psychiatric issues may precipitate ingestion for self-harm.[19] Superwarfarins lead to potent vitamin K epoxide reductase (VKOR) inhibitors with longer half-lives, prompting their use as potent rodenticides.[20] Vitamin K_1 has been crucial in treating warfarin overdoses since 1930s. It is rapidly absorbed, especially when administered intravenously, with a half-life that facilitates quick action against excessive anticoagulation.

Synonyms

Vitamin K_1, Konakion MM[21]

Dose Formulations

- *Injection*: 2 mg/0.2 mL; 10 mg/mL adult dose of 10–20 mg slow IV over 30 minutes
- *Tablet*: 1 mg, 1–2 mg orally. It can be raised to 10 mg if severe coagulopathy is present. Menadiol diphosphate (vitamin K analog) is available as 10 mg tablets.

Synthesis and Biological Action[21]

Vitamin K1 is essential for synthesizing clotting factors II, VII, IX, and X in the liver.[22] Vitamin K occurs in two bioactive forms: (1) vitamin K_1 and (2) vitamin K_2. Vitamin K_1 (phylloquinone) is a product of plant synthesis. It is most prevalent in green leafy vegetables because it is directly involved in photosynthesis.[21]

Vitamin K_2 is created in the gut by bacteria. Gut flora converts Vitamin K_1 into vitamin K_2 (menaquinone); function of vitamin K_2 in the body is to add carboxylic acid groups to glutamate residues to form gamma-carboxyglutamate residues.[23] This is an important step required for the creation of clotting factors. The compound with two carboxylic acid groups on the gamma-carboxyglutamate residue allows chelation of calcium ions. Calcium ions binding is a crucial step for vitamin K-dependent clotting factors to trigger clotting cascades. Vitamin K is responsible as a factor in synthesizing prothrombin and factors VII, IX, and X.[21 23]

Absorption and Pharmacokinetics[24]

- *Absorption*: Well absorbed orally; also available in IV and IM forms
- *Distribution*: Distributed primarily to the liver
- *Metabolism*: Metabolized in the liver
- *Elimination*: Excreted in bile and urine
- *Half-life*: 1–2 hours for vitamin K_1; longer for vitamin K_2

Indications

- Poisoning with coumarin-type anticoagulants (e.g., warfarin) and anticoagulant rodenticides, especially superwarfarins. Oral anticoagulants have been rarely used for self-harm purpose, but their accidental/unintentional overdose is common. Superwarfarins are common agent used successfully for self-harm purpose.[24]
- Vitamin K is indicated in deficiency state and bleeding disorders, especially related to liver dysfunction.

Dosage[24]

- *Active bleeding or life-threatening hemorrhage:*
  - *Nonanticoagulant therapy patients:* 10–20 mg IV for adults (250 µg/kg for children, maximum 10 mg)
  - *Anticoagulant therapy patients:* 5–10 mg IV for adults (100 µg/kg for children, maximum 10 mg). Adjust based on clinical response and international normalized ratio (INR) levels
  - *Prothrombin complex concentrate:* 25–50 units/kg IV or fresh frozen plasma (15 mL/kg) if available
- *No active bleeding:*
  - *Nonanticoagulant therapy patients:* 5–10 mg IV for adults (100 µg/kg for children, maximum 10 mg)
  - *Anticoagulant therapy patients:*
    - *INR ≥8.0 (≥5.0 for long-acting anticoagulant rodenticides)*: 1.0–3.0 mg IV for adults (15–30 µg/kg for children, maximum 1 mg)
    - *INR <8.0 but more than therapeutic range (or <5.0 for long-acting rodenticides):* Stop anticoagulant therapy and monitor INR daily. Restart cautiously once INR is in the therapeutic range
    - *Long-acting anticoagulants:* Treatment may be needed for weeks or months. Monitor INR for 2 weeks post-treatment

Contraindications

Administration of vitamin K requires caution in neonates, patients with hereditary hypoprothrombinemia, renal impairment, cases of overanticoagulation due to heparin, and hypersensitivity to vitamin K.[24]

Side Effects

Side effects are rare, but may include anaphylactic reactions (particularly with IV administration), flushing, and taste disturbances.[25]

Folinic Acid (as Calcium Folinate or Disodium Folinate)

Folinic acid (5-formyltetrahydrofolic acid) is a naturally occurring, biologically active, reduced form of folic acid. It is found in green leafy vegetables. It is a potent antidote to folic acid antagonist such as methotrexate.[26] It was first introduced for methotrexate toxicity in 1950. Folinic acid acts rapidly by bypassing metabolic blocks induced by methotrexate. It is administered intravenously for immediate effect, with a metabolism independent of the pathways blocked by methotrexate. Folinic acid has become important in clinical practice, mainly because humans cannot synthesize folates de novo.[26]

Ingredients

- *Calcium folinate*: 3 (10 mL ampoule), 7.5 (2 mL ampoule), and 10 mg/mL (5, 10, 20, 30, and 35 mL ampoules)
- *Disodium folinate*: 50 mg/mL (2 or 8 mL ampoules)

Synthesis and Biological Action

Folinic acid, also known as leucovorin, is a form of folate (vitamin B9) synthesized chemically from p-aminobenzoic acid and dihydrofolate or derived from natural sources.[27] It bypasses the need for dihydrofolate reductase, directly replenishing reduced folate levels essential for DNA synthesis and repair.[27] Folinic acid counteracts the effects of folic acid antagonists. This is possible because folinic acid enters cells through reduced folate carrier to get converted to tetrahydrofolate in spite of methotrexate being there. Thereby, it is "rescuing" these cells from methotrexate toxicity. It also enhances the impact of fluoropyrimidines.[28]

Absorption and Pharmacokinetics[26]

- *Absorption:* Well absorbed orally; also available in IV and IM forms
- *Distribution:* Widely distributed in body tissues
- *Metabolism:* Rapidly converted to active forms of folate
- *Elimination:* Primarily excreted in urine
- *Half-life:* Approximately 6 hours

Indications

- Methotrexate and pyrimethamine toxicity. "Leucovorin rescue" is the term used when high-dose folinic acid is used to manage the toxic effects of methotrexate overdose/therapy.[27]
- Formic acid, formalin, and formaldehyde poisoning
- Methanol poisoning (formate is important component needing therapy)
- Folate deficiency (megaloblastic anemia)
- Patients with repeated nitrous oxide exposure or requiring treatment with long-term nitrous oxide may benefit from folinic acid prophylaxis to prevent bone marrow suppression.

Dosage[27,29]

- *Methotrexate toxicity*:
  - *Rescue therapy:* 100 mg/m² IV every 6 hours until methotrexate levels are known. Adjust according to methotrexate concentration:
    - 50 µmol/L: 1,000 mg/m² IV every 6 hours
    - 5–50 µmol/L: 100 mg/m² IV every 6 hours
    - 0.5–5 µmol/L: 30 mg/m² IV/oral every 6 hours
    - $<$0.5 µmol/L: 10 mg/m² IV/oral every 6 hours
    - $<$0.05 µmol/L or undetectable: Folinic acid is not required
- *Formic acid/formaldehyde*: 30 mg IV every 6 hours for 48 hours
- *Methanol poisoning*: 30 mg IV every 6 hours for 48 hours
- *Trimethoprim or pyrimethamine*: Give 5–15 mg orally, IM, or IV daily until the restoration of hematopoiesis[30]
- *Folate deficiency*: 1–5 mg orally daily

Cautions

Folic acid cannot substitute for folinic acid in methotrexate toxicity as folic acid's biological availability relies on dihydrofolate reductase, which is inhibited by methotrexate.[29]

Contraindications

Contraindications can be pernicious anemia or other vitamin B_{12} deficiency states.

Side Effects

The most commonly reported adverse reactions are nausea, vomiting, diarrhea, leukopenia, alopecia, and stomatitis. Some patients may also experience erythema, pruritus, skin rash, and urticaria. Anaphylactic reactions are possible but rare.[31]

Hydroxocobalamin

Hydroxocobalamin is a synthetic form of vitamin B12. It is used to treat vitamin B_{12} deficiency, but most importantly is used as an effective antidote for cyanide poisoning.[32] It binds cyanide ions and forms cyanocobalamin. This is nontoxic and readily excreted renally. Its introduction in the 1960s significantly improved the treatment of accidental cyanide poisoning, especially the type seen in fire accident or smoke inhalation victims.[33]

Synonyms

Cyanokit[32]

Ingredients

Hydroxocobalamin is available as a powder for IV infusion. Vials come in 2.5 (reconstituted with 100 mL diluent) and 5 g (reconstituted with 200 mL diluent), using sodium chloride 9 mg/mL solution. Reconstituted solution contains 25 mg/mL hydroxocobalamin.[34]

Indications

Chelating antidote for cyanide poisoning is seen in exposure to cyanide gas, smoke inhalation, or in fire accident victims.[32]

Dosage

- *Adult:* 5 g IV over 15 minutes; repeat if necessary
- *Child:* 70 mg/kg (not exceeding 5 g) IV over 15 minutes; repeat if necessary

Pharmacology

Hydroxocobalamin is a precursor of methylcobalamin and adenosylcobalamin, which are the active forms of vitamin B_{12}. The methylcobalamin component in hydroxocobalamin plays a role in the development of the nervous system during childhood and hematopoiesis.[33,34] Adenosylcobalamin is involved with the metabolism of carbohydrates, amino acids, and fatty acids and is, thus, involved in myelin formation. Therefore, the role of vitamin B_{12} highlights the clinical features that may present in vitamin B_{12} deficiency and the indications for the use of hydroxocobalamin.[33] Methylcobalamin is a cofactor for the enzyme methionine synthase, an essential enzyme

TABLE 3: Summary of vitamin antidotes.

Vitamins	*Indications*	*Dosage*	*Contraindications*	*Complications/side effects*
B_6 (pyridoxine)	Isoniazid poisoning	• *Adult:* 1 g IV per gram of isoniazid ingested (maximum 5 g). • *Pediatric:* 70 mg/kg (maximum 5 g)	Hypersensitivity to pyridoxine	Sensory neuropathy at high doses
K_1 (phytomenadione)	Warfarin overdose, rodenticide poisoning	• *Active bleeding:* 10–20 mg IV (adults) and 250 µg/kg (children) • *No active bleeding:* Adjust dose based on INR	Hypersensitivity to vitamin K components	Anaphylactic reactions, flushing, and taste disturbances
Folinic acid	Methotrexate toxicity, methanol, and formic acid poisoning	• *Methotrexate toxicity:* 100 mg/m^2 IV every 6 hours, adjust based on levels • *Other poisonings:* 30 mg IV every 6 hours for 48 hours	Pernicious anemia, other B12 deficiency states	Allergic reactions, GI disturbances
Hydroxocobalamin	Cyanide poisoning	• *Adult:* 5 g IV over 15 minutes; may repeat if necessary • *Child:* 70 mg/kg IV over 15 minutes; may repeat if necessary	Hypersensitivity to hydroxocobalamin or cobalt	Red discoloration of skin and urine, potential hypertension, and acute kidney injury

(GI: gastrointestinal; INR: international normalized ratio; IV: intravenous)

in the formation of methionine from homocysteine. This reaction is critical in the synthesis of purines and pyrimidines needed for DNA synthesis and red blood cell formation.[34]

Adverse Reactions[35]

- Red discoloration of skin and urine for up to 35 days
- Potential for hypertension and acute kidney injury; monitor renal function post-treatment.

Contraindications

Contraindications can be hypersensitivity to hydroxocobalamin or cobalt.[35]

CONCLUSION

Vitamins such as pyridoxine, vitamin K, hydroxocobalamin, and folinic acid are used to treat specific types of poisonings. This specificity not only increases the efficacy of these antidotes but also highlights the broader shift in medical treatments toward more personalized and precise interventions in the form of specific antidotes. Easy availability and nontoxic nature of these natural/synthetic supplements make them ideal antidotes **(Table 3)**.

REFERENCES

1. Parojcic D, Stupar D, Mirica M. Theriac: medicine and antidote. Vesalius. 2003;9(1):28-32.
2. Tsatsakis AM, Vassilopoulou L, Kovatsi L, Tsitsimpikou C, Karamanou M, Leon G, et al. The dose response principle from philosophy to modern toxicology: the impact of ancient philosophy and medicine in modern toxicology science. Toxicol Rep. 2018;5:1107-13.
3. Galen. (2013). On Theriac to Piso, A critical edition with translation and commentary. Submitted by Robert Adam Leigh to the University of Exeter as a thesis for the degree of Doctor of Philosophy in Classics in July 2013. 136-8. [online] Available from https://ore.exeter.ac.uk/repository/bitstream/10871/13641/1/LeighR.pdf. [Last accessed February, 2025].
4. King H. "First behead your viper": acquiring knowledge in Galen's poison stories. In: Grell OP, Cunningham A, Arrizabalaga J (Eds). "It All Depends on the Dose" Poisons and Medicines in European History, 1st edition. London: Routledge; 2018, pp. 25-42.
5. Michaleas SN, Laios K, Tsoucalas G, Androutsos G. Theophrastus Bombastus Von Hohenheim (Paracelsus) (1493–1541): the eminent physician and pioneer of toxicology. Toxicol Rep. 2018;8:411-4.
6. Michaleas SN, Pantos C, Chatzipanagiotou S, Samonis G, Karamanou M. Theophrastus Bombastus Von Hohenheim: theological reformer, philosopher and physician. J Relig Health. 2021;60(6):3907-14.
7. Meischner N. History of a case of severe affection from the bite of a viper. Lond Med Phys J. 1820;43(253):196-7.
8. Walsh JHT. Strychnine as an antidote to snake-poison. Ind Med Gaz. 1893;28(12):430.
9. Some account of the Tanjore antidotes for the bite of a mad dog; and also for the bite of venomous serpents. Lond Med J. 1789;10(Pt 3):283-95.
10. Meillier A, Heller C. Acute cyanide poisoning: hydroxocobalamin and sodium thiosulfate treatments with two outcomes following one exposure event. Case Rep Med. 2015;2015:217951.
11. Daly JS, Cooney DO. Interference by tannic acid with the effectiveness of activated charcoal in "universal antidote". Clin Toxicol. 1978;12(5):515-22.
12. Magowska A. The natural history of the concept of antidote. Toxicol Rep. 2021;8:1305-9.
13. NHS. (2020). Overview: vitamins and minerals. [online] Available from www.nhs.uk/conditions/vitamins-and-minerals/. [Last accessed February, 2025].
14. Lheureux P, Penaloza A, Gris M. Pyridoxine in clinical toxicology: a review. Eur J Emerg Med. 2005;12(2):78-85.
15. Rabincowitch JC, Snell EE. The vitamin B6 group; microbiological and natural occurrence of pyridoxamine phosphate. J Biol Chem. 1947;169(3):643-50.
16. Ebadi M. Regulation and function of pyridoxal phosphate in CNS. Neurochem Int. 1981;3(3-4):181-205.
17. Clayton PT. B6-responsive disorders: a model of vitamin dependency. J Inherit Metab Dis. 2006;29(2-3):317-26.
18. Bendich A, Cohen M. Vitamin B6 safety issues. Ann N Y Acad Sci. 1990;585:321-30.
19. O'Reilly RA, Aggeler PM. Covert anticoagulant ingestion: study of 25 patients and review of world literature. Medicine (Baltimore). 1976;55(5):389-99.
20. Hadler MR, Shadbolt RS. Novel 4-hydroxycoumarin anticoagulants active against resistant rats. Nature. 1975;253(5489):275-7.
21. McKeown NM, Jacques PF, Gundberg CM, Peterson JW, Tucker KL, Kiel DP, et al. Dietary and nondietary determinants of vitamin K biochemical measures in men and women. J Nutr. 2002;132(6):1329-34.
22. Tie JK, Stafford DW. Structural and functional insights into enzymes of the vitamin K cycle. J Thromb Haemost. 2016;14(2):236-47.
23. Thijssen HHW, Vervoort LMT, Schurgers LJ, Shearer MJ. Menadione is a metabolite of oral vitamin K. Br J Nutr. 2006;95(2):260-6.
24. Wojciechowski VV, Calina D, Tsarouhas K, Pivnik AV, Sergievich AA, Kodintsev VV, et al. A guide to acquired vitamin K coagulopathy diagnosis and treatment: the Russian perspective. Daru. 2017;25(1):10.
25. Britt RB, Brown JN. Characterizing the severe reactions of parenteral vitamin K1. Clin Appl Thromb Hemost. 2018;24(1):5-12.

26. Scaglione F, Panzavolta G. Folate, folic acid and 5-methyltetrahydrofolate are not the same thing. Xenobiotica. 2014;44(5):480-8.
27. Howard SC, McCormick J, Pui CH, Buddington RK, Harvey RD. Preventing and managing toxicities of high-dose methotrexate. Oncologist. 2016;21(12):1471-82.
28. Shiroky JB, Neville C, Esdaile JM, Choquette D, Zummer M, Hazeltine M, et al. Low-dose methotrexate with leucovorin (folinic acid) in the management of rheumatoid arthritis. Results of a multicenter randomized, double-blind, placebo-controlled trial. Arthritis Rheum. 1993;36(6):795-803.
29. Jardine LF, Ingram LC, Bleyer WA. Intrathecal leucovorin after intrathecal methotrexate overdose. J Pediatr Hematol Oncol. 1996;18(3):302-4.
30. Greiner PO, Zittoun J, Marquet J, Cheron JM. Pharmacokinetics of (-)-folinic acid after oral and intravenous administration of the racemate. Br J Clin Pharmacol. 1989;28(3):289-95.
31. Benchalal M, Yahchouchy-Chouillard E, Fouere S, Fingerhut A. Anaphylactic shock secondary to intravenous administration of folinic acid: a first report. Ann Oncol. 2002;13(3):480-1.
32. Thakkar K, Billa G. Treatment of vitamin B12 deficiency-methylcobalamine? Cyancobalamine? Hydroxocobalamin?-clearing the confusion. Eur J Clin Nutr. 2015;69(1):1-2.
33. Pott JWR, Wong KH. Leber's hereditary optic neuropathy and vitamin B12 deficiency. Graefes Arch Clin Exp Ophthalmol. 2006;244(10):1357-9.
34. Oh R, Brown DL. Vitamin B12 deficiency. Am Fam Physician. 2003;67(5):979-86.
35. James J, Warin RP. Sensitivity to cyanocobalamin and hydroxocobalamin. Br Med J. 1971;2(5756):262.

4.16 Calcium Gluconate

Sheila Nainan Myatra, Abhisheksingh R Rajput, Keyurkumar B Shah

INTRODUCTION

Calcium gluconate is a calcium salt of gluconic acid. Calcium gluconate plays an important role as an antidote by treating the hypocalcemia that occurs due to molecule toxicity and by functional antagonism and action at a postreceptor level in various other conditions. In this chapter, we describe the role of calcium gluconate in various conditions, including contraindications, drug interactions, precautions, and specific monitoring required during its use.

PHARMACOLOGY

Calcium gluconate is a transparent, colorless, and slightly yellow-colored solution. One gram of calcium gluconate is equivalent to 4.64 mEq or 2.32 mmol or 93 mg of elemental calcium. Initially, it was believed that calcium gluconate has a low bioavailability and requires gluconate metabolism in the liver to release ionized calcium.[1] However, later, it was shown that the simple dissociation of calcium from gluconate is responsible for the release of calcium rather than hepatic metabolism.[2] Due to the lower risk of tissue necrosis in case of extravasation of the drug, calcium gluconate is often preferred over calcium chloride.[3]

ROLE AS AN ANTIDOTE

Calcium gluconate acts as an antidote in the following ways:

- To treat hypocalcemia that occurs due to molecule toxicity, e.g., hydrofluoric acid exposure, citrate toxicity, and ethylene glycol toxicity.[4]
- Functional antagonism and/or action at postreceptor level, e.g., hyperkalemia, hypermagnesemia, calcium channel blocker (CCB) toxicity, and beta-blocker overdose.[4-7]

ROLE IN VARIOUS CONDITIONS

Hydrofluoric Acid Exposure

Hydrofluoric acid toxicity occurs through the dermal, gastrointestinal, and inhalational routes.[8] Ammonium, sodium, potassium, and other soluble fluoride and bifluoride salts can produce the toxicity of hydrofluoric acid.

Mechanism of Action

Fluoride toxicity occurs due to the release of hydrogen ions, increase in permeability of the cell membrane to potassium and complexation of fluoride with calcium and magnesium and, therefore, interference with various enzyme systems.[9,10] This leads to hypocalcemia and hypomagnesemia. Calcium is the mainstay of treatment for hydrofluoric acid burns, because it binds to fluoride ions, effectively neutralizing them and preventing additional toxicity. Additionally, calcium gluconate will replenish ionized calcium in case hypocalcemia develops, which is very common in this situation. Calcium gluconate may be administered in the following ways:

- *Local application:* A 2.5% calcium gluconate gel is commercially available. In case of unavailability, it can be prepared by mixing 25–30 mL of calcium gluconate solution with 75–100 mL of water-soluble jelly or glycerol.
- *Intradermal or subcutaneous route:* If pain is persistent, calcium gluconate 1 g/10 mL can be injected intradermally or subcutaneously. It is important to note that calcium chloride cannot be used in place of calcium gluconate for subcutaneous or intradermal injection as the chloride salts can lead to tissue necrosis.
- *Bier's block:* If pain persists or if there is a large burn, Bier's block may be utilized. In 40 mL of 0.9% saline, inject 1 g (10 mL) of calcium gluconate and administer over 20 minutes.[7,11]
- *Intra-arterial infusion:* As a last resort, 10–15 mL of 10% calcium gluconate can be mixed with 40 mL of Ringer's lactate and injected into the artery that supplies the burned area over a 3-hour period.
- *Inhalational exposure:* A 2.5% calcium gluconate solution may be used for nebulization. To prepare this solution of nebulized calcium gluconate, combine 1.5 mL of 10% calcium gluconate solution with 4.5 mL of sterile water or 0.9% sodium chloride.
- *Management of hypocalcemia:*
    - *Severe hypocalcemia* (seizure, tetany, laryngospasm, and ionic calcium <4 mg/dL): 1–2 g (100–200 mg elemental calcium) (10–20 mL) of 10% calcium gluconate diluted in 50–100 mL of dextrose or normal saline should be given over 10 minutes and repeated every 10 minutes to an hour until symptoms resolve.[12] In pediatric population, the dose is 0.6 mL/kg of a 10% solution infused over 5–10 minutes. Rhythm monitoring with an electrocardiography (EKG) is advised during intravenous (IV) calcium bolus administration (IV push lasting 10 minutes). After this, steps to manage moderate hypocalcemia are followed.
    - *Moderate-to-severe hypocalcemia* (ionized calcium 4 mg/dL in the absence of seizures or tetany): Adults can receive an infusion of elemental calcium at a rate of approximately 100 mg/h over several hours. Patients with persistent hypocalcemia can receive a continuous infusion of calcium gluconate ranging from 5 to 20 mg/kg/h.
    - *Mild hypocalcemia* (ionized calcium level >4–5 mg/dL): 1–2 g calcium gluconate IV over 2 hours. Asymptomatic patients can take calcium orally.

Citrate Toxicity

Risk factors for citrate toxicity are massive transfusions (citrate is used as a preservative in the blood bags), regional citrate anticoagulation during continuous renal replacement therapy (CRRT), liver failure, and cardiogenic shock. Citrate toxicity manifests as a high anion gap metabolic acidosis or metabolic alkalosis based on liver function and hypocalcemia.[13,14] Total calcium will be normal or high with low ionized calcium. Total calcium is normal or high, because instruments that detect calcium will also detect citrate–calcium complexes in the serum and consider it as total calcium. The management of citrate toxicity during CRRT includes decreasing the citrate infusion rate, decreasing blood pump speed, and increasing the dialysate flow rate. Calcium gluconate can be used to treat severe hypocalcemia as described above.

Ethylene Glycol Toxicity

Oxalic acid produced during the metabolism of ethylene glycol metabolism chelates calcium, leading to hypocalcemia.[15,16] Such patients should be closely monitored for signs and symptoms of hypocalcemia such as QT prolongation, hyperreflexia, muscle spasms, tetany, and seizures. Calcium gluconate can be used in such cases as described above.

Calcium Channel Blocker Toxicity

To counteract the cardiovascular effects of CCB, calcium gluconate is frequently employed. Nevertheless, calcium salt therapy is frequently unsuccessful. This is due to CCB poisoning, interfering with the intracellular handling of calcium as well as its serum concentration. The role of calcium against CCB toxicity is to overwhelm the calcium receptors in order to competitively antagonize the CCB. Serum concentration remains normal in CCB overdose. It is an adjunct to the main therapy of CCB overdose that includes high-dose insulin therapy, glucagon, and atropine. The dose required is 0.6 mL/kg (60 mg/kg) of 10% calcium gluconate solution given as a bolus, followed by a continuous infusion of 0.6–1.5 mL/kg/h (60–150 mg/kg/h). The ionized calcium levels must be tracked throughout the process, so as to achieve a calcium level twice that of normal.[6]

Beta-blocker Toxicity

In vitro studies suggest that beta-blocker negative inotropic action is related to interference with both forward and reverse calcium transport in the sarcoplasmic reticulum as well as inhibition of microsomal and mitochondrial calcium uptake.[17,18] Calcium entry into the cardiac cell leads to contraction of myofibrils, leading to a positive cardiac inotropy effect. Calcium administration is used when hemodynamic instability is refractory to other measures. A 10% calcium gluconate solution should be given intravenously at 0.6–1.2 mL/kg (60–120 mg/kg) over 5–10 minutes and repeated every 10–20 minutes for three to four times, followed by a continuous infusion at 0.65 mL/kg/h.[4] Many times, beta-blocker and/or CCB overdose occur along with cardioactive steroid such as digoxin toxicity. In such a case, it is a myth that administration of calcium for hyperkalemia in the presence of digoxin toxicity may lead to stone heart syndrome. This is based on the result of case series of five patients in a single-center retrospective study. Therefore, needed calcium administration should be undertaken with due care to counteract the CCB and/or beta-blocker component of toxicity.

Hyperkalemia

Modest hyperkalemia leads to less negative resting membrane potential (RMP) (e.g., from -90 to -80) and threshold potential (e.g., from -75 to -70). The effect is more pronounced on the RMP compared to the threshold potential. This leads to cardiac hyperexcitability. Administration of calcium in this condition will lead to a more positive threshold potential and thereby restore the difference between RMP and threshold potential. Thus, cardiac myocyte membrane potential gets stabilized.[19] When there is severe hyperkalemia, voltage-gated sodium channels become inactivated and cannot be depolarized, regardless of the strength of the impulse. Calcium turns the voltage sensor of the sodium channels from inactive to closed, allowing the sodium channel to open with depolarization.[20]

For treatment of hyperkalemia, 10–20 mL of a 10% solution of calcium gluconate is given intravenously over 2–5 minutes to stabilize cardiac cell membranes. Its action typically starts in 3 minutes and lasts for 20–60 minutes. During this time, EKG findings of hyperkalemia should improve. However, if the EKG findings persist or worsen, another dose of calcium gluconate should be administered.[21]

Hypermagnesemia

Hypermagnesemia leads to the blockade of calcium and potassium channels both intracellularly and extracellularly. This will manifest as neuromuscular blockade, cardiopulmonary arrest, and ventilatory failure. Calcium acts as a physiologic competitive antagonist of this hypermagnesemia toxicity.[5,22] The dose is the same as what is described in the section under hyperkalemia.

ADVERSE EFFECTS AND TOXICITY

Extravasation of calcium formulations may lead to tissue necrosis. This occurs due to the calcium-induced vasoconstriction of capillaries and intracellular fluid retention. Calcium gluconate has a lesser propensity to cause tissue necrosis compared to chloride formulation. Calcinosis cutis, dermal deposits of calcium salts, can develop at a later stage and lead to ulceration.[2] If extravasation occurs, stop the infusion and gently aspirate the extravasated fluid. Elevate the area with extravasation and apply cold dry compresses. Hyaluronidase can be intradermally or subcutaneously into the border of area with extravasation and into the catheter.[23] Some patients may develop systemic toxicity because of hypercalcemia. This is usually observed in CCB or beta-blocker toxicity where aggressive calcium infusion is used.[24] Clinical manifestations of hypercalcemia include, but are not limited to, nausea, vomiting, ileus, cognitive alteration, dysrhythmias, and nephrolithiasis.[25]

CONTRAINDICATIONS AND DRUG INTERACTIONS

Calcium gluconate should be used with caution in patients with hyperphosphatemia, as it will lead to the formation of calcium phosphate crystals, which will get deposited in the kidney and blood vessels. Likewise, it should not be combined with phosphate-containing solution during infusion.[2] Calcium gluconate should be avoided in patients with hypercalcemia and sarcoidosis.

Calcium gluconate infusion should be avoided along with bicarbonate infusion in the same intravenous line, as it will form calcium carbonate crystals, which may precipitate. In addition, when given along with the antibiotic ceftriaxone, the resultant calcium ceftriaxone complex will precipitate and may embolize; hence, the two drugs should not be mixed.[2] Administration of calcium gluconate with the antibiotic minocycline renders minocycline ineffective and, therefore, should be avoided.[2]

MONITORING

Close monitoring is required, especially while treating CCB and beta-blocker toxicity, as the dose of calcium used is high and frequent. This is to avoid hypercalcemia. The target is twice the upper limit of normal in these cases.[6] Ionized calcium should be measured every 1–4 hours during the administration of a calcium gluconate infusion.

CONCLUSION

- Calcium gluconate is preferred over calcium chloride for peripheral administration as extravasation-related tissue injury is less common compared to chloride salts.
- It is used via different routes such as intradermal, subcutaneous, topical, intravenous, intra-arterial, and nebulization (in case of hydrofluoric and fluoric acid salt exposure) depending on the site of exposure.
- It is used to treat hypocalcemia that develops during citrate toxicity, hydrofluoric acid exposure, and ethylene glycol toxicity.
- Calcium gluconate works as a physiologic antagonist in case of hyperkalemia and hypermagnesemia.
- It is used as an adjunct to the primary therapy in case of toxicity with a CCB or a beta-blocker.
- Frequent monitoring is required to avoid hypercalcemia during calcium administration.

REFERENCES

1. White RD, Goldsmith RS, Rodriguez R, Moffitt EA, Pluth JR. Plasmic ionic calcium levels following injection of chloride, gluconate, and gluceptate salts of calcium. J Thorac Cardiovasc Surg. 1976;71:609-13.
2. Kabi F. Calcium gluconate injection, for intravenous use. Lake Zurich, IL: Fresenius Kabi; 2017.
3. French S, Subauste J, Geraci S. Calcium abnormalities in hospitalized patients. South Med J. 2012;105(4):231-7.
4. Hoek TLV, Morrison LJ, Shuster M, Donnino M, Sinz E, Lavonas EJ, et al. Part 12: cardiac arrest in special situations: 2010 American Heart Association guidelines for cardiopulmonary resuscitation and emergency cardiovascular care. Circulation. 2010;122(18 Suppl 3):S829-61.
5. McDonnell NJ, Muchatuta NA, Paech MJ. Acute magnesium toxicity in an obstetric patient undergoing general anaesthesia for caesarean delivery. Int J Obstet Anesth. 2010;19(2):226-31.
6. Shah SK, Goswami SK, Babu RV, Sharma G, Duarte AG. Management of calcium channel antagonist overdose with hyperinsulinemia-euglycemia therapy: case series and review of the literature. Case Rep Crit Care. 2012:927040.
7. Hatzifotis M, Williams A, Muller M, Pegg S. Hydrofluoric acid burns. Burns. 2004;30(2):156-9.
8. Chan KM, Svancarek WP, Creer M. Fatality due to acute hydrofluoric acid exposure. J Toxicol Clin Toxicol. 1987;25:333-9.
9. Caravati EM. Acute hydrofluoric acid exposure. Am J Emerg Med. 1988;6:143-50.
10. Edinburg M, Swift R. Hydrofluoric acid burns of the hands: a case report and suggested management. Aust N Z J Surg. 1989;59:88-91.
11. Lin TM, Tsai CC, Lin SD, Lai CS. Continuous intra-arterial infusion therapy in hydrofluoric acid burns. J Occup Environ Med. 2000;42:892-7.
12. Cooper MS, Gittoes NJ. Diagnosis and management of hypocalcaemia. BMJ. 2008;336(7656):1298-302.
13. Auffant RA, Downs JB, Amick R. Ionized calcium concentration and cardiovascular function after cardiopulmonary bypass. Arch Surg. 1981;116:1072-6.
14. Dzik WH, Kirkley SA. Citrate toxicity during massive blood transfusion. Transfus Med Rev. 1988;2:76-94.
15. Introna F, Smialek JE. Antifreeze (ethylene glycol) intoxications in Baltimore. Report of six cases. Acta Morphol Hung. 1989;37:245-63.
16. Parry MF, Wallach R. Ethylene glycol poisoning. Am J Med. 1974;57:143-50.
17. Langemeijer J, de Wildt D, de Groot G, Sangster B. Calcium interferes with the cardiodepressive effects of beta-blocker overdose in isolated rat hearts. J Toxicol Clin Toxicol. 1986;24:111-33.
18. Noack E, Kurzmack M, Verjovski-Almeida S, Inesi G. The effect of propranolol and its analogs on Ca^{++} transport by sarcoplasmic reticulum vesicles. J Pharmacol Exp Ther. 1978;206:281-8.
19. Meroney WH, Herndon RF. The management of acute renal insufficiency. J Am Med Assoc. 1954;155:877-83.
20. Hofer CA, Smith JK, Tenholder MF. Verapamil intoxication: a literature review of overdoses and discussion of therapeutic options. Am J Med. 1993;95:431-8.
21. Long B, Warix JR, Koyfman A. Controversies in management of hyperkalemia. J Emerg Med. 2018;55(2):192-205.

22. Agus ZS, Morad M. Modulation of cardiac ion channels by magnesium. Annu Rev Physiol. 1991;53:299-307.
23. Reynolds PM, MacLaren R, Mueller SW, Fish DN, Kiser TH. Management of extravasation injuries: a focused evaluation of noncytotoxic medications. Pharmacotherapy. 2014;34(6):617-32.
24. Sim MT, Stevenson FT. A fatal case of iatrogenic hypercalcemia after calcium channel blocker overdose. J Med Toxicol. 2008;4:25-29.
25. Turner JJO. Hypercalcaemia—presentation and management. Clin Med (Lond). 2017;17:270-3.

4.17 Glucagon

JV Divatia, Veer Thakkar

INTRODUCTION

Glucagon is a peptide hormone secreted by α-cells of the islets of Langerhans located in the pancreas. It consists of 29 amino acids. Hypoglycemia is the main stimulus for the release of glucagon from these α-cells. It acts as an antagonist to insulin. Glucagon and insulin play a crucial role in regulating fuel metabolism. The main actions of glucagon are on glucose metabolism: It promotes glycogenolysis and gluconeogenesis. It also acts on lipid and protein metabolism, food intake, and satiety modulation.

GLUCOSE METABOLISM

Glucagon is a hyperglycemic agent. Initial research into the pathogenesis of diabetes mellitus suggested that it was due to the relative or absolute decrease in insulin levels. Unsurprisingly, increased levels of glucagon are found in all forms of diabetes. Various theories have established that there is dysregulation of insulin and glucagon. These include insulinocentric, bihormonal, and glucagonocentric.

PHARMACOKINETICS

Absorption

Glucagon is readily absorbed when administered as 1 mg dose subcutaneously. The peak plasma concentration is achieved within 10–15 minutes. When 1 mg is administered intramuscularly, the peak plasma concentration is achieved in 10 minutes. The peak plasma concentration achieved with 1 mg dose is 3,391 pg/mL.

Metabolism

Glucagon is rapidly metabolized in the liver, kidney, and plasma. It has a half-life of approximately 40 minutes following subcutaneous administration and 26 minutes following intramuscular (IM) administration.

PHARMACODYNAMICS

Intravenous

Intravenous (IV) glucagon, administration in the dose of 0.25–0.5 mg, achieves peak glucose concentration in 5–20 minutes. It also produces smooth muscle relaxation of the gastrointestinal tract within 45 seconds, and the effect may last from 9 to 17 minutes.

Intramuscular

When injected IM (1 mg), it achieves a peak glucose concentration within 30 minutes. IM injection also produces smooth muscle relaxation of the gastrointestinal tract within 8–10 minutes and it lasts for 12–27 minutes.

INDICATIONS FOR USE

Hypoglycemia

Glucagon is used in the immediate treatment of hypoglycemia caused by excess insulin. These include hyperinsulinism, surreptitious insulin administration, or sulfonylurea ingestion. It is not effective in other causes of hypoglycemia.

Children

In a hypoglycemic child presenting with altered mental status and difficult IV access, glucagon is administered to acutely increase the plasma glucose. The recommended dose is 0.5 (<25 kg) or 1 mg (>25 kg) intramuscularly.

Adults

A hypoglycemic patient with altered consciousness can be administered glucagon intranasally, subcutaneously, or intramuscularly in the absence of an IV access. After administration of glucagon, the recovery of consciousness usually happens within 15 minutes, but it may be accompanied with side effects such as nausea and vomiting. This can be averted by oral intake of concentrated carbohydrates, immediately after the patient gains consciousness.

Glucagon is not a substitute for dextrose; dextrose is to be administered to hypoglycemic patients at the earliest.

OTHER INDICATIONS AS AN ANTIDOTE

Beta-blocker Poisoning

The use of glucagon for the treatment of beta-blocker overdose was first described in a case series published in the early 1980s. The authors postulated that glucagon increases heart rate and myocardial contractility and improves atrioventricular conduction. These actions may bypass the beta-adrenergic receptor site, which is blocked in the presence of beta-blockers. Thus, glucagon may be considered as an alternative therapy for profound beta-blocker intoxications associated with bradycardia and hypotension not responding to isoproterenol and atropine.[1]

The dose of glucagon recommended to reverse severe beta-blockade is 50 μg/kg IV loading dose, followed by a continuous infusion of 1–15 mg/h. Glucagon at such high doses may lead to side effects such as nausea, vomiting, hypokalemia, and hyperglycemia.

In 2020, a systematic review was conducted to evaluate the effects of treatment for beta-blocker poisoning. The authors concluded that glucagon was associated with minor improvements in hemodynamics through an increase in heart rate in two case series, nine case reports, and five animal studies.[2] These studies need to be substantiated with robust clinical trials in human subjects.

Calcium Channel Blocker Poisoning

Glucagon increases the intracellular levels of cyclic adenosine monophosphate, and, thus, in animal models, it has been shown to increase the heart rate in calcium channel blocker poisoning. Nonetheless, it has minimal effects on the mean arterial pressure. It has been used effectively in humans as well in cases refractory to conventional therapy for calcium channel blocker poisoning.[3-5] The dose of glucagon used for this is 5 mg IV bolus and may be repeated at 10-minute interval or an infusion may be started titrated to the desired response.

Because of the logistical difficulties associated with obtaining large amounts of glucagon needed for infusion, the recommendation is that high-dose insulin euglycemic therapy (HIET) and catecholamine therapy be optimized before adding glucagon infusion, unless readily available in adequate quantities. Calcium channel blocker overdose can also receive treatment with glucagon; glucagon is a second-line therapy behind calcium, epinephrine, high-dose insulin, and dextrose.[6,7]

DOSAGE FORMS AVAILABLE

Glucagon is available as a formulation to be administered intravenously (bolus or infusion), intramuscularly, subcutaneously, and intranasally.[8,9] A formulation as dehydrated powder is to be reconstituted with supplied sterile water or as a purpose-formulated intranasal spray. A prefilled glucagon autoinjector has been approved but is not yet commercially available. The intranasal powder essentially can be administered directly into the patient's nose as a spar, without any preparation. It is important to hold the other nostril closed while administering. There are no dosage alterations required for any major organ dysfunction in special populations (pregnancy, elderly).

ADVERSE EFFECTS

The frequently encountered adverse effect is nausea, most commonly observed with IV administration. It is noted in as much as one-third of patients where it is administered. Hypertension is noted within 2 hours following administration. It is attributed to the positive inotropic effects of glucagon. Severe anaphylaxis has been reported due to its nature as a foreign protein. This may manifest with hypotension, rash, and vomiting. Hypersensitivity reactions are rarely reported.

Less common adverse effects are rebound hypoglycemia, especially in the presence of undetected/suspected insulinoma. Worsening hyperglycemia is reported in the presence of pancreatic glucagon-secreting lesions.

It may precipitate severe hypertension if administered inadvertently to patients with pheochromocytoma.

Except for documented allergy or allergic reaction, there is no absolute contraindication to its use.

In case of an overdose of glucagon, which may manifest with severe hypertension, treatment with alpha-blocking agents and vasodilators will help mitigate the problem.

CONCLUSION

Glucagon is an important agent and should always be available in the emergency department as an antidote. Not only it helps in reversing refractory hypoglycemia, it also helps in reversing the calcium channel and beta-blocker toxicity. The cost is a major factor in precuring this important antidote, nevertheless, it can be life saving in many life threatening poisonings.

REFERENCES

1. Peterson CD, Leeder JS, Sterner S. Glucagon therapy for beta-blocker overdose. Drug Intell Clin Pharm. 1984;18(5):394-8.
2. Rotella JA, Greene SL, Koutsogiannis Z, Graudins A, Leang YH, Kuan K, et al. Treatment for beta-blocker poisoning: a systematic review. Clin Toxicol (Phila). 2020;58(10):943-83.
3. Mahr NC, Valdes A, Lamas G. Use of glucagon for acute intravenous diltiazem toxicity. Am J Cardiol. 1997;79:1570-1.
4. Walter FG, Frye G, Mullen JT, Ekins BR, Khasigian PA. Amelioration of nifedipine poisoning associated with glucagon therapy. Ann Emerg Med. 1993;22:1234-7.
5. Doyon S, Roberts JR. The use of glucagon in a case of calcium channel blocker overdose. Ann Emerg Med. 1993;22:1229-33.
6. Graudins A, Lee HM, Druda D. Calcium channel antagonist and beta-blocker overdose: antidotes and adjunct therapies. Br J Clin Pharmacol. 2016;81(3):453-61.
7. Shepherd G. Treatment of poisoning caused by beta-adrenergic and calcium-channel blockers. Am J Health Syst Pharm. 2006;63(19):1828-35.
8. Reno FE, Edwards CN, Jensen MB, Török-Bathó M, Esdaile DJ, Piché C, et al. Needle-free nasal delivery of glucagon for treatment of diabetes-related severe hypoglycemia: toxicology of polypropylene resin used in delivery device. Cutan Ocul Toxicol. 2016;35(3):242-7.
9. Rickels MR, Ruedy KJ, Foster NC, Piché CA, Dulude H, Sherr JL, et al. Intranasal glucagon for treatment of insulin-induced hypoglycemia in adults with type 1 diabetes: a randomized crossover noninferiority study. Diabetes Care. 2016;39(2):264-70.

4.18 Sodium Bicarbonate

Prabakaran Parameswaran, Balaji Venkatachalam, Nagarajan Ramakrishnan

INTRODUCTION

Bicarbonate (HCO_3) is one of the important buffers, which regulates the acid-base homeostasis.[1] Carbon dioxide (CO_2) is one of the products of metabolism, which combines with water (H_2O) to produce carbonic acid (H_2CO_3), catalyzed by carbonic anhydrase.[2] Later, H_2CO_3 dissociates into HCO_3 and hydrogen ions, which are excreted by the kidneys.

$$\text{Dissolved } CO_2 + H_2O \leftrightarrow H_2CO_3 \leftrightarrow HCO_3^- + H+$$

The above equation can move bidirectional, and H_2CO_3 may also dissociate into CO_2 and H_2O. The dissolved CO_2 is excreted through the lungs, underscoring the importance of adequate respiration after HCO_3 administration.

Providing additional sodium ions and *alkaline molecules* are the major mechanisms by which sodium bicarbonate ($NaHCO_3$) exerts its therapeutic efficacy. HCO_3 excreted by the kidneys increases urine pH and alters the elimination kinetics of some xenobiotics, which may have therapeutic applications in toxicology.

Sodium bicarbonate has limited therapeutic applications in critical care, because its adverse effects may outweigh the benefits. Further, due to the lack of high-quality randomized controlled trials (RCTs) on the utility of $NaHCO_3$ in critical care toxicology, most recommendations are based only on level III clinical data and animal studies.

Sodium bicarbonate is available in oral as well as intravenous (IV) forms as 4.2%, 7.5%, and 8.4% solutions **(Table 1)**. IV forms are more commonly used in critical care toxicology. Therapeutic administration of $NaHCO_3$ may alter the pharmacokinetics and pharmacodynamics (Pk/Pd) of the xenobiotic or toxin, reducing its volume of distribution or facilitating its renal excretion.[3]

Although $NaHCO_3$ is used in various clinical scenarios, it has potential adverse effects such as ionized hypocalcemia,

TABLE 1: Commonly used sodium bicarbonate products and their composition.

Percentage	*mEq*	*mEq/mL*	*mOsm*
8.4	50	1	2
7.5	44.6	0.9	1.79
4.2	5	0.5	1

hypervolemia, hypernatremia, hypercapnia, hyperosmolarity, hypokalemia, intracellular acidosis, paradoxical acidosis in the cerebrospinal fluid (CSF), and rebound acidosis.[4,5] Most of the data on the utility of $NaHCO_3$ in toxicology are from sodium channel blocker toxicity, salicylate overdose, and methanol and ethylene glycol toxicity, and these are discussed below in further detail.

SODIUM CHANNEL BLOCKER TOXICITY

Sodium channels are transcellular proteins that have a major role in cardiac and neuronal membrane stabilization.[6] When these fast sodium channels are blocked, depolarization is impaired, predisposing the myocardium to ventricular arrhythmias. Drugs, which act on these sodium channels, are used in conditions such as mood disorders, seizure disorders, and pain management.[7-9] Drugs acting on sodium channels include many antiarrhythmics (quinidine, procainamide, lidocaine, flecainide, propafenone, and amiodarone), antiepileptics (phenytoin, lamotrigine, and carbamazepine), selective serotonin reuptake inhibitors (SSRIs), (escitalopram, venlafaxine), local anesthetics, tricyclic antidepressants (TCAs) (amitriptyline and nortriptyline), and miscellaneous drugs (hydroxychloroquine, phenothiazines, and thioridazine).

Tricyclic antidepressants are a class of drugs, which have utility in psychological disorders such as depression, anxiety, psychosomatic disorders, and peripheral neuropathy. TCAs have a narrow therapeutic index, which leads to toxicity either due to intentional or accidental overdosing or due to altered Pk/Pd in patients with renal and hepatic dysfunction. TCA toxicity may cause severe metabolic acidosis; electrocardiogram (ECG) changes such as QRS widening (>100 ms), QTc prolongation, right axis deviation, R wave in aVR, and fatal ventricular arrhythmias; and neurotoxicity, including seizures and coma.

Sodium bicarbonate is the standard initial therapy for hypotension or arrhythmia due to TCA toxicity. Administration of $NaHCO_3$ leads to metabolic alkalosis, alkalinization of the receptor with decreased receptor binding, increase in extracellular fluid (ECF) sodium (which reduces the active form of TCA), and increased protein binding of the drug. This increase in ECF sodium creates an electrochemical gradient in cardiac cell membrane and inhibits TCA-mediated sodium channel blockade.[10,11]

In TCA toxicity, 1–2 mEq/kg of $NaHCO_3$ (8.4%) may be given as a bolus followed by infusion. The initial bolus dose is important, as studies and case reports have shown a beneficial effect of HCO_3 with bolus doses.[12] The response is assessed on ECG, which would demonstrate narrowing of QRS complex, resolution of arrhythmia, and improvement in hemodynamics. Once QRS narrowing is achieved, a continuous infusion may be initiated. The infusion is tapered over the next few hours to days based on stabilization of ECG findings. Frequent blood gases may be required to assess the response. Repeat bolus HCO_3 doses may be considered if QRS widens again.

The end points of $NaHCO_3$ therapy in TCA are given as follows:[8]

- Narrowing of QRS complex <120 ms (most important). Duration of QRS complex correlates with seizures and ventricular dysrhythmias.
- pH 7.50–7.55
- R/S ratio <0.7 in aVR on ECG

Avoid serum sodium levels increasing beyond 155 mmol/L during treatment.

SALICYLATE TOXICITY

Salicylic acids are the class of drugs, which have a wide array of indications in cardiovascular disease, rheumatology, and pain medicine. A few examples are aspirin (antiplatelets), bismuth subsalicylate (antidiarrheal),[13] methyl salicylate (ingredients in topical ointments for musculoskeletal pain), and topical keratolytic in dermatology.

Mechanism of Salicylate Toxicity

Salicylates act by inhibition of cyclooxygenase (COX) enzyme, resulting in reduced concentration of thromboxane A2 and prostaglandins. At higher concentrations, they may cause uncoupling of oxidative phosphorylation.[14] Salicylates are weak acids remaining in both charged and uncharged forms. Whenever blood pH decreases (acidosis), the concentration of the uncharged form increases, which easily diffuses across the blood–brain barrier, causing central nervous system (CNS) manifestations.[14]

Signs and Symptoms

Patients with salicylate toxicity often present with nausea, vomiting, giddiness, hyperthermia, altered sensorium, and tachypnea.

Alkalinization of the blood with $NaHCO_3$ is recommended in salicylate poisoning.[15] Inducing metabolic alkalosis with $NaHCO_3$ leads to a reduction in unionized form of salicylate, thereby preventing these ions from crossing blood-brain barrier and subsequently increasing renal clearance.[15]

The dose of HCO_3 is 1–2 mEq/kg bolus followed by infusion.

Titrate the $NaHCO_3$ infusion rate to maintain a urine pH ≥7.5. Increases in serum pH up to 7.55–7.6 are well tolerated in patients with normal kidney function. Frequent arterial blood gases may be required to ensure serum pH between 7.5 and 7.55. Onset of acute kidney injury (AKI) warrants renal replacement therapy (RRT).

The end points for alkalization in salicylate poisoning are given as follows:

- Serum salicylate concentration <40 mg/dL
- Resolution of metabolic acidosis
- Urine pH >7.5
- Resolution of symptoms with normal respiratory rate and effort

METHANOL AND ETHYLENE GLYCOL POISONING

Methanol and ethylene glycol are found in cleaning liquids, some industrial chemicals, and also in illicit liquor. They are metabolized by alcohol dehydrogenase and aldehyde dehydrogenase with end products such as formic acid and oxalic acid, respectively.[16] Formic acid may lead to retinal toxicity, and oxalic acid causes nephrotoxicity.

Clinical manifestations of toxicity include headache, oliguria, blindness, altered sensorium, and seizures. Blood investigations may reveal high anion gap metabolic acidosis (HAGMA), osmolar gap >10, and hypocalcemia.[17]

Treatment

Fomepizole (4-methylpyrazole) is the specific antidote for methanol toxicity, which may not be readily available in intensive care units (ICUs). Ethanol may be used as an antidote, as it is a competitive (enzyme) antagonist for methanol toxicity.

Sodium bicarbonate may be used along with other supportive measures, as alkalosis reduces the uncharged form of these alcohols. $NaHCO_3$ therapy should be considered when serum pH <7.30.[18]

The recommended dose is 1–2 mEq/kg of $NaHCO_3$ bolus, followed by maintenance infusion 150–250 mL/h (133 mEq of $NaHCO_3$ in 1 L of 5% dextrose). When pH >7.3, infusion may be discontinued.

ROLE OF SODIUM BICARBONATE TO ENHANCE URINARY ELIMINATION OF XENOBIOTICS AND SNAKE VENOM

Bicarbonate may also be used for urinary elimination of acidic compounds, in addition to direct toxin—xenobiotic antagonism (due to the alkaline nature of the HCO_3).

When the urine is alkalinized with HCO_3 infusion, the higher pH traps the ionized toxin or xenobiotic in the urine, preventing its reabsorption, which is ultimately excreted. Also, the rise in serum pH, which happens during HCO_3 therapy, prevents penetration of toxins to other compartments such as CNS.[15]

Conventionally and historically, HCO_3 infusion is coupled with forced diuresis (fluids and diuretics), which has no evidence base. A simple alkaline therapy coupled with maintenance of euvolemia (without forced diuresis) may help in elimination of these toxins.

Alkaline therapy may also serve as a bridge when emergency hemodialysis is not available. The prerequisites for successful urinary alkalinization therapy are adequate renal perfusion and kidney function.

Urinary alkalinization may have a role in the management of certain xenobiotic toxicities (such as salicylates, barbiturates, chlorophenoxy herbicides, methotrexate, chlorine gas, and uranium toxicity) and snake bite (Viperidae—Russell's viper, pit viper, and *Echis carinatus*). Viper venom is vasculotoxic with hemorrhagic proteins, causing bleeding complications, hemolysis, disseminated intravascular coagulation (DIC), rhabdomyolysis, and AKI.[19] Early administration of HCO_3 with appropriate volume expansion (urinary alkalinization) may prevent deposition of cast (heme pigment) in the renal tubules and AKI in viper snake bite.[20] This may also increase the risk of calcium phosphate deposition in the tubules when there is hyperphosphatemia secondary to rhabdomyolysis. It would also be essential to monitor for alkalosis, hypokalemia, and hypocalcemia while giving HCO_3 infusion.

Dose

About 150 mEq of $NaHCO_3$ in 1 L of water or 5% dextrose may be started at the rate of 200–250 mL/h. The goal is to achieve a urine pH of >6.5.

Indicators of Successful Bicarbonate Therapy

- Serum pH >7.5
- Urine pH >6.5
- Creatine kinase levels <5,000 units/L

BOX 1: Indications for bicarbonate therapy in critical care.

- Prevention and treatment of contrast-associated nephropathy[3]
- Severe metabolic acidosis (pH <6.9)[5]
- Overdose or toxicity with sodium channel blockers (tricyclic antidepressants)[10]
- Salicylate poisoning[14]
- Poisoning or overdose with methotrexate, metformin, phenobarbital, chlorpropamide, and fluoride, neuroleptics, antiepileptics, antihistamines, propoxyphene, chloroquine, hydroxychloroquine, quinine, cocaine, beta-blockers (propranolol, labetalol, acebutolol), metformin, and copper sulfate[15]
- Methanol and ethylene glycol poisoning[17]
- Snake bite, particularly Viperidae species[20]
- Refractory hyperkalemia (if associated with severe metabolic acidosis along with insulin–dextrose infusion and beta-2 agonist nebulization)[22]

Urinary alkalinization is a promising therapeutic tool in certain poisoning and toxicities, but the evidence base is weak. Forced alkaline diuresis (FAD) is not superior to saline diuresis in preventing rhabdomyolysis induced AKI.[21]

Appropriate and judicious use of HCO_3 with careful monitoring to avoid complications is essential in the management of specific toxins and xenobiotics. The indications of $NaHCO_3$ in critical care toxicology are summarized in **Box 1**.

CONCLUSION

Sodium bicarbonate may have a role in the management of specific poisonings. The high sodium content and alkaline nature of the molecule are the reasons for its therapeutic effects. Careful monitoring of blood gases, pH (blood and urine), electrolytes (sodium, potassium, and calcium), and ECG should be done when $NaHCO_3$ is used.

REFERENCES

1. Alka K, Casey JR. Bicarbonate transport in health and disease. IUBMB Life. 2014;66(9):596-615.
2. Mirrakhimov AE, Ayach T, Barbaryan A, Talari G, Chadha R, Gray A. The role of sodium bicarbonate in the management of some toxic ingestions. Int J Nephrol. 2017;2017:1-8.
3. Weisbord SD, Gallagher M, Jneid H, Garcia S, Cass A, Thwin SS, et al. Outcomes after angiography with sodium bicarbonate and acetylcysteine. J Vasc Surg. 2018;68(4):1271.
4. Forsythe SM, Schmidt GA. Sodium bicarbonate for the treatment of lactic acidosis. Chest. 2000;117(1):260-7.
5. Viallon A, Zeni F, Lafond P, Venet C, Tardy B, Page Y, et al. Does bicarbonate therapy improve the management of severe diabetic ketoacidosis? Crit Care Med. 1999; 27(12):2690-3.
6. Peters CH, Ruben PC. Introduction to Sodium Channels: Voltage Gated Sodium Channels. Berlin Heidelberg: Springer; 2014. pp. 1-6.
7. The Sicilian gambit. A new approach to the classification of antiarrhythmic drugs based on their actions on arrhythmogenic mechanisms. Task Force of the Working Group on Arrhythmias of the European Society of Cardiology. Circulation. 1991;84(4):1831-51.
8. Stafstrom CE. Mechanisms of action of antiepileptic drugs: the search for synergy. Curr Opin Neurol. 2010;23(2):157-63.
9. Dupuy JM, Ostacher MJ, Huffman J, Perlis RH, Nierenberg AA. A critical review of pharmacotherapy for major depressive disorder. Int J Neuropsychopharmacol. 2011; 14(10):1417-31.
10. Glassman AH. Cardiovascular effects of tricyclic antidepressants. Annu Rev Med. 1984;35(1):503-11.
11. Sasyniuk B, Jhamandas V, Valois M. Experimental amitriptyline intoxication: treatment of cardiac toxicity by administration of sodium bicarbonate. Ann Emerg Med. 1986;15(1):93.
12. Isoardi KZ, Chiew AL. Too much of a good thing: bicarbonate toxicity following treatment of sodium channel blocker overdose. Emerg Med Australas. 2022;34(4):639-41.
13. Feldman S, Chen SL, Pickering LK, Cleary TG, Ericsson CD, Hülse M. Salicylate absorption from a bismuth subsalicylate preparation. Clin Pharmacol Ther. 1981;29(6):788-92.
14. O'Malley GF. Emergency department management of the salicylate-poisoned patient. Emerg Med Clin North Am. 2007;25(2):333-46.
15. Proudfoot AT, Krenzelok EP, Vale JA. Position paper on urine alkalinization. J Toxicol Clin Toxicol. 2004;42(1):1-26.
16. Kraut JA. Diagnosis of toxic alcohols: limitations of present methods. Clin Toxicol. 2015;53(7):589-95.
17. Miller H, Barceloux DG, Krenzelok EP, Olson K, Watson W. American Academy of Clinical Toxicology practice guidelines on the treatment of ethylene glycol poisoning. J Toxicol Clin Toxicol. 1999;37(5):537-60.
18. Barceloux DG, Bond GR, Krenzelok EP, Cooper H, Vale JA. American Academy of Clinical Toxicology practice guidelines on the treatment of methanol poisoning. J Toxicol Clin Toxicol. 2002;40(4):415-46.
19. Isbister GK, O'Leary MA, Elliott M, Brown SGA. Tiger snake (Notechis spp.) envenoming: Australian Snakebite Project (ASP-13). Med J Aust. 2012;197(3):173-7.
20. Basavaraj A, Giri P. Prevention of acute kidney injury in vasculotoxic snake bite with forced alkaline diuresis. Int J Sci Res. 2019:8(1).
21. Huerta-Alardín AL, Varon J, Marik PE. Bench-to-bedside review: rhabdomyolysis—an overview for clinicians. Crit Care. 2005;9(2):158-69.
22. Ngugi NN, McLigeyo SO, Kayima JK. Treatment of hyperkalaemia by altering the transcellular gradient in patients with renal failure: effect of various therapeutic approaches. East African Med J. 1997;73:503-9.

4.19 Cyanide Antidote Kit

YP Singh, Saurabh Jain, Gaurav Pratap Singh

INTRODUCTION

Cyanide, a deadly poison with rapid and severe toxic effects, necessitates prompt and effective intervention in cases of exposure. The development and deployment of cyanide poison kits have emerged as critical tools in emergency situations where immediate counteraction is imperative to save lives.

ETIOLOGY

Although cyanide poisoning can result from various types of exposures such as structural fires, medical exposure (sodium nitroprusside), industrial exposure, and certain foods, domestic fire remains the most common cause of toxicity.

Cyanide has multiple industrial applications, e.g., electroplating production, photography, plastics and rubber manufacturing, and pesticides, and poses an occupational hazard. Toxic levels of cyanide have been found in patients who receive prolonged infusions of sodium nitroprusside.[1-3]

PATHOPHYSIOLOGY

Onset of signs and symptoms is rapid with intravenous and inhalation exposure but can be more insidious with oral or transdermal exposure.

Cyanide is a cytochrome C oxidase inhibitor, producing a histotoxic type of hypoxia **(Fig. 1)**, because it interferes with oxidative phosphorylation. It interferes with aerobic respiration and blocks the mitochondrial electron transport chain, resulting in cellular hypoxia and ATP depletion leading to severe metabolic acidosis.[4,5]

DIAGNOSIS

Keeping a high index of suspicion with regard to the circumstances of presentation is important.

Multiple causalities may present after a major fire outbreak, and mass hysteria has been reported as a finding after cyanide exposure. Bitter almond odor is reported by many patients exposed to cyanide. Patient with a history of depression may present with sudden collapse from intentional cyanide poisoning. Iatrogenic cyanide poisoning should be suspected in patients with lactic acidosis, tachyphylaxis, and new-onset altered sensorium on prolonged nitroprusside infusion.

Negative physical findings and the absence of lactic acidosis rule out cyanide poisoning as a diagnosis.

Under appropriate circumstances (residential fire), lactate concentration >10 mmol/L at the time of hospital admission defines a blood cyanide concentration of >40 μmol/L, and a lactate level >6 mmol/L suggests significant cyanide exposure.[6,7] Plasma lactate concentration at the time of admission correlates more closely with cyanide levels than carbon monoxide levels in patients with residential fire.

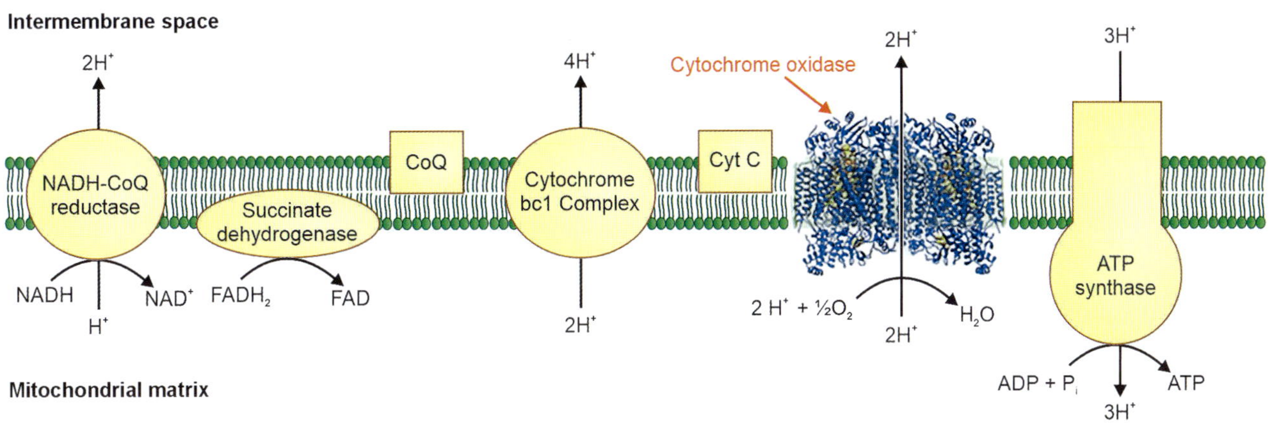

Fig. 1: Mitochondrial function in cyanide poisoning. Cyanide inhibits cytochrome oxidase, disrupting the electron transport chain.

It is to be kept in mind that lactate alone cannot be considered diagnostic of cyanide poisoning, because lactic acidosis can be multifactorial representing various causes of mitochondrial dysfunction.

Cyanide and thiocyanate assays done with liquid chromatography-tandem mass spectrometry (LC-MS/MS) are considered specific tests.[8] Since cyanide has a short half-life, the main metabolite, thiocyanate, is typically measured to determine exposure.

TREATMENT

Supportive measures to ensure patent airway, breathing, and circulation are the cornerstone for treatment. Cyanide antidote should be administered on strong suspicion of cyanide toxicity, without waiting for laboratory confirmation. Cyanide has various antidotes, with different mechanisms of action and variable clinical and risk profiles. There is a lack of consensus among the medical community regarding the antidote or antidotes with the best reward-to-risk ratio.

ANTICYANIDE KIT

Anticyanide kit is an antidote kit containing amyl nitrite, sodium nitrite, and sodium thiosulfate. This is the traditional method to treat cyanide poisoning and has been advocated as an essential fixture in any industry using cyanide in any form (cyanide gas/hydrogen cyanide liquid). The nitrites (amyl and sodium) in the kit are administered with an aim to iatrogenically induce methemoglobinemia. Cyanide is known to have a higher affinity for methemoglobin; therefore, it will preferentially bind to methemoglobin, leaving the mitochondria intact. This will help the mitochondria to start functioning normally and resume oxidative phosphorylation. This prevents cytotoxic hypoxia and resultant organ dysfunction. Once cyanide binds to methemoglobin, sodium thiosulfate is injected. Sodium thiosulfate here will act as a sulfhydryl donor for the enzyme rhodanese. This enzyme then converts cyanide to the less toxic thiocyanate, which gets excreted renally.

Amyl Nitrite (Inhalational)

Amyl nitrite is available in the anticyanide kit as glass ampules, which need to be broken for inhalation. As soon as cyanide exposure is suspected, the patient should be removed from the source. One should not wait for the signs of toxicity to appear. The amyl nitrite ampules are broken inside a folded piece of cloth, and the victim is asked to inhale amyl nitrite. Amyl nitrite has a rapid onset of action and a short half-life. Amyl nitrite primarily works by converting hemoglobin to methemoglobin, which binds to cyanide and allows cytochrome oxidase a3 to reactivate the electron transport chain. Methemoglobin reversibly binds to cyanide to form cyanmethemoglobin, a nontoxic compound.

Although it has been used as a first-aid measure, it is no longer available in cyanide antidote kits in the United States and is no longer considered an acceptable initial response.

Sodium Nitrite and Sodium Thiosulfate

These two drugs are often used in combination. They are available in the anticyanide kit as ampules for injection. Although they are cheap and very effective, they are now considered as second-line agents after hydroxocobalamin.[9]

Intravenous (IV) sodium nitrite is the second agent to be used. It is administered as a rapid IV bolus after exposure. It further promotes the conversion of hemoglobin to methemoglobin like amyl nitrite. Although it is rapidly effective, it may result in life-threatening toxicity.

Intravenous sodium thiosulfate is the next agent to be used. It is administered as a slow IV infusion. It helps in enhancing the detoxification process by converting cyanide to the less toxic thiocyanate. Sodium thiocyanate is nontoxic and is excreted in the urine. It poorly penetrates into the mitochondria and has a slow onset of action.[9] Due to its short half-life and delayed onset of action, sodium thiosulfate must always be given in combination with other therapies.[10]

It should not be used in patients with smoke inhalation unless their carboxyhemoglobin concentration is very low (<10%). The induction of methemoglobinemia multiplies the effect of any existing carboxyhemoglobin, which may significantly decrease the oxygen-carrying capacity of blood.[11] Hemodynamic collapse secondary to vasodilation is another serious side effect.

Dose and Administration

Currently available kit contains amyl nitrite, sodium nitrite, and sodium thiosulfate. Sodium nitrite 300 mg ampule is available. A dose of 10 mg/kg is given IV bolus over 3–5 minutes in adults. This is followed by sodium thiosulfate. Sodium thiosulfate is available as one ampule or 12.5 g in 50 mL. This is injected intravenously over 30 minutes in adults.

Efficacy

Many animal studies have shown the administration of anticyanide kit as a lifesaving intervention; however, there are no randomized trials. Most of the data on efficacy have been extrapolated from its use in various case reports.[12]

Adverse Effects

Cyanide kit administration has various side effects. The most common being are severe hypotension, methemoglobinemia, and hypersensitivity reactions.[13] Methemoglobinemia may further worsen the tissue oxygenation by binding to oxygen. This may compromise the effects of anticyanide kit administration.

HYDROXOCOBALAMIN (CYANOKIT)

Hydroxocobalamin has been used for treating acute cyanide poisoning for over 30 years.[13]

Hydroxocobalamin, a form of vitamin B_{12}, binds with cyanide to form cyanocobalamin, which is nontoxic and renally eliminated.[14] Cyanide has a greater affinity to bind with hydroxocobalamin rather than cytochrome oxidase a3 forming cyanocobalamin, thereby sparing the mitochondrial function. Alternatively, cyanide may dissociate from cyanocobalamin at a very slow rate undergoing detoxification by mitochondrial enzyme rhodanese.[15]

Hydroxocobalamin is clinically safe in antidotal doses without any significant toxicity compared with other cyanide antidotes. Owing to its rapid onset of action and feasibility of prehospital use (tolerability and safety profiles), it is considered the drug of choice in Europe and Australia and is also approved by the US Food and Drug Administration (FDA). Coadministration of sodium thiosulfate (through a separate line or sequentially) has been suggested to have a synergistic effect on detoxification.

Dose and Administration

- About 5 g of hydroxocobalamin is administered by IV infusion over 15 minutes.
- Depending upon the severity and clinical response, a second dose of 5 g may be administered by IV infusion up to a total dose of 10 g.

Efficacy

The efficacy of hydroxocobalamin has been proven in retrospective as well as prospective studies.[5] Many animal studies have displayed improved mortality with treatment.[16] The evidence, thus, available has been sufficient to recommend hydroxocobalamin for the treatment of acute cyanide poisoning. This has now become the standard of care in most settings.

Adverse Effects[17]

- Transient hypertension (a benefit in hypotensive patients)

TABLE 1: Antidotes to cyanide poisoning.

Drugs	***Mechanism***	***Administration***	***Comment***
Hydroxocobalamin	Combines with unbound cyanide to form cyanocobalamin (nontoxic, undergoes renal elimination)	5 g for adults, administered for 15 minutes; repeat a dose if needed	• First-line therapy • Minimal side effects
Amyl nitrite	Induces methemoglobinemia, which binds cyanide	• Crushed 0.3 mL ampule inhaled for 15 seconds • May repeat 3–5 minutes until intravenous access established	• No longer recommended as first aid • Poor risk reward profile
Sodium nitrite	Induces methemoglobinemia, which binds cyanide	300 mg (10 mL in a 3% solution) or 10 mg/kg given intravenously for 3–5 minutes	Given as a part of anticyanide kit along with sodium thiosulfate
Sodium thiosulfate	Combines with unbound cyanide to form renally excreted thiocyanate	1 ampule or 12.5 g in 50 mL, given intravenously for 30 minutes in adults	• Given as a part of anticyanide kit along with sodium nitrite • Can also be given in sequence with hydroxocobalamin

- Reddish-brown skin, mucous membrane, and urine discoloration
- Anaphylaxis and anaphylactoid reactions (rare)
- Worsening of renal function has been reported, and it is recommended to monitor renal function for 7 days following therapy.

CONCLUSION

Cyanide toxicity is a rapidly fatal condition if not detected and treated early. Lack of rapid detection modalities and nonspecific clinical presentation make the diagnosis more challenging.

The development and utilization of cyanide antidote kits represent a pivotal advancement in the field of emergency medicine.

Hydroxocobalamin is currently the first-line therapy for suspected or confirmed cyanide poisoning but may not be available always. Sodium thiosulfate and sodium nitrite are the parts of commercially available anticyanide kit but can also be ordered separately. This is a must have antidote in hospitals, which are in the vicinity of industries utilizing cyanide gas or hydrocyanic acid. It is also mandatory to store anticyanide kit in hospitals bordering areas prone to fire-related disasters[18] **(Table 1)**.

REFERENCES

1. Pruthi S, Shah S, Gambhir HS. Laundry blues: a case of methemoglobinemia with laundry detergent and tylenol ingestion. QJM. 2017;110(9):595-6.
2. Zacarias CH, Esteban C, Rodrigues GL, Nascimento ES. Occupational exposure to hydrogen cyanide during large-scale cassava processing, in Alagoas State, Brazil. Cad Saude Publica. 2017;33(7):e00073416.
3. Netto AB, Netto CM, Mahadevan A, Taly AB, Agadi JB. Tropical ataxic neuropathy—a century old enigma. Neurol India. 2016;64(6):1151-9.
4. Pauluhn J. Risk assessment in combustion toxicology: should carbon dioxide be recognized as a modifier of toxicity or separate toxicological entity? Toxicol Lett. 2016;262:142-15.
5. Huzar TF, George T, Cross JM. Carbon monoxide and cyanide toxicity: etiology, pathophysiology and treatment in inhalation injury. Expert Rev Respir Med. 2013;7(2):159-70.
6. Baud FJ, Barriot P, Toffis V, Riou B, Vicaut E, Lecarpentier Y, et al. Elevated blood cyanide concentrations in victims of smoke inhalation. N Engl J Med. 1991;325:1761-6.
7. Reade MC, Davies SR, Morley PT, Dennett J, Jacobs IC. Review article: management of cyanide poisoning. Emerg Med Australas. 2012;24(3):225-38.
8. Alluhayb AH, Severance C, Hendry-Hofer T, Bebarta VS, Logue BA. Concurrent determination of cyanide and thiocyanate in human and swine antemortem and postmortem blood by high-performance liquid chromatography–tandem mass spectrometry. Anal Bioanal Chem. 2023;415:6595-609.
9. Hall AH, Saiers J, Baud F. Which cyanide antidote? Crit Rev Toxicol. 2009;39(7):541-52.
10. Gracia R, Shepherd G. Cyanide poisoning and its treatment. Pharmacotherapy. 2004;24(10):1358-65.
11. Kirk MA, Gerace R, Kulig KW. Cyanide and methemoglobin kinetics in smoke inhalation victims treated with the cyanide antidote kit. Ann Emerg Med. 1993;22(9):1413-8.
12. Hall AH, Dart R, Bogdan G. Sodium thiosulfate or hydroxocobalamin for the empiric treatment of cyanide poisoning? Ann Emerg Med. 2007;49(6):806-13.
13. Hamel J. A review of acute cyanide poisoning with a treatment update. Crit Care Nurse. 2011;31(1):72-82.
14. Anseeuw K, Delvau N, Burillo-Putze G, de Laco F, Geldner G, Holmström P, et al. Cyanide poisoning by fire smoke inhalation: a European expert consensus. Eur J Emerg Med. 2013;20(1):2-9.
15. Thompson JP, Marrs TC. Hydroxocobalamin in cyanide poisoning. Clin Toxicol (Phila). 2012;50(10):875-85.
16. Bebarta VS, Pitotti RL, Dixon P, Lairet JR, Bush A, Tanen DA. Hydroxocobalamin versus sodium thiosulfate for the treatment of acute cyanide toxicity in a swine (*Sus scrofa*) model. Ann Emerg Med. 2012;59(6):532-9.
17. Barillo DJ. Diagnosis and treatment of cyanide toxicity. J Burn Care Res. 2009;30(1):148-52.
18. Dart RC, Goldfrank LR, Erstad BL, Huang DT, Todd KH, Weitz J, et al. Expert consensus guidelines for stocking of antidotes in hospitals that provide emergency care. Ann Emerg Med. 2018;71(3):314-25.

4.20 Anticoagulant Drugs and Their Reversal: Mechanisms, Agents, and Clinical Strategies

Charanpreet Singh

INTRODUCTION

There is a growing armamentarium of medications, which can be used for anticoagulation. The use of traditional agents such as unfractionated heparin (UFH), low-molecular-weight heparin (LMWH), and vitamin K antagonists (VKAs) is being supplanted by newer agents, collectively known as direct-acting oral anticoagulant agents (DOACs). While the use of DOACs is now recommended for patients with most indications requiring anticoagulation, laboratory tests to assess their efficacy and toxicity are not easily available. Management of a patient with suspected DOAC and anticoagulant toxicity is thus an important skill set for physicians. Through this chapter, we will give a brief introduction of the different classes of anticoagulants, as well as their reversal agents, before discussing management of patients with anticoagulant toxicity.

ANTICOAGULANTS

Heparin

Unfractionated heparin functions by enhancing the activity of antithrombin III (AT III), thereby increasing its ability to inhibit thrombin (factor IIa) and factor Xa, which prevents the formation of fibrin clots. Additionally, UFH inhibits other coagulation factors, such as factors IXa, XIa, and XIIa, contributing to its overall anticoagulant effect. Due to its large and heterogeneous molecular structure, UFH exhibits variable pharmacokinetics, necessitating careful monitoring via activated partial thromboplastin time (aPTT) to ensure therapeutic efficacy and minimize the risk of bleeding.

Low-molecular-weight heparin, derived from UFH through a process of depolymerization, similarly enhances the activity of AT III but predominantly inhibits factor Xa due to its shorter polysaccharide chains. This specificity is due to LMWH chains being insufficiently long to bind both AT III and thrombin simultaneously. LMWH offers more predictable pharmacokinetics and a longer half-life compared to UFH, allowing for once or twice daily subcutaneous administration without the need for routine laboratory monitoring, thereby making it more convenient for outpatient management.

In summary, while both UFH and LMWH exert their anticoagulant effects by enhancing AT III, UFH has a broader range of activity, whereas LMWH is more specific to factor Xa and provides easier and more predictable dosing.

Vitamin K Antagonists

Vitamin K antagonists, such as warfarin, are a class of anticoagulants that prevent blood clot formation by inhibiting the enzyme vitamin K epoxide reductase complex 1 (VKORC1).[1] This inhibition impedes the conversion of vitamin K epoxide back to its active form, vitamin K hydroquinone, which is necessary for the carboxylation and activation of clotting factors II, VII, IX, and X, as well as proteins C and S. As a result, VKAs reduce the overall ability of blood to clot. Warfarin is the most commonly used VKA. Its effect requires several days to manifest fully, as it depends on the degradation of existing active clotting factors. The pharmacokinetics of VKAs can vary widely among individuals due to factors such as genetic differences, dietary vitamin K intake, and interactions with certain foods and other medications. Therefore, regular monitoring and dose adjustments are necessary to maintain the therapeutic range, typically measured using the international normalized ratio (INR), with a common target range of 2.0–3.0.

Direct-acting Oral Anticoagulants

Direct-acting oral anticoagulant agents directly inhibit specific coagulation factors, offering rapid onset of action and fixed dosing without the need for routine laboratory monitoring. The two main categories of DOACs are direct thrombin inhibitors and direct factor Xa inhibitors.[2] Direct thrombin inhibitors, such as dabigatran, bind directly to thrombin (factor IIa) and inhibit its ability to convert fibrinogen to fibrin, thus preventing clot formation. Direct factor Xa inhibitors, including rivaroxaban, apixaban, and edoxaban, target and inhibit factor Xa, a key enzyme in the coagulation cascade responsible for the conversion of prothrombin to thrombin.

Direct-acting oral anticoagulant agents offer several advantages over traditional anticoagulants. They have more predictable pharmacokinetics and pharmacodynamics, allowing for fixed dosing without the need for frequent INR monitoring. DOACs may prolong either prothrombin time (PT) or aPTT depending on their mechanism of action (i.e., direct thrombin inhibitors or factor Xa inhibitors). However, the prolongation is not indicative of a specific level, and specialized tests are required to monitor the same, and that too in special occasions where toxicity is suspected, such as in a bleeding patient. Additionally, DOACs have fewer dietary restrictions and drug interactions compared to warfarin. Their rapid onset of action allows for quick initiation of anticoagulation, and their relatively short half-lives can be beneficial in situations requiring temporary discontinuation of therapy.

ANTICOAGULANT REVERSAL AGENTS

Protamine

Protamine is a positively charged protein and is essential for neutralizing the effects of heparin. By forming stable complexes with heparin molecules, protamine reverses their anticoagulant properties. The pharmacokinetics of protamine involves its rapid action upon intravenous administration. It begins neutralizing heparin almost immediately, with its effects typically manifesting within 5 minutes. Protamine's half-life is approximately 7 minutes, and it is metabolized and cleared from the bloodstream relatively quickly, primarily by the kidneys. Protamine dosing must be carefully calculated based on the amount of heparin that needs to be neutralized, and excessive dosing can lead to complications such as hypotension and bradycardia. Protamine is highly effective in reversing the anticoagulant effects of UFH. It can neutralize UFH almost completely, making it the preferred choice in situations where rapid reversal is critical. However, its efficacy in reversing LMWH is less pronounced. Protamine can neutralize about 60–75% of LMWH's anticoagulant activity, necessitating additional consideration and monitoring when managing patients on LMWH.

Vitamin K

Vitamin K plays a pivotal role in the reversal of anticoagulation, particularly in the context of managing patients on VKAs. Vitamin K can be administered orally or intravenously, with the route of administration chosen based on the urgency of reversal. Oral vitamin K is typically used for less urgent situations, as it has a slower onset of action. Intravenous vitamin K, on the other hand, acts more rapidly and is used in emergency scenarios where immediate correction of coagulopathy is necessary. It is important to note that while vitamin K effectively reverses the anticoagulant effects of VKAs, the process can take several hours, as the synthesis of clotting factors is not instantaneous. In cases of severe bleeding, additional measures such as the administration of prothrombin complex concentrates (PCC) (discussed below) may be required to provide immediate hemostatic support until vitamin K takes full effect.

Prothrombin Complex Concentrate and Activated Prothrombin Complex Concentrate

Prothrombin complex concentrate (PCC) and activated prothrombin complex concentrate (aPCC) are critical agents used in the reversal of anticoagulant-associated bleeding, particularly for patients on VKAs and certain DOACs. These concentrates contain various clotting factors that are essential for restoring hemostasis in bleeding patients.

Prothrombin complex concentrates contain a combination of clotting factors II, VII, IX, and X, which are the factors inhibited by VKAs. PCC is available as 3-factor and 4-factor PCC, with 4-factor PCC being the preferred agent for treatment of VKA-associated bleeds.[3] The administration of PCC rapidly replenishes these factors, providing an immediate increase in the levels of functional clotting factors in the bloodstream. This makes PCC an effective choice for urgent reversal of VKA-induced anticoagulation, especially in life-threatening bleeding or prior to emergency surgical procedures. PCC is administered intravenously, and dosing is based on the patient's body weight and the degree of anticoagulation required. One of the main advantages of PCC over fresh frozen plasma (FFP) is the lower volume required, reducing the risk of volume overload in patients.

Activated prothrombin complex concentrates, such as FEIBA (factor VIII inhibitor bypassing activity), contain activated clotting factors II, IX, and X, along with factor VII in its activated form. The action of aPCC is rapid, similar to PCC, and it is administered intravenously. The typical dosing for aPCC in the context of bleeding is 50–100 U/kg, with adjustments made based on the clinical scenario and the patient's response. Both PCC and aPCC have been associated with thromboembolic risks, necessitating careful monitoring during administration.

Idarucizumab

Idarucizumab is a monoclonal antibody fragment specifically designed to reverse the anticoagulant effects of dabigatran, a direct thrombin inhibitor.[4] It binds to dabigatran with high affinity, neutralizing its anticoagulant activity almost immediately. Idarucizumab is used in situations where rapid reversal is required, such as in cases of life-threatening bleeding or urgent surgical procedures. The recommended dose is 5 g, administered as two consecutive 2.5-g infusions over 5–10 minutes each.

Andexanet Alfa

Andexanet alfa is a recombinant modified human factor Xa protein designed to reverse the anticoagulant effects of factor Xa inhibitors, such as apixaban and rivaroxaban.[5] By acting as a decoy receptor, andexanet alfa binds to factor Xa inhibitors with high affinity, effectively neutralizing their anticoagulant effects. Dosing is dependent on the specific factor Xa inhibitor and the timing of the last dose.

REVERSAL OF ANTICOAGULATION[6,7]

The strategy for reversal of anticoagulation depends on multiple factors—the presence or absence of bleed, the type of bleed (major vs. nonmajor), and the anticoagulant being used. A major bleed is defined as any bleed which is either at a critical site [such as the central nervous system (CNS), airway, retroperitoneum, and pericardium] or causes hemodynamic compromise or a drop in hemoglobin by ≥2 g/dL.

Heparin

Nonmajor Bleed

With either UFH or LMWH, if the patient has a nonmajor bleed, just general supportive measures are indicated, which may include use of tranexamic acid or withholding UFH or LMWH if clinically indicated.[8] Reversal agents are not usually recommended in this scenario.

Major Bleed

For patients with a major bleed on continuous UFH infusion, it is recommended to stop the infusion and administer a reversal agent, i.e., protamine. It is given at a dose of 1 mg/100 U of UFH administered in the past 2–3 hours, with the dosing being capped at 50 mg usually and monitoring the aPTT after 15 minutes. If the aPTT is still supratherapeutic, an additional dose of 0.5 mg/100 U of UFH administered in the past 2–3 hours may be given.

For patients on therapeutic dosing of LMWH, it is recommended to stop the LMWH and administer protamine. If the last dose of LMWH is within 8 hours of the bleed, it is advised to give 1 mg protamine/1 mg of LMWH, with the dosing being capped at 50 mg. If the last dose of LMWH is between 8 and 12 hours of bleed, 0.5 mg protamine per 1 mg of LMWH (maximum dose 50 mg) administered is recommended. If the last dose of LMWH is >12 hours from bleed, administration of protamine is unlikely to be useful.

Vitamin K Antagonists

Supratherapeutic INR with no Bleed

Patients with a supratherapeutic INR with no bleed are generally instructed to stop the VKA with daily monitoring of the INR till it is back in the therapeutic range. There is no consensus among different guidelines regarding use of vitamin K in this scenario. However, a low dose of oral vitamin K (2.5–5 mg) should be given if the INR is >10. For patients with an INR between 4.5 and 10, use of vitamin K is more controversial, with a meta-analysis of six studies not showing any benefit. However, it is given as an optional agent in most guidelines. If for any reason oral vitamin K cannot be given, intravenous vitamin K 1 mg can be considered for patients with an INR >10.[9,10]

Increased INR with Bleed

In patients with a bleed, the type and severity of the bleed define the management necessitated. In patients with a nonmajor bleed, supportive measures such as withholding VKAs, administration of vitamin K, and daily monitoring of INR are recommended. However, a patient with a major bleed would require the administration of PCC along with the above measures. Intravenous 4-factor PCC is usually recommended, 1,500–2,000 U is given intravenously over 10 minutes along with intravenous vitamin K 10 mg. The dose of vitamin K is higher to completely neutralize the effect of VKAs in comparison to the lower dose of vitamin K utilized in patients with asymptomatic rise in INR, where the goal of therapy is just to bring the INR to a therapeutic level. INR is rechecked after 15–30 minutes, and if still supratherapeutic, repeat dosing may be considered. Cost often makes utilization of PCC difficult in our setting. If PCC is not available, FFP at a dose of 10–15 mL/kg should be given in addition to intravenous vitamin K.

Direct-acting Oral Anticoagulant Agents

For patients on DOACs, management of a bleeding patient is further complicated by the fact that tests for checking levels are not easily available. Usual coagulation parameters such as PT and aPTT may be elevated with these drugs but may be normal, and there is also no linear correlation of increased times with drug efficacy and levels in the body. As such, clinical suspicion and history are vital for early treatment initiation and management.

For patients with minor bleeds, conservative measures such as administration of tranexamic acid and stopping of culprit drug are usually recommended. Individual reversal agents are not usually given in these settings.

For patients with major bleeds, universal measures include use of PCC or aPCC. In addition, activated charcoal ingestion can also be done if the last dose was taken within the last 2 hours of presentation/bleed. For patients on dabigatran, dialysis may also be tried to help in the removal of the drug from the body.[11]

Specific reversal agents are also now available for these agents. For patients on dabigatran, idarucizumab may be given to patients with a major bleed. The dose is 2.5 g given as two doses, with an additional 5 g dose if hemostasis is not achieved.

For patients on oral factor Xa inhibitors, such as rivaroxaban and apixaban, the specific reversal agent, which is recommended, is andexanet alfa. However, a recent study in patients with an intracerebral hemorrhage found that while andexanet alfa was associated with an increased rate of hematoma control, it was also associated with an increased risk of thrombosis, especially ischemic stroke.[12]

What is important to note is that all reversal agents, such as andexanet, PCC, and aPCC are associated with an increased risk of thrombosis. Hence, the overall condition of the patient and risk for thrombosis versus risk of increasing bleed by not administering the reversal agent needs to be taken into consideration before giving the drug.

The different reversal agents and treatments are summarized in **Table 1**.

TABLE 1: Reversal and management strategies for patients with anticoagulant toxicity.

Heparin (UFH and LMWH)		
Nonmajor bleed		• Supportive measures • May withhold drug if clinically warranted • No specific reversal agent is required
Major bleed	UFH	• Stop infusion • Protamine administration • Check aPTT after 15 minutes and redose with protamine if needed
	LMWH	• Stop LMWH • Protamine administration • Check anti-Xa levels if available after 15–30 minutes and consider redosing
Vitamin K antagonists		
No bleed with INR <4.5		Omit/lower dose and recheck INR daily
No bleed with INR 4.5–10		• Omit/lower dose and recheck INR daily • May give low-dose oral vitamin K
No bleed with INR >10		• Omit/lower dose and recheck INR daily • Low-dose oral vitamin K
Nonmajor bleed		• Conservative measures • May consider stopping warfarin • May consider IV vitamin K
Major bleed		• Stop drug • Supportive measures • IV vitamin K • Use PCC/aPCC/FFP • Recheck INR after 30 minutes of PCC/aPCC administration
Dabigatran		
Nonmajor bleed		• Consider stopping the drug • Supportive measures
Major bleed		• Idarucizumab administration • If unavailable, consider PCC/aPCC • Consider activated charcoal if the last intake is within 2 hours • Consider hemodialysis
Apixaban/rivaroxaban		
Nonmajor bleed		• Consider stopping the drug • Supportive measures
Major bleed		• PCC/aPCC administration • Can give andexanet alfa as well • Consider activated charcoal if the last intake is within 2 hours

(aPCC: activated prothrombin complex concentrate; aPTT; activated partial thromboplastin time; FFP: fresh frozen plasma; INR: international normalized ratio; IV: intravenous; LMWH: low-molecular-weight heparin; PCC: prothrombin complex concentrate; UFH: unfractionated heparin)

CONCLUSION

The effective management of anticoagulant therapy requires a comprehensive understanding of the mechanisms, indications, and potential complications associated with these drugs. The availability and appropriate use of reversal agents are crucial for mitigating bleeding risks and ensuring patient safety, particularly in urgent or emergent situations. Vitamin K, PCCs, idarucizumab, and andexanet alfa represent essential tools for the rapid and effective reversal of anticoagulant effects. As the field of anticoagulation continues to evolve, emerging therapies and personalized approaches hold promise for enhancing treatment outcomes and reducing adverse events. Ongoing research and adherence to evidence-based guidelines will be vital in optimizing the balance between preventing thromboembolism and managing bleeding risks, ultimately improving the care of patients on anticoagulant therapy.

REFERENCES

1. Ansell J, Hirsh J, Hylek E, Jacobson A, Crowther M, Palareti G. Pharmacology and management of the vitamin K antagonists: American College of Chest Physicians Evidence-Based Clinical Practice Guidelines. Chest. 2008;133(6 Suppl.):160S-98S.
2. Yeh CH, Fredenburgh JC, Weitz JI. Oral direct factor Xa inhibitors. Circ Res. 2012;111(8):1069-78.
3. Voils SA, Baird B. Systematic review: 3-factor versus 4-factor prothrombin complex concentrate for warfarin reversal: does it matter? Thromb Res. 2012;130(6):833-40.
4. Pollack CV, Reilly PA, van Ryn J, Eikelboom JW, Glund S, Bernstein RA, et al. Idarucizumab for dabigatran reversal. N Engl J Med. 2015;373(6):511-20.
5. Connolly SJ, Milling TJ, Eikelboom JW, Gibson CM, Curnutte JT, Gold A, et al. Andexanet alfa for acute major bleeding associated with factor Xa inhibitors. N Engl J Med. 2016;375(12):1131-41.
6. Holbrook A, Schulman S, Witt DM, Vandvik PO, Fish J, Kovacs MJ, et al. Evidence-based management of anticoagulant therapy: antithrombotic therapy and prevention of thrombosis, 9th ed: American College of Chest Physicians Evidence-Based Clinical Practice Guidelines. Chest. 2012;141(2 Suppl.):e152S-84S.
7. Tomaselli GF, Mahaffey KW, Cuker A, Dobesh PP, Doherty JU, Eikelboom JW, et al. 2017 ACC expert consensus decision pathway on management of bleeding in patients on oral anticoagulants: a report of the American College of Cardiology Task Force on expert's consensus decisions pathways. J Am Coll Cardiol. 2017;70(24): 3042-67.
8. Makris M, Van Veen JJ, Tait CR, Mumford AD, Laffan M. Guideline on the management of bleeding in patients on antithrombotic agents. Br J Haematol. 160(1):35-46.
9. Khatib R, Ludwikowska M, Witt DM, Ansell J, Clark NP, Holbrook A, et al. Vitamin K for reversal of excessive vitamin K antagonist anticoagulation: a systematic review and meta-analysis. Blood Adv. 2019;3(5):789-96.
10. Lubetsky A, Yonath H, Olchovsky D, Loebstein R, Halkin H, Ezra D. Comparison of oral vs intravenous phytonadione (vitamin K1) in patients with excessive anticoagulation: a prospective randomized controlled study. Arch Intern Med. 2003;163(20):2469-73.
11. Kim B, Garcia DA. What is the role of hemodialysis for dabigatran-associated major bleeding? Hematology. 2014(1);514-7.
12. Connolly SJ, Sharma M, Cohen AT, Demchuk AM, Czlonkowska A, Lindgren AG, et al. Andexanet for factor Xa inhibitor-associated acute intracerebral hemorrhage. N Engl J Med. 2024;390:1745-55.

Index

Page numbers followed by *b* refer to box, *f* refer to figure, *fc* refer to flowchart, and *t* refer to table.

A

B

C

Q

R

S

T

U

V

W

X

Y

Z